# Lippincott's
# Illustrated Reviews:
# Microbiology
## Second Edition

# Lippincott's Illustrated Reviews: Microbiology
## Second Edition

**Richard A. Harvey, Ph.D.**

Department of Biochemistry
University of Medicine and Dentistry of New Jersey–
Robert Wood Johnson Medical School
Piscataway, New Jersey

**Pamela C. Champe, Ph.D.**

Department of Biochemistry
University of Medicine and Dentistry of New Jersey–
Robert Wood Johnson Medical School
Piscataway, New Jersey

**Bruce D. Fisher, M.D.**

Clinical Professor of Medicine
University of Medicine and Dentistry of New Jersey–
Robert Wood Johnson Medical School
Medical Director, QualCare, Inc.
Piscataway, New Jersey

LIPPINCOTT WILLIAMS & WILKINS
A **Wolters Kluwer** Company
Philadelphia • Baltimore • New York • London
Buenos Aires • Hong Kong • Sydney • Tokyo

This book is dedicated to the
memory of Harriet Rouse, whose
dedication to her students and
love of microbiology made her the
consummate teacher and mentor.

v

## Contributors (first and second editions):

**Sewell P. Champe, Ph.D. (deceased)**
Waksman Institute
Rutgers University
Piscataway, New Jersey

**Donald Dubin, M.D.**
Department of Molecular Genetics and Microbiology
University of Medicine and Dentistry of New Jersey–
Robert Wood Johnson Medical School
Piscataway, New Jersey

**Florence Kimball, Ph.D.**
Department of Molecular Genetics and Microbiology
University of Medicine and Dentistry of New Jersey–
Robert Wood Johnson Medical School
Piscataway, New Jersey

**Harriet Rouse, Ph.D. (deceased)**
Department of Molecular Genetics and Microbiology
University of Medicine and Dentistry of New Jersey–
Robert Wood Johnson Medical School
Piscataway, New Jersey

**William A. Strohl, Ph.D.**
Department of Molecular Genetics and Microbiology
University of Medicine and Dentistry of New Jersey–
Robert Wood Johnson Medical School
Piscataway, New Jersey

**Victor Stollar, M.D.**
Department of Molecular Genetics and Microbiology
University of Medicine and Dentistry of New Jersey–
Robert Wood Johnson Medical School
Piscataway, New Jersey

**William E. Winter, M.D.**
Department of Pathology
University of Florida College of Medicine
Gainesville, Florida

## Graphics:

**Michael Cooper**
Cooper Graphics
www.cooper247.com

*Acquisitions Editor:* Betty Sun
*Development Editor:* Kathleen H. Scogna
*Marketing Manager:* Jennifer Kuklinski
*Production Editor:* Jennifer D. Glazer
*Printer:* R.R. Donnelley & Sons-Willard

351 West Camden Street
Baltimore, MD 21201

530 Walnut Street
Philadelphia, PA 19106

The publisher is not responsible (as a matter of product liability, negligence, or otherwise) for any injury resulting from any material contained herein. This publication contains information relating to general principles of medical care that should not be construed as specific instructions for individual patients. Manufacturers' product information and package inserts should be reviewed for current information, including contraindications, dosages, and precautions.

*Printed in the United States of America*

First Edition, 2001

ISBN-13: 978-0-7817-8215-9

ISBN-10: 0-7817-8215-5

**Library of Congress Cataloging-in-Publication Data is available**

*The publishers have made every effort to trace the copyright holders for borrowed material. If they have inadvertently overlooked any, they will be pleased to make the necessary arrangements at the first opportunity.*

To purchase additional copies of this book, call our customer service department at **(800) 638-3030** or fax orders to **(301) 223-2320.** International customers should call **(301) 223-2300.**

To send comments to the authors, e-mail: **richardaharvey@gmail.com**

***Visit Lippincott Williams & Wilkins on the Internet: http://www.LWW.com.***
Lippincott Williams & Wilkins customer service representatives are available from 8:30 AM to 6:00 PM, EST.

07  08  09  10
2  3  4  5  6  7  8  9  10

# Acknowledgments

We are grateful to the many friends and colleagues who generously contributed their time and effort to help us make this book as accurate and useful as possible. The support of our other colleagues at the University of Medicine and Dentistry of New Jersey–Robert Wood Johnson Medical School is highly valued. Richard A, Harvey and Pamela C. Champe owe special thanks to Dr. Masayori Inouye, who has encouraged us over the years in this and other teaching projects.

Bruce D. Fisher offers a special thanks to his wife, Doris, who has always supported his work, and to Donald Armstrong, MD, MACP—a gifted clinician and scholar, mentor and friend.

Without talented artists, an Illustrated Review would be impossible, and we have been particularly fortunate in working with Michael Cooper throughout this project. His artistic sense and computer graphics expertise have greatly added to our ability to bring microbiology "stories" alive for our readers. We are also highly appreciative of Dr. Hae Sook Kim and Linda Duckenfield, SM/MT (ASCP), for assistance in preparing photomicrographs.

The editors and production staff of Lippincott Williams & Wilkins were a constant source of encouragement and discipline. We particularly want to acknowledge the tremendously supportive and creative contributions of our editor, Betty Sun, whose imagination and positive attitude helped us bring this complex project to completion. The design, content, editing, and assembly of the book have been greatly enhanced through the efforts of Kathleen Scogna and Jennifer Glazer.

# Unique Clinical Features

## Summaries of bacteria and their diseases

## Summary of common diseases

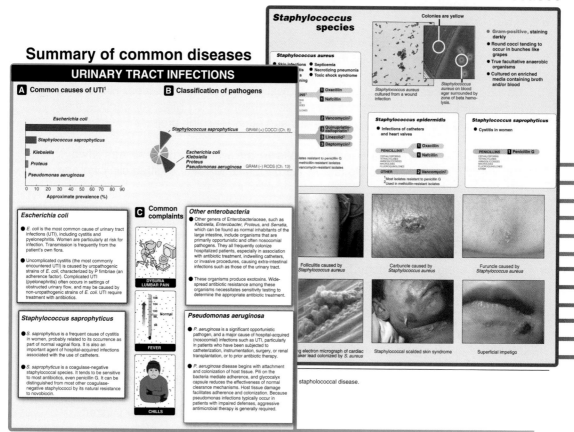

**Figure 33.4** (continued)
Disease summary of urinary tract infections. [1]Uncomplicated cystitis.

## Illustrated Case Studies

### Case 1: Man with necrosis of the great toe

This 63-year-old man with a long history of diabetes mellitus was seen in consultation because of an abrupt deterioration in his clinical status. He was admitted to the hospital for treatment of an ulcer, which had been present on his left great toe for several months. Figure 34.1 shows a typical example of perforating ulcer in a diabetic man.

Because of the inability of medical therapy (multiple courses of oral antibiotics) to resolve the ulcer, he underwent amputation of his left leg below the knee. On the first postoperative day he developed a temperature of 101°F, and on the

second postoperative day he became disoriented and his temperature reached 105.2°F. His amputation stump was mottled with many areas of purplish discoloration, and the most distal areas were quite obviously necrotic (dead). Crepitus (the sensation of displacing gas when an area is pressed with the fingers) was palpable up to his patella. An X-ray of the left lower extremity showed gas in the soft tissues, extending beyond the knee to the area of the distal femur. A Gram stain of a swab from the necrotic tissue is sh

**Figure 34.1**
Perforating ulcer of the great toe.

**Figure 34.2**
Gram stain of material swabbed from deep within a crepitant area. There are numerous polymorpho-nuclear leukocytes, and many large gram-positive bacilli, as well as a few gram-negative bacilli and cocci.

## Quick Review

### Herpesviridae
Epstein-Barr virus
Herpes simplex virus, Type 1
Herpes simplex virus, Type 2
Human cytomegalovirus
Human herpesvirus, Type 8
Varicella-zoster virus

### Common characteristics

- Linear, double-stranded DNA genome
- Replicate in the nucleus
- Envelope contains antigenic, species-specific glycoproteins
- In the tegument between the envelope and capsid are a number of virus-coded enzymes and transcription factors essential for initiation of the infectious cycle
- All herpesviruses can enter a latent state following primary infection, to be reactivated at a later time

# Contents

"She's the most effective of our emerging new pathogens."

# Introduction to Microbiology

# 1

## I. OVERVIEW

Microorganisms can be found in every ecosystem and in close association with every type of multicellular organism. They populate the healthy human body by the billions as benign passengers (normal flora, see p. 7) and even as participants in bodily functions, for example, bacteria play a role in the degradation of intestinal contents. In this volume, we primarily consider the role of microorganisms—bacteria, fungi, protozoa, helminths, and viruses—in the initiation and spread of human diseases. Those relatively few species of microorganisms that are harmful to humans, either by production of toxic compounds or by direct infection, are characterized as pathogens.

Most infectious disease is initiated by colonization (that is, the establishment of proliferating microorganisms on the skin or mucous membranes, Figure 1.1). The major exceptions are diseases caused by introduction of organisms directly into the bloodstream or internal organs. Microbial colonization may result in: 1) elimination of the microorganism without affecting the host, or 2) infection in which the organisms multiply and cause the host to react by making an immune or other type of response. Infectious disease occurs when the organism causes tissue damage and impairment of body function.

## II. PROKARYOTIC PATHOGENS

All prokaryotic organisms are classified as bacteria, whereas eukaryotic organisms include fungi, protozoa, and helminths, as well as humans. Prokaryotic organisms are divided into two major groups: the eubacteria, which include all bacteria of medical importance, and the archaebacteria, a collection of evolutionarily distinct organisms. Cells of prokaryotic and eukaryotic organisms differ in several significant structural features as illustrated in Figure 1.2.

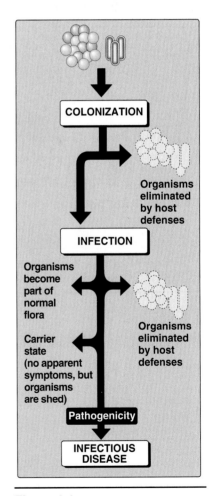

**Figure 1.1**
Some possible outcomes following exposure to microorganisms.

1

**Figure 1.2**
Comparison of prokaryotic and eukaryotic cells.

### A. Typical bacteria

Most bacteria have shapes that can be described as either a rod, sphere, or corkscrew. Prokaryotic cells are smaller than eukaryotic cells (Figure 1.3). Nearly all bacteria, with the exception of the mycoplasma, have a rigid cell wall surrounding the cell membrane that determines the shape of the organism. The cell wall also determines whether the bacterium is classified as gram-positive or gram-negative (see p. 21). External to the cell wall may be flagella, pili, and/or a capsule. Bacterial cells divide by binary fission. However, many bacteria exchange genetic information carried on plasmids—small, specialized genetic elements capable of self-replication—including the information necessary for establishment of antibiotic-resistance. Bacterial structure, metabolism, and genetics, and the wide variety of human diseases caused by bacteria are described in detail in Unit II, beginning on p. 49.

### B. Atypical bacteria

Atypical bacteria include groups of organisms such as *Mycoplasma*, *Chlamydia*, and *Rickettsia* that, although prokaryotic, lack significant characteristic structural components or metabolic capabilities that separate them from the larger group of typical bacteria.

## III. FUNGI

Fungi are nonphotosynthetic, generally saprophytic, eukaryotic organisms. Some fungi are filamentous, and are commonly called molds, whereas others—the yeasts—are unicellular (see p. 203). Fungal reproduction may be asexual, sexual, or both, and all fungi produce spores. Pathogenic fungi can cause diseases, ranging from skin infections (superficial mycoses) to serious, systemic infections (deep mycoses).

## IV. PROTOZOA

Protozoa are single-celled, nonphotosynthetic, eukaryotic organisms that come in various shapes and sizes. Many protozoa are free-living, but others are among the most clinically important parasites of humans. Members of this group infect all major tissues and organs of the body. They can be intracellular parasites, or extracellular parasites in the blood, urogenital region, or intestine. Transmission is generally by ingestion of an infective stage of the parasite or by insect bite. Protozoa cause a variety of diseases that are discussed in Chapter 21, p. 217.

## V. HELMINTHS

Helminths are groups of worms that live as parasites. They are multicellular, eukaryotic organisms with complex body organization. They are divided into three main groups: tapeworms (cestodes), flukes (trematodes), and roundworms (nematodes). Helminths are parasitic, receiving nutrients by ingesting or absorbing digestive contents, or ingesting or absorbing body fluids or tissues. Almost any organ in the body can be parasitized. All major groups of helminths can cause disease in humans, as described in Chapter 22, p. 227.

# VI. VIRUSES

Viruses are obligate intracellular parasites that do not have a cellular structure. Rather, a virus consists of molecule(s) of DNA (DNA virus) or RNA (RNA virus), but not both, surrounded by a protein coat. A virus may also have an envelope derived from the plasma membrane of the host cell from which the virus is released. Viruses contain the genetic information necessary for directing their own replication, but require the host's cellular structures and enzymatic machinery to complete the process of their own reproduction. The fate of the host cell following viral infection ranges from rapid lysis releasing many progeny virions, to gradual, prolonged release of viral particles. Viruses cause a broad spectrum of diseases (see Unit IV, beginning on p. 233).

# VII. ORGANIZING THE MICROORGANISMS

Trying to assimilate the names and characteristics of pathogenic organisms can be an overwhelming experience unless the flood of information is organized into logical groupings. In addition, it is helpful if these relationships can be visualized, using a consistent color-coding system. To this end, the authors have adopted several graphic formats that are used throughout this book.

## A. Hierarchical organization

The first is a hierarchical organization that resembles a family tree (Figures 1.4 and 1.5). These graphs provide a summary of the major characteristics of a particular microorganism. For example, tracing the lineage of staphylococci reveals that they have rigid cell walls and are simple, unicellular, free-living organisms that are gram-positive cocci.

## B. Pie chart organization: bacteria and viruses

A second, simpler format represents selected groups of bacteria or viruses as wedges of a pie chart. These pie charts focus on the most important defining characteristics of a particular organism. For example, bacteria are organized into eight groups according to Gram staining, morphology, and biochemical or other characteristics. The ninth section of the bacterial pie chart, labeled "Other", is used to represent any organism not included in one of the other eight categories (Figure 1.6). In a similar way, viral pathogens are organized into seven groups based on the nature of their genome, symmetry of organization, and the presence or absence of a lipid envelope (Figure 1.7).

## C. Taxonomy

This book uses a taxonomic hierarchy for the classification of bacteria, fungi, protozoans, and helminths. [Note: The classification of viruses is described on p. 234.] Kingdoms are divided into evolutionarily related phyla, classes, orders, families, genera, and species. The first letter of the genus name is always capitalized, and the species name begins with a lower case letter. Both names are printed in italics.

**Figure 1.3**
Relative size of organisms and molecules.

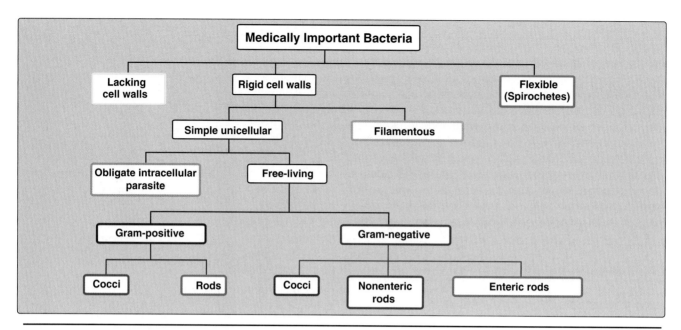

**Figure 1.4**
Classification of medically important bacterial families.

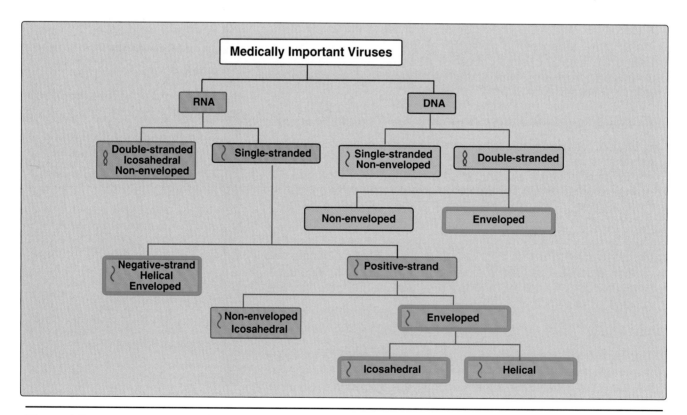

**Figure 1.5**
Classification of medically important virus families.

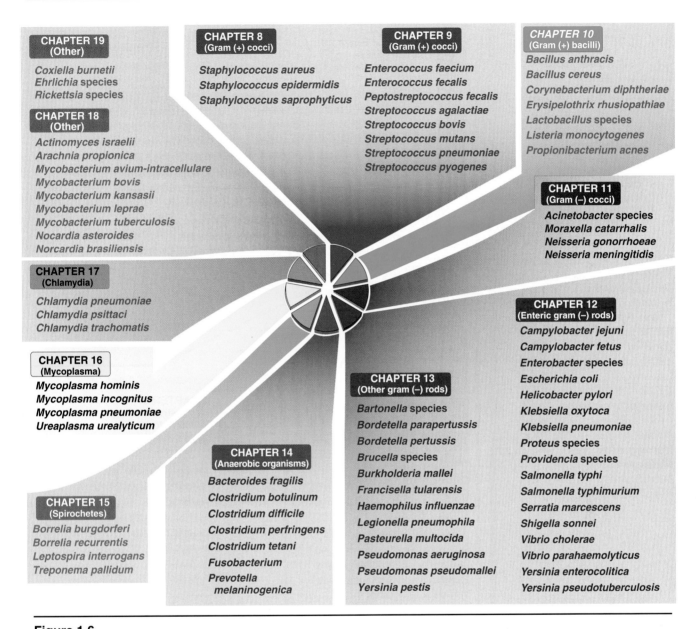

**CHAPTER 19**
**(Other)**

Coxiella burnetii
Ehrlichia species
Rickettsia species

**CHAPTER 18**
**(Other)**

Actinomyces israelii
Arachnia propionica
Mycobacterium avium-intracellulare
Mycobacterium bovis
Mycobacterium kansasii
Mycobacterium leprae
Mycobacterium tuberculosis
Nocardia asteroides
Norcardia brasiliensis

**CHAPTER 17**
**(Chlamydia)**

Chlamydia pneumoniae
Chlamydia psittaci
Chlamydia trachomatis

**CHAPTER 16**
**(Mycoplasma)**

Mycoplasma hominis
Mycoplasma incognitus
Mycoplasma pneumoniae
Ureaplasma urealyticum

**CHAPTER 15**
**(Spirochetes)**

Borrelia burgdorferi
Borrelia recurrentis
Leptospira interrogans
Treponema pallidum

**CHAPTER 8**
**(Gram (+) cocci)**

Staphylococcus aureus
Staphylococcus epidermidis
Staphylococcus saprophyticus

**CHAPTER 14**
**(Anaerobic organisms)**

Bacteroides fragilis
Clostridium botulinum
Clostridium difficile
Clostridium perfringens
Clostridium tetani
Fusobacterium
Prevotella
   melaninogenica

**CHAPTER 9**
**(Gram (+) cocci)**

Enterococcus faecium
Enterococcus fecalis
Peptostreptococcus fecalis
Streptococcus agalactiae
Streptococcus bovis
Streptococcus mutans
Streptococcus pneumoniae
Streptococcus pyogenes

**CHAPTER 13**
**(Other gram (–) rods)**

Bartonella species
Bordetella parapertussis
Bordetella pertussis
Brucella species
Burkholderia mallei
Francisella tularensis
Haemophilus influenzae
Legionella pneumophila
Pasteurella multocida
Pseudomonas aeruginosa
Pseudomonas pseudomallei
Yersinia pestis

**CHAPTER 10**
**(Gram (+) bacilli)**

Bacillus anthracis
Bacillus cereus
Corynebacterium diphtheriae
Erysipelothrix rhusiopathiae
Lactobacillus species
Listeria monocytogenes
Propionibacterium acnes

**CHAPTER 11**
**(Gram (–) cocci)**

Acinetobacter species
Moraxella catarrhalis
Neisseria gonorrhoeae
Neisseria meningitidis

**CHAPTER 12**
**(Enteric gram (–) rods)**

Campylobacter jejuni
Campylobacter fetus
Enterobacter species
Escherichia coli
Helicobacter pylori
Klebsiella oxytoca
Klebsiella pneumoniae
Proteus species
Providencia species
Salmonella typhi
Salmonella typhimurium
Serratia marcescens
Shigella sonnei
Vibrio cholerae
Vibrio parahaemolyticus
Yersinia enterocolitica
Yersinia pseudotuberculosis

**Figure 1.6**
Medically important bacteria discussed in this book, organized into similar groups based on morphology, biochemistry, and/or staining properties.

**Figure 1.7**
Medically important viruses discussed in this book, organized into similar groups based on the nature of the genome and the presence or absence of a lipid envelope.

# Normal Flora

# 2

## I. OVERVIEW

The human body is continuously inhabited by many different micro-organisms—mostly bacteria, but also fungi and other microorganisms—which under normal circumstances in a healthy individual are harmless, and may even be beneficial. These microorganisms are termed "normal flora." The normal flora are also termed commensals, which literally means "organisms that dine together." Except for occasional transient invaders, the internal organs and systems are sterile, including the spleen, pancreas, liver, bladder, central nervous system, and blood. A healthy newborn enters the world in essentially sterile condition, but, after birth, it rapidly acquires normal flora from food and the environment, including from other humans. The species contained in normal flora cannot be rigidly defined for all humans, because those species vary from individual to individual, as a result of physiologic differences, diet, age, and geographic habitat. It is useful to be aware of the normal types and distribution of resident flora, because such knowledge provides an understanding of the possible infections that result from injury to a particular body site, and places in perspective the possible sources and significance of microorganisms isolated from the site of an infection.

> Although bacteria and other microorganisms have not been considered plants for many years, the term "flora" is still widely used to describe microbial inhabitants of the human body.

## II. DISTRIBUTION OF NORMAL FLORA IN THE BODY

The most common sites of the body inhabited by normal flora are, as one might expect, those in contact or communication with the outside world, namely, the skin, eye, mouth, upper respiratory tract, gastrointestinal tract, and urogenital tract.

### A. Skin

Skin can acquire any bacteria that happen to be in the immediate environment, but this transient flora either dies or is removable by washing (Figure 2.1). The skin surface does not provide a favorable environment for colonization by microorganisms; for example, it is

**Figure 2.1**
A. Examples of bacteria that inhabit the skin. B. Arm of individual who injects drugs by "skin popping."

**Figure 2.2**
Examples of bacteria that inhabit the conjunctival sac.

generally dry (moist regions of the skin are more conducive to bacterial growth than dry regions), it has a slightly acidic pH, and the sweat glands produce a liquid containing a high concentration of sodium chloride that causes a hyperosmotic environment on the skin surface. Nevertheless, the skin supports a permanent bacterial population (resident flora), residing in multiple layers of the skin (see Figure 2.1). The resident flora regenerate even after vigorous scrubbing. Most common among the skin colonizers ($10^3$ to $10^4$ per $cm^2$) are aerobic *Staphylococcus epidermidis* and other coagulase-negative staphylococci (see p. 76) that reside in the outer layers of the skin, and account for some ninety percent of the skin aerobes. Anaerobic organisms, such as *Propionibacterium acnes*, reside in deeper skin layers, hair follicles, and sweat and sebaceous glands. Skin inhabitants are generally harmless, although *S. epidermidis* can attach to and colonize plastic catheters and medical devices that penetrate the skin, sometimes resulting in serious bloodstream infections.

## B. Eye

The conjunctiva of the eye is colonized primarily by *S. epidermidis*, followed by *Staphylococcus aureus*, aerobic corynebacteria (diphtheroids), and *Streptococcus pneumoniae*. Other organisms that normally inhabit the skin are also present, but at a lower frequency (Figure 2.2). Tears, which contain the antimicrobial enzyme lysozyme, help limit the bacterial population of the conjunctiva.

## C. Mouth and nose

The mouth and nose harbor many microorganisms, both aerobic and anaerobic (Figure 2.3). Among the most common are diphtheroids (aerobic *Corynebacterium* species), *S. aureus*, and *S. epidermidis*. In addition, the teeth and surrounding gingival tissue are colonized by their own particular species, such as *Streptococcus mutans*. [Note: *S. mutans* can enter the bloodstream following dental surgery, and colonize damaged or prosthetic heart valves, leading to potentially fatal infective endocarditis.] Some normal residents of the nasopharynx can also cause disease; for example, *S. pneumoniae*, found in the naso-

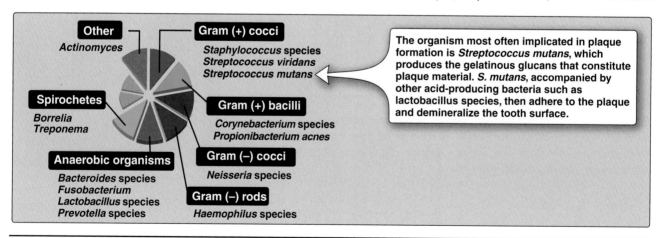

**Figure 2.3**
Examples of bacteria that inhabit the mouth.

pharynx of many healthy individuals, can cause acute bacterial pneumonia, especially in the aged and those whose resistance is impaired. [Note: Pneumonia is frequently preceded by an upper or middle respiratory viral infection, which predisposes the individual to *S. pneumoniae* infection of the pulmonary parenchyma.]

### D. Intestinal tract

In an adult, the density of microorganisms in the stomach is relatively low ($10^3$ to $10^5$ per gram of contents) due to gastric enzymes and acidic pH. The density of organisms increases along the alimentary canal, reaching $10^8$ to $10^{10}$ bacteria per gram of contents in the ileum, and $10^{11}$ per gram of contents in the large intestine. Some twenty percent of the fecal mass consists of many different species of bacteria, more than 99 percent of which are anaerobes (Figure 2.4). *Bacterioides* species constitute a significant percentage of bacteria in the large intestine.

> *Escherichia coli*, a facultatively anaerobic organism, constitutes less than 0.1 percent of the total population of bacteria in the intestinal tract. However, this endogenous *E. coli* is a major cause of urinary tract infections.

### E. Urogenital tract

The low pH of the adult vagina is maintained by the presence of *Lactobacillus* species, which are the primary components of normal flora. If the lactobacillus population in the vagina is decreased, for example, by antibiotic therapy, the pH rises and potential pathogens can overgrow. The most common example of such overgrowth is the yeast-like fungus, *Candida albicans* (see p. 213), which itself is a minor member of the normal flora of the vagina, mouth, and small intestine. The urine in the kidney and bladder is sterile, but can become contaminated in the lower urethra by the same organisms that inhabit the outer layer of the skin and perineum (Figure 2.5).

## III. BENEFICIAL FUNCTIONS OF NORMAL FLORA

Normal flora can provide some definite benefits to the host. First, the sheer number of harmless bacteria in the lower bowel and mouth make it unlikely that, in a healthy person, an invading pathogen could compete for nutrients and receptor sites. Second, some bacteria of the bowel produce antimicrobial substances to which the producers themselves are immune. Third, bacterial colonization of a newborn infant acts as a powerful stimulus for the development of the immune system. Fourth, bacteria of the gut provide important nutrients, such as vitamin K, and aid in digestion and absorption of nutrients. [Note: Although humans can obtain vitamin K from food sources, bacteria can be an important supplemental source if nutrition is impaired.]

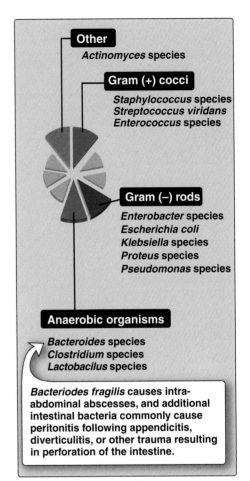

**Other**
*Actinomyces* species

**Gram (+) cocci**
*Staphylococcus* species
*Streptococcus viridans*
*Enterococcus* species

**Gram (−) rods**
*Enterobacter* species
*Escherichia coli*
*Klebsiella* species
*Proteus* species
*Pseudomonas* species

**Anaerobic organisms**
*Bacteroides* species
*Clostridium* species
*Lactobacilus* species

*Bacteriodes fragilis* causes intra-abdominal abscesses, and additional intestinal bacteria commonly cause peritonitis following appendicitis, diverticulitis, or other trauma resulting in perforation of the intestine.

**Figure 2.4**
Examples of bacteria that inhabit the gastrointestinal tract.

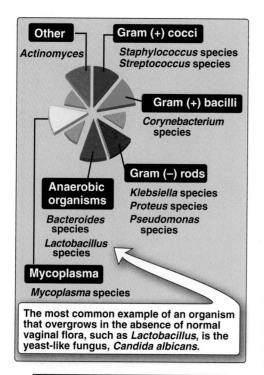

**Figure 2.5**
Examples of bacteria that inhabit
the vagina.

# IV. HARMFUL EFFECTS OF NORMAL FLORA

Clinical problems caused by normal flora arise under the following conditions: 1) When the organisms are displaced from their normal site in the body to an abnormal site. An example already mentioned is the introduction of the normal skin bacterium, *S. epidermidis*, into the bloodstream where it can colonize catheters and heart valves, resulting in bacterial endocarditis. 2) When potential pathogens gain a competitive advantage due to diminished populations of harmless competitors. For example, when normal bowel flora is depleted by antibiotic therapy leading to overgrowth by the resistant *C. difficile*, which can cause severe colitis. 3) When harmless, commonly ingested food substances are converted into carcinogenic derivatives by bacteria in the colon. A well-known example is the conversion by bacterial sulfatases of the sweetener cyclamate into the bladder carcinogen cyclohexamine. 4) When individuals are immunocompromised, normal flora can overgrow and become pathogenic. [Note: Colonization by normal, but potentially harmful, flora should be distinguished from the carrier state in which a true pathogen is carried by a healthy (asymptomatic) individual and passed to other individuals where it results in disease. Typhoid fever is an example of a disease that can be acquired from a carrier (see p. 116).]

## Study Questions

**Choose the ONE correct answer**

2.1 The primary effect of lactobacilli in the adult vagina is to

    A. maintain an alkaline environment.

    B. maintain an acidic environment.

    C. produce a protective mucus layer.

    D. increase fertility.

    E. keep the menstrual cycle regular.

> Correct answer = B. Lactobacilli produce acid that, in turn, inhibits the growth of potential pathogenic bacteria and fungi. None of the other answers are known to be attributed to lactobacilli.

2.2 A patient presents with severe colitis associated with an overgrowth of *Clostridium difficile* in the lower bowel. The most likely cause of this condition is

    A. botulinum food poisoning.

    B. a stomach ulcer.

    C. a compromised immune system.

    D. antibiotic therapy.

    E. mechanical blockage of the large intestine.

> Correct answer = D. Antibiotic therapy can reduce normal flora in the bowel, allowing pathogenic organisms normally present in low numbers to overgrow. None of the other answers explains the overgrowth of *C. difficile*.

2.3 The predominant bacterial species that colonizes the human skin is

    A. *Lactobacillus*.

    B. *Candida albicans*.

    C. *Streptococcus pneumoniae*.

    D. *Staphylococcus epidermidis*.

    E. *Bacterioides fragilis*.

> Correct answer = D. Human skin normally contains up to 10,000 *S. epidermidis* per cm$^2$. Other colonizing bacteria may be present but in much lower numbers. *C. albicans* is a yeast-like fungus, not a bacterium.

# Pathogenicity of Microorganisms

# 3

## I. OVERVIEW

A pathogenic microorganism is defined as one that causes or is capable of causing disease. Some microorganisms are unequivocally pathogenic, whereas others (the majority) are generally harmless. Further, some pathogens cause disease only under certain conditions (for example, being introduced into a normally sterile body site, or infection of an immunocompromised host). This chapter considers factors that influence whether a microorganism is a pathogen.

## II. BACTERIAL PATHOGENESIS

The infectious process can, in general, be divided into several stages: 1) entry into the host, with evasion of host primary defenses; 2) adhesion of the microorganism to host cells; 3) propagation of the organism; 4) damage to host cells by bacterial toxins or an inflammatory response of the host; and 5) evasion of host secondary defenses. Pathogenicity of a microorganism depends on its success in completing some or all of these stages. The terms "virulence" and "pathogenicity" are often used interchangeably. For example, virulence can be quantified by how many organisms are required to cause disease in fifty percent of those exposed to the pathogen ($ID_{50}$, where I = Infectious and D = Dose), or to kill fifty percent of test animals ($LD_{50}$, where L = Lethal; Figure 3.1).

### A. Virulence factors

Virulence factors are those characteristics of a bacterium that enhance its pathogenicity, that is, the ability to cause disease. Some of the more important classes of virulence factors are reviewed below.

1. **Entry into the host:** The first step of the infectious process is the entry of the microorganism into the host by one of several ports: the respiratory tract, gastrointestinal tract (GI), urogenital tract, or skin that has been cut, punctured, or burned. Once entry is achieved, the pathogen must overcome a diversity of host defenses before it can establish itself. These include phagocytosis, the acidic environments of the stomach and urogenital tract, and various hydrolytic and proteolytic enzymes found in the saliva, stomach, and small intestine. Bacteria that have an outer poly-

**Figure 3.1**
$ID_{50}$ (I = infectious, D = dose) versus $LD_{50}$ (L = lethal, D = dose).

## A Fimbrial (Pilus) Adhesion

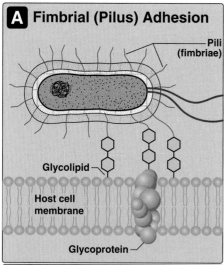

Pili (fimbriae)

Glycolipid

Host cell membrane

Glycoprotein

## B Afimbrial Adhesion

Cell Wall

Cell surface adhesion molecule

## C Hydrophobic Adhesion

Cell Wall

Hydrophobic interaction between bacterial cell wall and host cell membrane

**Figure 3.2**
Bacterial adhesion to host cell membranes.

saccharide capsule (for example, *Streptococcus pneumoniae* and *Neisseria meningitidis*) have a better chance of surviving these primary host defenses.

2. **Adherence to host cells:** Some bacteria (for example, *Escherichia coli*, see p. 111) use pili to adhere to the surface of host cells. Group A streptococci have similar structures (fimbriae, see p. 80). Other bacteria have cell surface adhesion molecules or particularly hydrophobic cell walls that allow them to adhere to the host cell membrane (Figure 3.2). In each case, adherence enhances virulence by preventing the bacteria from being carried away by mucus, or washed from organs with significant fluid flow, such as the urinary and the GI tracts. Adherence also allows each attached bacterial cell to form a microcolony. A striking example of the importance of adhesion is that of *Neisseria gonorrhoeae* in which strains that lack pili are not pathogenic (see p. 110).

3. **Invasiveness:** Invasive bacteria are those that can enter host cells or penetrate mucosal surfaces, spreading from the initial site of infection. Invasiveness is facilitated by several bacterial enzymes, the most notable of which are collagenase and hyaluronidase. These enzymes degrade components of the extracellular matrix, providing the bacteria with easier access to host cell surfaces. Invasion is followed by inflammation, which can be either pyogenic (involving pus formation) or granulomatous (having nodular inflammatory lesions), depending on the organism.

> The pus of pyogenic inflammations contains mostly neutrophils, whereas granulomatous lesions contain fibroblasts, lymphocytes, and macrophages.

4. **Bacterial toxins:** Some bacteria cause disease by producing toxins, of which there are two general types: the exotoxins and the endotoxins. Exotoxins, which are proteins, are secreted by both gram-positive and gram-negative bacteria. In contrast, endotoxins, which are lipopolysaccharides, are not secreted, but instead are integral components of the cell walls of gram-negative bacteria.

a. **Exotoxins:** These include some of the most poisonous substances known. It is estimated that as little as one microgram of tetanus exotoxin can kill an adult human. Exotoxin proteins generally have two polypeptide components (Figure 3.3); one is responsible for binding the protein to the host cell, and one is responsible for the toxic effect. In several cases, the precise target for the toxin has been identified. For example, diphtheria toxin is an enzyme that blocks protein synthesis. It does so by attaching an ADP-ribosyl group to human protein elongation factor EF-2,[1] inactivating it (see p. 92). Most exotoxins are

[1]See p. 439 in *Lippincott's Illustrated Reviews: Biochemistry* (3rd ed.) for a discussion of elongation factors in protein synthesis.

rapidly inactivated by moderate heating (60°C), notable exceptions being staphylococcal enterotoxin and *E. coli* heat-stable toxin (ST). In addition, treatment with dilute formaldehyde destroys the toxic activity of most exotoxins but does not affect their antigenicity. Formaldehyde-inactivated toxins, called toxoids, are useful in preparing vaccines (see p. 36). Exotoxin proteins are, in many cases, encoded by genes carried on plasmids or temperate bacteriophages. An example is the diphtheria exotoxin that is encoded by the *Tox* gene of a temperate bacteriophage that can lysogenize *Corynebacterium diphtheriae*. Strains of *C. diphtheriae* that carry this phage are pathogenic, whereas those that lack the phage are nonpathogenic).

**b. Endotoxins:** These are heat-stable, lipopolysaccharide (LPS) components of the outer membranes of gram-negative—but not gram-positive—bacteria. They are released into the host's circulation following bacterial cell lysis. LPS consists of polysaccharide O (somatic antigen), which protrudes from the exterior cell surface, a core polysaccharide, and a lipid component called lipid A that faces the cell interior. The lipid A moiety is responsible for the toxicity of this molecule. The main physiologic effects of LPS endotoxins are fever, shock, hypotension, and thrombosis, collectively referred to as septic shock. These effects are produced indirectly by activation of macrophages, with the release of cytokines, activation of complement, and activation of the coagulation cascade. Death can result from multiple organ failure. Although gram-positive bacteria do not contain LPS, their cell wall peptidoglycan can elicit a shock syndrome similar to that caused by LPS, but usually not as severe. Because the peptidoglycan fragments of gram-positive bacteria are chemically so different from LPS, and are also less potent, they are generally not considered to be endotoxins.

> Elimination of the causative bacteria by antibiotics can initially exacerbate the symptoms by causing sudden massive release of endotoxin into the circulation.

## B. Antigenic switching

A successful pathogen must evade the host's immune system that recognizes bacterial surface antigens. One important evasive strategy for the pathogen is to change its surface antigens. This is accomplished by several mechanisms. One mechanism, called phase variation, is the genetically reversible ability of certain bacteria to turn off and turn on the expression of genes coding for surface antigens. A second mechanism, called antigenic variation, involves the modification of the gene for an expressed surface antigen by genetic recombination with one of many variable unexpressed DNA sequences. In this manner, the expressed surface antigen can assume many different antigenic structures (see Figure 11.3, p. 102).

**Figure 3.3**
Action of exotoxins.

## C. Which is the pathogen?

If a particular microorganism is isolated from infected tissue (for example, a necrotic skin lesion), one cannot conclude that the isolated organism caused the lesion. The organism could, for example, be a harmless member of the normal skin flora (see p. 7) that happened to be in the vicinity. Alternatively, the organism may not be a natural resident of the skin, but an opportunistic pathogen that secondarily infected the necrotic lesion. [Note: An opportunistic pathogen is an organism that is unable to cause disease in healthy, immunocompetent individuals, but can infect people whose defenses have been impaired.] A nineteenth century German microbiologist, Robert Koch, recognized this dilemma, and defined a series of criteria (Koch's postulates) by which the identity of the causative microbial agent of a disease can be confirmed (Figure 3.4). [Note: Whereas this protocol has been successful in establishing the etiology of most infections, it fails if the causative organism cannot be cultured *in vitro*.]

## D. Infections in human populations

Bacterial diseases may be communicable from person-to-person or noncommunicable. For example, cholera is highly communicable (the disease-causing organism, *Vibrio cholerae*, is easily spread), whereas botulism is noncommunicable because only those people who ingest the botulinum exotoxin are affected. Highly communicable diseases, such as cholera, are said to be contagious, and tend to occur as localized epidemics in which the disease frequency is higher than normal. When an epidemic becomes worldwide, it is called a pandemic. Pandemics, such as the 1918 influenza pandemic, arise because the human population has never been exposed to, and, thus, has no immunity against, the specific strain of influenza virus.

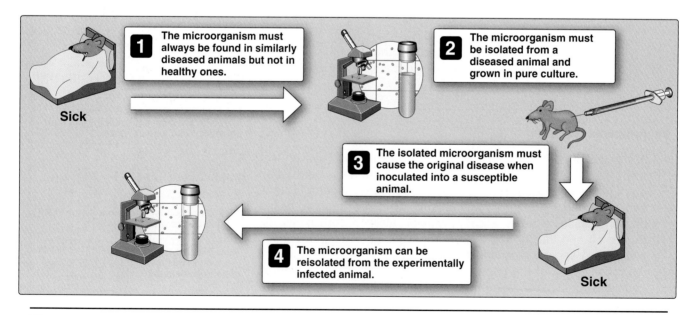

**Figure 3.4**
Koch's postulates.

# III. VIRAL PATHOGENESIS

Viruses can replicate only inside living cells. Consequently, the first pathogenic manifestations of viral infection are seen at the cellular level. The course of events following initial exposure to some viruses may include rapid onset of observable symptoms, which is referred to as an acute infection. Alternatively, the initial infection by other viruses may be mild or asymptomatic. Following the initial infection, the most common outcome is that the virus is cleared completely from the body by the immune system.

> For some viruses the initial infection is followed by either a persistent infection or a latent infection.

## A. Viral pathogenesis at the cellular level

Cells show a variety of different responses to viral infection, depending on the cell type and virus. Many viral infections cause no apparent morphologic or functional changes in the cell. When changes do occur, several (potentially overlapping) responses can be recognized (Figure 3.5).

1. **Cell death:** A cell can be directly killed by the virus. In most cases, this is due to the inhibition of synthesis of cellular DNA, RNA, and protein. Some viruses have specific genes responsible for this inhibition. Dead or dying cells release a brood of progeny viruses that repeat the replication process. Examples of viruses that kill their host cells are adenovirus (see p. 250) and poliovirus (see p. 283).

2. **Transformation:** Some viruses transform normal cells into malignant cells. In many ways, this is the opposite of cell death, because malignant cells have less fastidious growth requirements than do normal cells, and they have an indefinitely extended lifetime. Transformation is an irreversible genetic process caused by the integration of viral DNA into the host's DNA (see p. 243).

3. **Cell fusion:** Infection of cells with certain viruses causes the cells to fuse, producing giant, multinucleate cells. Viruses with this property include herpesviruses (see p. 257) and paramyxoviruses (see p. 309). The ability of infected cells to fuse is apparently due to virus-induced changes in the structure of the cell membrane.

4. **Cytopathic effect (CPE):** CPE is a catch-all term that refers to any visible change in appearance of an infected cell, for example, cell rounding, production of patches of stainable viral proteins inside the cell, and cell disintegration. Some viruses can be roughly identified by the time of onset and pattern of CPE in cell culture, as well as by the types of cells in which these viruses cause CPE.

**Figure 3.5**
Types of viral pathogenesis at the cellular level.

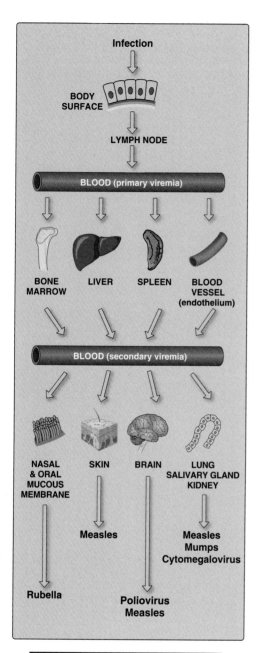

**Figure 3.6**
Examples of dissemination of virus to secondary sites in the body.

## B. Initial infections

Following initial multiplication at the primary site of entry, the viral infection may remain localized or become disseminated. The infection may be asymptomatic (unapparent). Alternatively, typical symptoms of disease may occur, often in two temporally distinct forms: 1) early symptoms at the primary site of infection; and 2) delayed symptoms due to dissemination from the primary site, causing infection of secondary sites.

> Virus transmission can occur before symptoms of the generalized illness are apparent, making it difficult to control the spread of viral diseases.

1. **Routes of entry and dissemination to secondary sites:** Common routes by which viruses enter the body are essentially the same as for bacterial infections (that is, through the skin, respiratory tract, GI tract, or urogenital tract). In each case, some viruses remain localized and cause disease that is largely restricted to the primary site of infection. Other viruses undergo multiplication in cells at the primary site, which may be accompanied by symptoms, followed by invasion of the lymphatic system and the blood. [Note: The presence of virus in the blood is termed "viremia".] Virus is, thereby, disseminated throughout the body, and can infect cells at secondary sites characteristic for each specific virus type, thus causing the disease typically associated with that species (Figure 3.6).

2. **Typical secondary sites of localization:** Secondary sites of infection determine the nature of the delayed symptoms, and usually the major characteristics associated with the resulting disease. Viruses frequently exhibit tropism for specific cell types and tissues. This specificity is usually caused by the presence of specific host cell surface receptors recognized by particular viruses. Whereas any tissue or organ system is a potential target for virus infection, the fetus represents an important site for secondary localization of virus infections. Virus from the maternal circulation infects cells of the placenta, thereby gaining access to the fetal circulation, and ultimately to all tissues of the developing fetus (Figure 3.7). Fetal death or developmental abnormalities are often the result. Neonatal infection can also occur during birth when the fetus comes in contact with infected genital secretions of the mother or breast-feeds.

3. **Virus shedding and mode of transmission:** The mode of transmission of a viral disease is largely determined by the tissues that produce progeny virus, and/or the fluids into which they are released. These are not necessarily the secondary sites of infection, but, in fact, are often the site of primary infection at a time before symptoms are apparent. Tissues commonly involved in viral shedding are the skin, respiratory tract, the GI tract, and bodily fluids.

4. **Factors involved in termination of acute infection:** In a typical, uncomplicated, acute infection, virus is totally eliminated from the host in two to three weeks. This outcome is primarily a function of the host's immune system, with involvement of both cell-mediated and humoral responses. The relative importance of these two responses depends on the virus and the nature of the disease.

   a. **Cell-mediated responses:** The earliest immune system responses to virus infection are a generalized inflammatory response, accompanied by nonspecific killing of infected cells by natural killer cells. This latter activity, enhanced by interferon and other cytokines, begins well before the virus-specific immune response. Later, cytolysis by virus-specific cytotoxic T lymphocytes that recognize virus peptides displayed on the cell surface also eliminates infected cells. These cellular responses are especially significant in that they help limit the spread of the infection by killing infected cells before they have released progeny virus.

   > Cell surface immunodeterminants recognized by T cells are often derived from nonstructural or internal proteins of the virus. Thus, this response complements the inactivation of free virus by humoral antibody, which is directed against capsid or envelope proteins.

   b. **Humoral response:** Whereas circulating antibodies may be directed against any virus protein, those that are of greatest significance in controlling an infection react specifically with epitopes on the surface of the virion, and result in inactivation of the virus's infectivity. The process is called neutralization. This response is of primary importance in suppressing diseases that involve a viremic stage, but secretory antibodies (IgA) also play an important protective role in primary infections of the respiratory and GI tracts. Humoral antibodies also take part in killing infected cells by two mechanisms: 1) antibody-dependent, cell-mediated cytotoxicity, in which natural killer cells and other leukocytes bearing Fc receptors bind to the Fc portions of antibodies that are complexed to virus antigens on the surface of the infected cell and kill it; and 2) complement-mediated lysis of infected cells to which virus-specific antibody has bound.

---

## A Modes of virus transmission

**Infected mothers can transmit viral infections to their offspring by three routes:**

**1** In utero by transplacental spread

Virus

**2** During delivery through an infected birth canal

**3** After birth by ingestion of breast milk

Virus in milk

## B Some viruses transmitted mother to infant

Herpes simplex virus types 1 and 2
Human cytomegalovirus
Human immunodeficiency virus
Rubella virus

**Figure 3.7**
Mother-to-infant (vertical) transmission of viral infections.

## Study Questions

**Choose the ONE correct answer.**

3.1 Endotoxins belong to a class of biological molecules called

    A. mucopolysaccharides.
    B. lipopolysaccharides.
    C. nucleic acids.
    D. proteins.
    E. peptidoglycans.

> Correct answer = B. Endotoxins are integral lipopolysaccharide constituents of the outer membrane of gram-negative bacteria. The peptidoglycans, present in large amounts in gram-positive bacteria, can be toxic, but are not considered to be endotoxins.

3.2 Exotoxins belong to a class of biologic molecules called

    A. mucopolysaccharides.
    B. lipopolysaccharides.
    C. nucleic acids.
    D. proteins.
    E. peptidoglycans.

> Correct answer = D. Exotoxins are secreted toxic proteins that, in many cases, have a well-defined cellular site of action.

3.3 The mechanism of action of diphtheria toxin is to

    A. disrupt the cell membrane.
    B. block nucleic acid synthesis.
    C. block protein synthesis.
    D. interfere with neurotransmission.
    E. destroy the cell nucleus.

> Correct answer = C. Diphtheria toxin inactivates the polypeptide elongation factor EF-2, blocking protein synthesis. Tetanus toxin interferes with neurotransmission.

3.4 A 48-year-old woman presented at the emergency room complaining of urinary urgency and flank pain. Microscopic examination of a urine sample revealed gram-negative rods. Prior to initiation of antibiotic therapy, she abruptly developed fever, chills, and delirium. Hypotension and hyperventilation rapidly followed. These observations suggest that the patient is responding to the release of bacterial

    A. collagenase.
    B. exotoxin.
    C. hyaluronidase.
    D. lipopolysaccharide (LPS).
    E. peptidoglycan.

> Correct answer = D. The patient is most likely suffering from septic shock. In two thirds of patients, septic shock results from infection with gram-negative bacteria, such as *Escherichia coli*, *Klebsiella*, *Enterobacter*, *Proteus*, *Pseudomonas*, or *Bacteroides*. Septicemia is more common in persons whose resistance is already compromised by an existing condition. The gram-negative bacteria release endotoxins—heat-stable, lipopolysaccharide (LPS) components of the outer membranes. The main physiologic effects of LPS endotoxins are fever, hypotension, and thrombosis, collectively referred to as septic shock. Death can result from multiple organ failure. Gram-positive bacteria release exotoxins that can elicit a shock syndrome, but response is usually not as severe as that of gram-negative septic shock.

And what makes you think you'd be such a good assassin, Mr T?

JOE'S MERCENARIES HIRING

*"As each disease is finally eradicated, redundant lymphocytes increasingly find themselves looking for other work."*

# Diagnostic Microbiology

# 4

## I. OVERVIEW

Identification of the organism causing an infectious process is usually essential for effective antimicrobial and supportive therapy. Initial treatment may be empiric, based on the microbiologic epidemiology of the infection and the patient's symptoms. However, definitive microbiologic diagnosis of an infectious disease usually involves one or more of the following five basic laboratory techniques, which guide the physician along a narrowing path of possible causative organisms: 1) direct microscopic visualization of the organism; 2) cultivation and identification of the organism; 3) detection of microbial antigens; 4) detection of microbial DNA or RNA; and 5) detection of an inflammatory or host immune response to the microorganism (Figure 4.1).

## II. SENSITIVITY AND SPECIFICITY OF TEST RESULTS

Interpretation of laboratory tests is influenced by the reliability of the results. Ideally, a diagnostic test is positive in the presence of a pathogen (true-positive) and negative in the absence of a pathogen (true-negative). However, in practice, no laboratory test is perfect. An assay may give negative results in the presence of a pathogen (false-negative) or positive results in the absence of a pathogen (false-positive). Thus, it is useful to define the reliability of a diagnostic procedure in terms of its sensitivity and specificity. The sensitivity of a test is the probability that it will be positive in the presence of a pathogen:

$$\text{Sensitivity} = \frac{\text{True-positives}}{\text{True-positives} + \text{False-negatives}} \times 100 \text{ percent}$$

As the number of false-negatives approaches zero, the sensitivity approaches 100 percent (that is, all infected patients are detected). Specificity is the probability that a test will be negative if the pathogen is not present:

$$\text{Specificity} = \frac{\text{True-negatives}}{\text{True-negatives} + \text{False-positives}} \times 100 \text{ percent}$$

As the number of false-positives approaches zero, the specificity approaches 100 percent (that is, all positive patients are actually

**Figure 4.1**
Laboratory techniques that are useful in diagnosis of microbial diseases.

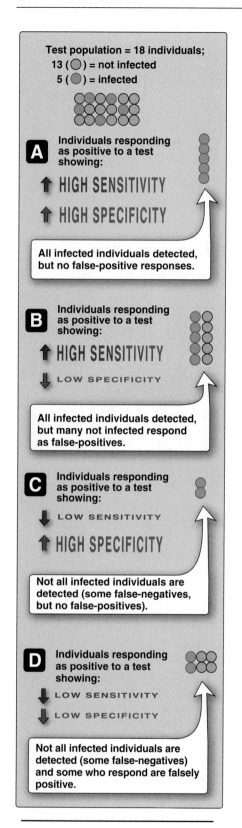

**Figure 4.2**
Effect of sensitivity and specificity of a test on the presence of false-positives and false-negatives.

infected). Figure 4.2 shows the results obtained with tests of high and low sensitivity/specificity.

## III. PATIENT HISTORY AND PHYSICAL EXAMINATION

A clinical history is the most important part of the evaluation of patients. For example, a history of cough points to the possibility of respiratory tract infection; dysuria suggests urinary tract infection. A history of travel to developing countries may implicate exotic organisms. For example, a patient who recently swam in the Nile has an increased risk of schistosomiasis. Patient occupations may suggest exposure to certain pathogens, such as brucellosis in a butcher or anthrax in farmers. Even the age of the patient can sometimes guide the clinician in predicting the identity of pathogens, for example, a gram-positive coccus in the spinal fluid of a newborn infant is unlikely to be *Streptococcus pneumoniae* (pneumococcus), but most likely to be *S. agalactiae* (Group B). This organism is sensitive to penicillin G. By contrast, a gram-positive coccus in the spinal fluid of a forty-year-old is most likely to be *Streptococcus pneumoniae*. This organism is frequently resistant to penicillin G, and often requires treatment with a third generation cephalosporin (such as cefotaxime or ceftriaxone) or vancomycin. The etiology implied by the patient's age may thus guide initial therapy. A physical examination often provides confirmatory clues to the presence and extent (localized or disseminated) of disease. For example, erythema migrans (a large skin lesion with a bright red outer border and partially clear central area, see p. 165) indicates early localized Lyme disease. Clues to the presence of bacteremia (a disseminated infection) may include chills, fever (or sometimes hypothermia), or cardiovascular instability heralding septic shock. Physical signs of pulmonary consolidation suggest pneumonia. If one adds stupor and stiff neck to this constellation of findings, the organism causing the pneumonia may have spread to the meninges, warranting a further search for it in the cerebrospinal fluid.

> All laboratory studies must be directed by the patient's history and physical examination and then evaluated, taking into consideration the sensitivity and specificity of the test.

## IV. DIRECT VISUALIZATION OF THE ORGANISM

In many infectious diseases, pathogenic organisms can often be directly visualized by microscopic examination of patient specimens, such as sputum, urine, or cerebrospinal fluid. The organism's microscopic morphology and staining characteristics can provide the first screening step in arriving at a specific identification. The organisms to be examined need be neither alive nor able to multiply. Microscopy gives rapid and inexpensive results, and may allow the clinician to initiate treatment without waiting for the results of a culture, as noted in the spinal fluid example in the previous paragraph.

## A. Gram stain

Because unstained bacteria are difficult to detect with the light microscope, most patient material is stained prior to microscopic evaluation. The most common and useful staining procedure—the Gram stain—separates bacteria into two classifications according to the composition of their cell walls. If a clinical specimen on a microscope slide is treated with a solution of crystal violet and then iodine, the bacterial cells will stain purple. If the stained cells are then treated with a solvent, such as alcohol or acetone, gram-positive organisms retain the stain, whereas gram-negative species lose the stain, becoming colorless (Figure 4.3). Addition of the counterstain safranin stains the clear, gram-negative bacteria pink or red. Most, but not all, bacteria are stainable and fall into one of these two groups. [Note: Microorganisms that lack cell walls, such as mycoplasma, cannot be identified using the Gram stain.]

1. **Applications of the Gram stain:** The Gram stain is important therapeutically because gram-positive and gram-negative bacteria have differing susceptibilities to various antibiotics, and the Gram stain may, therefore, be used to guide initial therapy until definitive identification of the microorganism can be obtained. In addition, the morphology of the stained bacteria can sometimes be diagnostic; for example, gram-negative intracellular diplococci in urethral pus provides a presumptive diagnosis of gonorrhea. Gram stains of specimens submitted for culture are often invaluable aids in the interpretation of culture results. For example, a specimen may show organisms under the microscope, but appear sterile in culture media. This discrepancy may suggest: 1) fastidious organisms (bacteria with complex nutrient requirements) that are unable to grow on the culture media employed; or 2) fragile organisms, such as gonococcus or anaerobic organisms, that may not survive transport. In these cases, direct visualization with the Gram stain may provide the only clue to the nature, variety, and relative number of infecting organisms.

2. **Limitations of the Gram stain:** The number of microorganisms required is relatively high—visualization with the Gram stain requires greater than $10^4$ organisms/mL. Liquid samples with low

1 Heat-fix specimen to slide. Flood slide with crystal violet solution; allow to act for 1 minute.

Crystal violet solution

2 Rinse the slide, then flood with iodine solution; allow iodine to act for 1 minute. Before acetone decolorization (next step), all organisms appear purple, that is, gram-positive.

Iodine solution

3 Rinse off excess iodine. Decolorize with acetone, approximately 5 seconds (time depends on density of specimen).

Acetone

4 Wash slide immediately in water. After acetone decolorization, those organisms that are gram-negative are no longer visible.

5 Apply safranin counterstain for 30 seconds.

Safranin

6 Wash in water, blot, and dry in air. Gram-negative organisms are visualized after application of the counterstain.

**Figure 4.3**
Steps in Gram stain method.
Key:  ● = Gram-positive violet.  ⬤▬ = Gram-negative red.  ⬭ = Colorless.

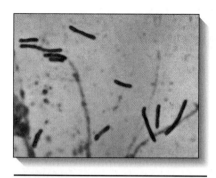

**Figure 4.4**
*Mycobacterium tuberculosis* stained with acid-fast stain.

**Figure 4.5**
India ink preparation of *Cryptococcus neoformans* in cerebrospinal fluid. These yeast cells are identified by large transparent capsules that exclude the India ink particles.

**Figure 4.6**
Fungi in unstained nasal sinus exudate, made distinct from other materials (such as cells) with potassium hydroxide.

numbers of microorganisms (for example, in cerebrospinal fluid), require centrifugation to concentrate the pathogens. The pellet is then examined after staining.

### B. Acid-fast stain

Stains such as Ziehl-Neelsen (the classic acid-fast stain) are used to identify organisms that have waxy material (mycolic acids) in their cell walls. Most bacteria that have been stained with carbolfuchsin can be decolorized by washing with acidic alcohol. However, certain acid-fast bacteria, retain the carbolfuchsin stain after being washed with an acidic solution. The most clinically important acid-fast bacterium is *Mycobacterium tuberculosis*, which appears pink, often beaded, and slightly curved (Figure 4.4). Acid-fast staining is reserved for clinical samples from patients suspected of having mycobacterial infection.

### C. India ink preparation

This is one of the simplest microscopic methods. It is useful in detecting *Cryptococcus neoformans* in cerebrospinal fluid (Figure 4.5). One drop of centrifuged cerebrospinal fluid is mixed with one drop of India ink on a microscope slide beneath a glass cover slip. Cryptococci are identified by their large, transparent capsules that displace the India ink particles.

### D. Potassium hydroxide (KOH) preparation

Treatment with KOH dissolves host cells and bacteria, sparing fungi (Figure 4.6). One drop of sputum or skin scraping is treated with ten percent KOH, and the specimen is examined for fungal forms.

## V. GROWING BACTERIA IN CULTURE

Culturing is routine for most bacterial and fungal infections, but is rarely used to identify helminths or protozoa. Culturing of many pathogens is straightforward, for example, streaking a throat swab onto a blood agar plate in search of group A β-hemolytic streptococcus. However, certain pathogens are very slow growing (for example, *Mycobacterium tuberculosis*), or are cultured only with difficulty (for example, *Bartonella henselae*). Microorganisms isolated in culture are identified using such characteristics as colony size, shape, color, Gram stain, hemolytic reactions on solid media, odor, and metabolic properties. In addition, pure cultures provide samples for antimicrobial susceptibility testing (see p. 30). The success of culturing depends on appropriate collection and transport techniques, and on selection of appropriate culture media, because some organisms may require special nutrients. Also, some media are used to suppress the growth of certain organisms in the process of identifying others (see p. 23)

### A. Collection of specimens

Many organisms are fragile and must be transported to the laboratory with minimal delay; for example, gonococci and pneumococci are very sensitive to heating or drying. Samples must be cultured promptly or, if this is not possible, transport media must be used to extend the viability of the organism to be cultured. When anaerobic organisms are suspected, the patient's specimen must be protected from the toxic effect of oxygen (Figure 4.7).

## B. Growth requirements

All clinically important bacteria are heterotrophs (that is, they require organic carbon for growth). Heterotrophs may have complex or simple requirements for organic molecules. [Note: Organisms that can reduce carbon dioxide and, thus, do not require organic compounds for cell growth, are called autotrophs.] Most bacteria require varying numbers of growth factors, which are organic compounds required by the cell to grow, but which the organism cannot itself synthesize (for example, vitamins). Organisms that require either a large number of growth factors or must be supplied with very specific ones are referred to as fastidious.

## C. Oxygen requirement:

Bacteria can be categorized according to their growth responses in the presence and absence of oxygen. Aerobic bacteria (aerobes) such as *M. tuberculosis*, grow in the presence of oxygen, and can use oxygen as the terminal electron acceptor in energy production (see p. 185). Obligate aerobes have an absolute requirement for oxygen. Facultative organisms, such as *Escherichia coli*, grow in the presence or absence of oxygen. The "true" facultatives use oxygen preferentially as the terminal electron acceptor when it is present, whereas microaerophilic organisms, such as *Campylobacter jejuni*, require or tolerate oxygen, but at an oxygen partial pressure lower than that of the atmosphere. Anaerobic bacteria such as *Clostridium botulinum* can grow in the absence of oxygen, producing energy by fermentation (see p. 153), whereas obligate anaerobes grow only in the absence of oxygen and may, in fact, be killed by small amounts of oxygen.

## D. Media

Two general strategies are used to isolate pathogenic bacteria, depending on the nature of the clinical sample. The first method uses enriched media to promote the nonselective growth of any bacteria that may be present. The second approach employs selective media that only allow growth of specific bacterial species from specimens that normally contain large numbers of bacteria (for example, stool, genital tract secretions, or sputum).

|| Isolation of a bacterium is usually performed on solid medium. Liquid medium is used to grow larger quantities of a culture of bacteria that has already been isolated as a pure culture).

**1. Enriched media:** Media fortified with blood, yeast extracts, or brain or heart infusions are useful in growing fastidious organisms. For

**Figure 4.7**
Anaerobic transport media containing a nonnutritive medium that retards diffusion of oxygen after addition of the specimen. Microorganisms may remain viable for up to 72 hours. It is important to use an airless syringe for liquid specimens such as pus, rather than a swab in a tube— especially when transport medium is not available. Also, if promptly transported in a syringe, one has the advantage of seeing the relative proportions of each morphology in mixed infections.

example, sheep blood agar contains protein sources, sodium chloride, and five percent sheep blood, and supports the growth of most gram-positive and gram-negative bacteria isolated from human sources (see p. 89). However, *Haemophilus influenzae* and *Neisseria gonorrhoeae*, among others, are highly fastidious organisms. They require chocolate agar, which contains red blood cells that have been lysed (see p. 131). This releases intracellular nutrients, such as hemoglobin, hemin ("X" factor), and $NAD^+$ ("V" factor), required by these organisms. Enriched media are useful for culturing normally sterile body fluids, such as blood or cerebrospinal fluid, in which the finding of any organisms provides reasonable evidence for infection due to that organism.

> Failure to culture an organism may indicate that the culture medium is inadequate, or the incubation conditions do not support bacterial growth.

**Figure 4.8**
Lactose-fermenting, gram-negative rods produce pink colonies on MacConkey agar.

2. **Selective media:** The most commonly used selective medium is MacConkey agar (see p. 115), which supports the growth of most gram-negative rods, especially the Enterobacteriaceae, but inhibits growth of gram-positive organisms and some fastidious gram-negative bacteria, such as *Haemophilus* and *Neisseria* species. Growth on blood agar and chocolate agar, but not MacConkey agar suggests a gram-positive isolate or a fastidious gram-negative species. In contrast, most gram-negative rods often form distinctive colonies on MacConkey agar. This agar is also used to detect organisms able to metabolize lactose (Figure 4.8). Clinical samples are routinely plated on blood agar, chocolate agar, and MacConkey agar. Hektoen enteric agar is also a selective medium that differentiates lactose/sucrose fermenters and nonfermenters, as well as $H_2S$ producers and nonproducers. It is often used to culture *Salmonella* and *Shigella* species. Thayer-Martin agar is another selective medium composed of chocolate agar supplemented with several antibiotics that suppress the growth of nonpathogenic *Neisseria* and other normal and abnormal flora. This medium is normally used to isolate gonococci.

> When submitting samples for culture, the physician must alert the laboratory to likely pathogens whenever possible, especially when unusual organisms are suspected. This allows inclusion of selective media that might not be used routinely. It also alerts the laboratory to hold specimens longer, if a slow-growing organism, such as *Nocardia*, is suspected.

Bacteria that ferment lactose produce acids that decrease the pH of agar. The acidity causes a pH indicator in the agar to turn pink.

# VI. IDENTIFICATION OF BACTERIA

The most widely used identification scheme involves determining the morphologic and metabolic properties of the unknown bacterium, and comparing these with properties of known microorganisms. Alternate identification schemes using nucleic acid–based methods are discussed on p. 29. Immunologic methods used in diagnosis are described on p. 26. It is essential to start identification tests with pure bacterial isolates grown from a single colony.

## A. Single-enzyme tests

Different bacteria produce varying spectra of enzymes. For example, some enzymes are necessary for the bacterium's individual metabolism and some facilitate the bacterium's ability to compete with other bacteria or establish an infection. Tests that measure single bacterial enzymes are simple, rapid, and generally easy to interpret. They can be performed on organisms already grown in culture, and often provide presumptive identification.

1. **Catalase test:** The enzyme catalase catalyzes the degradation of hydrogen peroxide to water and molecular oxygen ($H_2O_2 \rightarrow H_2O + O_2$). Catalase-positive organisms rapidly produce bubbles when exposed to a solution containing hydrogen peroxide (Figure 4.9). The catalase test is key in differentiating between many gram-positive organisms; for example, staphylococci are catalase-positive, whereas streptococci and enterococci are catalase-negative.

2. **Oxidase test:** The enzyme cytochrome oxidase is part of electron transport and nitrate metabolism in some bacteria. The enzyme can accept electrons from artificial substrates, such as a phenylenediamine derivative, producing a dark, oxidized product (see Figure 4.9). This test assists in differentiating between groups of gram-negative bacteria. *Pseudomonas aeruginosa*, for example, is oxidase-positive.

3. **Urease:** The enzyme urease hydrolyzes urea to ammonia and carbon dioxide ($NH_2CONH_2 + H_2O \rightarrow 2NH_3 + CO_2$). The ammonia produced can be detected with pH indicators that change color in response to the increased alkalinity (see Figure 4.9). The test helps to identify certain species of Enterobacteriaceae, *Corynebacterium urealyticum* and *Helicobacter pylori*.

4. **Coagulase test:** Coagulase is an enzyme that causes a clot to form when bacteria are incubated with plasma. The test is used to differentiate *Staphylococcus aureus* (coagulase-positive) from coagulase-negative staphylococci.

## B. Tests based on the presence of metabolic pathways

These tests measure the presence of a metabolic pathway in a bacterial isolate, rather than a single enzyme. Commonly used assays include those for oxidation and fermentation of different carbohydrates, the ability to degrade amino acids, and use of specific sub-

**Catalase test**

Bubbles indicate production of oxygen gas by catalase.

**Oxidase test**

Dark, oxidized product results from cytochrome oxidase activity.

**Urease test**

pH indicator in agar turns dark due to production of $NH_3$ by urease.

Coagulase-positive bacteria promote clotting of serum.

**Coagulase test**

**Figure 4.9**
Tests commonly used in identifying bacteria.

**Figure 4.10**
Rapid manual biochemical system for bacterial identification. Different appearances of the upper and lower pairs of wells indicate the positive or negative ability of a bacterium to utilize each substrate.

**Figure 4.11**
A. Vitek test card containing test wells.
B. Color of well changes with time.

strates. A widely used manual system for rapid identification of members of the family Enterobacteriaceae and other gram-negative bacteria makes use of twenty microtubes containing substrates for various biochemical pathways. The test substrates in the microtubes are inoculated with the bacterial isolate to be identified, and, after five hours' incubation, the metabolic profile of the organism is constructed from color changes in the microtubes. These color changes indicate the presence or absence of the bacteria's ability to metabolize a particular substrate. The results are compared with a data bank containing test results from known bacteria (Figure 4.10). The probability of a match between the test organism and known pathogens is then calculated.

### C. Automated systems

Microbiology laboratories are increasingly using automated methods to identify bacterial pathogens. For example, in the Vitek System, small plastic reagent cards containing microliter quantities of various biochemical test media in thirty wells provide a biochemical profile that allows for organism identification (Figure 4.11). An inoculum derived from cultured samples is automatically transferred into the card, and a photometer intermittently measures color changes in the card that result from the metabolic activity of the organism. The data are analyzed, stored, and printed in a computerized data base.

## VII. IMMUNOLOGIC DETECTION OF MICROORGANISMS

In the diagnosis of infectious diseases, immunologic methods take advantage of the specificity of antigen-antibody binding. For example, known antigens and antibodies are used as diagnostic tools in identifying microorganisms. In addition, serologic detection of a patient's immune response to infection, or antigenic or nucleic acid evidence of a pathogen in a patient's body fluids, is frequently useful. Immunologic methods are useful when the infecting microorganism is difficult or impossible to isolate, or when a previous infection needs to be documented. Most methods for determining whether antibodies or antigens are present in patients' sera or other body fluids require some type of immunoassay procedure, such as those described in this section.

## A. Detection of microbial antigen with known antiserum

These methods of identification are often rapid, and show favorable sensitivity and specificity (see Figure 4.2, p. 20). However, unlike microbial culturing techniques, these immunologic methods do not permit further characterization of the microorganism, such as determining its antibiotic sensitivity, or characteristic metabolic patterns.

1. **Capsular swelling reaction:** Some bacteria having capsules can be identified directly in clinical specimens by a swelling reaction that occurs when the organisms are treated with serum containing specific antibodies (see Figure 9.10, p. 86). This method, sometimes called the Quellung reaction, can be used for all serotypes of *S. pneumoniae*, *H. influenzae* type b, and *Neisseria meningitidis* groups A and C.

2. **Slide agglutination test:** Some microorganisms, such as *Salmonella* and *Shigella* species, can be identified by agglutination (clumping) of a suspension of bacterial cells on a microscopic slide. Agglutination occurs when a specific antibody directed against the microbial antigen is added to the suspension, causing cross-linking of the bacteria.

## B. Identification of serum antibodies

Detection in a patient's serum of antibodies that are directed against microbial antigens provides evidence for a current or past infection with a specific pathogen. A discussion of the general interpretation of antibody responses includes the following rules: 1) antibody may not be detectable early in an infection; 2) the presence of antibodies in a patient's serum cannot differentiate between a present and a prior infection; and 3) a rise in antibody titer over a seven-to-ten day period does distinguish between a present or prior infection. Techniques such as complement fixation and agglutination can be used to quantitate antimicrobial antibodies.

1. **Complement fixation:** One older but still useful method for detecting serum antibody directed against a specific pathogen employs the ability of antibody to bind complement (Figure 4.12). A patient's serum is first incubated with antigen specific for the suspected infectious agent, followed by the addition of complement. If the patient's serum does contain IgG or IgM antibodies that target the specific antigen (indicating past or current infection), then the added complement will be sequestered in an antigen-antibody-complement complex ("complement fixation"). Next, sensitized (antibody-coated) indicator sheep red blood cells are added to the solution. If complement has been fixed (because the patient's serum contained antibodies against the added antigen), then little complement will be available to bind to the antibody–red blood cell complexes, and the cells will not lyse. If complement has not been depleted by initial antigen-antibody complexes (because the patient's serum does not contain antibodies to the specific antigen), the complement will bind to the antibody–red blood cell complexes, causing the cells to lyse. As hemolyzed red blood cells release hemoglobin, the reaction can be monitored with a spectrophotometer.

**Figure 4.12**
Complement fixation.

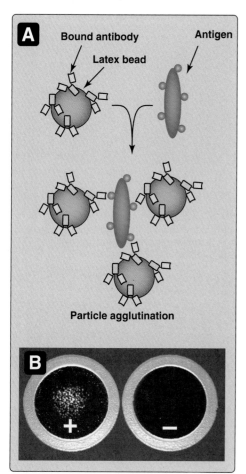

**Figure 4.13**
A. Schematic representation of antigens agglutinating latex beads with bound antibody. B. Photograph of agglutination reaction.

2. **Direct agglutination:** "Febrile agglutinins" is a test panel sometimes ordered to evaluate patients with fever of unknown origin, or when a suspected organism is difficult or dangerous to culture in the laboratory. This test measures the ability of a patient's serum antibody to directly agglutinate specific killed (yet intact) microorganisms. This test is used to evaluate patients suspected of being infected by *Brucella abortus* or *Francisella tularensis*, among others.

3. **Direct hemagglutination:** Antibodies directed against red blood cells can arise during the course of various infections. For example, such antibodies are typically found during infectious mononucleosis caused by Epstein-Barr virus (see p. 268). When uncoated (native) animal or human red blood cells are used in agglutination reactions with serum from a patient infected with such an organism, antibodies to red blood cell antigens can be detected (the patient's antibodies cause the red blood cells to clump). This test is, therefore, a direct hemagglutination reaction. In the case of some diseases, including pneumonia caused by *Mycoplasma pneumoniae*, IgM autoantibodies may develop that agglutinate human red blood cells at 4°C but not at 37°C. This is termed the "cold agglutinins" test.

C. **Other tests used to identify serum antigens or antibodies**

1. **Latex agglutination test:** Latex and other particles can be readily coated with either antibody (for antigen detection) or antigen (for antibody detection). Addition of antigen to antibody-coated latex beads causes agglutination that can be visually observed (Figure 4.13). For example, such methods are used to rapidly test cerebral spinal fluid for antigens associated with common forms of bacterial or fungal meningitis. When antigen is coated onto the latex bead, antibody from a patient's serum can be detected.

> Latex agglutination tests are widely used for the identification of β-hemolytic streptococci group A.

2. **Enzyme-linked immunosorbent assay (ELISA):** In this diagnostic technique, antibody specific for an antigen of interest is bound to the walls of a plastic microtiter well (Figure 4.14). Patient serum is then incubated in the wells, and any antigen in the serum is bound by the antibody on the well walls. The wells are then washed, and a second antibody is added—this one also specific for the antigen, but recognizing epitopes different from those bound by the first antibody. After incubation, the wells are again washed, removing any unattached antibody. Attached to the second antibody is an enzyme, which, when presented with its substrate, produces a colored product, the intensity of the color produced being proportional to the amount of bound antigen. ELISAs can also be used to detect or quantitate antibody in a patient's serum. In this instance, the wells are coated with antigen

specific for the antibody in question. The patient's serum is allowed to react with the bound antigen, the wells are washed, and a secondary antibody (that recognizes the initial antibody) conjugated to a color product-producing enzyme is added to the well. After a final washing, substrate for the bound enzyme is added to the well, and the intensity of the colored product can be measured.

3. **Fluorescent-antibody tests:** Organisms in clinical samples can be detected directly by specific antibodies coupled to a fluorescent compound, such as fluorescein. In the direct immunofluorescence antibody technique, a sample of concentrated body fluid (for example, CSF or serum), tissue scraping (for example, skin), or cells in tissue culture is incubated with a fluorescein-labeled antibody directed against a specific pathogen. The labeled antibody bound to the microorganism absorbs ultraviolet light, and emits visible fluorescence that can be detected by the human eye, using a fluorescence microscope. A variation of the technique, the indirect immunofluorescence antibody technique, involves the use of two antibodies. The first, unlabeled antibody (the target antibody) binds a specific microbial antigen in a sample such as those described above. This clinical sample is subsequently stained with a fluorescent antibody that recognizes the target antibody. Because a number of labeled antibodies can bind to each target antibody, the fluorescence from the stained microorganism is intensified.

# VIII. DETECTION OF MICROBIAL DNA OR RNA

A highly specific method of pathogen detection involves identification of its DNA or RNA in a patient sample. The basic strategy is to detect a relatively short sequence of nucleotide bases of DNA or RNA (target sequence) that is unique to the pathogen. This is done by hybridization with a complementary sequence of bases, referred to as the probe. [Note: In bacteria, DNA sequences coding for 16S ribosomal RNA sequences (rRNA) are commonly used targets, because each microorganism contains multiple copies of its specific rRNA gene, thus increasing the sensitivity of the assay.] The methods for detecting microbial DNA or RNA fall into two categories: direct hybridization, and amplification methods using the polymerase chain reaction[1] or one its variations.

## A. Direct hybridization methods

These methods use a probe—a single-stranded piece of DNA, usually labeled with an enzyme, fluorescent molecule, radioactive label, or some other detectable molecule. The nucleotide sequence of the probe is complementary to the DNA of interest (the target DNA). To obtain the target DNA, an appropriate sample from the patient is cultured to increase the number of the presumptive disease-causing microorganisms, and then treated, so that the

1 Antibody specific for an antigen of interest is bound to the walls of a plastic microtiter well.

← Antigen

2 Patient serum is incubated in the well. Any antigen in the serum is bound by the antibody on the well walls.

Wash wells to remove unbound antigen

← Enzyme

← Antibody

Add second, enzyme-labeled antibody specific for a different epitope on the antigen

3 Enzyme-labeled antibody is added to the well and binds to the antigen.

Wash wells; unbound antibody is thus removed.

Add substrate for attached enzyme.

Substrate → Product

4 Enzyme makes colored product from added substrate. Intensity of color produced is proportional to the amount of bound antigen.

**Figure 4.14**
Principle of enzyme-linked immunosorbent assay (ELISA).

[1]See ***Lippincott's Illustrated Reviews: Biochemistry*** (3rd ed.), Chapter 32, p. 445 for a more detailed presentation of the techniques used in molecular biology.

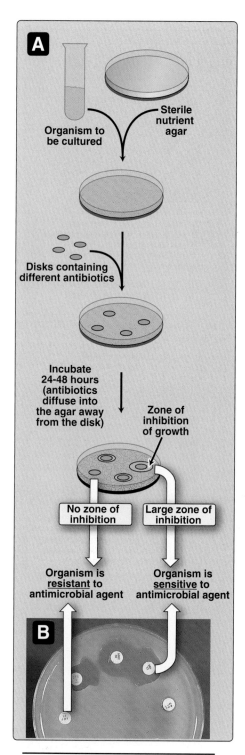

microorganisms lyse, releasing DNA. Single-stranded DNA, produced by alkaline denaturation of the double-stranded DNA, is first bound to a solid support such as a nitrocellulose membrane. The immobilized DNA strands are then available for hybridization to the microorganism-specific, labeled probe. Unbound probe is removed by washing the filter, and the extent of hybridization is then measured by the retention of the labeled probe on the filter.

## B. Amplification methods

Methods employing nucleic acid amplification techniques, such as the polymerase chain reaction (PCR[2]), have a major advantage over direct detection with nucleic acid probes because amplification methods allow specific DNA or RNA target sequences of the pathogen to be amplified millions of times without having to culture the microorganism itself for extended periods.

> Nucleic acid amplification methods are sensitive, specific for the target organism, and are unaffected by the prior administration of antibiotics.

1. **Applications:** Nucleic acid amplification techniques are generally quick, easy, and accurate. A major use of these techniques is for the detection of organisms that cannot be grown *in vitro*, or for which current culture techniques are insensitive. Further, they are useful in the detection of organisms that require complex media or cell cultures and/or prolonged incubation times.

2. **Detection:** Amplified sequences are detected by various methods; for example, agarose gel electrophoresis or blotting the product onto a membrane such as a nitrocellulose filter, followed by probe hybridization (as described above). Newer detection methods capture the amplified target sequences in a well, using a complementary strand of DNA that has been fixed to the surface of the well.

3. **Limitations:** PCR amplification is limited by the occurrence of spurious false-positives due to cross-contamination with other microorganisms' nucleic acid. PCR tests are often costly.

## IX. SUSCEPTIBILITY TESTING

After a pathogen is cultured, its sensitivity to specific antibiotics serves as a guide in choosing antimicrobial therapy. Some pathogens, such as *Streptococcus pyogenes* and *Neisseria meningitidis*, usually have predictable sensitivity patterns to certain antibiotics. In contrast, most gram-negative bacilli, enterococci, and staphylococcal species show unpredictable sensitivity patterns to various antibiotics, and require susceptibility testing to determine appropriate antimicrobial therapy.

**Figure 4.15**
A. Outline of disk diffusion method for determining the sensitivity of bacteria to antimicrobial agents.
B. Photograph of culture plate with antibiotic-impregnated disks.

[2]See p. 459 in *Lippincott's Illustrated Reviews: Biochemistry* (3rd ed.) for a descripton fo the polymerase chain reaction.

## A. Disk-diffusion method

The classic qualitative method to test susceptibility to antibiotics has been the Kirby-Bauer disk-diffusion method, in which disks with exact amounts of different antimicrobial agents are placed on culture dishes inoculated with the microorganism to be tested. The organism's growth (resistance to the drug) or lack of growth (sensitivity to the drug) is then monitored (Figure 4.15). In addition, the size of the zone of growth inhibition is influenced by the concentration and rate of diffusion of the antibiotic on the disk.

> The disk-diffusion method is useful when susceptibility to an unusual antibiotic, not available in automated systems, is to be determined.

## B. Minimal inhibitory concentration

Quantitative testing uses a dilution technique, in which tubes containing serial dilutions of an antibiotic are inoculated with the organism whose sensitivity to that antibiotic is to be tested. The tubes are incubated and later observed to determine the minimal inhibitory concentration (MIC) of the antibiotic necessary to prevent bacterial growth (Figure 4.16). To provide effective antimicrobial therapy, the clinically obtainable antibiotic concentration in body fluids should be greater than the MIC. Quantitative susceptibility testing may be necessary for patients who either fail to respond to antimicrobial therapy, or who relapse during therapy. In some clinical cases, the minimum bactericidal concentration may need to be determined. This is the lowest concentration of antibiotic that kills 100 percent of the bacteria, rather than simply inhibiting growth.

## C. Bacteriostatic vs. bactericidal drugs

As noted above, antimicrobial drugs may be bacteriostatic or bactericidal. Bacteriostatic drugs arrest the growth and replication of bacteria at serum levels achievable in the patient, thus limiting the spread of infection while the body's immune system attacks, immobilizes, and eliminates the pathogens. If the drug is removed before the immune system has scavenged the organisms, enough viable organisms may remain to begin a second cycle of infection. For example, Figure 4.17 shows a laboratory experiment in which the growth of bacteria is arrested by the addition of a bacteriostatic agent. Note that viable organisms remain, even in the presence of the bacteriostatic drug. By contrast, addition of a bactericidal agent kills bacteria, and the total number of viable organisms decreases. Although practical, this classification may be too simplistic because it is possible for an antibiotic to be bacteriostatic for one organism and bactericidal for another (for example, chloramphenicol is bacteriostatic against gram-negative rods and bactericidal against pneumococci).

**Figure 4.16**
Determination of minimal inhibitory concentration (MIC) of an antibiotic.

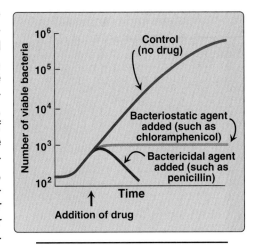

**Figure 4.17**
Effects of bactericidal and bacteriostatic drugs on the growth of bacteria *in vitro*.

## Study Questions

**Choose the ONE correct answer**

4.1  Among 100 employees at a hospital, five were infected with a particular pathogen. When the employees were tested for the presence of the pathogen, ten individuals gave a positive response. Subsequent evaluation by independent tests revealed that five of ten were, in fact, infected and five were not. Which one of the following best describes the original test?

A. High sensitivity, high specificity

B. High sensitivity, low specificity

C. Low sensitivity, high specificity

D. Low sensitivity, low specificity

E. Data do not allow a determination.

> Correct answer = B. All infected individuals were detected, but many false positives occurred.

4.2 Chose the item that correctly matches the microorganism with an appropriate stain or preparation.

A. *Mycobacterium tuberculosis* — India ink

B. Fungi — KOH

C. *Cryptococcus neoformans* in cerebrospinal fluid — Ziehl-Neelsen (classic acid-fast stain)

D. *Chlamydia* — Gram stain

E. *Escherichia coli* (gram-negative bacterium)—Crystal violet followed by treatment with acetone.

> Correct answer = B. Treatment with KOH dissolves host cells and bacteria, allowing fungi to be visualized. *My. tuberculosis* is stained by the Ziehl-Neelsen stain (the classic acid-fast stain). *C. neoformans* in cerebrospinal fluid is visualized with India ink. Organisms that are intracellular, such as chlamydia, or that lack a cell wall, such as mycoplasma or ureaplasma, are not readily detected by Gram stain. Most bacteria stain purple with crystal violet and iodine. If the stained cells are then treated with acetone, gram-positive organisms retain the stain, whereas gram-negative species, such as *E. coli*, lose the stain, becoming colorless. Visualization of *E. coli* requires the addition of the counterstain safranin, which stains gram-negative bacteria pink or red.

4.3 Which one of the following media is most suitable for identifying *Neisseria gonorrhoeae* in a cervical swab?

A. Sheep blood agar

B. Chocolate agar

C. MacConkey agar

D. Thayer-Martin medium

E. Hektoen enteric agar

*"Well, now that you have it, you can stop worrying about getting it"*

> Correct answer = D. Sheep blood agar supports the growth of most bacteria, both gram-positive and gram-negative. Chocolate agar provides the growth requirements for fastidious organisms such as *H. influenzae* or *N. gonorrhoeae*, as well as for most other less-fastidious bacteria. MacConkey agar supports most gram-negative rods, especially the Enterobacteriaeceae, but inhibits growth of gram-positive organisms and some fastidious gram-negative bacteria, such as haemophilus and neisseria species. Thayer-Martin medium, which is composed of chocolate agar supplemented with several antibiotics, suppresses the growth of nonpathogenic *Neisseria* and other normal and abnormal flora, but permits the growth of gonococcus. Hektoen enteric agar is also a selective medium often used to culture *Salmonella* and *Shigella* species.

# Vaccines and Antibiotics

# 5

## I. OVERVIEW

The availability of vaccines has resulted in the global eradication of smallpox and the virtual elimination of poliomyelitis, tetanus, and diphtheria in the United States (Figure 5.1). Protection of individuals from disease by vaccination can take two forms: passive and active immunization. Passive immunization is achieved by injecting a recipient with preformed immunoglobulins directed against an already present infection, whereas active immunization involves injection of modified or purified pathogens or their products. Both provide protective immune responses. Active and passive immunization differ in significant ways, and the situations under which one or the other or a combination (active-passive immunization) is preferred depends on the infecting microorganism, age of the patient, anticipated imminent contact with a pathogen, or time elapsed since contact. [Note: The reader is reminded of the common names for some childhood diseases discussed in this chapter: pertussis = whooping cough; rubella = german measles; rubeola = measles; varicella = chickenpox.]

## II. PASSIVE IMMUNIZATION

Passive immunization is achieved by injecting a recipient with preformed immunoglobulins obtained from human (or, occasionally, equine) serum. Passive immunization provides immediate protection to individuals who have been exposed to an infectious organism and who lack active immunity to that pathogen. Because passive immunization does not activate the immune system, it generates no memory response. Passive immunity is not permanent, but dissipates after a few weeks to months as the immunoglobulins are cleared from the recipient's serum.

### A. Types of immunoglobulins used to give passive immunity

Two basic formulations of prepared immunoglobulins have been developed: one from the serum of pooled human donors and one from serum obtained from hyperimmune donors (Figure 5.2).

1. **Nonspecific standard immunoglobulins:** This mixture of plasma proteins contains a broad spectrum of antibodies, with IgG predominating. These immunoglobulins (formerly, gamma globulins) contain a mixture of antibodies reflecting the previous exposures of the plasma donors to various antigens, either by natural infec-

**Figure 5.1**
Incidence of vaccine-preventable diseases in the United States at their highest incidence and in 2004. [Note: Y-axis is a logarithmic scale.]

STANDARD HUMAN IMMUNO-
GLOBULINS

Hepatitis A or measles

Used in individuals who may
have been exposed to these
viruses.

HYPERIMMUNE HUMAN
IMMUNOGLOBULINS

Hepatitis B

Used to prevent infection after
exposure to hepatitis virus, for
example, through contaminated
blood.

Rabies

Used in combination with rabies
vaccine to prevent rabies after
a bite from a rabid animal.

Tetanus

Used in combination with tetanus
booster vaccine to prevent tetanus
after a deep puncture wound.

Varicella-zoster

Used to prevent disseminated
disease in those who are immunosuppressed and may have been
exposed to the virus.

**Figure 5.2**
Immunoglobulins used for passive
immunization.

tion or by immunization. Standard immunoglobulin is used for prevention or attenuation of illnesses for which there is no specific
immunoglobulin preparation. This type of immunization is effective
when given immediately before or after exposure to an infectious
disease, such as hepatitis A.

2. **Hyperimmune human immunoglobulin:** This type of immunoglobulin contains high concentrations of antibodies directed against a
specific pathogen or toxin (for example, varicella-zoster
immunoglobulin or diphtheria antitoxin). These may be given to
patients who have recently been exposed to a specific pathogen.

### B. Adverse effects

There are risks associated with the injection of preformed antibody.
For example, the recipient can mount an adverse response to the
antigenic determinants of the foreign antibody, potentially leading to
systemic anaphylaxis. [Note: This is particularly true when the
immunoglobulins are obtained from a nonhuman source, such as a
horse.]

## III. ACTIVE IMMUNIZATION

Active immunization is achieved by injection of viable or nonviable
pathogens, or purified pathogen product, prompting the immune system
to respond as if the body were being attacked by an intact infectious
microorganism. Whereas passive immunization provides immediate
protection, active immunization may require several days to months to
become effective. Active immunization leads to prolonged immunity and
is generally preferred over the short-term immunity provided by passive
immunization with preformed immunoglobulins.

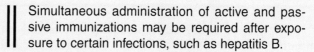

Simultaneous administration of active and passive immunizations may be required after exposure to certain infections, such as hepatitis B.

### A. Formulations for active immunization

Vaccines are made with 1) live, attenuated microorganisms; 2) killed
microorganisms; 3) microbial extracts; 4) vaccine conjugates; or 5)
inactivated toxins (toxoids). Both bacterial and viral pathogens are
targeted by these diverse means.

1. **Live pathogens:** When live pathogens are used, they are attenuated (weakened) to preclude clinical consequences of infection.
Attenuated microbes reproduce in the recipient, typically leading
to a more robust and long-lasting immune response than can be
obtained through vaccination with killed organisms. However, with
live, attenuated vaccines there is a possibility that the attenuated
vaccine strain will revert to an active pathogen after administration
to the patient. For example, vaccine-associated poliomyelitis
occurs following administration of approximately one of every 2.4

million doses of live polio vaccine. All recent cases of polio in the United States are vaccine-associated. Also, live, attenuated vaccines should not be given to immunocompromised individuals because there is the potential for a disseminated infection.

2. **Killed microorganisms:** Killed vaccines have the advantage over attenuated microorganisms in that they pose no risk of vaccine-associated infection. As noted above, killed organisms often provide a weak or short-lived immune response. Some vaccines, such as polio and typhoid vaccines, are available both in live and killed versions.

3. **Microbial extracts:** Instead of using whole organisms, vaccines can be composed of antigen molecules (often those located on the surface of the microorganism) extracted from the pathogen or prepared by recombinant DNA techniques. The efficacy of these vaccines varies. In some instances, the vaccine antigen is present on all strains of the organism, and the vaccine thus protects against infection by all strains. With other pathogens, such as pneumococcus, protective antibody is produced against only a specific capsular polysaccharide—one among more than eighty distinct types. Immunity to one polysaccharide type does not confer immunity to any other type. For this reason, the pneumococcal vaccine is composed of 23 different polysaccharides, comprising the antigens produced by the most common types of disease-causing pneumococci. Some pathogens, such as influenza virus, frequently change their antigenic determinants. Therefore, influenza virus vaccines must also change regularly to counter the different antigens of influenza A and B virus strains in circulation.

> In the case of rhinovirus infections—the leading cause of the common cold—at least 100 types of the virus are known. It is not practical to develop a vaccine that confers protection to this large number of antigenic types.

4. **Vaccine conjugates:** Vaccines can produce humoral immunity through B cell proliferation leading to antibody production, which may or may not involve helper T cells. For example, pneumococcal polysaccharide and the polysaccharide of *Haemophilus influenzae* type b induce B-cell type-specific protective antibody without involvement of helper T cells. These T cell–independent responses are characterized by low antibody titers, particularly in children younger than eighteen months. Thus, conventional *H. influenzae* polysaccharide vaccine does not provide protection for children three to eighteen months. Consequently, this organism has, in the past, produced severe infections in this age group. However, by covalently conjugating the *Haemophilus* polysaccharide to a protein antigen, such as diphtheria toxoid protein, *Haemophilus* vaccines produce a robust T cell–dependent antibody response even in three-month-old infants. Figure 5.3 shows the decreased inci-

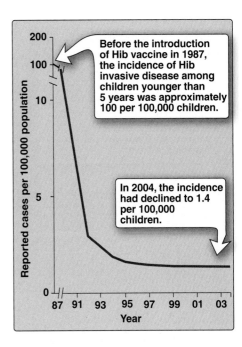

**Figure 5.3**
Incidence of infection in children due to *Haemophilus influenzae* type b (Hib) following introduction of conjugate vaccine in 1987.

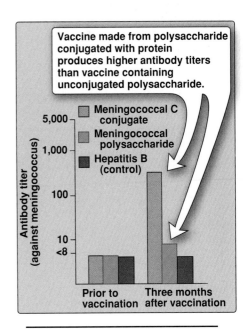

**Figure 5.4**
Serum bactericidal antibody response to vaccination with meningococcal C conjugate, meningococcal polysaccharide, and hepatitis B vaccine (control) in children, 15 to 23 months of age.

**Attenuated pathogen**

- Attenuated pathogen multiplies inside human host and provides continuous antigenic stimulation.

- Vaccine provides prolonged immunity (years to life), usually after a single dose.

- Vaccine often provides cell-mediated immunity.

**Killed pathogen**

- Killed pathogen does not multiply in the human host; the immune response is determined by the antigen content of the vaccine.

- Multiple doses of vaccine are required, with subsequent booster doses.

- Vaccine provides little cell-mediated immunity.

- Vaccine is administered by injection.

**Microbial extracts or products of pathogens**

- Instead of using whole organisms, vaccines can be composed of antigenic molecules extracted from the pathogen, from an acellular (noninfectious) filtrate of the culture medium in which the organism was grown, or produced by recombinant DNA techniques.

- Vaccines can be prepared against toxoids (derivatives of exotoxins). These are used when the pathogenicity of the organism is result of the secreted toxin.

| DISEASE OR VACCINE COMPONENTS | | |
| --- | --- | --- |
| **ATTENUATED PATHOGEN** | **KILLED PATHOGEN** | **MICROBIAL EXTRACTS OR PRODUCTS OF PATHOGENS** |
| **BACTERIAL DISEASES** Typhoid fever | Pertussis<br>Cholera<br>Plague<br>Typhoid fever<br>Q Fever | Acellular pertussis (*B. pertussis* antigen)<br>Anthrax (noninfectious filtrate from culture)<br>Diphtheria (toxoid)<br>Haemophilus influenzae type b infections<br>Lyme disease (recombinant vaccine)<br>Meningococcal infections<br>Pneumococcal infections<br>Tetanus (toxoid) |
| **VIRAL DISEASES** Rubeola<br>Mumps<br>Polio (Sabin)<br>Varicella-zoster<br>Adenovirus infections<br>Yellow fever<br>Rubella<br>Variola | Polio (Salk)<br>Hepatitis A<br>Influenza (whole virus)<br>Rabies<br>Japanese encephalitis | Hepatitis B (inactivated surface antigen; recombinant antigen) |

**Conjugated polysaccharide vaccines**

- Covalent binding (conjugation) of an antigenic polysaccharide to a protein enhances the immune response to these vaccines, particularly in children younger than 2 years.

**Figure 5.5**
Some diseases and their vaccines licensed for use in humans in the United States.

dence of *H. influenzae* disease following introduction of conjugated vaccine. A conjugate vaccine for *Streptococcus pneumoniae,* and one for *Neisseria meningitidis*, are also currently available. Figure 5.4 shows the favorable antibody response to conjugated polysaccharide obtained from *N. meningitidis.*

5. **Toxoids:** These are derivatives of bacterial exotoxins produced by chemically altering the natural toxin, or by engineering bacteria to produce harmless variants of the toxin. Vaccines containing toxoid are used when the pathogenicity of the organism is a result of the secreted toxin. Depending on the specific vaccine, administration is generally via intramuscular or subcutaneous routes. Figure 5.5 shows the formulation of some of the vaccines currently licensed in the United States. Details of the various vaccines are presented in the chapters in which the target microorganisms are discussed.

## B. Types of immune response to vaccines

Vaccines containing killed pathogens (such as hepatitis A or the Salk polio vaccine) or antigenic components of pathogens (such as hepatitis B subunit vaccine) do not enter host cells; therefore, they give rise to a primary B cell–mediated humoral response. These antibodies are ineffective in attacking intracellular organisms. By contrast, attenuated live vaccines (usually viruses) do penetrate cells. This results in the production of intracellular antigens that are displayed on the surface of the infected cell, prompting a cytotoxic T cell response, which is effective in eliminating intracellular pathogens.

## C. Effect of age on efficacy of immunization

1. **Passive immunity from mother:** Newborns receive serum IgG antibodies from their mothers, which gives them temporary protection against those diseases to which the mother was immune. In addition, maternal milk also contains secretory antibodies that provide some protection against intestinal and respiratory tract infections.

2. **Active immunization:** The infant's antibody-producing capacity develops slowly during the first year of life. Although the immune system is not fully developed, it is desirable to begin immunization at two months of age because diseases are common in this age group, and can be particularly severe (for example, whooping cough, *H. influenzae* meningitis). As with infants, the elderly have a reduced antibody response to vaccines.

## D. Adverse reactions to active vaccination

Adverse consequences of vaccinations range from mild to severe and even life-threatening (Figure 5.6). Symptoms vary among individuals and with the nature of the vaccination. Among the most common and mildest consequences of immunization are tenderness and swelling at the site of injection, and a mild fever.

# IV. BACTERIAL VACCINES

Vaccines against commonly encountered bacterial pathogens are summarized in Figure 5.7. The recommended childhood immunization schedule is shown in Figure 5.8. Vaccines with more specialized indications are described below.

## A. Less common bacterial pathogens

1. **Anthrax (*Bacillus anthracis*):** Anthrax vaccine consists of a noninfectious sterile filtrate from the culture of an attenuated strain of *B. anthracis* that contains no dead bacteria. The filtrate is adsorbed to an adjuvant, aluminum hydroxide. [Note: Adjuvants are substances that when injected with an antigen, serve to enhance the immunogencity of that antigen.] The incidence of all forms of naturally occurring anthrax is low, particularly the inhalation form of the disease. Thus, there is no opportunity to conduct field trials of the vaccine against inhalation anthrax, the form

**Figure 5.6**
Rare adverse effects associated with childhood vaccines.

## Pneumonia (*Streptococcus pneumoniae*)

● Two vaccines are available: Pneumococcal polysaccharide and pneumococcal polysaccharide–protein conjugate vaccines.

● Polysaccharide vaccine containing capsular polysaccharides is recommended for adults older than sixty years or persons with predisposing pathologies. The vaccine is not immunogenic in young children, and is not approved for children younger then two years.

● Pneumococcal conjugate vaccine is effective in children younger than two years. Vaccination is recommended for all children up to age 24 months.

## Lyme Disease (*Borrelia burgdorferi*)

● Noninfectious recombinant vaccine that contains lipoprotein OspA, an outer surface protein of *B. burgdorferi* is available.

● When a tick bites and ingests blood, antibodies present in the blood of an immunized individual kill *Borrelia burgdorferi* inside the tick and prevent entry into the circulation.

● Provides about 75 percent protection after three doses. Protection lasts less than one year. It is only effective against strains seen in the United States.

## Diphtheria (*Corynebacterium diphtheriae*)

● Vaccine contains diphtheria toxoid (formaldehyde-treated exotoxin), which stimulates antitoxin production.

● Indicated for use in young children as part of the DTaP vaccine.

● Prompt administration of equine diphtheria antitoxin can neutralize unbound toxin, preventing the disease from progressing. A conjugate vaccine that shows improved immunogenicity in children younger than two years is available.

## Meningitis (*Neisseria meningitidis*)

● Vaccine contains capsular polysaccharides of four important serotypes: A, C, W135, and Y.

● Vaccine is given to college students living in dormitories, military recruits entering boot camp, travelers visiting areas where meningitis is prevalent, and at times of outbreak.

Pie chart labels: Other, Gram (+) cocci *Streptococcus pneumoniae*, Chlamydia, Gram (+) bacilli *Corynebacterium diphtheriae*, Mycoplasma, Gram (–) cocci *Neisseria meningitidis*, Spirochetes, *Borrelia burgdorferi*, Gram (–) rods *Bordetella pertussis Haemophilus influenzae* type B, Anaerobic organisms *Clostridium tetani*

## Pertussis (*Bordetella pertussis*)

● An acellular pertussis vaccine containing purified proteins is replacing the traditional whole-cell pertussis vaccine used in the United States for the past fifty years. The acellular vaccine shows fewer adverse effects and has an efficacy equal to that of the whole cell preparation.

● Indicated for use in young children as part of the DTaP

## Tetanus (*Clostridium tetani*)

● Vaccine contains tetanus toxoid.

● Indicated for use in young children as part of the DTaP vaccine and for booster in adults.

● The vaccine is also given promptly after suspected infection and to under-immunized individuals.

## Meningitis (*Haemophilus influenzae* type b, Hib)

● Vaccine contains polysaccharide conjugated to diphtheria toxoid or other carrier protein.

● Indicated for use in young children in combination with the DTaP vaccine.

**Figure 5.7**
Summary of common vaccines against bacterial diseases. DTaP = diphtheria and tetanus toxoids and acellular pertussis vaccine.

| Age ▶ Vaccine ▼ | Birth | 1 Month | 2 Months | 4 Months | 6 Months | 12 Months | 15 Months | 18 Months | 24 Months | 4-6 Years | 11-12 Years | 13-14 Years | 15 Years | 16-18 Years |
|---|---|---|---|---|---|---|---|---|---|---|---|---|---|---|
| Hepatitis B | HepB | HepB | | HepB | | HepB | | | | HepB Series | | | | |
| Diphtheria, Tetanus, Pertussis | | | DTaP | DTaP | DTaP | | DTaP | | | DTaP | Tdap | | Tdap | |
| Haemophilus influenzae type b | | | Hib | Hib | Hib | Hib | | | | | | | | |
| Inactivated Poliovirus | | | IPV | IPV | | IPV | | | | IPV | | | | |
| Measles, Mumps, Rubella | | | | | | MMR #1 | | | | MMR #2 | | MMR #3 | | |
| Varicella | | | | | | Varicella | | | | Varicella | | | | |
| Meningoccal | | | | | | | | | | | MCV4 | | MCV4 | |
| | | | | | | | | | MPSV4 | | | MCV4 | | |
| Pneumococcal Conjugate | | | PCV | PCV | PCV | PCV | | | | PCV | PPV | | | |
| Influenza | | | | | | Influenza (Yearly) | | | | Influenza (Yearly) | | | | |
| Hepatitis A | | | | | | Hepatitis A Series | | | | Hepatitis A Series | | | | |

Vaccines within red line are for selected populations

| | Range of recommended ages | | Catch-up immunization | | 11-12 year old assessment |
|---|---|---|---|---|---|

**Figure 5.8**
Recommended childhood immunization schedule for 2006. [Note: Immunization schedules may change each year and clinicians should consult the Centers for Disease Control for details concerning current recommendations.] DTaP = diphtheria and tetanus toxoids and acellular pertussis vaccine. Hib = *Haemophilus influenzae* type b conjugate vaccine. MMR = measles-mumps-rubella vaccine. IPV = all-inactivate poliovirus vaccine.

most likely to be used in a biologic attack. Safety and efficacy of the vaccine are supported by studies in nonhuman primates where efficacy was close to 100 percent. Vaccine is recommended for goat hair and woolen mill workers, veterinarians, laboratory workers, and livestock handlers who are at risk as a result of occupational exposure.

2. **Cholera (*Vibrio cholerae*):** The vaccine contains killed bacteria and is given to travelers.

3. **Typhoid fever (*Salmonella typhi*):** The most commonly used vaccine contains an attenuated recombinant strain of *S. typhi*. It is given to individuals living in or traveling to high-risk areas, and to members of the military.

4. **Plague (*Yersinia pestis*):** The vaccine contains killed bacteria, and is given to high-risk individuals.

# V. VIRAL VACCINES

Immunity to viral infection requires an immune response to antigens located on the surface of the viral particles, or on virus-infected cells. For enveloped viruses, these antigens are often surface glycoproteins. The main limitation of viral vaccines occurs with viruses that show a genetically unstable antigenicity (that is, they exhibit antigenic determinants that continuously vary, such as with influenza viruses or the human immunodeficiency virus). Common viral pathogens for which there are vaccines include the following:

## A. Hepatitis A

Formalin-inactivated whole virus vaccine produces antibody levels in adults similar to those observed following natural infection, and approximately fifteen times those achieved by passive injection of immunoglobulin. Projections indicate that immunity from hepatitis A virus will probably last for approximately ten years after two doses of vaccine. The vaccine is indicated for travelers to endemic areas, homosexual men, injecting drug users, and day care workers.

> Currently in the United States, hepatitis A virus vaccine is not recommended for children younger than two years because residual anti-HAV passively acquired from the mother may interfere with vaccine immunogenicity.

## B. Hepatitis B

The current vaccine contains recombinant hepatitis surface antigen. Efficacy is 95 to 99 percent in healthy infants, children, and young adults. Its use is indicated for healthcare workers in contact with blood, and persons residing in an area with a high rate of endemic disease. Immunoglobulins obtained from hyperimmunized humans can provide passive immunity after accidental exposure (for example, a needlestick, or for the neonate of an infected mother). Active and passive treatments can be administered into different sites at the same time. Recommended uses of hepatitis A and B vaccines are shown in Figure 5.9.

## C. Varicella-zoster

This vaccine contains live, attenuated, temperature-sensitive varicella-zoster virus. Its efficacy in preventing chickenpox is approximately 85 to 100 percent in children, and this immunity is persistent. Anti–varicella-zoster immunoglobulin provides passive immunity for immunocompromised individuals at risk of infection.

## D. Polio

Vaccination is the only effective method of preventing poliomyelitis. Both the inactivated polio vaccine and the live, attenuated, orally administered polio vaccine have established efficacy in preventing poliovirus infection and paralytic poliomyelitis (see p. 285).

1. **Inactivated poliovirus (Salk) vaccine:** Because the inactivated vaccine cannot cause poliomyelitis, it is safe for use in immunocompromised persons and their contacts. The disadvantages of this inactivated vaccine are: 1) administration is by injection only; and 2) it provides less gastrointestinal immunity, resulting in the possibility of asymptomatic infection of the gastrointestinal tract with wild poliovirus, which could be transmitted to other persons.

---

**HEPATITIS A VACCINE**

**Routine immunization**

Children living in communities with high hepatitis A rates and periodic disease outbreaks

**Increased risk of hepatitis A**

International travelers to regions of endemic disease
Homosexual men with multiple sexual partners
User of illicit injectable drugs

**HEPATITIS B VACCINE**

**Routine immunization**

All infants and previously unvaccinated children by the age of 11 years

**Increased risk of hepatitis B**

People with multiple sexual partners
Sexual partner or household contacts of HBsAG-positive people
Homosexually active men
User of illicit injectable drug
Travelers to region of endemic disease
People occupationally exposed to blood or body fluids
Patients with renal failure
Patient receiving clotting-factor concentrates

**Figure 5.9**
Candidates for hepatitis immunization. HBsAg = hepatitis B surface antigen.

To eliminate the risk for vaccine-associated paralytic poliomyelitis (see next section), an all-inactivated poliovirus vaccine schedule is recommended for routine childhood vaccinations in the United States.

2. **Attenuated live poliovirus (Sabin) vaccine:** Advantages of this vaccine include: 1) it can be administered orally; 2) it provides life-long protection from poliovirus for more than 95 percent of recipients after the primary three-dose series; and 3) it provides early intestinal immunity. The main disadvantage of attenuated live virus vaccine is a small risk of infection, estimated to be 1 per 2.4 million doses.

## E. Influenza

The traditional "flu shot" vaccine contains formalin-inactivated virus. A live, attenuated influenza vaccine is administered intranasally. The vaccine provides peak protection about two weeks after its administration. Vaccine efficacy of seventy to ninety percent is generally achieved in young adults. The vaccine is recommended for adults older than 65, high-risk persons six months or older, and those who might transmit the virus to persons at high risk.

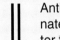 Antigenic drift requires that individuals be vaccinated against influenza annually prior to the winter flu season.

## F. Measles, mumps, and rubella (MMR)

This combination vaccine contains live, attenuated virus, and should be administered to young children prior to entering school. Measles vaccine should also be administered to individuals traveling in endemic areas.

## VI. DNA VACCINES

DNA vaccines represent a new approach to vaccination. The proposed mechanism for these vaccines can be summarized as follows: The gene for the antigen of interest is cloned into a bacterial plasmid that is engineered to increase the expression of the inserted gene in mammalian cells (Figure 5.10). After being injected, the plasmid enters a host cell where it remains in the nucleus as an episome (that is, it is not integrated into the cell's DNA). Using the host cell's protein synthesis machinery, the plasmid DNA in the episome directs the synthesis of the protein it encodes. This antigenic microbial protein may leave the cells and interact with T helper and B cells, or it may be cleaved into fragments and presented as MHC I antigen complex on the cell surface, resulting in activation of killer T cells. To date, the potency of DNA vaccines in humans has been disappointing.

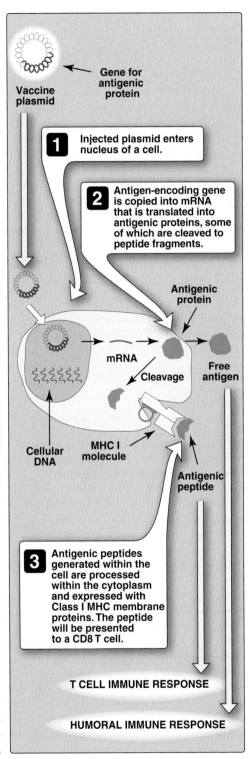

**Figure 5.10**
DNA vaccines produce antigen needed to generate immunity. MHC = Major histocompatibility complex.

**Figure 5.11**
A. Bar chart showing the six most commonly used drug families.
B. An example of the bar chart, with drugs of choice for the treatment of *Staphylococcus aureus* shown in bold print.

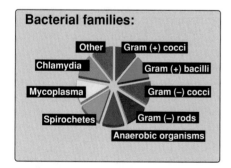

**Figure 5.12**
Organization of bacteria into nine families.

## VII. OVERVIEW OF ANTIBIOTICS

Antimicrobial drugs are effective in the treatment of infections because of their selective toxicity (that is, they have the ability to kill or injure an invading microorganism without harming the cells of the host). In most instances, the selective toxicity is relative, rather than absolute, requiring that the concentration of the drug be carefully controlled to attack the microorganism while still being tolerated by the host.

> Selective antimicrobial therapy takes advantage of the biochemical differences that exist between microorganisms and human beings.[1]

## VIII. AGENTS USED IN BACTERIAL INFECTIONS

In this book, the clinically useful antibacterial drugs are organized into six families—penicillins, cephalosporins, tetracyclines, aminoglycosides, macrolides, and fluoroquinolones, plus a seventh group labeled "Other" that is used to represent any drug not included in one of the other six drug families. Here and throughout the book, these seven groups are graphically presented as a bar chart ("drug stack," Figure 5.11A). The drug(s) of choice within each family that is/are used for treating a specific bacterial infection are shown in bold print, as illustrated for *S. aureus* in Figure 5.11B. [Note: As was introduced in Chapter 1 (see p. 4), the clinically important bacteria are also organized into groups based on Gram stain, morphology, and biochemical or other characteristics, and are represented as wedges of a "pie chart" (Figure 5.12). The ninth section of the bacterial pie chart, labeled "Other," is used to represent any organism not included in one of the other eight categories. In this chapter, the pie chart is used to illustrate the spectra of bacteria for which a particular class of antibiotics is therapeutically effective.] The general mechanisms of action and antibacterial spectra of the major groups of antibiotics are presented below.

### A. Penicillins

Penicillins are β-lactam antibiotics, named after the β-lactam ring that is essential to their activity. Penicillins selectively interfere with the synthesis of the bacterial cell wall (see p. 57)—a structure not found in mammalian cells. Penicillins are inactive against organisms devoid of a peptidoglycan cell wall, such as mycoplasma, protozoa, fungi, and viruses. To be maximally effective, penicillins require actively proliferating bacteria; they have little or no effect on bacteria that are not dividing. Their action is usually bactericidal (the bacteria die, see p. 31). Penicillins are the most widely effective antibiotics. For example, penicillin G is the cornerstone of therapy for infections caused by several infections (Figure 5.13). The major adverse reaction to penicillins is hypersensitivity. Unfortunately, many bacteria have developed resistance to these drugs.

 [1]See Unit VII in *Lippincott's Illustrated Reviews: Pharmacology* (3rd ed.) for a more detailed discussion of antimicrobial drugs.

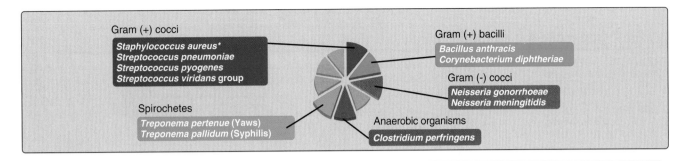

**Figure 5.13**
Summary of therapeutic applications of penicillin G. *Not producing β-lactamases or lacking penicillin-binding protein.

## B. Cephalosporins

Cephalosporins are β-lactam antibiotics that are closely related both structurally and functionally to the penicillins; they are also bactericidal. Cephalosporins have the same mode of action as the penicillins, but they tend to be more resistant than the penicillins to inactivation by β-lactamases produced by some bacteria. Cephalosporins are classified as first, second, third, or fourth generation, largely on the basis of bacterial susceptibility patterns and resistance to β-lactamases (see Figure 5.15). In this classification system, first-generation agents are active primarily against gram-positive organisms, including methicillin-sensitive *S. aureus*, and have limited activity against gram-negative bacilli. Second-generation agents have increased activity against gram-negative bacilli and variable activity against gram-positive cocci. Third-generation agents have significantly increased activity against gram-negative bacilli, with some of these agents active against *Pseudomonas aeruginosa*. [Note: Cefepime has been classified by some as fourth-generation because of its extended spectrum of activity against both gram-positive and gram-negative organisms that include *P. aeruginosa*.]

## C. Tetracyclines

A number of antibiotics, including tetracyclines, aminoglycosides, and macrolides, exert antimicrobial effects by targeting the bacterial ribosome, which has components that differ structurally from those of the mammalian cytoplasmic ribosomes. Binding of tetracyclines to the 30S subunit of the bacterial ribosome is believed to block access of the amino acyl-tRNA to the mRNA-ribosome complex at the acceptor site, thus inhibiting bacterial protein synthesis. Tetracyclines are broad-spectrum antibiotics (that is, many bacteria are sensitive to these drugs, Figure 5.14). Tetracyclines are generally bacteriostatic (the bacteria are prevented from multiplying, but are not killed by the drug, see p. 31).

## D. Aminoglycosides

Aminoglycosides inhibit bacterial protein synthesis. Susceptible organisms have an oxygen-dependent system that transports the antibiotic across the cell membrane. All aminoglycosides are bactericidal (that is, the bacteria are killed). They are effective only

**Figure 5.14**
Summary of therapeutic applications of tetracyclines and aminoglycosides.

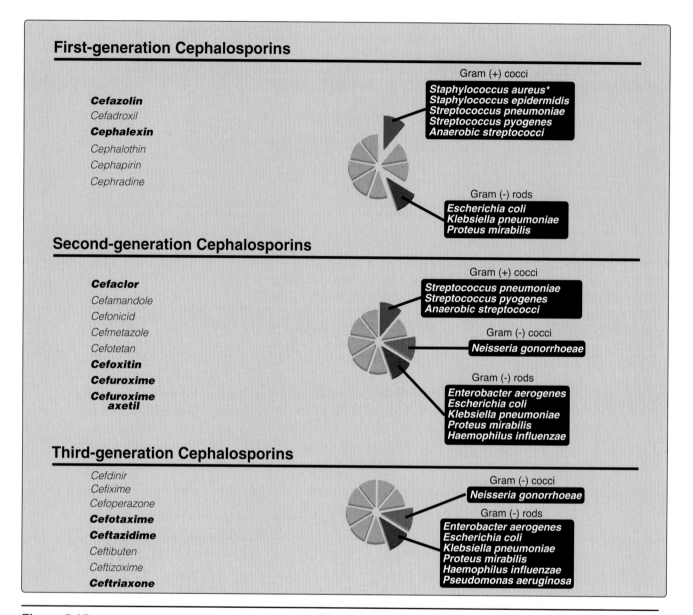

**Figure 5.15**
Summary of therapeutic applications of cephalosporins, with the more useful drugs shown in bold print. *Except methicillin-resistant *Staphylococcus aureus*.

against aerobic organisms because anaerobes lack the oxygen-requiring transport system. Gentamicin is used to treat a variety of infectious diseases including those caused by many of the Enterobacteriaceae (see Figure 5.14) and, in combination with penicillin, endocarditis caused by viridans group streptococci.

**E. Macrolides**

Macrolides are a group of antibiotics with a macrocyclic lactone structure. Erythromycin was the first of these to find clinical application, both as the drug of first choice, and as an alternative to penicillin in individuals who are allergic to β-lactam antibiotics. Newer macrolides, such clarithromycin and azithromycin, offer extended activity against some organisms and less severe adverse reactions.

The macrolides bind irreversibly to a site on the 50S subunit of the bacterial ribosome, thus inhibiting the translocation steps of protein synthesis. Generally considered to be bacteriostatic (see p. 31) they may be bactericidal at higher doses (Figure 5.16).

## F. Fluoroquinolones

Fluoroquinolones uniquely inhibit the replication of bacterial DNA by interfering with the action of DNA gyrase (topoisomerase II[2]) during bacterial growth and reproduction. Binding quinolone to both the enzyme and DNA to form a ternary complex inhibits the rejoining step, and thus can cause cell death by inducing cleavage of the DNA. Because DNA gyrase is a distinct target for antimicrobial therapy, cross-resistance with other more commonly used antimicrobial drugs is rare, but is increasing with multiple-drug–resistant organisms. All of the fluoroquinolones are bactericidal. Figure 5.16 shows some of the applications of the fluoroquinolone, ciprofloxacin.

## G. Other important antibacterial agents

1. **Vancomycin:** Vancomycin is a tricyclic glycopeptide that has become increasingly medically important because of its effectiveness against multiple drug-resistant organisms, such as methicillin-resistant staphylococci. Vancomycin inhibits synthesis of bacterial cell wall phospholipids as well as peptidoglycan polymerization at a site earlier than that inhibited by β-lactam antibiotics. Vancomycin is useful in patients with serious allergic reactions to β-lactam antibiotics and who have gram-positive infections. Vancomycin is also used for potentially life-threatening antibiotic-associated colitis caused by *Clostridium difficile* or staphylococci.

> ‖ To curtail the increase in vancomycin-resistant bacteria, use of this agent should be restricted to the treatment of serious infections caused by β-lactam-resistant gram-positive microorganisms.

2. **Trimethoprim-sulfamethoxazole**, a combination called co-trimoxazole, shows greater antimicrobial activity than equivalent quantities of either drug used alone (Figure 5.17). The synergistic antimicrobial activity of co-trimoxazole results from its inhibition of two sequential steps in the synthesis of tetrahydrofolic acid: sulfamethoxazole inhibits incorporation of PABA into folic acid, and trimethoprim prevents reduction of dihydrofolate to tetrahydrofolate.[3]

# IX. AGENTS USED IN VIRAL INFECTIONS

When viruses reproduce, they use much of the host's own metabolic machinery. Therefore, few drugs are selective enough to prevent viral replication without injury to the host. Viruses are also not affected by antibacterial agents. Nevertheless, some drugs sufficiently discriminate between

**Therapeutic applications of macrolides (erythromycin):**

Chlamydial species
*Mycoplasma pneumoniae*
*Ureaplasma urealyticum*
*Treponema pallidum*
*Corynebacterium diphtheriae*
*Legionella pneumophila*

**Therapeutic applications of fluoroquinolones (ciprofloxacin):**

*Enterbacteriaceae*
*Pseudomonas aeruginosa*

**Figure 5.16**
Summary of therapeutic applications of macrolides and fluoroquinolones.

**Therapeutic applications of trimethoprim-sulfamethoxazole**

*Pneumocystis jiroveci*
*Neisseria gonorrhoeae*
*Neisseria meningitidis*
*Clostridium difficile*
*Escherichia coli*
*Haemophilus influenzae*
*Legionella pneumophilia*
*Proteus mirabilis*
*Salmonella typhi*
*Shigella* species

**Figure 5.17**
Summary of therapeutic applications of trimethoprim-sulfamethoxazole.

[2]See p .399 in*Lippincott's Illustrated Reviews: Biochemistry* (3rd ed.) for a more detailed discussion of DNA gyrase.
[3]See p. 389 in *Lippincott's Illustrated Reviews: Pharmacology* (3rd ed.) for an explanation of how trimethoprim prevents the reduction of dihydrofolate.

cellular and viral reactions to be effective and yet relatively nontoxic. For example, efficient management strategies are available for infections due to herpes simplex virus, varicella-zoster virus, cytomegalovirus, influenza A and B viruses, and chronic hepatitis B and C.

## A. Organization of viruses

The clinically important viruses can be conveniently divided into seven groups based on the nature of their genome, symmetry of organization, and the presence or absence of a lipid envelope (Figure 5.18; see also Figure 23.3, p. 234). An organizational pie chart is presented throughout this book as a graphic aid in recalling the classification of the viruses. In Figure 5.19, the viral pie chart is used to summarize the therapeutic applications of selected antiviral agents, which are described below.

## B. Treatment of herpesvirus infections

Most antiviral agents used in treating herpesvirus infections are nucleoside analogues that require conversion to mono-, di-, and triphosphate forms by cellular kinases, viral kinases, or both, to selectively inhibit viral DNA synthesis. This class of antiviral agents includes acyclovir, cidofovir, famciclovir, ganciclovir, penciclovir, valacyclovir, and vidarabine. A second class of antiviral drugs with action against herpesviruses is represented by the pyrophosphate analogue, foscarnet.

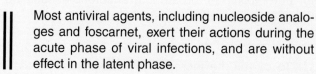

Most antiviral agents, including nucleoside analoges and foscarnet, exert their actions during the acute phase of viral infections, and are without effect in the latent phase.

## C. Treatment of acquired immunodeficiency syndrome (AIDS)

Antiretroviral drugs are divided into four main classes based on their mode of inhibition of viral replication. The first class represents nucleoside analogs that inhibit the viral RNA-dependent DNA polymerase (reverse transcriptase) of HIV. A second class of reverse transcriptase inhibitors is non-nucleoside analogs. The third class is protease inhibitors. The fourth class is a fusion inhibitor that prevents HIV from entering the host cell. Therapy with these antiretroviral agents, usually in combinations (a "cocktail" of drugs referred to as highly active anti-retroviral therapy, or HAART, see p. 304), may be beneficial in prolonging survival, to reduce the incidence and severity of opportunistic infections in patients with advanced HIV disease, and to delay disease progression in asymptomatic HIV-infected patients.

## D. Treatment of viral hepatitis

Prolonged (months) treatment with interferon-$\alpha$ has succeeded in reducing or eliminating indicators of hepatitis B virus replication in about one third of patients. However, recurrence of indications of the

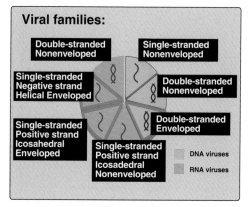

**Figure 5.18**
Organization of viruses into seven groups.

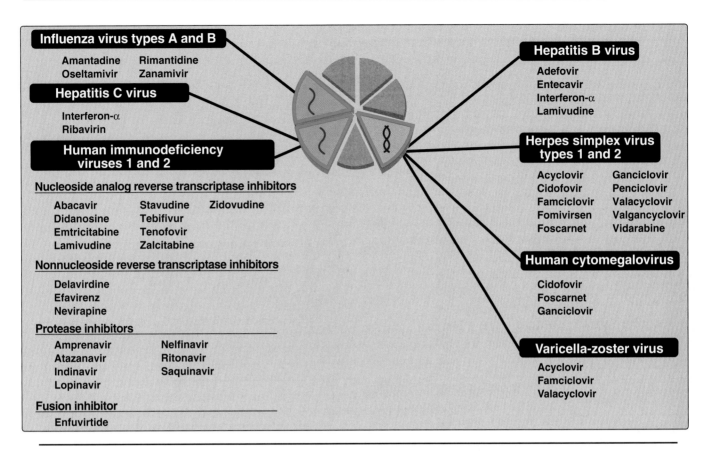

**Influenza virus types A and B**

Amantadine   Rimantidine
Oseltamivir  Zanamivir

**Hepatitis C virus**

Interferon-α
Ribavirin

**Human immunodeficiency viruses 1 and 2**

Nucleoside analog reverse transcriptase inhibitors

Abacavir      Stavudine      Zidovudine
Didanosine    Tebifivur
Emtricitabine Tenofovir
Lamivudine    Zalcitabine

Nonnucleoside reverse transcriptase inhibitors

Delavirdine
Efavirenz
Nevirapine

Protease inhibitors

Amprenavir    Nelfinavir
Atazanavir    Ritonavir
Indinavir     Saquinavir
Lopinavir

Fusion inhibitor

Enfuvirtide

**Hepatitis B virus**

Adefovir
Entecavir
Interferon-α
Lamivudine

**Herpes simplex virus types 1 and 2**

Acyclovir     Ganciclovir
Cidofovir     Penciclovir
Famciclovir   Valacyclovir
Fomivirsen    Valgancyclovir
Foscarnet     Vidarabine

**Human cytomegalovirus**

Cidofovir
Foscarnet
Ganciclovir

**Varicella-zoster virus**

Acyclovir
Famciclovir
Valacyclovir

**Figure 5.19**
Summary of therapeutic applications of selected antiviral agents.

infection may occur after discontinuance of the therapy. Lamivudine, an oral nucleoside analogue, is an effective treatment in patients with previously untreated chronic hepatitis B. However, only a minority of patients are cured or remain in remission after lamivudine therapy is withdrawn. Maintenance therapy may be indicated, but long-term use of lamivudine is limited by the appearance of viral polymerase gene mutants, which leads to reemergence of disease. The therapy of choice for hepatitis C is interferon-α in combination with ribavirin. The overall rate of response to this drug combination is three times greater than that seen with interferon-α monotherapy. However, anemia is a common adverse effect induced by ribavirin.

### E. Treatment of influenza

First-generation antiviral agents effective against influenza A include two related drugs, amantadine and rimantidine. Both stop viral uncoating by inhibition of the viral M2 membrane protein (see p. 319). These agents reduce both the duration and the severity of flu symptoms, but only if given early in infection. Given before the onset of symptoms, these drugs can also prevent disease, and are useful for treating high-risk groups. Second-generation antiviral agents effective against influenza A and B include zanamivir and oseltamivir. They inhibit viral neuraminidase, thereby preventing the release of virus from infected cells.

## Study Questions

**Choose the ONE correct answer**

5.1 Which one of the following most correctly describes vaccines containing live, attenuated pathogens?

   A. Pathogen does not multiply in human host
   B. Provides extended, sometimes life-long immunity
   C. No possibility for reversion to pathogenic form
   D. Provides little cell-mediated immunity
   E. Administered by injection

> Correct answer = B. Attenuated microbes reproduce in the recipient, typically leading to a more robust and longer-lasting immune response than can be obtained through vaccination with killed organisms.

5.2 Which one of the following best describes the components of vaccines against *Haemophilus influenzae* disease?

   A. Live, attenuated *H. influenzae*
   B. Killed *H. influenzae*
   C. Toxoid derived from *H. influenzae*
   D. Polysaccharide derived from *H. influenzae*
   E. Polysaccharide derived from *H. influenzae* conjugated to a protein antigen

> Correct answer = E. Covalent conjugates of capsular polysaccharide with diphtheria protein have been developed for *Haemophilus influenzae*. Unconjugated polysaccharide is weakly immunogenic in children younger than two. However, the conjugated vaccine produces higher of titers of antibody, superior responsiveness in children younger than two, and enhanced efficacy of booster administrations.

5.3 Which one of the following best describes the Sabin polio vaccine?

   A. Provides little gastrointestinal immunity
   B. Prepared with inactive virus
   C. Administered by injection
   D. Carries a small risk of causing disease
   E. Is an example of passive immunity

> Correct answer = D. The main disadvantage of attenuated live virus is the small risk of infection, estimated to be 1 per 2.4 million doses.

5.4 25-year-old woman whose blood tested positive for hepatitis B surface antigen (HBsAg) gave birth to a full-term child. Which of the following therapies would be most likely to minimize the transmission of hepatitis B to the neonate?

   A. Administer hepatitis B immunoglobulin
   B. Administer hepatitis B vaccine
   C. Administer hepatitis B immunoglobulin and hepatitis B vaccine.
   D. Bottle-feed the neonate

> Correct answer = C. Infants born to infected mothers are given hepatitis B immunoglobulin plus hepatitis B vaccine at birth, followed by additional doses of vaccine at one and six months. [Note: The two injections must be given at separate anatomical sites to prevent injected hepatitis B immunoglobulin from neutralizing the injected vaccine.] Perinatal infection of the neonate occurs at the time of delivery and is not related to consumption of breast milk.

*"It's a very effective dance when followed by a shot of penicillin"*

# Bacterial Structure, Growth, and Metabolism

# 6

## I. OVERVIEW

The cellular world is divided into two major groups, based on whether or not the cells have a nucleus (that is, an internal membrane-enclosed region that contains the genetic material). Cells that have a well-defined nucleus are called eukaryotic, whereas cells that lack a nucleus are called prokaryotic. All bacteria are prokaryotes. In addition, bacterial DNA is not organized into the elaborate multichromosomal structures of the eukaryotes, but typically is a single double-stranded molecule of DNA. Prokaryotes and eukaryotes employ very similar metabolic pathways to achieve cell growth and maintain viability. However, prokaryotes synthesize substances and structures that are unique to bacteria; for example, the bacterial cell wall. A generalized prokaryotic cell is shown in Figure 6.1.

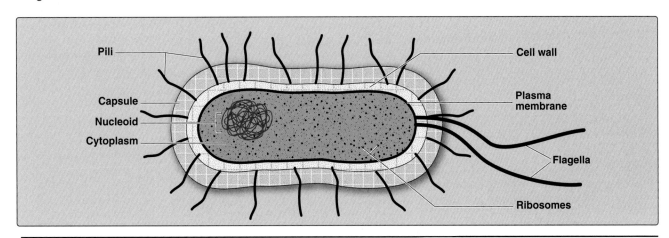

**Figure 6.1**
Generalized structure of a bacterial cell.

## II. THE CELL ENVELOPE

The bacterial "cell envelope" is a term applied to all material external to and enclosing the cytoplasm. It consists of several chemically and functionally distinct layers, the most prominent of which are cell wall and the cell membrane.

### A. Cell wall

The bacterial cell wall determines the shape of the cell. It is composed of a cross-linked polymeric mesh (peptidoglycan, Figure 6.2.) The glycan portion is a linear polymer of alternating monosaccharide subunits—N-acetylglucosamine (NAG) and N-acetylmuramic acid (NAM). This polymer is the carbohydrate "backbone" of the mesh. The "peptido" portion of the polymer is a short string of amino acids that serves to cross-link adjacent polysaccharide strands at the NAM subunits of the backbone, forming a network with high tensile strength (see Figure 6.2). [Note: The presence of D-amino acids helps render the bacterial wall resistant to host peptidases, such as those in the intestine.] A discussion of cell wall synthesis is presented on p. 55.

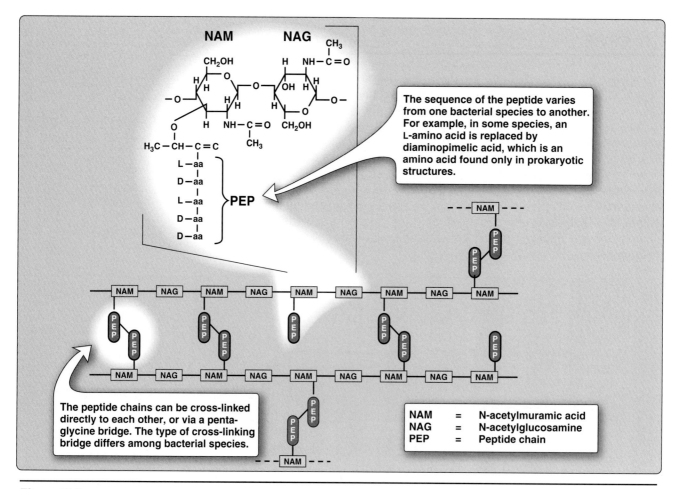

**Figure 6.2**
Structure of peptidoglycan, the major polymer of bacterial cell walls.

## B. Cell membrane

The cell membrane is composed of phospholipid, the molecules of which form two parallel surfaces (called a lipid bilayer) such that the polar phosphate groups are on the outside of the bilayer and the nonpolar lipid chains are on the inside. The membrane acts as a permeability barrier, restricting the kind and amount of molecules that enter and leave the cell.

## C. Differences between gram-positive and gram-negative species

The molecular details of the cell wall and membrane structures of gram-positive and gram-negative bacteria are shown in Figure 6.3. Additional surface layers, such as a capsule or glycocalyx, can be found in some species of gram-positive and gram-negative bacteria.

1. **Gram-positive organisms:** Gram-positive bacteria have thick, multilayered, peptidoglycan cell walls that are exterior to the membrane. The peptidoglycan in most gram-positive species is covalently linked to teichoic acid, which is essentially a polymer of substituted glycerol units linked by phosphodiester bonds. The teichoic acids are major cell surface antigens.

2. **Gram-negative organisms:** Gram-negative bacteria have two membranes—an outer membrane and an inner (cytoplasmic) membrane. The peptidoglycan layer is located between the two membranes (analogous to a slice of bread with butter on both sides) in what is called the periplasmic space. The periplasmic space also contains enzymes and various other substances. In contrast to gram-positive cells, the peptidoglycan layer of gram-negative cells is thin, and the cells are consequently more susceptible to physical damage. The outer membrane is distinguished by the presence of various embedded lipopolysaccharides. The polysaccharide portion (O-polysaccharide) is antigenic and can, therefore, be used to identify different strains and species. The lipid portion (called lipid A) is toxic to humans and animals. Because lipid A is an integral part of the membrane, it is called an endotoxin, as opposed to exotoxins, which are secreted substances.

> Do not confuse endo- or exotoxins with enterotoxins, which are exotoxins that are toxic for the mucosal membrane of the intestine. "Enterotoxin" denotes the site of action, rather than its origin.

## D. The external capsule and glycocalyx

Many bacteria secrete a sticky, viscous material that forms an extracellular coating around the cell. The material is usually a polysaccharide, however, in the case of pathogenic *Bacillus anthracis*, is poly-D-glutamic acid. If the material is tightly bound to the cell and has an organized structure, it is called a capsule (see Figure 6.1); if the material is loosely bound and amorphous, it is called a slime

**A** GRAM-POSITIVE

Peptidoglycan

Cytoplasmic membrane

**B** GRAM-NEGATIVE

The outer membrane contains O-polysaccharide, which is antigenic, and lipid A, an endotoxin.

Peptidoglycan

Outer membrane

Periplasmic space

Cytoplasmic membrane

**Figure 6.3**
Comparison of gram-positive and gram-negative bacterial cell walls.

**Figure 6.4**
The flagellum rotator machine.

layer or glycocalyx. The capsule and glycocalyx allow cells to adhere to surfaces, protect bacteria from antibodies and phagocytosis, and act as diffusion barriers against some antibiotics, thus contributing to the organisms' pathogenicity.

### E. Appendages

Many bacteria have hairlike appendages that project from the cell wall. There are of two kinds of appendages: flagella (singular, flagellum) and pili (singular, pilus).

1. **Flagella:** Prokaryotic flagella are long, semi-rigid, helical, hollow tubular structures composed of several thousand molecules of the protein flagellin. They enable bacteria to propel themselves, for example, in response to a chemotactic stimulus. Flagella are attached to the cell wall, cell membrane, or both by a basal body, which is a complex molecular machine that rotates the flagellum like the screw propeller of a ship (Figure 6.4). Cells may have one or many flagella. Flagella are highly antigenic.

> Bacteria that have flagella often do not form compact colonies on an agar surface, but instead swarm over the surface of the agar if it is sufficiently wet, producing a scumlike mat.

2. **Pili:** Pili (also called fimbriae), are shorter and thinner than flagella and function as attachment organs that promote specific cell-to-cell contact (see Figure 6.1). The attachment can be between the bacterial cell and the host eukaryotic cell, or between one bacterial cell and another.

## III. SPORES AND SPORULATION

To enhance survival during periods of environmental hostility (such as nutritional deprivation), some gram-positive rods undergo profound structural and metabolic changes. These result in the formation of a dormant cell called an endospore inside the original cell. Endospores can be released from the original cell as free spores (Figure 6.5). [Note: The terms "endospore" and "spore" are often used interchangeably.] Spores are the most resistant life-forms known. They are remarkably resistant to heat (they survive boiling), desiccation, ultraviolet light, and bacteriocidal chemical agents. In fact, sterilization procedures are assessed by their ability to kill spores.

### A. Sporulation

Sporulation can be thought of as repackaging a copy of bacterial DNA into a new form that contains very little water, has greatly reduced metabolic activity, does not divide, and has a restructured, highly impermeable, multilayered envelope. Spore formation begins with the invagination of the parent cell membrane, producing a double membrane that encapsulates and isolates a copy of the bacterial DNA in what will become the core of the spore. The mature spore retains the complete machinery for protein synthesis, and new spore-specific enzymes are synthesized in the core of the spore. At the same time, many enzymes of the original vegetative (nondividing) cell are degraded. When the endospore is completed, the parent cell lyses, releasing the spore.

### B. Spore germination

To return to the vegetative state, spores must first be subjected to a treatment that weakens the spore coat (such as heat or extremes of pH), thus allowing germination to occur. If the activated spore is in a nutritious environment, which it senses by monitoring various key metabolites, it begins to germinate. This process involves destruction of the cortex by lytic enzymes, followed by uptake of water, and release of dipicolinate from the cell.

### C. Medical significance of sporulation

Some of the most notorious pathogens are spore-formers, including *B. anthracis* (anthrax, see p. 94), *Bacillus cereus* (gastroenteritis, see p. 118), *Clostridium tetani* (tetanus, see p. 155), *Clostridium botulinum* (botulism, see p. 153), and *Clostridium perfringens* (gas gangrene, see p. 151). Spores of these organisms can remain viable for many years, and are generally not killed by boiling, but can be killed by autoclaving (that is, subjecting the spores to temperatures above 120°C at elevated pressure).

> In the absence of an autoclave, spores can be largely eliminated by a primary boiling to activate germination and, after a short period of vegetative growth, a second boiling.

## IV. GROWTH AND METABOLISM

All cells must accomplish certain metabolic tasks to maintain life. All cells, whether bacterial or human, accomplish these metabolic tasks by similar pathways. There are, however, some important differences that set bacteria apart metabolically from eukaryotic cells, and these differences can often be exploited in the development of antibacterial therapies.

### A. Characteristics of bacterial growth

If bacterial cells are suspended in a liquid nutrient medium, the increase in cell number or mass can be measured in several ways. Techniques include microscopically counting the cells in a given volume using a ruled slide, counting the number of appropriately diluted cells that are able to form colonies following transfer to a solid nutrient (agar) surface, or quantitating the turbidity—which is proportional to the cell mass—of a culture in liquid medium.

**Figure 6.5**
Formation of an endospore.

**Figure 6.6**
Kinetics of bacterial growth in liquid medium.

**Figure 6.7**
Growth of bacterial colonies on a solid, nutrient surface, for example, nutrient agar. [Note: The doubling time of bacteria is assumed to be 0.5 hr.]

1. **Stages of the bacterial growth cycle:** Because bacteria reproduce by binary fission (one becomes two, two become four, four become eight, etc.), the number of cells increases exponentially with time (the exponential or log phase of growth). Depending on the species, the minimum doubling time can be as short as twenty minutes or as long as several days. For example, for a rapidly growing species such as *E. coli* in a nutritionally complete medium, a single cell can give rise to some ten million cells in just eight hours. Eventually, growth slows and ceases entirely (stationary phase) as nutrients are depleted and toxic waste products accumulate. Most cells in a stationary phase are not dead, however. If they are diluted into fresh growth medium, exponential growth will resume after a lag phase. [Note: If held in stationary phase for an extended period, the cells will eventually die.] The phases of the growth cycle are illustrated in Figure 6.6.

2. **Surface growth:** If a single bacterial cell is placed on a solid nutrient agar surface, the progeny of this cell remain close to the site of deposition, and eventually form a compact macroscopic mass of cells (colony, Figure 6.7). For rapidly growing species, overnight incubation at 30° to 37°C is sufficient to produce visible colonies, each containing millions of cells. The gross characteristics of colonies (for example, color, shape, adherence, smell, and surface texture) can be useful guides for identification of the species of bacterium.

> Some species do not form compact circular colonies because the cells are capable of movement and swarm over the agar surface, especially if the surface is moist. Other species, particularly the actinomycetes, grow as long filaments of cells (mycelial growth).

## B. Energy production

A distinctive feature of bacterial metabolism is the variety of mechanisms used to generate energy from these carbon sources. According to the biochemical mechanism used, bacterial metabolism can be categorized into three types: aerobic respiration, anaerobic respiration, and fermentation (Figure 6.8).

1. **Aerobic respiration** (or simply, respiration) is the metabolic process in which molecular oxygen serves as the final electron acceptor of the electron transport chain. In this process, oxygen is reduced to water. Respiration is the energy-generating mode used by all aerobic bacteria.

2. **Anaerobic respiration** is the metabolic process in which inorganic compounds other than molecular oxygen serve as the final electron acceptors. Depending on the species, acceptors can be molecules such as nitrate or sulfate. Anaerobic respiration can be used as an alternative to aerobic respiration in some species (facultative organ-

isms), but is obligatory in other species (some obligate anaerobes). [Note: Other obligate anaerobes use fermentation as the main mode of energy metabolism. This is particularly true among the anaerobic bacteria of medical importance.]

3. **Fermentation** is an alternative anaerobic process exhibited by some species. It is the metabolic process by which an organic metabolic intermediate derived from a "fermentable" substrate serves as the final electron acceptor. The substrates that can be fermented and the final products depend on the species. Sugars are excellent fermentable substrates because they yield reducible intermediates. In fermentation of glucose to lactic acid, for example, the intermediate pyruvic acid is the final electron acceptor. Similarly, in fermentation of glucose to ethanol, acetaldehyde (a derivative of pyruvic acid) is the final electron acceptor.

## C. Cell wall synthesis

The bacterial cell wall, constructed on the surface of the cell membrane, is composed of a peptidoglycan polymer in which the repeating carbohydrate backbone subunit is NAG–NAM (see p. 50). These backbone chains are cross-linked by short peptides (PEP) to form a rigid meshwork (Figure 6.9).

1. **Activation of carbohydrate subunits:** As in all biologic polymerizations, NAM and NAG subunits are activated by attachment to a carrier; in this case, the nucleotide UDP.

2. **Synthesis of the linking peptide:** A pentapeptide is added to UDP–NAM by sequential transfer of amino acids, with the two terminal alanine residues added as a dipeptide. This pentapeptide may contain some nonstandard amino acids; for example, diaminopimelic acid (DAP, a metabolic precursor of lysine), and D-amino acids. As would be expected, the sequence is not dictated by an RNA template, but rather the specificity of the enzymes that form the peptide bonds.

3. **Transfer of the cell wall unit to bactoprenol phosphate:** The NAM–PEP moiety is transferred from the UDP carrier to another carrier, bactoprenol phosphate (BPP), located on the inner surface of the cell membrane. At this point, UDP–NAG transfers NAG to NAM–PEP, completing the peptidoglycan repeat unit now attached to the carrier BPP.

4. **Addition of the repeat unit to the existing peptidoglycan:** BPP carries the NAG–NAM–PEP repeat unit through the cell membrane to the outside surface where the peptidoglycan of the existing cell wall is located. The repeat unit is added to a free end of the existing peptidoglycan, increasing the length of the polymer by one repeat unit. Presumably, free ends are created by a limited hydrolytic loosening of the preexisting peptidoglycan.

5. **Cross-linking of the pentapeptide to the peptidoglycan backbone:** Although the N–terminal end of the pentapeptide is

**Figure 6.8**
Overview of respiration, fermentation, and energy production in bacteria. [Note: Compounds other than oxygen, such as nitrate and sulfate, can be used as terminal electron acceptors in anaerobic respiration.]

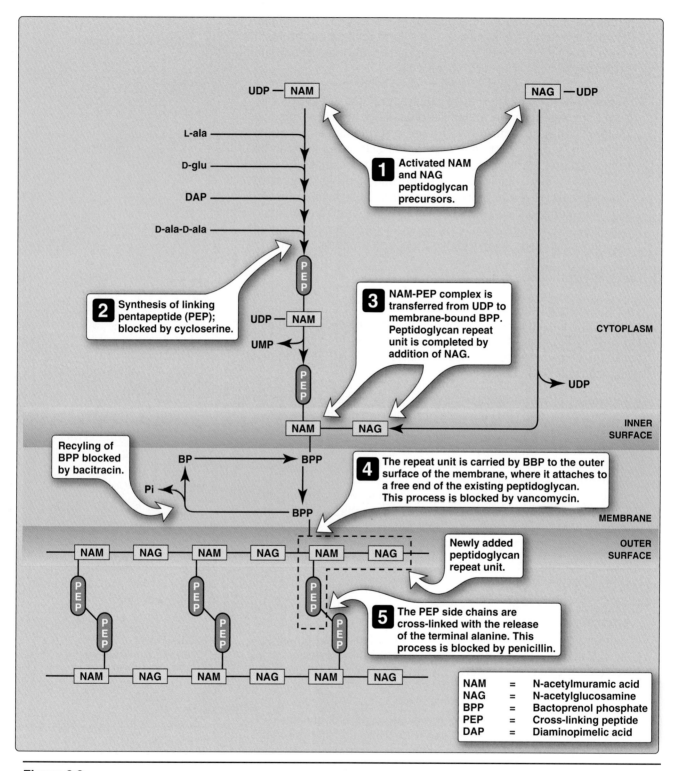

**Figure 6.9**
Synthesis of a bacterial cell wall.

attached to the NAM moieties of the backbone, the C–terminal end is dangling free. Cross-linking is brought about by a transpeptidation reaction that bonds DAP of the peptide in one chain to the alanine (ala) at position four of the peptide in an adjacent chain, causing the release of the terminal ala. This mode of direct cross-linking is characteristic of *E. coli* and many other gram-negative species. [Note: In gram-positive bacteria, such as *Staphylococcus aureus*, a glycine pentapeptide is usually interposed between lysine (lys) at position three of one PEP and ala at position four of the PEP to which the linkage is to be made (Figure 6.10.]

6. **Cell wall synthesis as a target of antibacterial agents:** Because many of the reactions involved in the synthesis of the bacterial cell wall do not occur in mammalian cells, bacterial cell wall synthesis is an ideal target for some highly specific antibacterial agents, particularly β-lactam antibiotics.

   a. **β-Lactam antibiotics:** Penicillins and cephalosporins inhibit the enzymes that catalyze transpeptidation and carboxypeptidation reactions of cell wall assembly. These enzymes are called penicillin-binding proteins (PBPs) because they all have active sites that bind β-lactam antibiotics. No single PBP species is the target of β-lactam antibiotics; rather their lethal effect on bacteria is the result of inactivation of multiple species of PBPs. Most PBPs are involved in bacterial cell wall synthesis. However, β-lactamases—enzymes that catalyze hydrolysis of the β-lactam ring—bind penicillin and are, therefore, also classified as PBPs. Most PBPs are membrane-bound except for β-lactamases, which may be either secreted or membrane-associated. Acquired resistance to β-lactam antibiotics may result from genetic modifications resulting in production of modified PBPs that have a lower affinity for β-lactam antibiotics (see p. 64).

   b. **Bacitracin, cycloserine, and vancomycin:** Other antibiotics that interfere with cell wall synthesis include bacitracin, which inhibits the recycling of bactoprenol phosphate; cycloserine, which inhibits synthesis of the D–ala–D–ala dipeptide that provides the two terminal residues of the pentapeptide; and vancomycin, which blocks incorporation of the NAG–NAM–PEP repeat unit into the growing peptidoglycan chain (see Figure 6.9).

**Figure 6.10**
A. Glycine bridge in the peptidoglycan of *Staphylococcus aureus*.
B. Organization of peptidoglycan layer in gram-positive cells.

## Study Questions

**Choose the ONE correct answer**

6.1 A bacterial culture with a starting density of $10^3$ cells/ml is incubated in liquid nutrient broth. If the bacteria have both a lag time and a generation time of ten minutes, what will the cell density be at thirty minutes?

    A. $1.0 \times 10^3$
    B. $2.0 \times 10^3$
    C. $3.0 \times 10^3$
    D. $4.0 \times 10^3$
    E. $6.0 \times 10^3$

> Correct answer = D. After a ten minute lag, the bacteria will double in number at twenty minutes and double again by thirty minutes.

6.2 Which of the following components are found in the cell walls of gram-positive bacteria, but not gram-negative bacteria?

    A. Cytoplasmic membrane
    B. Lipopolysaccharide
    C. Outer membrane
    D. Peptidoglycan
    E. Teichoic acid

> Correct answer = E. Gram-positive bacteria have thick, multilayered, peptidoglycan cell walls that are exterior to the membrane. The peptidoglycan in most gram-positive species is covalently linked to teichoic acid, which is essentially a polymer of substituted glycerol units linked by phosphodiester bonds. All gram-positive species also have teichoic acid in their membranes, where it is covalently linked to glycolipid. Teichoic acids are major cell surface antigens. Gram-negative bacteria have two membranes—an outer membrane and an inner (cytoplasmic) membrane. Their peptidoglycan layer is located between the two membranes in the periplasmic space. The periplasmic space also contains enzymes and various other substances. The outer membrane is distinguished by the presence of various embedded lipopolysaccharides.

6.3 In 1998, a large botulism outbreak occurred in El Paso, Texas. The foodborne illness was shown to be caused by foil-wrapped baked potatoes that were held at room temperature for several days before their use in dips at a Greek restaurant. The dip yielded botulinum toxin type A, as did stool and, in some cases serum samples from 18 of the 30 affected patients. Four patients required mechanical ventilation; none died. What would be the expected outcome if the potatoes had been reheated to 100°C for 10 minutes before being served? [Hint: See pp. 153–154 for properties of *Clostridium botulinum* toxin].

    A. Heat would kill the spores of *C. botulinum*.
    B. Heat would promote the vegetative state.
    C. Heat would inactivate the toxin in the potato dip.
    D. Heat would increase the number of toxin-producing bacteria.
    E. Heat would not alter the outcome.

> Correct answer = C. *C. botulinum* spores are commonly found on raw potatoes and generally are not killed if the potatoes are baked in foil, which holds in moisture and thus keeps the potatoes' surface temperature at 100°C (below the temperature required for spore killing of >120°C). During storage at room temperature in the anaerobic environment provided by the foil, spores germinate and toxin forms. Heating at 100°C would kill most *C. botulinum* because the bacterium is large in its vulnerable, vegative state. Heat would also inactivate toxin produced during room-temperature storage. However, any remaining spores would not be killed.

*"That pill they advertise all the time on TV. I'm not sure what it is, but I want it!"*

# Bacterial Genetics

# 7

## I. OVERVIEW

Because a single type of molecule, DNA, is the genetic material of all cellular organisms from bacteria to humans, basic genetic phenomena—gene mutation, gene replication, and gene recombination—are much the same for all life forms. The prototypic organism used in microbial genetic studies for the past fifty years is the enteric, gram-negative *Escherichia coli* (see p. 111). An aspect of microbial genetics of great clinical importance is the ability of bacteria to transfer genes, especially genes for antibiotic resistance, to other bacteria both within and between species. Such transfer allows the flow of antibiotic resistance genes from nonpathogenic bacterial populations to pathogenic populations, with potentially dire consequences for public health.

## II. THE BACTERIAL GENOME

The genome of an organism is defined as the totality of its genetic material. For bacteria, the genome consists of a single chromosome that carries all of the essential genes and one or more varieties of plasmid that generally carry nonessential genes (Figure 7.1).

### A. The chromosome

All of the essential genes and many nonessential genes of the bacterium are carried on a single, long piece of circular, double-stranded DNA. This molecular structure is called the "chromosome" by analogy with the heredity-carriers of eukaryotic cells. Most bacteria have chromosomes that contain 2000 to 4000 genes.

### B. Plasmids

Typically, bacteria contain small DNA circles (plasmids), which range in size from 1.5 kilobase (kb) pairs to 120 kb pairs (less than one-tenth the size of the bacterial chromosome). Plasmids repli-

**CHROMOSOME**
- Circular, double-stranded DNA
- 3000 genes (3000 kilobases)
- Single copy per cell
- Highly folded in cell

Cell wall

**BACTERIUM**

**PLASMID**
- Circular, double-stranded DNA
- 5-100 genes (5-100 kilobases)
- 1-20 copies per cell

**Figure 7.1**
The bacterial genome. [Note: Helical double-stranded DNA is shown as two concentric circles.]

**1** Attachment of phage to cell surface receptor

← Bacteriophage

Cell wall of bacterium

0 MINUTES

**2** Injection of phage DNA into cell

DNA

1 MINUTE

**3** Synthesis of new phage DNA and phage proteins

10 MINUTES

Phage proteins

**4** Assembly of new phage particles

25 MINUTES

Complete phage particle

**5** Lysis of cell and release of progeny phage

30 MINUTES

**Figure 7.2**
Bacteriophage replication. Clock indicates total elapsed time starting with attachment at t = 0. [Note: Bacterial chromosome and plasmid are not shown.]

cate independently of the chromosome, and can exist in the cell as one copy or as many copies. Plasmids can carry genes for toxins and for proteins that promote the transfer of the plasmid to other cells, but usually do not include genes that are essential for cell growth or replication. Many plasmids contain mobile DNA sequences (transposons) that can move between plasmids, and between plasmids and the chromosome (see pp. 63–64).

> Transposons, the repository for many antibiotic resistance genes, are responsible for the ability of some plasmids to integrate into the chromosome.

## III. BACTERIOPHAGE

A bacteriophage (phage) is a virus that replicates inside a bacterial cell; it consists of nothing more than a piece of nucleic acid encapsulated in a protective protein coat. Depending on the phage, the nucleic acid can be DNA or RNA, double-stranded or single-stranded, and range in size from about 3000 bases (3 genes) to about 200,000 bases (200 genes). The typical replicative cycle (Figure 7.2) begins with attachment of the phage to receptors on the cell surface, followed by injection of the nucleic acid into the bacterial cell, leaving all or most of the protein outside the cell. [Note: This is in contrast to viral infection of vertebrate cells, in which the entire virus is taken up by the cell, and its nucleic acid released intracellularly (see pp. 236–237).] The phage nucleic acid takes over the cell's biosynthetic machinery to replicate its own genetic material, and to synthesize phage-specific proteins. When sufficient coat proteins and new phage DNA have accumulated, these components self-assemble into mature phage particles, with the DNA encapsulated by the phage coat. Release of new phage particles is accomplished by a phage-specific enzyme (lysozyme) that dissolves the bacterial cell wall. The number of phage particles in a sample can be determined by a simple and rapid plaque assay. If a single phage particle is immobilized in a confluent bacterial lawn growing on a nutrient agar surface, this phage, within a few hours, will produce millions of progeny at the expense of neighboring bacterial cells, leaving a visible "hole" or plaque in the otherwise opaque lawn (Figure 7.3).

### A. Virulent phage

Phage are classified as virulent or temperate depending on the nature of their relationship to the host bacterium. Infection of a bacterium with a virulent phage inevitably results in the death of the cell by lysis, with release of newly replicated phage particles. Under optimal conditions, a bacterial cell infected with only one phage particle can produce hundreds of progeny in twenty minutes. [Note: Generally, phage that attack one bactrial species do not attack other bacterial species.]

## B. Temperate phage

A bacterium infected with a temperate phage can have the same fate as a bacterium infected with a virulent phage (lysis rapidly following infection). However, an alternative outcome is also possible, namely, after entering the cell, the phage DNA, rather than replicating autonomously, can fuse or integrate with the chromosome of the host cell. In this state (prophage), the expression of phage genes is repressed indefinitely by a protein (repressor) encoded within the phage genome. No new phage particles are produced, the host cell survives, and the phage DNA replicates as part of the host chromosome.

## C. Lysogenic bacteria

Lysogenic bacteria carry a prophage; the phenomenon is termed lysogeny, and the bacterial cell is said to be lysogenized. Nonlysogenic bacteria can be made lysogenic by infection with a temperate phage. The association of prophage and bacterial cell is highly stable, but can be destabilized by various treatments, such as exposure to ultraviolet light, that damage the host DNA. When DNA damage occurs, repression of phage genes is lifted, the prophage excises from the host chromosome, replicates autonomously, and produces progeny phage particles. The host cell is lysed just as with a virulent phage. The emergence of the virus from its latent prophage state is called induction. The acquisition by bacteria of properties due to the presence of a prophage is called lysogenic conversion.

# IV. GENE TRANSFER

Genes can be transferred from one bacterial cell to another by three distinct mechanisms: conjugation, transduction, and transformation. Because the transferred DNA usually does not contain an origin of replication, these genes will be passed on to succeeding generations only if the transferred DNA becomes incorporated into the recipient chromosome, which has an origin of replication.

## A. Conjugation

Conjugation is the process by which bacteria transfer genes from one cell to another by cell-to-cell contact. The donor (male) and recipient (female) cells must have the proper genetic constitution to adhere to each other, and form a cytoplasmic bridge between the cells through which DNA can pass. Specifically, the process requires the presence on the donor cell of hairlike projections called sex pili that make contact with specific receptor sites on the surface of the recipient cell. This contact results in the formation of a relatively stable cell pair, and the initiation of DNA transfer (Figure 7.4).

Mixture of $10^8$ uninfected bacterial cells and a single phage-infected cell in melted agar.

Solidification of top agar layer immobilizes all cells.

Infected cell

12 hours

Phage replicate in the infected cell. The cell lyses, releasing progeny that infect adjacent cells. These cells lyse, and the cycle repeats.

Top view of agar plate

Growth of uninfected bacteria creates an opaque lawn except at the location of the original infected cell, where there is a plaque (hole) containing millions of phage.

**Figure 7.3**
Visual detection of bacteriophage by the plaque method.

**Figure 7.4**
Cell-to-cell transfer of a conjugative plasmid (Chromosomal DNA is not shown).

**B. Transduction**

Transduction refers to transfer of genes from one cell to another via a phage vector without cell-to-cell contact. There are two ways in which this can occur: generalized transduction and specialized transduction. In each case, the transducing phage is a temperate phage, so that the recipient cell survives the phage infection.

1. **Generalized transduction:** In generalized transduction, a random fragment of bacterial DNA, resulting from phage-induced cleavage of the bacterial chromosome, is accidentally encapsulated in a phage protein coat in place of the phage DNA (Figure 7.5A). When this rare phage particle infects a cell, it injects the bacterial DNA fragment into the cell. If this fragment becomes integrated into the recipient chromosome by recombination, the recipient cell will be stably transduced.

2. **Specialized transduction:** In specialized transduction, only certain bacterial genes, located on the bacterial chromosome in close proximity to the prophage insertion site of the transducing phage, are transduced (Figure 7.5B). The phage acquires the bacterial genes by a rare, abnormal excision from the bacterial chromosome. In general, a specialized transducing phage particle contains both phage and bacterial DNA joined together as a single molecule. After infecting another cell, this joint molecule integrates into the recipient chromosome just as phage DNA normally does in the process of becoming a prophage.

**C. Transformation**

Transformation is the transfer of genes from one cell to another by means of naked DNA. The discovery of transformation in 1928, one of the most important in all of biology, led eventually to the identification of DNA as the genetic material.

1. **Transformation process:** Studies of the transformation phenomenon itself revealed that the ability of a cell to be transformed (called competence) depends on a transitory physiologic state of the cell that allows DNA to cross the cell membrane. As free, double-stranded DNA enters the recipient cell, one of the two strands is destroyed by nucleases. The remaining single strand invades the resident chromosome, seeking a region of sequence homology. If such a sequence is found, the invading strand replaces one of the two resident strands by a complex cut-and-paste process. Transformation probably has only a minor effect on gene flow in natural bacterial populations, but it is useful experimentally for introducing a cloned gene (for example, the human gene for insulin) into bacterial cells.

## V. GENETIC VARIATION

Although all of the cells in a "pure" bacterial culture are derived from a single original cell, the culture typically contains rare cells that differ from the originating cell. The majority, if not all, of such variants (mutants) are due to changes (mutations) in their DNA.

**Figure 7.5**
Certain phage can package bacterial genes and transfer them to other bacteria (transduction). By one mechanism (A) any bacterial gene can be transferred; by a second mechanism (B) only certain genes can be transferred, namely those in close proximity to a prophage.

## A. Mutations

Strictly speaking, any change in the structure of genetic material or, more specifically, any change in the base sequence of DNA, is called a mutation. Some mutations are unstable (that is, they frequently revert back to their original state), and others do not noticeably affect the organism. Mutations that come under study are usually those that are stable, and that cause some change in the characteristics of the organism. Mutations can be classified according to the kind of chemical change that occurs in the DNA or, when the mutation affects a protein-coding gene, by the effect the mutation has on the translation of the message.[1]

## B. Mobile genetic elements

In recent years, it has been recognized that the arrangement of genes in the genome of bacteria—and probably all organisms—is

[1]See p. 431 in *Lippincott's Illustrated Reviews: Biochemistry* (3rd ed.) for a discussion of different types of mutations.

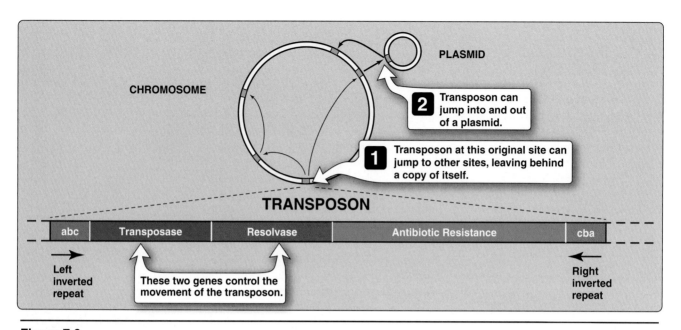

**Figure 7.6**
A transposon can move from place to place in the chromosome, leaving a copy of itself behind at the previous site.

not entirely static. Certain DNA segments, called transposons, have the ability to move from place to place on the chromosome and into and out of plasmids. Transposons do not exist as segments free of the genome but only as segments within the genome. There are two general types of transposons: replicative and nonreplicative. A replicative transposon leaves a copy of itself at the original location. Thus, the transposition process doubles the number of copies of the transposon. A nonreplicative transposon does not leave a copy of itself at the original location. If transposition inserts a transposon into a functional gene, the function of the gene is generally destroyed; this was the original basis by which transposons were discovered. Transposons can thus be viewed as internal mutagenic agents. The transposition process and the structure of a typical replicative transposon are shown in Figure 7.6. This transposon has three genes and a length of about five kilobases. The transposase and resolvase genes code for enzymes involved in the transposition process, whereas the antibiotic resistance gene is a "passenger." The transposon is bounded by short (about fifty bases), inverted repeats. These inverted repeats are the elements recognized by the transposase as it initiates the transposition. Mobile genetic elements are probably responsible for most of the genetic variability in natural bacterial populations, and for the spread of antibiotic resistance genes.

## C. Mechanisms of acquired antibiotic resistance

Acquired antibiotic resistance requires a temporary or permanent gain or alteration of bacterial genetic information. Most resistance genes are plasmid-mediated; however, plasmid-mediated traits can interchange with chromosomal elements. Transfer of genetic material from plasmid to chromosome can occur by simple recombinational events, but the process is greatly facilitated by transposons. Many resistance genes, such as plasmid-mediated β-lactamases, tetracycline-resis-tance genes, and aminoglycoside-modifying enzymes, are organized on transposons. Resistance to antibiotics is accomplished by three principal mechanisms (Figure 7.7):

1. **Decreased uptake (or increased efflux) of antibiotic:** For exam-ple, gram-negative organisms can limit the penetration of certain agents, including β-lactam antibiotics, tetracyclines, and chloram-phenicol, as a result of alteration in the number and structure of porins (proteins that form chanels) in the outer membrane.

2. **Alteration of the target site for antibiotic:** For example, *Staphylococcus pneumoniae* resistance to β-lactam antibiotics involves alterations in one or more of the major bacterial peni-cillin-binding proteins (see p. 75), which results in decreased bind-ing of the antibiotic to its target.

3. **Acquisition of the ability to destroy or modify the antibiotic:** Examples of antibiotic inactivating enzymes include: 1) β-lacta-mases that hydrolytically inactivate the β-lactam ring of penicillins, cephalosporins, and related drugs; 2) acetyltransferases that transfer an acetyl group to the antibiotic, inactivating chloram-phenicol or aminoglycosides; 3) esterases that hydrolyze the lac-tone ring of macrolides.

## VI. GENE REGULATION

In general, bacteria can manufacture most of the organic compounds (amino acids, nucleotides, carbohydrates, lipids) that they need; in this regard they are more versatile than higher organisms. This metabolic resourcefulness is a distinct advantage when the organism is in a nutri-tionally poor environment, but is extremely wasteful in a nutritious envi-ronment if the bacterium must keep all of the unneeded biosynthetic enzymes ready at hand. Bacteria, therefore, have evolved various mechanisms for producing certain metabolic enzymes only when they are needed.

> Most metabolite regulatory mechanisms involve control of transcription of the gene into messen-ger RNA, rather than control of translation of the messenger.

### A. Negative control (repression)

Lactose is a disaccharide composed of glucose and galactose, which is found in dairy products. The first step in lactose metabolism is cleavage into monosaccharide units, a job performed by the enzyme β-galactosidase. To avoid being wasteful, bacteria synthe-size β-galactosidase only when lactose is present in the growth medium. Bacteria accomplish this control by producing a repressor protein that, when lactose is absent, binds to a specific site on the DNA (operator site) near the start of the β-galactosidase gene (Figure 7.8A). When repressor is bound, RNA polymerase—which

**Figure 7.7**
Three common mechanisms of antibiotic resistance.

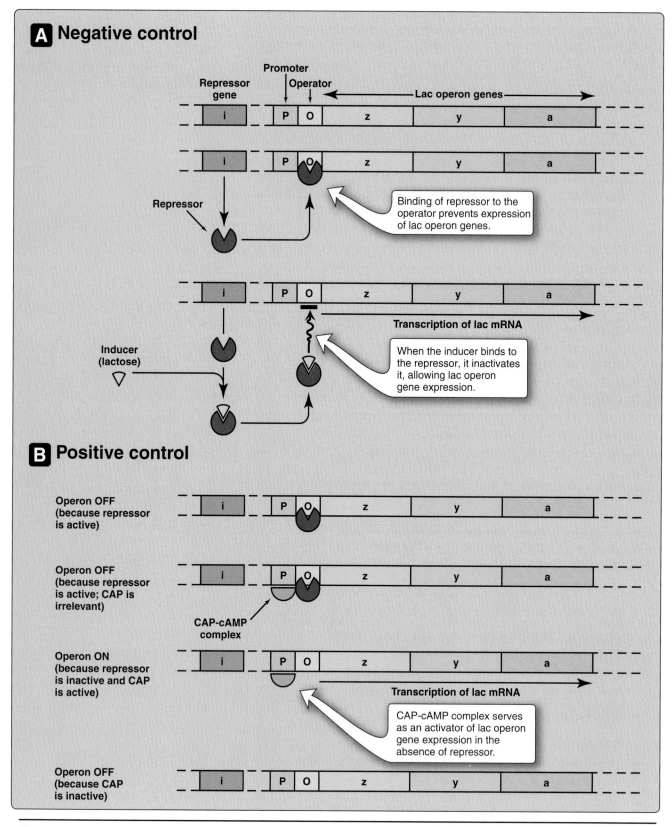

**Figure 7.8**
Bacterial genes can be controlled negatively by repressors or positively by activators.

recognizes the promoter region that is upstream from the operator site—is blocked from initiating transcription of the genes. When lactose is present, it binds to the repressor protein, preventing the repressor from binding to the DNA, and allowing transcription of the genes. The β-galactosidase gene is actually one of a set of three contiguous genes, the other two are a lactose permease, and β-galactoside transacetylase. Together, these three genes, all of which are controlled by the same repressor, comprise the lac operon. This mechanism is called negative control because the controlling element—the repressor—acts to prevent transcription. In this example, lactose is an inducer of the lac operon. [Note: In other cases, the free repressor does not repress unless it is combined with another compound (corepressor). For example, the repressor for the tryptophan operon is active only when it binds tryptophan.]

## B. Positive control (catabolite activation)

If bacteria are grown in medium containing glucose and another sugar, the bacteria use glucose exclusively as an energy source. This is because transcription of all of the operons for use of sugars other than glucose fails to occur, even though the inducing sugars are present. The reason for this failure is that the sugar-utilization operons, of which the lac operon is an example, must be activated by a specific protein called catabolite activator protein (CAP), which, in turn, is only functional as an activator when complexed with cyclic AMP. [Note: CAP is also called CRP (cyclic AMP receptor protein).] Glucose, in turn, regulates CAP activity by regulating the level of cyclic AMP. When glucose is present at a high level, cyclic AMP is at a low level, and sugar-utilization operons are not activated. When glucose is absent or at a low level, cyclic AMP is at a high level and sugar utilization operons are activated (Figure 7.8B).

> Catabolite activation is a global regulatory mechanism by which many operons, each under individual control, are regulated by a single activator protein.

## C. Modifications of RNA polymerase specificity

Microorganisms are often compelled to switch on or off large groups of genes in response to stressful environmental conditions. For example, under starvation conditions, many species sporulate, a process that requires major changes in metabolic pathways. Similarly, sudden exposure to elevated temperature ("heat shock") elicits formation of many new proteins. In both cases, the shift in gene expression results from a modification of the RNA polymerase, specifically, a replacement of the normal σ (sigma) subunit with an alternative subunit that recognizes a different set of promoters.[2]

[2]See p. 415 in *Lippincott's Illustrated Reviews: Biochemistry* (3rd ed.) for a discussion of the role of sigma factor in the activity of RNA polymerase.

## Study Questions

**Choose the ONE correct answer**

7.1  A lysogenic bacterium

    A. carries a prophage.

    B. causes lysis of other bacteria on contact.

    C. cannot support the replication of a virulent phage.

    D. is often a human pathogen.

    E. is usually not capable of conjugal genetic transfer.

Correct answer = A. A lysogenic bacterium can generate phage because it carries phage genes in a latent state (prophage). Lysogenicity does not impart any special lytic properties to the bacterium nor, in general, does it affect conjugal transfer or the ability to support the replication of other unrelated phage. The presence of a prophage can convert certain bacteria to human pathogens, but such cases are rare.

7.2  Which one of the following statements concerning plasmids is true?

    A. All plasmids can be transfered between bacteria by conjugation.

    B. Much of the information coded in the plasmid is essential to the survival of the bacteria cell.

    C. R plasmids carry genes for antibiotic resistance.

    D. R plasmids cannot be transferred to other bacterial cells.

    E. Plasmids lack an origin of replication.

Correct answer = C. Plasmids are small, circular, supercoiled DNA molecules found in some bacteria. They usually do not carry essential genes, but some plasmids, such as R (resistance) plasmids, carry genes coding for antibiotic resistance. All plasmids have their own origin of replication, so that they are replicated along with the host chromosome and passed along to progeny cells. Only some plasmids possess genes that allow for transmittal to other bacteria by the process of conjugation.

7.3  What occurs when a temperate bacteriophage enters a state called "lysogeny"?

    A. Most viral genes are expressed.

    B. The bacterial cell is lysed.

    C. Many new viruses are produced.

    D. Most normal bacterial functions are turned off.

    E. The virus may become integrated into the host genome.

Correct answer = E. There are two types of bacteriophages: lytic and temperate. The distinction is made according to the life cycle of the bacteriophage. On entering a bacterium, lytic phages produce phage nucleic acids and proteins, assemble many new phage particles, lyse the cell, and release the progeny phage. Temperate phages, however, can penetrate the bacterium and enter a dormant state called lysogeny; in which most viral genes are repressed. Bacterial functions remain active and the bacterium is not harmed. Some dormant phages replicate as plasmids; others, such as phage lambda, become integrated into the host genome as prophages. The prophage DNA is replicated along with the host DNA as the bacterium grows and divides.

*Pssst! Hey kid! Wanna be a Superbug..? Stick some of this into your genome... Even penicillin won't be able to harm you..!*

*"It was on a short-cut through the hospital kitchens that Albert was first approached by a member of the Antibiotic Resistance."*

# Staphylococci

# 8

## I. OVERVIEW

Staphylococci and streptococci (see Chapter 9) constitute the main groups of medically important gram-positive cocci. Staphylococcal infections range from the trivial to the rapidly fatal. They can be very difficult to treat, especially those contracted in hospitals, because of the remarkable ability of staphylococci to become resistant to antibiotics. Staphylococci are ubiquitous in nature, with about a dozen species occurring as part of human flora. The most virulent of the genus, *Staphylococcus aureus*, is one of the most common causes of bacterial infections, and is also an important cause of food poisoning and toxic shock syndrome. Among less virulent staphylococcal species, *Staphylococcus epidermidis* is an important cause of prosthetic implant infections, whereas *Staphylococcus saprophyticus* causes urinary tract infections, especially cystitis in women. Figure 8.1 summarizes the staphylococci described in this chapter.

## II. GENERAL FEATURES

Staphylococci generally stain darkly gram-positive (Figure 8.2). They are round rather than oval, and tend to occur in bunches like grapes. Staphylococci are rather fastidious, requiring various amino acids and other growth factors, and are routinely cultured on enriched media containing broth and/or blood (see p. 23). Staphylococci are true facultatively anaerobic organisms. They produce catalase, which is one feature that distinguishes them from the catalase-negative streptococci. The most virulent species of staphylococcus is *S. aureus*, almost all isolates of which secrete coagulase—an enzyme that causes citrated plasma to clot. There are other species that occasionally cause disease; these lack coagulase and are often referred to as coagulase-negative staphylococci.

> Staphylococci are hardy, being resistant to heat and drying, and thus can persist for long periods on fomites (inanimate objects), which can then serve as sources of infection. Frequent hand washing before and after contact with food or potentially infected individuals decreases the transmission of staphylococcal disease.

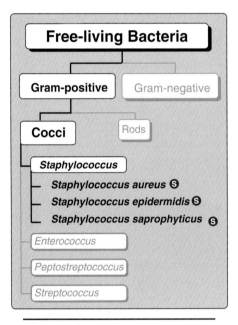

**Figure 8.1**
Classification of Staphylococci.
Ⓢ See p. 331 for a summaries of these organisms.

**Figure 8.2**
Gram stain of *Staphylococcus aureus.*
Streptococcus

69

**Figure 8.3**
Causes of disease resulting from
infection with *Staphylococcus
aureus*.

## III. STAPHYLOCOCCUS AUREUS

Generally, significant host compromise is required for *S. aureus* infection, such as a break in the skin or insertion of a foreign body (for example, wounds, surgical infections, or central venous catheters), an obstructed hair follicle (folliculitis), or a compromised immune system. *S. aureus* disease may be: 1) largely or wholly the result of actual invasive infection (that is, colonization), overcoming host defense mechanisms, and the production of extracellular substances which facilitate invasion; 2) a result of toxins in the absence of invasive infection ("pure" toxinoses); or 3) a combination of invasive infection and intoxication (Figure 8.3).

### A. Epidemiology

*S. aureus* is frequently carried by healthy individuals on the skin and mucous membranes. Carriers serve as a source of infection to themselves and others; for example, by direct contact, by contamination of fomites (objects such as a doorknob, which in turn can be a source of infection) or food, which can then result in food poisoning.

### B. Pathogenesis

Pathogenic virulence factors are the genetic, biochemical, or structural features that enable an organism to produce disease. The clinical outcome of an infection depends on the virulence of the pathogen and the opposing effectiveness of the host defense mechanisms. *S. aureus* expresses many potential virulence factors (Figure 8.4). [Note: Coagulase is generally not considered a virulence factor because coagulase-negative mutants are as virulent as the corresponding parental strains; the association between coagulase positivity and virulence in nature is probably fortuitous.]

For the majority of diseases caused by S. aureus, pathogenesis depends on the combined actions of several virulence factors, so it is difficult to determine precisely the role of any given factor.

1. **Cell wall virulence factors:**

   a. **Protein A** is a major component of the *S. aureus* cell wall. It binds to the Fc moiety of IgG, exerting an antiopsonin (and therefore strongly antiphagocytic) effect.

   b. **Fibronectin-binding protein (FnBP)** and other staphylococcal surface proteins promote binding to mucosal cells and tissue matrices.

2. **Cytolytic exotoxins:** α, β, γ, and δ toxins attack mammalian cell (including red blood cell) membranes, and are often referred to as hemolysins. α-Toxin is the best studied, and is chromosomally encoded. It polymerizes into tubes that pierce membranes, resulting in the loss of important molecules and, eventually, in osmotic lysis.

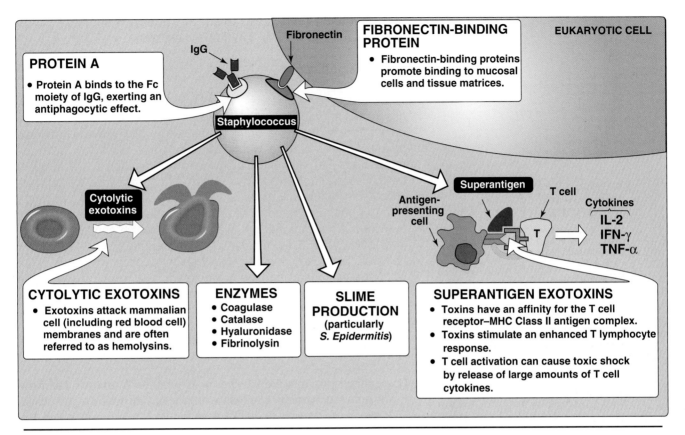

**Figure 8.4**
Virulence factors that may play a role in the pathogenesis of staphylococcal infections.

3. **Superantigen exotoxins:** These toxins have an affinity for the T cell receptor–MHC Class II antigen complex. They stimulate enhanced T lymphocyte response (as many as twenty percent of T cells respond, compared with 0.01 percent responding to the usual processed antigens). This difference is a result of their ability to recognize a relatively conserved region of the T cell receptor. This major T cell activation can cause toxic shock syndrome, primarily by release into the circulation of inordinately large amounts of T cell cytokines, such as interleukin-2 (IL-2), interferon-γ (IFN-γ), and tumor necrosis factor-α (TNF-α).

   a. **Enterotoxins:** Enterotoxins (six major antigenic types: A, B, C, D, E, and G) are produced by approximately half of all *S. aureus* isolates. When these bacteria contaminate food and are allowed to grow, they secrete enterotoxin, ingestion of which can cause food poisoning. [Note: The toxin stimulates the vomiting center in the brain by binding to neural receptors in the upper gastrointestinal (GI) tract.] Enterotoxins are superantigens that are even more heat-stable than *S. aureus*; therefore, organisms are not always recovered from incriminated food.

   b. **Toxic shock syndrome toxin (TSST–1)** is the classic cause of toxic shock syndrome. Because of similarities in molecular structure, it is sometimes referred to as staphylococcal enterotoxin F (SEF), although it does not cause food poisoning when ingested.

**c. Exfoliatin (exfoliative toxin, ET)** is also a superantigen. It causes scalded skin syndrome in children.

## C. Clinical significance

*S. aureus* causes disease by infecting tissues—typically creating abscesses and/or by producing toxins (Figure 8.5). A common entry point into the body is a break in the skin, which may be a minute needlestick or a surgical wound. Another portal of entry is the respiratory tract. For example, staphylococcal pneumonia is a frequent complication of influenza. The localized host response to staphylococcal infection is inflammation, characterized by swelling, accumulation of pus, and necrosis of tissue. Fibroblasts and their products may form a wall around the inflamed area, which contains bacteria and leukocytes. This creates a characteristic, pus-filled boil or abscess. Serious consequences of staphylococcal infections occur when the bacteria invade the bloodstream. The resulting septicemia (the presence and persistence of pathogenic microorganisms or their toxins in the blood) may be rapidly fatal. Bacteremia (the presence of viable bacteria circulating in the bloodstream) may result in seeding internal abscesses, skin lesions, or infections in the lung, kidney, heart, skeletal muscle, or meninges.

1. **Localized skin infections:** The most common *S. aureus* infections are small, superficial abscesses involving hair follicles (folliculitis) or sweat or sebaceous glands (see Figure 8.12). For example, the common sty (external hordeolum) is created by infection of an eyelash follicle. Subcutaneous abscesses called furuncles (boils) often form around foreign bodies, such as splinters. These generally respond to local therapy, that is, removal of the foreign body, soaking, and drainage as indicated. Carbuncles are larger, deeper, multiloculated skin infections that can lead to bacteremia and require antibiotic therapy and debridement. Impetigo is usually a localized, superficial, spreading crusty skin lesion generally seen in children. It can be caused by *S. aureus*, although more commonly by *Streptococcus pyogenes* (see p. 80), or both organisms together.

 Human staphylococcal infections usually remain localized at the portal of entry by normal host defenses.

2. **Deep, localized infections:** These may be metastatic from superficial infections or skin carriage, or may result from trauma. *S. aureus* is the most common cause of acute and chronic infection of bone marrow. *S. aureus* is also the most common cause of acute infection of joint space in children (septic joint). [Note: Septic joints are medical emergencies because pus can rapidly cause irreparable cartilage damage. They must be treated promptly with drainage and an antibiotic.]

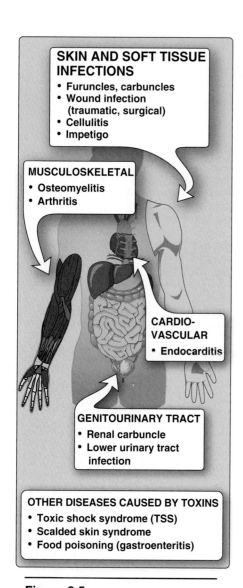

**SKIN AND SOFT TISSUE INFECTIONS**
- Furuncles, carbuncles
- Wound infection (traumatic, surgical)
- Cellulitis
- Impetigo

**MUSCULOSKELETAL**
- Osteomyelitis
- Arthritis

**CARDIO-VASCULAR**
- Endocarditis

**GENITOURINARY TRACT**
- Renal carbuncle
- Lower urinary tract infection

**OTHER DISEASES CAUSED BY TOXINS**
- Toxic shock syndrome (TSS)
- Scalded skin syndrome
- Food poisoning (gastroenteritis)

**Figure 8.5**
Diseases caused by *Staphylococcus aureus*.

3. **Acute endocarditis**, generally associated with intravenous drug abuse, is caused by injection of contaminated preparations or by needles contaminated with *S. aureus*. *S. aureus* also colonizes the skin around the injection site, and if the skin is not sterilized before injection, the bacteria can be introduced into soft tissues and the bloodstream, even when a sterilized needle is used.

> || An abscess in any organ or tissue should make you suspect S. aureus.

4. **Septicemia** is a generalized infection with sepsis or bacteremia that may be associated with a known focus (for example, a septic joint) or not (an occult focus).

5. **Pneumonia:** *S. aureus* is a cause of severe, necrotizing pneumonia.

6. **Nosocomial infections:** *S. aureus* is one of the most common causes of hospital-acquired infections, often of wounds (surgical, decubital) or bacteremia associated with catheters (see Figure 8.10). Progression to septicemia is often a terminal event.

7. **Toxinoses** are diseases caused by the action of a toxin, frequently when the organism that secreted the toxin is undetectable. Toxinoses caused by *S. aureus* include:

   a. **Toxic shock syndrome**, which results in high fever, rash (resembling a sunburn, with diffuse erythema followed by desquamation), vomiting, diarrhea, hypotension, and multiorgan involvement (especially GI, renal, and/or hepatic damage). An outbreak of toxic shock syndrome occurred in the late 1970s among menstruating women. It was shown to be related to the use of hyperabsorbant tampons by women who happened to be vaginally colonized by toxic shock syndrome toxin–(TSST)–positive strains of *S. aureus*. [Note: These tampons stimulated TSST expression, resulting in entry of the toxin into the circulation in the absence of true infection.] The incidence has decreased markedly since such tampons were removed from the market. Of the few cases of toxic shock syndrome that occur currently, approximately half are associated with ordinary *S. aureus* infections; of the latter, many result from a circulating enterotoxin rather than TSST. Figure 8.6 shows the desquamation (peeling or scaling of the skin) seen in toxic shock syndrome.

   b. **Staphylococcal gastroenteritis** is caused by ingestion of food contaminated with enterotoxin-producing *S. aureus*. Often contaminated by a food-handler, these foods tend to be protein-rich (for example, egg salad, cream pastry) and improperly refrigerated. Symptoms, such as nausea, vomiting, and diarrhea, are acute following a short incubation period (less than six hours), and are triggered by local actions of the toxin on the GI tract rather than from infection. See p. 372 for a summary of food poisoning.

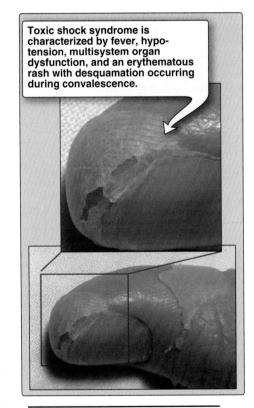

Toxic shock syndrome is characterized by fever, hypotension, multisystem organ dysfunction, and an erythematous rash with desquamation occurring during convalescence.

**Figure 8.6**
Desquamation of skin in toxic shock syndrome.

> The short incubation period of staphylococcal food poisoning occurs because the toxin in the food has already been formed by the staphylococci before the food is ingested.

    **c. Scalded skin syndrome** involves the appearance of superficial bullae resulting from the action of an exfoliative toxin that attacks the intercellular adhesive of the stratum granulosum, causing marked epithelial desquamation (see Figure 8.12). The bullae may be infected or may result from toxin produced by organisms infecting a different site.

### D. Laboratory identification

Identification of an isolate as a staphylococcus relies largely on microscopic and colony morphology, and catalase positivity (Figure 8.7). Bacteria stain strongly gram-positive, and are frequently seen in grapelike clusters (see Figure 8.2). *S. aureus* is distinguished from the coagulase-negative staphylococci primarily by coagulase positivity. In addition, *S. aureus* colonies tend to be yellow (hence "aureus," meaning golden) and hemolytic (see Figure 8.12), rather than gray and nonhemolytic like the coagulase-negative staphylococci. *S. aureus* is also distinguished from most coagulase-negative staphylococci by being mannitol-positive.

### E. Immunity

*S. aureus* infections do not elicit strong or long-lasting immunity, as demonstrated by the continuing susceptibility of individuals to *S. aureus* infections throughout life.

### F. Treatment

Serious *S. aureus* infections require aggressive treatment, including incision and drainage of localized lesions, as well as systemic antibiotics. Choice of antibiotics is complicated by the frequent presence of acquired antibiotic resistance determinants (see p. 64). Virtually all community- and hospital-acquired *S. aureus* infections are now resistant to penicillin G due to penicillinase-encoding plasmids or transposons (Figure 8.8). This has required the replacement of the initial agent of choice, penicillin G, by β-lactamase-resistant penicillins, such as methicillin or oxacillin. However, increased use of methicillin and related antibiotics has resulted in methicillin-resistant *S. aureus.*

1. **Hospital-acquired methicillin-resistant *S. aureus* (MRSA):** In recent decades, a high percentage (often in the range of fifty percent) of hospital *S. aureus* isolates has been found to be also resistant to methicillin (see Figure 8.8) or oxacillin. Antibiotic resistance is caused by chromosomal acquisition of the gene for a modified penicillin-binding protein (PBP, see p. 57), PBP-2a. This protein codes for a new peptidoglycan transpeptidase with a low

**Figure 8.7**
Catalase-positive culture of *Staphylococcus aureus*.

The test for catalase is performed by adding 3% hydrogen peroxide to a colony on an agar plate. Catalase-positive cultures produce O₂ and bubble immediately.

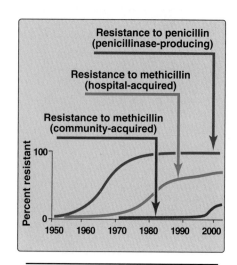

**Figure 8.8**
Trends in the prevalence of drug-resistant strains of *Staphylococcus aureus.*

affinity for all currently available β-lactam antibiotics, and thus renders infections with methicillin-resistant *S. aureus* unresponsive to β-lactam therapy. Compared with methicilllin-sensitive *S. aureus*, MRSA infections are associated with worse outcomes, including longer hospital and ICU stays, longer durations of mechanical ventilation, and higher mortality rates. MRSA strains are also frequently resistant to many other antibiotics, some being sensitive only to glycopeptides such as vancomycin.

2. **Community-acquired MRSA (CA-MRSA)** infections were documented in the mid-1990s, occurring in individuals who have no previous risk factors for MRSA infections, such as exposure to hospitals (see Figure 8.8). The most common clinical manifestations of CA-MRSA are skin and soft tissue infections such as abscesses or cellulitis (Figure 8.9). Less commonly, CA-MRSA can also cause severe diseases such as necrotizing pneumonia, osteomyelitis, and septicemia. Community-acquired MRSA has a number of characteristics that help distinguish it from hospital-associated MRSA. For example, CA-MRSA has a characteristic pattern of DNA fragments obtained upon enzymic cleavage and electrophoresis, and it produces specific toxins. CA-MRSA also exhibits a unique antibiotic resistance pattern, that is, CA-MRSA is sensitive to many antibiotics that do not show much activity against hospital-associated MRSA. These antibiotics include ciprofloxacin and clindamycin, with some CA-MRSA even sensitive to erythromycin, gentamicin, rifampin, tetracycline, and/or trimethoprim-sulfamethoxazole).

3. **Vancomycin resistance:** Vancomycin has been the agent of choice for empiric treatment of life-threatening *S. aureus* infections. Unfortunately, in 1997, several MRSAs were isolated that had also acquired low-level vancomycin resistance.

The incidence of vancomycin resistance has increased steadily, prompting the use of alternative drugs such as quinupristin-dalfopristin, linezolid, and daptomycin. These agents have good *in vitro* activity against MRSA and most other clinically important gram-positive bacterial pathogens.

> Emerging antibiotic-resistant strains of *S. aureus* that infect otherwise healthy individuals (community-acquired infections) are often more virulent than the more common strains that originate in hospitals.

## G. Prevention

There is no effective vaccine against *S. aureus*. Infection control procedures, such as barrier precautions and disinfection of hands and fomites, are important in the control of nosocomial *S. aureus* epidemics.

**Figure 8.9**
Comparison of the incidence of hospital-aquired and community-acquired methicillin-resistant *Staphylococcus aureus* infections.

## IV. COAGULASE-NEGATIVE STAPHYLOCOCCI

Of twelve coagulase-negative staphylococcal species that have been recovered as normal commensals of human skin and anterior nares, the most abundant and important is *S. epidermidis*. For this reason some clinical laboratories designate all coagulase-negative staphylococci as *S. epidermidis*, a practice that is not encouraged. The second most important coagulase-negative staphylococcus is *S. saprophyticus*, which has a special medical niche. Coagulase-negative staphylococcal species are important agents of hospital-acquired infections associated with the use of implanted prosthetic devices and catheters.

### A. Staphylococcus epidermidis

*S. epidermidis* is present in large numbers as part of the normal flora of the skin (see p. 7). As such, it is frequently recovered from blood cultures, generally as a contaminant from skin. Despite its low virulence, it is a common cause of infection of implants such as heart valves and catheters (Figure 8.10). Acquired drug resistance by *S. epidermidis* is even more frequent than by *S. aureus*. Vancomycin sensitivity remains the rule, but vancomycin-resistant isolates have been reported.

**Figure 8.10**
*Staphylococcus epidermidis* growing on extracellar slime on surface of colonized catheter.

> *S. epidermidis* produces an extracellular polysaccharide material (sometimes called "slime") that facilitates adherence to bioprosthetic material surfaces, such as intravenous catheters, and acts as a barrier to antimicrobial agents.

### B. Staphylococcus saprophyticus

This organism is a frequent cause of cystitis in women, probably related to its occurrence as part of normal vaginal flora (see p. 10). It tends to be sensitive to most antibiotics, even penicillin G. *S. saprophyticus* can be distinguished from *S. epidermidis* and most other coagulase-negative staphylococci by its natural resistance to novobiocin (Figure 8.11). [Note: Urinary coagulase-negative staphylococcus is often presumed to be *S. saprophyticus*; novobiocin resistance can be used for confirmation.]. Figure 8.12 presents a summary of diseases caused by staphylococcus.

| Species | Frequency of disease | Coagulase | Color of colonies | Mannitol fermentation | Novobiocin resistance |
|---|---|---|---|---|---|
| *S. aureus* | Common | + | Golden yellow | + | − |
| *S. epidermidis* | Common | − | White | − | − |
| *S. saprophyticus* | Occasional | − | Variable | − | + |

**Figure 8.11**
Summary of various species of staphylococci.

# *Staphylococcus* species

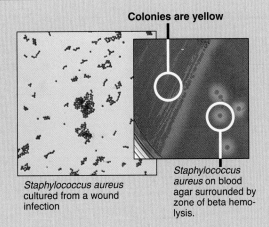

Colonies are yellow

*Staphylococcus aureus* cultured from a wound infection

*Staphylococcus aureus* on blood agar surrounded by zone of beta hemolysis.

- **Gram-positive**, staining darkly
- Round cocci tending to occur in bunches like grapes
- True facultative anaerobic organisms
- Cultured on enriched media containing broth and/or blood

## *Staphylococcus aureus*

- Skin infections
- Osteomyelitis
- Endocarditis
- Food poisoning
- Septicemia
- Necrotizing pneumonia
- Toxic shock syndrome

PENICILLINS[1]
- **1** Oxacillin
- **1** Nafcillin

CEPHALOSPORINS
TETRACYCLINES
AMINOGLYCOSIDES
MACROLIDES
FLUOROQUINOLONES

OTHER
- **2** Vancomycin[2]

OTHER
- **3** Quinupristin-dalfopristin[3]
- **3** Linezolid[3]
- **3** Daptomycin[3]

[1]Most isolates resistant to penicillin G
[2]Used in methicillin-resistant isolates
[3]Used in vancomycin-resistant isolates

## *Staphylococcus epidermidis*

- Infections of catheters and heart valves

PENICILLINS[1]
- **1** Oxacillin
- **1** Nafcillin

CEPHALOSPORINS
TETRACYCLINES
AMINOGLYCOSIDES
MACROLIDES
FLUOROQUINOLONES

OTHER
- **2** Vancomycin[2]

[1]Most isolates resistant to penicillin G
[2]Used in methicillin-resistant isolates

## *Staphylococcus saprophyticus*

- Cystitis in women

PENICILLINS
- **1** Penicillin G

CEPHALOSPORINS
TETRACYCLINES
AMINOGLYCOSIDES
MACROLIDES
FLUOROQUINOLONES
OTHER

Folliculitis caused by *Staphylococcus aureus*

Carbuncle caused by *Staphylococcus aureus*

Furuncle caused by *Staphylococcus aureus*

Scanning electron micrograph of cardiac pacemaker lead colonized by *S. aureus*

Staphylococcal scalded skin syndrome

Superficial impetigo

**Figure 8.12**
Summary of stapholococcal disease.

## Study Questions

Choose the ONE best answer

8.1 A 32-year-old woman became ill four days after the onset of her menstrual period. She presented in the emergency room with fever (104°F; normal = 98.6°F), elevated white blood cell count (16,000/mm$^3$; normal = 4,000 to 10,000/mm$^3$), and a rash on her trunk and extremities. She complained of fatigue, vomiting, and diarrhea. She had recently eaten at a fast-food restaurant, but otherwise had prepared all her meals at home. The patient described most likely has:

A. staphylococcal food poisoning.

B. scalded skin syndrome.

C. infection with a *Staphylococcus saprophyticus*.

D. chickenpox.

E. toxic shock syndrome.

Correct answer = E. The patient shows signs of toxic shock syndrome. Toxic shock syndrome as defined in the outbreak of the late '70s and early '80s included an erythematous/peeling rash (not purpuric) and was caused by overproduction of TSST-1 by colonizing *S. aureus* triggered by something in hyperabsorbent tampons. Many signs and symptoms are the results of the super-antigen activity of TSST, which activates a whole subclass of T cells, causing overproduction of cytokines. *S. saprophyticus* is a frequent cause of cystitis in women, but is not associated with toxic shock syndrome.

8.2 A 57-year-old man arrives at the emergency room complaining of weakness, fatigue, and intermittent fever that has recurred for several weeks. The patient had a cardiac valvular prosthesis implanted five years earlier. Physical examination reveals petechiae (pinpoint, nonraised, purplish-red spots caused by intradermal hemorrhage) on the chest and stomach. Blood cultures grew catalase-positive, coagulase-negative, cocci. The gram-positive organisms failed to ferment mannitol, and their growth was inhibited by novobiocin. What is the most likely infectious agent?

A. *Staphylococcus aureus*

B. *Staphylococcus epidermidis*

C. *Staphylococcus saprophyticus*

D. *Streptococcus pneumoniae*

E. *Streptococcus agalactiae*

Correct answer = B. The patient is probably suffering from bacterial endocarditis caused by *S. epidermidis* infection of the prosthetic heart valve. *S. epidermidis* is a coagulase- negative organism that is unable to ferment mannitol, and is sensitive to novobiocin but usually resistant to penicillin. Patients with congenital heart malformations, acquired valvular defects (for example, rheumatic heart disease), prosthetic valves, and previous bacterial endocarditis show an increased incidence of bacterial endocarditis. Intravenous drug users also have a high risk for infection. *S. pneumoniae* and *S. agalactiae* can be ruled out, because streptococci are catalase-negative, which is a feature that distinguishes them from catalase-positive staphyococci.

*"MOSES, ALL TESTS INDICATE YOU HAVE A STAFF INFECTION."*

# Streptococci

# 9

## I. OVERVIEW

Streptococci and staphylococci (see Chapter 8) constitute the main groups of medically important gram-positive cocci. Streptococci are gram-positive, nonmotile, and catalase-negative. Clinically important genera include *Streptococcus* and *Enterococcus* (Figure 9.1). They are ovoid to spherical in shape, and occur as pairs or chains (see Figure 9.15). Most are facultative anaerobes (capable of growing in the absence or presence of oxygen), but grow fermentatively even in the presence of oxygen. Because of their complex nutritional requirements, blood-enriched medium is generally used for their isolation. Diseases caused by this group of organisms include acute infections of the throat and skin caused by Group A streptococci (*Streptococcus pyogenes*); female genital tract colonization, resulting in neonatal sepsis caused by Group B streptococci (*Streptococcus agalactiae*); pneumonia, otitis media, and meningitis caused by *Streptococcus pneumoniae*; and endocarditis caused by the viridans group of streptococci.

## II. CLASSIFICATION OF STREPTOCOCCI

Streptococci can be classified by several schemes, for example, by the hemolytic properties of the organisms, and according to the presence of specific surface antigens determined by immunologic assays.

### A. Hemolytic properties on blood agar

α-Hemolytic streptococci cause a chemical change in the hemoglobin of red cells in blood agar, resulting in the appearance of a green pigment that forms a ring around the colony (see Figure 9.15). β-Hemolytic streptococci cause gross lysis of red blood cells, resulting in a clear ring around the colony (see Figure 9.15). γ-Hemolytic is a term applied to streptococci that cause no color change or lysis of red blood cells.

> The traditional division of streptococci based on the ability of the bacterial colony to hemolyze erythrocytes in the blood agar medium is still considered the first step in the classification of streptococci.

**Figure 9.1**
Classification of streptococci.
Ⓢ See p. 331 for summaries of these organisms.

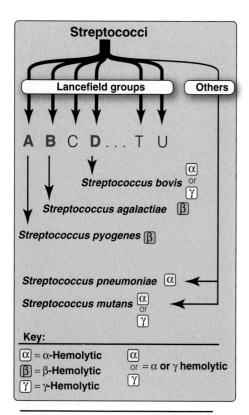

**Figure 9.2**
Classification schemes for streptococci.

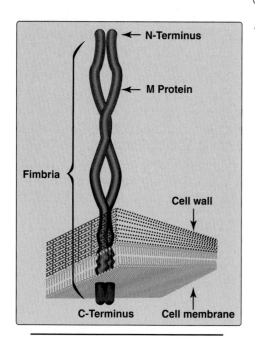

**Figure 9.3**
Schematic representation of the streptococcal M protein.

## B. Serologic (Lancefield) groupings

Many species of streptococci have a polysaccharide in their cell walls known as C-carbohydrate, which is antigenic and easily extractable with dilute acid. The Lancefield scheme classifies primarily β-hemolytic streptococci into Groups A through U on the basis of their C-carbohydrate. The clinically most important groups of β-hemolytic streptococci are types A and B (Figure 9.2). Commercial kits in which group-specific antisera are coupled to latex beads are now widely used for identification of β-hemolytic streptococci.

## III. GROUP A β-HEMOLYTIC STREPTOCOCCI

*S. pyogenes*, the most clinically important member of this group of gram-positive cocci, is one of the most frequently encountered bacterial pathogens of humans worldwide. It can invade apparently intact skin or mucous membranes, causing some of the most rapidly progressive infections known. A low inoculum suffices for infection. Some strains of *S. pyogenes* cause postinfectious sequelae, including rheumatic fever and acute glomerulonephritis. Nasopharyngeal carriage is common especially in colder months and particularly among children.

> Unlike staphylococcal species, *S. pyogenes* does not survive well in the environment. Instead, its habitat is infected patients, and also normal human carriers in whom the organism resides on skin and mucous membranes.

## A. Structure and physiology

*S. pyogenes* occur as long chains when recovered from liquid culture (see Figure 9.15), but may appear as individual cocci, pairs, or clusters of cells in Gram stains of samples from infected tissue. Structural features involved in the pathology or identification of Group A streptococci include:

1. **Capsule:** Hyaluronic acid,[1] identical to that found in human connective tissue, forms the outermost layer of the cell. This capsule is not recognized as foreign by the body and, therefore, is nonimmunogenic.

2. **Cell wall:** The cell wall contains a number of clinically important components. Beginning with the outer layer of the cell wall, these components include the following (Figure 9.3):

   a. **Fimbriae:** *S. pyogenes* cells are surrounded by a fringe of fimbriae (pilus-like structures). The fimbriae contain the major *S. pyogenes* virulence factor, the M protein. [Note: The bacterium is not infectious in the absence of M protein.] M proteins extend from an anchor in the cell membrane, through the cell wall and then the capsule, with the N-terminal end of the protein exposed on the surface of the bacterium. M proteins are highly variable,

[1]See p. 157 in *Lippincott's Illustrated Reviews: Biochemistry* (3rd ed.) for a discussion of hyaluronic acid.

especially the N-terminal regions, resulting in over eighty different antigenic types. Thus, individuals may have many *S. pyogenes* infections throughout their lives, as they encounter new M protein types for which they have no antibodies.

    **b. Group A-specific C-carbohydrate** is composed of rhamnose and N-acetylglucosamine. [Note: All group A streptococci, by definition, contain this antigen.]

    **c. Protein F (fibronectin-binding protein)** mediates attachment to fibronectin in the pharyngeal epithelium.

  **3. Extracellular products:** Like *Staphylococcus aureus* (see p. 70), *S. pyogenes* secretes a wide range of exotoxins that often vary from one strain to another, and that play roles in the pathogenesis of disease caused by these organisms (Figure 9.4).

## B. Epidemiology

The only known reservoir for *S. pyogenes* in nature is the skin and mucous membranes of the human host. Respiratory droplets or skin contact spread Group A streptococcal infection from person to person, especially in crowded environments such as classrooms or children's play areas.

## C. Pathology

*S. pyogenes* cells, perhaps in an inhaled droplet, attach to the pharyngeal mucosa via actions of protein F, lipoteichoic acid, and M protein. The bacteria may simply colonize (that is, replicate only sufficiently to maintain themselves without causing injury); the patient is then considered colonized. Alternatively, bacteria may grow and secrete toxins, causing damage to surrounding cells, invading the mucosa, and eliciting an inflammatory response with attendant influx of white cells, fluid leakage, and pus formation. The patient then has streptococcal pharyngitis. Occasionally, there is sufficient spread that the bloodstream is significantly invaded, possibly resulting in septicemia and/or seeding of distant sites, where cellulitis (acute inflammation of subcutaneous tissue), fasciitis (inflammation of the tissue under the skin that covers a surface of underlying tissue), or myonecrosis (death of muscle cells) may develop rapidly or insidiously.

## D. Clinical significance

*S. pyogenes* is a major cause of cellulitis. More specific syndromes include:

  **1. Acute pharyngitis or pharyngotonsilitis:** Pharyngitis is the most common type of *S. pyogenes* infection. *S. pyogenes* pharyngitis ("strep throat") is associated with severe, purulent inflammation of the posterior oropharynx and tonsillar areas (see Figure 9.15). [Note: If a sunburnlike rash develops on the neck, trunk, and extremities in response to the release of pyrogenic exotoxin to which the patient does not have antibodies, the syndrome is designated scarlet fever.]

**Streptococcus pyogenes**

Cytokines → **Pyrogenic exotoxins**

Cause various effects, including the rash seen in scarlet fever and streptococcal toxic shock disease.

**Streptolysin O Streptolysin S**

Damage mammalian cells, resulting in cell lysis and release of lysosomal enzymes.

Fibrin clot — Plasmin → **Streptokinase**

Catalyzes conversion of plasminogen to plasmin, causing lysis of clots, facilitating the rapid spread of organisms.

C5a → ~~C5a~~ **C5a peptidase**

Inactivates complement component C5a.

DNA → **Streptodornases**

DNAses that degrade the viscous DNA in necrotizing tissue or exudates, aiding the spread of infection.

Hyaluronic acid → **Hyaluronidase**

Disrupts the organization of ground substance, facilitating the spread of infection.

**Figure 9.4**
Cytolytic toxins and other exoenzymes produced by *Streptococcus pyogenes*.

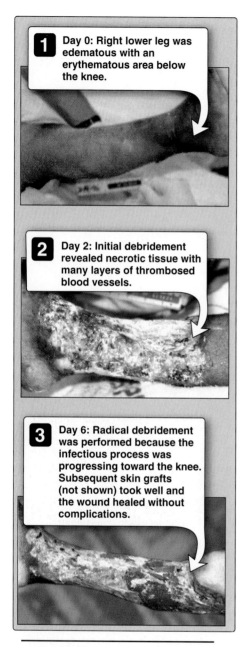

**1** Day 0: Right lower leg was edematous with an erythematous area below the knee.

**2** Day 2: Initial debridement revealed necrotic tissue with many layers of thrombosed blood vessels.

**3** Day 6: Radical debridement was performed because the infectious process was progressing toward the knee. Subsequent skin grafts (not shown) took well and the wound healed without complications.

**Figure 9.5**
Necrotizing fasciitis in a 59-year-old woman.

Many strep throats are mild, and many sore throats caused by viruses are severe. Hence, laboratory confirmation is important for accurate diagnosis and treatment of streptococcal pharyngitis, particularly for the prevention of subsequent acute rheumatic fever and rheumatic heart disease.

2. **Impetigo:** Although *S. aureus* is recovered from most contemporary cases of impetigo (see p. 72), *S. pyogenes* is the classic cause of this syndrome. The disease begins on any exposed surface (most commonly, the legs). Typically affecting children, it can cause severe and extensive lesions on the face and limbs (see Figure 9.15). Impetigo is treated with a topical agent such as mupirocin, or systemically with penicillin or a first-generation cephalosporin such as cephalexin, which are effective against both *S. aureus* and *S. pyogenes*.

3. **Erysipelas:** Affecting all age groups, patients with erysipelas experience a fiery red, advancing erythema, especially on the face or lower limbs (see Figure 9.15).

4. **Puerperal sepsis:** This infection is initiated during, or following soon after, the delivery of a newborn. It is caused by exogenous transmission (for example, by nasal droplets from an infected carrier, or from contaminated instruments), or endogenously, from the mother's vaginal flora. This is a disease of the uterine endometrium in which patients experience a purulent vaginal discharge, and are systemically ill.

5. **Invasive group A streptococcal (GAS) disease:** Common during the first half of the century, invasive GAS disease became rare until its resurgence during the past decade. Patients may have a deep local invasion without necrosis (cellulitis) or with it (necrotizing fasciitis/myositis, Figure 9.5). [Note: The latter disease led to the term "flesh-eating bacteria."] Invasive GAS disease often spreads rapidly, even in otherwise healthy individuals, leading to bacteremia and sepsis. Symptoms may include a toxic shock-like syndrome, fever, hypotension, multiorgan involvement, a sunburn-like rash, or a combination of these symptoms.

6. **Acute rheumatic fever:** This autoimmune disease occurs two to three weeks after the initiation of pharyngitis. It is caused by cross-reactions between antigens of the heart and joint tissues, and the streptococcal antigen (especially the M protein epitopes). It is characterized by fever, rash, carditis, and arthritis. Rheumatic fever is preventable if the patient is treated within the first ten days following initiation of acute pharyngitis.

7. **Acute glomerulonephritis:** This rare, postinfectious sequela occurs as soon as one week after impetigo or pharyngitis ensues, due to a few nephritogenic strains of group A streptococci.

Antigen-antibody complexes on the basement membrane of the glomerulus initiate the disease. There is no evidence that penicillin treatment of the streptococcal skin disease or pharyngitis (to eradicate the infection) can prevent acute glomerulonephritis.

8. **Streptococcal toxic shock syndrome:** This syndrome is defined as isolation of group A β-hemolytic streptococci from blood or another normally sterile body site in the presence of shock and multiorgan failure. The syndrome is mediated by production of streptococcal pyrogenic exotoxins that function as superantigens causing massive, nonspecific T cell activation and cytokine release. Patients may initially present with flulike symptoms, followed shortly by necrotizing soft tissue infection, shock, adult respiratory distress syndrome, and renal failure. Treatment must be prompt and includes antistreptococcal antibiotics, usually consisting of high-dose penicillin G plus clindamycin).

### E. Laboratory identification

Rapid latex antigen kits for direct detection of group A streptococci in patient samples are widely used. In a positive test, the latex particles clump together; in a negative test, they stay separate, giving the suspension a milky appearance (Figure 9.6). These tests have high specificity but variable sensitivity compared with culture techniques. Specimens from patients with clinical signs of pharyngitis and a negative antigen detection test should undergo routine culturing for streptococcal identification. Depending on the form of the disease, specimens for laboratory analysis can be obtained from throat swabs, pus and lesion samples, sputum, blood, or spinal fluid. *S. pyogenes* forms characteristic small, opalescent colonies surrounded by a large zone of β hemolysis on sheep blood agar (see Figure 9.15). [Note: Hemolysis of the blood cells is caused by steptolysin S, which damages mammalian cells resulting in cell lysis.] This organism is highly sensitive to bacitracin, and diagnostic disks with a very low concentration of the antibiotic inhibit growth in culture. Group A C-carbohydrate can be identified by the precipitin reaction. Serologic tests detect a patient's antibody titer to streptolysin-O (ASO test) after group A streptococcal infection. Anti-DNase B titers (ADB test) are particularly elevated following streptococcal infections of the skin.

### F. Treatment

Antibiotics are used for all Group A streptococcal infections. *S. pyogenes* has not acquired resistance to penicillin G, which remains the antibiotic of choice for acute streptococcal disease. In a penicillin-allergic patient, a macrolide such as clarithromycin or azithromycin is the preferred drug (see Figure 9.15). Penicillin G plus clindamycin are used in treating necrotizing fasciitis and in streptococcal toxic shock syndrome.

### G. Prevention

Rheumatic fever is prevented by rapid eradication of the infecting organism. Prolonged prophylactic antibiotic therapy is indicated after

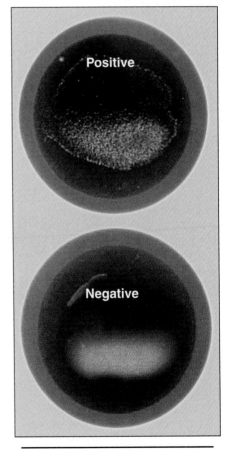

**Figure 9.6**
Latex agglutination for identification of group A β-hemolytic streptococci.

an episode of rheumatic fever, because having had one episode of this autoimmune disease in the past is a major risk factor for subsequent episodes if the patient is again infected with *S. pyogenes*.

## IV. GROUP B β-HEMOLYTIC STREPTOCOCCI

Group B streptococci, represented by the pathogen *S. agalactiae*, are gram-positive, catalase-negative organisms. *S. agalactiae* is found in the vaginocervical tract of female carriers, and the urethral mucous membranes of male carriers, as well as in the GI tract. Transmission occurs from an infected mother to her infant at birth, and venereally (propagated by sexual contact) among adults. Group B streptococci are a leading cause of meningitis and septicemia in neonates, with a high mortality rate. They are also an occasional cause of infections in postpartum women (endometritis) and individuals with impaired immune systems, in whom the organism may cause septicemia or pneumonia. Samples of blood, cervical swabs, sputum, or spinal fluid can be obtained for culture on blood agar. ELISA tests can also demonstrate the presence of bacterial antigen in these samples. Group B streptococci are β-hemolytic, with larger colonies and less hemolysis than group A. Most isolates remain sensitive to penicillin G and ampicillin, which are still the antibiotics of choice (see Figure 9.15). In life-threatening infections, an aminoglycoside can be added to the regimen. [Note: Pregnant carriers should be treated with ampicillin during labor if risk factors such as premature rupture of membranes or prolonged labor are present.]

> Intrapartum prophylaxis of group B streptococcal carriers and selective administration of antibiotics to newborns reduce neonatal group B streptococcal sepsis by as much as ninety percent.

## V. STREPTOCOCCUS PNEUMONIAE (PNEUMOCOCCUS)

*S. pneumoniae* are gram-positive, nonmotile, encapsulated cocci (Figure 9.7). They are lancet-shaped, and their tendency to occur in pairs accounts for their earlier designation as *Diplococcus pneumoniae*.

> *S. pneumoniae* is the most common cause of pneumonia and otitis media and an important cause of meningitis and bacteremia/sepsis.

**Figure 9.7**
*Streptoccus pneumoniae* are gram-positive, nonmotile, encapsulated lancet-shaped cocci.

The risk of disease is highest among young children, older adults, smokers, and persons with certain chronic illnesses. Like other streptococci, *S. pneumoniae* is fastidious and routinely cultured on blood agar. It releases an α-hemolysin that damages red cell membranes, causing colonies to be α-hemolytic.

## A. Epidemiology

*S. pneumoniae* is an obligate parasite of humans, and can be found in the nasopharynx of many healthy individuals. This organism is extremely sensitive to environmental agents. Pneumococcal infections can be either endogenous or exogenous. For example, endogenous infection involves the spread of *S. pneumoniae* residing in the nasopharynx of a carrier who develops impaired resistance to the organism. Susceptibility to the infection may result from, for example, general debilitation such as that caused by malnutrition or alcoholism, to respiratory damage following a prior viral infection, or to a depressed immune system. Patients with sickle cell disease or those who have had their spleens removed are particularly at risk for *S. pneumoniae* infection. Infection can also be exogenous, for example, by droplets from the nose of a carrier. Individuals such as those described above as susceptible to endogenous infection are also most likely to be infected by the exogenous route.

## B. Pathogenesis

The bacterial capsule of *S. pneumoniae* is the most important virulence factor, and is the basis for the classification of serotypes of this organism. Cell-associated enzymes, pneumolysin, and autolysin contribute to its pathogenicity (Figure 9.8).

1. **Capsule:** The *S. pneumoniae* polysaccharide capsule is both antiphagocytic and antigenic. Antiphagocytic properties of the capsule protect the bacteria from polymorphonuclear leukocyte attack, facilitating growth of the bacteria prior to the appearance of anticapsular antibodies. There are approximately 85 distinct capsular serotypes, some of which endow strains with greater virulence than others, as reflected by the fact that about twenty serotypes account for the vast majority of pneumococcal infections.

2. **Autolysin:** This peptidoglycan hydrolase is present in the bacterial cell wall, and is normally inactive. However, it is readily triggered (for example, by surface-active agents, β-lactam antibiotics, or aging), resulting in cell lysis. Autolysin is thus responsible for the release of intracellular virulence factors (notably, pneumolysin).

3. **Pneumolysin:** Although retained within the cytosol of intact pneumococci, pneumolysin is thought to be an important virulence factor by virtue of its ability to attack mammalian cell membranes, causing lysis once it is released by autolysin from the interior of the bacterium.

## C. Clinical significance

1. **Acute bacterial pneumonia:** A leading cause of death, especially in the aged and those whose resistance is impaired, this disease is caused most frequently by *S. pneumoniae* (Figure 9.9). Pneumonia is frequently preceded by an upper or middle respiratory viral infection, which predisposes to *S. pneumoniae* infection of pulmonary parenchyma. Mechanisms by which virus infection

**Figure 9.8**
Cytolytic toxins produced by *Streptococcus pneumoniae*.

**Figure 9.9**
Age-specific rates of community-acquired pneumonia caused by specific pathogens.

**Inhibition by optochin**
Growth of colonies of *Streptococcus pneumoniae* is inhibited by optochin contained in the disk applied to the blood agar plate.

**A**

Optochin disk

**Quellung reaction**
Capsules of *Streptococcus pneumoniae* swell in the presence of specific pneumococcal antiserum.

**B**

Negative          Positive

**C**

Negative          Positive

**Lysis by bile acids**
Bile acids, such as sodium deoxycholate, dissolve *Streptococcus pneumoniae* and clear the turbidity of a heavy inoculum of organisms.

**Figure 9.10**
Laboratory tests useful in the identification of *Streptococcus pneumoniae*. A. Optochin disk test. B. Quellung reaction. C. Lysis by bile acids.

predisposes an individual to streptococcal pneumonia include increased volume and viscosity of secretions that are more difficult to clear, and secondary inhibition of the action of bronchial cilia by viral infection.

2. **Otitis media:** The most common bacterial infection of children, this disease (which is characterized by earache) is most frequently caused by pneumococcus, followed by *Haemophilus influenza* and *Moraxella catarrhalis* (see p. 391). The traditional empiric treatment of pneumococcal otitis media with a β-lactam antibiotic (with or without a penicillinase-inhibitor) has been threatened by the spread of penicillin-resistant pneumococci.

3. **Bacteremia/sepsis** in the absence of a focus of infection is commonly caused by pneumococcus, especially in splenectomized individuals.

4. **Meningitis:** *H. influenzae* was formerly the leading cause of bacterial meningitis in the United States. After a vaccine was developed against this organism, *S. pneumoniae* became the most common cause of bacterial meningitis (see p. 377). This disease has a high mortality rate, even when treated appropriately.

## D.  Laboratory identification

Specimens for laboratory evaluation can be obtained from a nasopharyngeal swab, blood, pus, sputum, or spinal fluid. α-Hemolytic colonies appear when *S. pneumoniae* is grown on blood agar overnight under aerobic conditions at 37°C. Lancet-shaped, gram-positive diplococci are observed on a Gram stain of the sample. Growth of these bacteria is inhibited by low concentrations of the surfactant, optochin, and the cells are lysed by bile acids (Figure 9.10). Capsular swelling is observed when the pneumococci are treated with type-specific antisera (the Quellung reaction).

## E.  Treatment

*S. pneumoniae* isolates were highly sensitive to penicillin G, the initial agent of choice, until the late 1980s. Since then, the incidence of penicillin resistance has been increasing worldwide. The mechanism of this resistance is an alteration of one or more of the bacterium's penicillin-binding proteins (PBPs, see p. 57) rather than production of β-lactamase. Modified PBPs have a much reduced affinity for penicillin G, and for some, but not all, of the other β-lactams. Most resistant strains remain sensitive to third generation cephalosporins (such as cefotaxime or ceftriaxone), and all are still sensitive to vancomycin; these antibiotics are therefore the agents of choice for invasive infections by penicillin-resistant strains of *S. pneumoniae* (see Figure 9.15).

## F.  Prevention

There are two types of pneumococcal vaccine: pneumococcal polysaccharide vaccine (PPV) and pneumococcal conjugate vaccine (PCV7).

1. **PPV:** Introduced in the United States in 1983, PPV immunizes against 23 serotypes of *S. pneumoniae* and is indicated for the protection of high-risk individuals older than two years. This vaccine protects against the pneumococcal strains responsible for 85 to 90 percent of infections, including prominent penicillin-resistant strains.

2. **PCV7:** The heptavalent pneumococcal conjugate vaccine (PCV7), licensed in the United States in 2000, is effective in infants and toddlers (six weeks to five years of age). It is made up of seven pneumococcal antigens conjugated to CRM197–a mutant nontoxic diphtheria toxin. Significant declines in the incidence of invasive pneumococcal disease occurred through 2003 in the age group targeted for vaccination and among older children and adults (Figure 9.11). In addition, the vaccine prevented greater numbers of invasive pneumococcal cases through indirect effects on pneumococcal transmission (that is, herd immunity) than through its direct effect of protecting vaccinated children.

> Young children show a weak immunologic response to an oligosaccharide-only vaccine. However, if the oligosaccharide is conjugated to a protein, a protective immune response occurs.

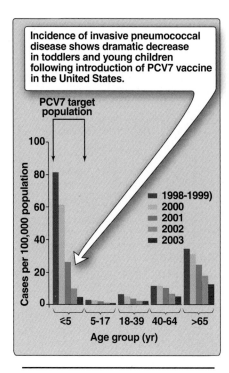

**Figure 9.11**
Incidence of vaccine-type invasive pneumococcal disease before and after the introduction of pneumococcal conjugate vaccine (PCV7), by age and year.

# VI. ENTEROCOCCI

Enterococci contain a C-carbohydrate that reacts with group D antisera. Therefore, in the past, they were considered group D streptococci. Today, DNA analysis and other properties have placed them in their own genus, *Enterococcus*. The clinically most important species are *E. faecalis* and *E. faecium*. Enterococci can be α-, β-, or non-hemolytic. As a rule, enterococci are not very virulent, but they have become prominent as a cause of nosocomial infections as a result of their multiple antibiotic resistance. Figure 9.12 shows the microscopic appearance of *E. faecalis*.

## A. Epidemiology

Enterococci are part of the normal fecal flora. However, they can also colonize oral mucous membranes and skin, especially in hospital settings. These organisms are highly resistant to environmental and chemical agents, and can persist on fomites.

## B. Diseases

Enterococci seldom cause disease in normal, healthy individuals. However, under conditions in which host resistance is lowered or the integrity of the gastrointestinal or genitourinary tract has been disrupted (for example, by instrumentation), enterococci can spread to normally sterile sites, causing urinary tract infections, bacteremia-sepsis, subacute bacterial endocarditis, biliary tract infection, or intra-abdominal abscesses.

**Figure 9.12**
*Enterococcus fecalis* showing chain formation characteristic of *Streptococcus*.

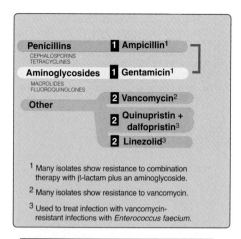

**Figure 9.13**
Antimicrobial agents useful in treating infections caused by Enterococci.

### C. Laboratory identification

Enterococci are distinguished from the non–Group D streptococci by their ability to survive in the presence of bile, and to hydrolyze the polysaccharide esculin. Unlike nonenterococcal group D strepto-cocci, enterococci grow in 6.5 percent NaCl, and yield a positive pyrazin amidase (PYR) test. *E. faecalis* can be distinguished from *E. faecium* by their fermentation patterns, which are commonly evaluated in clinical laboratories.

### D. Treatment

Enterococci are naturally resistant to β-lactam antibiotics and aminoglycosides, but are sensitive to the synergistic action of a combination of these classes. In the past, the initial regimens of choice were penicillin +/– streptomycin, or ampicillin +/– gentamicin (Figure 9.13). However, acquired resistance determinants in many current strains negate this synergy. In addition, isolates frequently have natural or acquired resistances to many other antibiotic classes, including glycopeptide, such as vancomycin. Newer antibiotics, such as the combination of quinupristin and dalfopristin, are used to treat vancomycin-resistant infections. However, some enterococcal strains are resistant to all commercially available antibiotics. [Note: *E. faecium* is more likely to be vancomycin- or multiply-resistant than *E. faecalis*.]

### E. Prevention

The rise of nosocomial infections by multiple drug-resistant enterococci is largely the result of selection due to high antibiotic usage in hospitals. Judicious use of antibiotics is an important factor in controlling the emergence of these infections.

## VII. NONENTEROCOCCAL GROUP D STREPTOCOCCI

*Streptococcus bovis* is the most clinically important of the nonenterococcus group D streptococci. Part of normal fecal flora, they are either α– or nonhemolytic. *S. bovis* occasionally causes urinary tract infections and subacute bacterial endocarditis, the latter especially in association with colon cancer. The organism is bile- and esculin-positive, but is PYR-negative, and does not grow in 6.5 percent salt (unlike the enterococci). It tends to be sensitive to penicillin and other antibiotics.

## VIII. VIRIDANS STREPTOCOCCI

The viridans group of streptococci includes many gram-positive, catalase-negative, α– or γ–hemolytic species that constitute the main facultative oral flora. The viridans streptococci are relatively avirulent, but *Streptococcus mutans* and other members of the viridans group cause dental caries. In patients with abnormal or damaged heart valves, they can also infect these valves during a bacteremia, causing subacute bacterial endocarditis (Figure 9.14). Therefore, at-risk patients with rheumatic, congenital, or arteriosclerotic valvular disease should receive prophylactic penicillin before undergoing dental procedures.

**Figure 9.14**
Streptococcal endocarditis showing vegetation of the mitral valve leaflet. [Note: Vegetation is a tissue outgrowth composed of fibrin, bacteria, and aggregated blood platelets adherent to a diseased heart valve.]

Gram (+) cocci

## Streptococcus species

- **Gram-positive**
- Ovoid to spherical in shape, occurring as pairs or chains
- Nonmotile, catalase-negative
- Most are facultative anaerobes, but grow fermentatively even in the presence of oxygen
- Culture on blood agar

α-Hemolytic streptococci on blood agar

*Streptococcus pyogenes* (Gram stain)

β-Hemolytic streptococci on blood agar

### *Streptococcus pyogenes*
(Group A, β-hemolytic)

- Acute pharyngitis or pharyngotonsillitis
- Acute rheumatic fever
- Erysipelas
- Puerperal sepsis
- Invasive group A streptococcal (GAS) disease

PENICILLINS [1] Penicillin G[1]
CEPHALOSPORINS
TETRACYCLINES
AMINOGLYCOSIDES

MACROLIDES [2] Clarithromycin or azithromycin[2]
FLUOROQUINOLONES
OTHER

[1] *S. pyogenes* has not acquired resistance to penicillin G.
[2] For penicillin-allergic patient

### *Streptococcus agalactiae*
(Group B, β-hemolytic)

- Meningitis and septicemia in neonates
- Endometritis
- Septicemia or pneumonia in individuals with impaired immune systems
- Diabetic foot infections

PENICILLINS [1] Penicillin G[3]
CEPHALOSPORINS
TETRACYCLINES

AMINOGLYCOSIDES [2] An aminoglycoside[4]

MACROLIDES
FLUOROQUINOLONES
OTHER

[3] All isolates remain sensitive to penicillin G and ampicillin.
[4] In life-threatening infections, an aminoglycoside can be added to the regimen.

### *Streptococcus pneumoniae*
(α-hemolytic)

- Acute bacterial pneumonia
- Otitis media
- Meningitis

PENICILLINS [1] Penicillin G[5]

Cephalosporins [1] Cefotaxime
[1] Ceftriaxone
CEPHALOSPORINS
TETRACYCLINES
AMINOGLYCOSIDES
MACROLIDES
FLUOROQUINOLONES

OTHER [2] Vancomycin[6]

[5] Penicillin G has been the drug of choice, but resistant strains are regularly seen.
[6] Most resistant strains remain sensitive to vancomycin.

Facial erysipelas

Impetigo

Streptococcal pharyngitis

**Figure 9.15**
Summary of streptococcal disease.

## Study Questions

**Choose the ONE correct answer**

9.6 A 52-year-old man, generally in good health, is diagnosed with carcinoma and is scheduled for surgery. While waiting for his HMO to arrange for a bed, he develops persistent low-grade fever and constitutional symptoms. Physical examination is unremarkable other than a heart murmur not previously present. Outpatient blood cultures yield gram-positive, α-hemolytic cocci. The most likely cause for the clinical picture is:

A. spread of carcinoma.

B. anxiety, with skin flora contamination of the blood cultures.

C. subacute endocarditis caused by *Streptococcus bovis*.

D. subacute endocarditis caused by Group B streptococci.

E. AIDS.

> Correct answer = C. *S. bovis*, a member of normal fecal flora, is hemolytic and a not uncommon cause of subacute endocarditis seen in association with bowel neoplasms.

9.7 A 55-year-old man was admitted to a local hospital with fever and chills. The patient was HIV positive and had received multiple courses of antibiotics. Blood cultures grew gram-positive cocci, which tested positive with Group D streptococcal antisera. The isolate was resistant to penicillin and vancomycin. Which one of the following is the most likely pathogen?

A. *Streptococcus pneumoniae*

B. *Enterococcus faecium*

C. *Streptococcus pyogenes*

D. *Streptococcus agalactiae*

E. *Enterococcus faecalis*

> Correct answer = B. *E. faecium* is most likely to be vancomycin- or multiply drug-resistant.

"I'm sorry, this is never easy. It's strep"

# Gram-positive Rods

# 10

## I. OVERVIEW

The gram-positive rods discussed in this chapter (Figure 10.1) are not closely related, nor do they cause similar clinical conditions. The genus *Corynebacterium* includes *Corynebacterium diphtheriae*, the cause of the prototypic toxin-mediated disease diphtheria, as well as several usually harmless human commensals. *Bacillus* is a large genus of spore-forming bacteria, principally of soil origin; however anthrax is caused by *Bacillus anthracis*. *Listeria monocytogenes* causes various types of infection in populations such as newborns, pregnant women, and the immunocompromised.

## II. CORYNEBACTERIA

Corynebacteria are small, slender, pleomorphic, gram-positive rods of distinctive morphology that tend to stain unevenly. They are non-motile, unencapsulated, and do not form spores. *Corynebacterium* is a large genus of diverse habitat. Most species are facultative anaerobes, and those found associated with humans, including the pathogen *C. diphtheriae*, grow aerobically on standard laboratory media such as blood agar.

### A. Corynebacterium diphtheriae

Diphtheria, caused by *C. diphtheriae*, is an acute respiratory or cutaneous disease and may be a life-threatening illness. The development of effective vaccination protocols and widespread immunization beginning in early childhood has made the disease rare in developed countries. Thus, few present-day American clinicians have seen a case of the disease. However, diphtheria is a serious disease throughout the world, particularly in those countries where the population has not been immunized.

1. **Epidemiology:** *C. diphtheriae* is found in the throat and nasopharynx of carriers and in patients with diphtheria. This disease is a local infection, usually of the throat. Therefore, the organism is

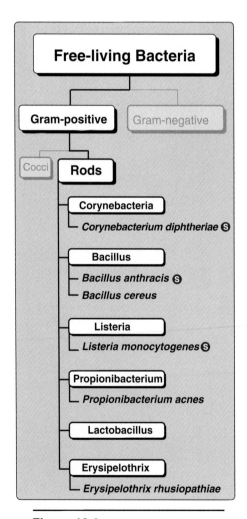

**Figure 10.1**
Classification of gram-positive rods.
Ⓢ See p. 331 for summaries of these organisms.

**Figure 10.2**
Action of diphtheria toxin.

1. A membrane receptor recognizes and binds a portion of the toxin (fragment B).

Diphtheria toxin

Cell membrane

CELL

Receptor for toxin

2. The toxin enters the cell by receptor-mediated endocytosis and dissociates into fragments A and B.

Active fragment of toxin

3. The A fragment is translocated to the cytosol where it catalyzes the transfer of adenosine diphosphate ribose (ADPR) from NAD$^+$ to EF-2.

NAD$^+$

Nicotinamide

EF-2 → EF-2 – ADPR

4. The ADPR-elongation factor complex is inactivated, and peptide synthesis stops.

primarily spread by respiratory droplets, usually by convalescent or asymptomatic carriers. It is less frequently spread by direct contact with an infected individual or a contaminated fomite.

2. **Pathogenesis:** Diphtheria is caused by the local and systemic effects of a single exotoxin that inhibits eukaryotic protein synthesis. The toxin molecule is a heat-labile polypeptide that is composed of two fragments, A and B. Fragment B binds to susceptible cell membranes and mediates the delivery of fragment A to its target. Inside the cell, fragment A separates from fragment B, and catalyzes a reaction between nicotine adenine dinucleotide (NAD$^+$) and the eukaryotic polypeptide chain elongation factor, EF-2[1] (Figure 10.2).

3. **Clinical significance**

   Infection may result in clinical disease which has two forms—respiratory and cutaneous—or in an asymptomatic carrier state.

   a. **Upper respiratory tract infection:** Diphtheria consists of a strictly local infection, usually of the throat. The infection produces a distinctive thick, grayish, adherent exudate (pseudomembrane) that is composed of cell debris from the mucosa and inflammatory products (see Figure 10.5). It coats the throat, and may extend into the nasal passages or downward in the respiratory tract, where the exudate sometimes obstructs the airways, even leading to suffocation. As the disease progresses, generalized symptoms occur caused by production and absorption of toxin (Figure 10.3). Although all human cells are sensitive to diphtheria toxin, the major clinical effects involve the heart and peripheral nerves. Cardiac conduction defects and myocarditis may lead to congestive heart failure and permanent heart damage. Neuritis of cranial nerves and paralysis of muscle groups, such as those that control movement of the palate or the eye, are seen late in the disease.

   b. **Cutaneous diphtheria:** A puncture wound or cut in the skin can result in introduction of *C. diphtheriae* into the subcutaneous tissue, leading to a chronic, nonhealing ulcer with a gray membrane. Rarely, exotoxin production leads to tissue degeneration and death.

4. **Immunity:** Diphtheria toxin is antigenic and stimulates the production of antibodies that neutralize the toxin's activity. [Note: Formalin treatment of the toxin produces a toxoid that retains the antigenicity but not the toxicity of the molecule. This is the material used for immunization against the disease (see p. 36).]

[1]See p. 436 in *Lippincott's Illustrated Reviews: Biochemistry* (3rd ed.) for a discussion of polypeptide chain elongation.

5. **Laboratory identification:** The presumptive diagnosis and decision to treat for diphtheria must be based on initial clinical observation. Diphtheria should be considered in patients with pharyngitis, low-grade fever, and cervical adenopathy (swelling of the neck). Erythema of the pharynx progressing to adherent gray pseudomembranes increases suspicion of diphtheria. However, a definitive diagnosis requires isolation of the organism, which must then be tested for virulence using an immunologic precipitin reaction to demonstrate toxin production. *C. diphtheriae* can be isolated most easily from a selective medium, such as Tinsdale's agar (see Figure 10.5), which contains potassium tellurite, an inhibitor of other respiratory flora, and on which the organism produces several distinctive black colonies with halos (see Figure 10.5). *C. diphtheriae* from clinical material or culture has a distinctive morphology when stained, for example, with methylene blue. This morphology includes characteristic bands and reddish (polychromatic) granules that are often seen in thin, sometimes club-shaped rods that appear in clumps, suggestive of Chinese characters or picket fences (see Figure 10.4).

**Figure 10.3**
Diphtheria with marked swelling of the lymph nodes in the neck.

> Initial decision to treat for diphtheria must be based on clinical observation. Culture and assay for toxin production are required for confirmation of the diagnosis.

6. **Treatment:** Treatment of diphtheria requires prompt neutralization of toxin, followed by eradication of the organism. A single dose of horse serum antitoxin inactivates any circulating toxin, although it does not affect toxin already bound to a cell-surface receptor. [Note: Serum sickness caused by a reaction to the horse protein may cause complications in approximately ten percent of patients.] *C. diphtheriae* is sensitive to several antibiotics, such as erythromycin or penicillin (Figure 10.5). Antibiotic treatment slows the spread of infection and, by killing the organism, prevents further toxin production.

**Figure 10.4**
*Corynbacterium diphtheriae.*

7. **Prevention:** The cornerstone of diphtheria prevention is immunization with toxoid, usually administered in the DPT triple vaccine, together with tetanus toxoid and pertussis antigens (see p. 38). The initial series of injections should be started in infancy. Booster injections of diphtheria toxoid (with tetanus toxoid) should be given at approximately ten-year intervals throughout life. The control of an epidemic outbreak of diphtheria involves rigorous immunization and a search for healthy carriers among patient contacts.

## B. Diphtheroids

Several other corynebacterium species that morphologically resemble the type species, *C. diphtheriae*, are common commensals of the nose, throat, nasopharynx, skin, urinary tract, and conjunctiva.

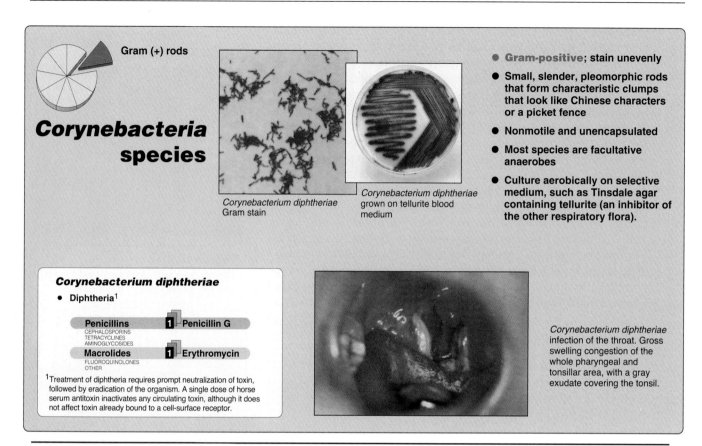

**Figure 10.5**
Summary of *Corynebacterium diphtheriae* disease.

They are therefore called diphtheroids, and are generally unable to produce exotoxin, but a few cause disease in rare circumstances, such as in immunosuppressed individuals.

## III. BACILLUS SPECIES

Species of the genus *Bacillus* are gram-positive, form endospores, and are either strictly or facultatively aerobic (that is, they can grow in the presence of oxygen, but do not require it). Most of the seventy or so species of *Bacillus* are found in soil and water, and are usually encountered in the medical laboratory as airborne contaminants. *B. anthracis*, the cause of the disease anthrax, is clinically the most important member of this genus.

### A. Bacillus anthracis

Anthrax is a rare disease in the United States. For example, from 1984 to 1997, only three case of cutaneous anthrax were reported. However, in 2001, twenty new cases occurred—eleven cutaneous and eleven inhalation anthrax. These infections resulted from probable exposure to *B. anthracis* powder sent through the mail. The source of these organisms remains unknown.

1. **Epidemiology:** Anthrax is an enzootic disease of worldwide occurrence. [Note: An enzootic disease is endemic to a population of animals (that is, its occurrence changes little over time). This is as compared to an epizootic disease, which attacks a large number of animals at the same time (similar to a human epidemic).] Anthrax affects principally domestic herbivores—sheep, goats, and horses—and is transmitted to humans by contact with infected animal products or contaminated dust (Figure 10.6). Infection is usually initiated by the subcutaneous inoculation of spores through incidental skin abrasions. Less frequently, the inhalation of spore-laden dust causes a pulmonary form of anthrax. [Note: Sometimes an occupational hazard, this form of pneumonia is known as "woolsorter's disease."] *B. anthracis* spores may remain viable for many years in contaminated pastures, or in bones, wool, hair, hides, or other animal materials. These spores, like those of clostridia (see p. 53), are highly resistant to physical and chemical agents. In the United States, a veterinary vaccine in widespread use makes domestic animal sources of the disease quite rare. Contaminated agricultural imports may account for the few cases seen, and lead occasionally to the quarantine of goods from endemic areas.

> *B. anthracis* is a potential bioterrorism agent because it can be easily grown in large quantities, is resistant to destruction, and can be formulated into an aerosol for wide dissemination. Physicians must be prepared to recognized anthrax even though it is rarely seen in the United States.

2. **Pathogenesis:** *B. anthracis* possesses a capsule that is antiphagocytic and is essential for full virulence. The organism also produces three plasmid-coded exotoxins: edema factor, a calmodulin-dependent adenylate cyclase, causes elevation of intracellular cAMP, and is responsible for the severe edema usually seen in *B. anthracis* infections; lethal toxin is responsible for tissue necrosis; protective antigen (so named because of its use in producing protective anthrax vaccines) mediates cell entry of edema factor and lethal toxin

3. **Clinical significance**

   a. **Cutaneous anthrax:** About 95 percent of human cases of anthrax are cutaneous. Upon introduction of organisms or spores that germinate, a papule develops. It rapidly evolves into a painless, black, severely swollen "malignant pustule," which eventually crusts over. The organisms may invade regional lymph nodes and then the general circulation, leading to fatal septicemia. Although some cases remain localized and

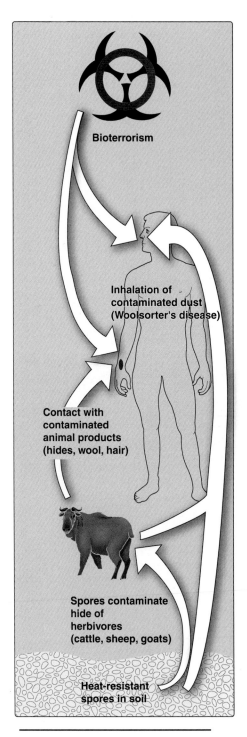

**Figure 10.6**
Anthrax in animal and human hosts.

heal, the overall mortality in untreated cutaneous anthrax is about twenty percent.

b. **Pulmonary anthrax (woolsorter's disease)** is caused by inhalation of spores. It is characterized by progressive hemorrhagic lymphadenitis (inflammation of the lymph nodes), and has a mortality rate approaching 100 percent if left untreated.

4. **Laboratory identification:** *B. anthracis* is easily recovered from clinical materials, where it is often present in massive numbers. Microscopically, the organisms appear as blunt-ended bacilli that occur singly, in pairs, or frequently in long chains (Figure 10.7). They do not sporulate often in clinical samples, but do so in culture. The spores are oval and centrally located. On blood agar, the colonies are large, grayish, and nonhemolytic, with an irregular border. Unlike many bacillus species, *B. anthracis* is nonmotile and is encapsulated *in vivo*. A direct immunofluorescence assay aids in identification of the organism.

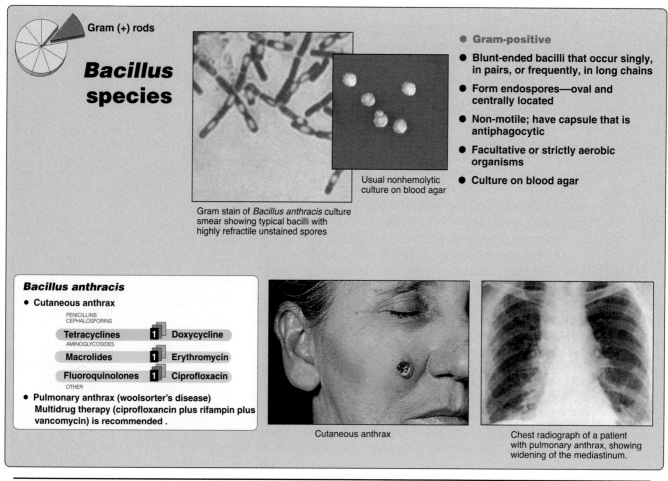

**Gram (+) rods**

*Bacillus species*

Gram stain of *Bacillus anthracis* culture smear showing typical bacilli with highly refractile unstained spores

Usual nonhemolytic culture on blood agar

- **Gram-positive**
- **Blunt-ended bacilli that occur singly, in pairs, or frequently, in long chains**
- **Form endospores—oval and centrally located**
- **Non-motile; have capsule that is antiphagocytic**
- **Facultative or strictly aerobic organisms**
- **Culture on blood agar**

**Bacillus anthracis**
- **Cutaneous anthrax**

PENICILLINS
CEPHALOSPORINS

| Tetracyclines | 1 | Doxycycline |

AMINOGLYCOSIDES

| Macrolides | 1 | Erythromycin |

| Fluoroquinolones | 1 | Ciprofloxacin |

OTHER

- **Pulmonary anthrax (woolsorter's disease)**
  Multidrug therapy (ciprofloxancin plus rifampin plus vancomycin) is recommended .

Cutaneous anthrax

Chest radiograph of a patient with pulmonary anthrax, showing widening of the mediastinum.

**Figure 10.7**
Summary of anthrax disease.

**5. Treatment:** *B. anthracis* is sensitive to a variety of antibiotics. Cutaneous anthrax responds to doxcycline, ciprofloxacin, or erythromycin (see Figure 10.7). Penicillin is not recommended because of inducible β-lactamase in *B. anthracis*. Multidrug therapy (for example, ciprofloxacin plus rifampin plus vancomycin) is recommended for inhalation anthrax.

> Aggressive therapy is indicated for inhalation anthrax both because of the severity of the disease and the fact that the disease is often not diagnosed until late in the course of the illness.

**6. Prevention:** A cell-free vaccine is available for workers in high risk occupations (see p. 37). Postexposure prophylaxis with ciprofloxacin or doxycycline is recommended. [Note: Because of the resistance of endospores to chemical disinfectants, autoclaving is the most reliable means of decontamination.

## B. Other species of bacillus

Uncommonly, other species of bacillus are implicated in opportunistic lesions, particularly following trauma or the placement of artificial devices and catheters. A commonly identified species is *Bacillus cereus*. Strains of this species produce a tissue-destructive exotoxin. *B. cereus* also causes food poisoning by means of enterotoxins with either emetic or diarrheal effects.

## IV. LISTERIA

*Listeria* species are slender, short, gram-positive rods (see Figure 10.9). They do not form spores. Sometimes they occur as diplobacilli or in short chains, and they are avid intracellular parasites that may be seen within host cells in tissue samples. *Listeria* species are catalase-positive, and display a distinctive tumbling motility by light microscopy in liquid medium, which is most active after growth at 25°C; these characteristics distinguish it from streptococcus (catalase-negative) or corynebacterium (nonmotile) species, both of which may be confused morphologically with listeria. *Listeria* species grow facultatively on a variety of enriched media.

## A. Epidemiology

*Listeria monocytogenes* is the only species that infects humans, although the *Listeria* species are widespread among animals in nature. Listeria infections, which may occur as sporadic cases or in small epidemics, are usually foodborne. For example, studies have shown that two to three percent of processed dairy products (including ice cream and cheese), twenty to thirty percent of ground meats, and a majority of retail poultry samples are contaminated with *L. monocytogenes*. [Note: *L. monocytogenes* is capable of growth at

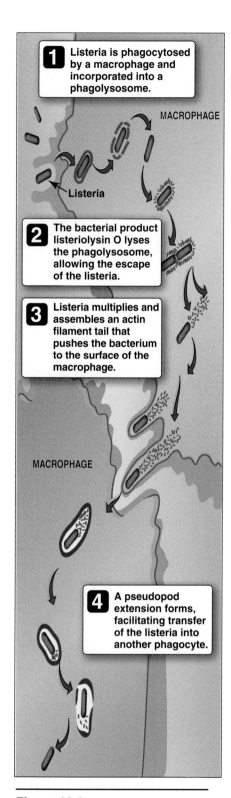

**1** Listeria is phagocytosed by a macrophage and incorporated into a phagolysosome.

MACROPHAGE

Listeria

**2** The bacterial product listeriolysin O lyses the phagolysosome, allowing the escape of the listeria.

**3** Listeria multiplies and assembles an actin filament tail that pushes the bacterium to the surface of the macrophage.

MACROPHAGE

**4** A pseudopod extension forms, facilitating transfer of the listeria into another phagocyte.

**Figure 10.8**
Life cycle of *Listeria monocytogenes* in host macrophages.

4°C, thus refrigeration does not reliably suppress its growth in food.] One to fifteen percent of healthy humans are asymptomatic intestinal carriers of the organism. Listeria infections are most common in pregnant women, fetuses or newborns, and in immunocompromised individuals, such as the elderly or patients receiving corticosteroids. In the United States, some 2000 cases are reported each year, with 450 deaths and 100 stillbirths.

> Blood cultures are indicated in pregnant febrile women when no alternate pathology (for example, urinary tract infection) is readily detected.

### B. Pathogenesis

*L. monocytogenes* is a facultative, intracellular parasite that has been used extensively to study phagocytosis and immune activation of macrophages. The organism attaches to and enters a variety of mammalian cells, apparently by normal phagocytosis; once internalized, it escapes from the phagocytic vacuole by elaborating a membrane-damaging toxin called listeriolysin O. [Note: Mutants lacking a functional listeriolysin O are avirulent.] *L. monocytogenes* grows in the cytosol and stimulates changes in cell function that facilitate its direct passage from cell to cell. The organisms induce a reorganization of cellular actin such that short filaments and actin-binding proteins cohere to the bacteria, creating a cometlike "tail." This complex appears to propel the organisms through the cell to pseudopods in contact with adjacent cells. Bacterium-produced membrane-degrading phospholipases then mediate the passage of the organism directly to a neighboring cell, allowing avoidance of the intercellular milieu, including cells of the immune system (Figure 10.8).

### C. Clinical significance

Septicemia and meningitis are the most commonly reported forms of *L. monocytogenes* infection (listeriosis). A variety of focal lesions are less frequently seen, such as granulomatous skin lesions. Pregnant women, usually in the third trimester, may have a milder "flulike" illness. In this as well as in asymptomatic vaginal colonization, the organism can be transmitted to a newborn (*L. monocytogenes* is a relatively common cause of newborn meningitis) or to the fetus and initiate abortion. Immunocompromised individuals, especially those with defects in cellular immunity, are susceptible to serious generalized infections.

### D. Laboratory identification

The organism can be isolated from blood, cerebrospinal fluid, and other clinical specimens by standard bacteriologic procedures. On blood agar, *L. monocytogenes* produces a small colony surrounded by a narrow zone of β hemolysis (Figure 10.9). *Listeria* species can be distinguished from various streptococci by morphology, positive motility, and the production of catalase.

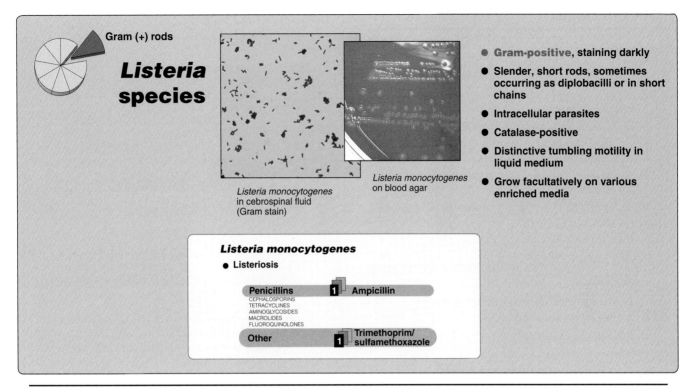

**Figure 10.9**
Summary of *Listeria* species.

### E. Treatment and prevention

A variety of antibiotics have been successfully used to treat *L. monocytogenes* infections, including ampicillin and trimethoprim/sulfamethoxazole (Figure 10.9). Prevention of *L. monocytogenes* infections can be accomplished by proper food preparation and handling.

## V. OTHER NON-SPORE-FORMING, GRAM-POSITIVE RODS

*Propionibacterium* is a genus of anaerobic or microaerophilic rods of diphtheroidlike morphology. They are common inhabitants of normal skin, and, in rare instances, have been reported as causes of endocarditis or infections of plastic implants. *P. acnes*, often a strict anaerobe, has been implicated as a contributing cause of acne. Various species of *Lactobacillus* are part of the commensal flora of human mucous membranes. They produce quantities of lactic acid during fermentation, and have been thought to assist in maintaining the acid pH of normal mucous epithelia. However, acid production by oral lactobacilli may play a role in the production of dental caries. *Erysipelothrix rhusiopathiae* is a filamentous, gram-positive rod that causes disease in animals and, rarely, a skin infection called erysipeloid in people who commonly handle animal products, for example, butchers, veterinarians, and fishermen.

## Study questions

**Choose the ONE correct answer**

10.1 A diagnosis of diphtheria is confirmed by:

    A. microscopic appearance of organisms stained with methylene blue.

    B. isolation of a typical colony on Tinsdale's agar.

    C. isolation of typical organisms from materials such as blood, showing invasiveness.

    D. detection of β phage plaques in cultures of suspicious isolates.

    E. demonstration of toxin production by a suspicious isolate.

> Correct answer = E. Observation of diphtheria toxin production (E) is required to prove the diagnosis. Items A and B are presumptive indicators. β phage (D) is a temperate phage, and lytic activity is not observed. *C. diphtheriae* is noninvasive, and the organism (but not the toxin) is recovered only from surface infections such as those of the oropharynx and skin lesions.

10.2 *Listeria monocytogenes* shows which of the following characteristics?

    A. It can grow at refrigerator temperatures (4°C).

    B. It is an extracellular pathogen.

    C. It is catalase-negative.

    D. It is a gram-negative coccus.

    E. It is strictly a human pathogen.

> Correct answer = A. *L. monocytogenes* grows optimally at 30 to 37°C, but is capable of growth at 4°C. Thus, refrigeration does not reliably suppress its growth in food. *L. monocytogenes* is a catalase-positive, gram-positive, obligate intracellular pathogen. These organisms are found in cattle, other warmblooded animals, and fish, where they can cause disease.

10.3 A 26-year-old woman, eight months pregnant, visits her obstetrician complaining of fever, myalagia and backache of recent onset. Three weeks earlier, the patient had been a weekend guest at a rural farmhouse, where all the food was reported to be "unprocessed" and "natural." A culture of the patient's blood shows gram-positive rods that are catalase-positive and display a distinctive tumbling motility in liquid medium. What is the most likely source of the woman's infection?

    A. Well-done roast beef

    B. Fresh, raw cow's milk

    C. Home-baked bread

    D. Homemade apple sauce

    E. Baked apple pie

> Correct answer = B. The woman is most likely experiencing listerosis. *Listeriae* are common in the GI tract and milk of cattle, but are normally killed by pasteurization. Unpasteurized milk was presumably consumed at the farm.

*". . .striking, as it does, every fourth person."*

# Neisseriae

# 11

## I. OVERVIEW

The genus *Neisseria* consists of gram-negative, aerobic cocci. Two *Neisseria* species are pathogenic for humans—*Neisseria gonorrhoeae* (commonly called gonococcus), the causal agent of gonorrhea; and *Neisseria meningitidis* (commonly called meningococcus), a frequent cause of meningitis. Gonococci and meningococci are nonmotile diplococci that cannot be distinguished from each other under the microscope. However, they can be differentiated in the laboratory by sugar use patterns, and the sites of their primary infections. Both bacteria are classified as pyogenic cocci because infections by these organisms are also characterized by the production of purulent (puslike) material comprised largely of white blood cells. Neisseriae and organisms that are easily confused with them are discussed in this chapter (Figure 11.1.)

## II. NEISSERIA GONORRHOEAE

Gonorrhea is one of the most frequently reported infectious diseases in the United States. The causal agent, *N. gonorrhoeae*, a gram-negative diplococcus, is frequently observed inside polymorphonuclear leukocytes of clinical samples obtained from infected patients (Figure 11.2). *N. gonorrhoeae* is usually transmitted during sexual contact or, more rarely, during the passage of a baby through an infected birth canal. It does not survive long outside the human body because it is highly sensitive to dehydration.

### A. Structure

Gonococci are unencapsulated (unlike meningococci, see p. 104), piliated, and nonmotile, and resemble a pair of kidney beans.

1. **Pili:** These hairlike surface appendages are made of helical aggregates of repeating peptide subunits called pilin. Pili enhance attachment of the organism to host epithelial and mucosal cell surfaces and confer resistance to phagocytosis; they are, therefore, among the most important virulence factors. Pili are also antigenic. At least twenty gonococcal genes code for pilin, most of which are not expressed at any given time because they lack promoters[1] (that is, they are "silent"). By shuffling and recombining chromosomal regions of these genes, a single strain of *N. gonorrhoeae* can, at different times, synthesize ("express") multiple

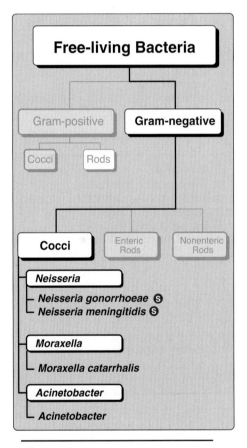

**Figure 11.1**
Classification of *Neisseria* and related organisms. ⑤ See pp. 331 for summaries of these organisms.

[1] See p. 421 in ***Lippincott's Illustrated Reviews: Biochemistry*** (3rd ed.) for a discussion of promoters.

**Figure 11.2**
A. Presence of *Neisseria gonorrhoeae* in polymorphonuclear leukocytes in urethral discharge. B. Gonococcus (electron microscope) showing pili.

**Figure 11.3**
Antigenic variation in the gonococcus.

pilins that have different amino acid sequences. This process, known as gene conversion, allows the organism to produce antigenically different pilin molecules over time (Figure 11.3).

2. **Lipooligosaccharide:** Gonococcal lipooligosaccharides (LOS) have shorter, more highly branched, nonrepeat O-antigenic side chains than do lipopolysaccharides found in other gram-negative bacteria (LPS, see p. 13). The bactericidal antibodies in normal human serum are IgM molecules directed against LOS antigens.

3. **Outer membrane proteins (OMPs):** OMP I, functioning as a porin in complex with OMP III, is antigenically diverse in different strains of gonococci. OMP II is referred to as the "opacity protein" because its presence renders gonococcal colonies less translucent. OMP II, along with pili, mediates attachment of the organism to a host cell. Because of OMP II's ability to undergo extensive antigenic variation, it also contributes significantly to the ability of the organism to evade the immune response and cause repeated infections.

### B. Pathogenesis

Pili and OMP II facilitate adhesion of the gonococcus to epithelial cells of the urethra, rectum, cervix, pharynx, or conjunctiva, and, therefore, make colonization possible. Pili also enable the bacterium to resist phagocytosis. [Note: Only piliated gonococci are virulent.] In addition, both gonococci and meningococci produce an IgA protease that cleaves IgA$_1$, helping the pathogen to evade immunoglobulins of this subclass.

### C. Clinical significance

Gonococci most often colonize the mucous membrane of the genitourinary tract or rectum (for example, Figure 11.4 shows gonococci growing in the fallopian tube). There the organisms may cause a localized infection with the production of pus, or may lead to tissue invasion, chronic inflammation, and fibrosis. A higher proportion of females than males are generally asymptomatic; these individuals act as the reservoir for maintaining and transmitting gonococcal infections. [Note: More than one sexually transmitted disease may be acquired at the same time; for example, gonorrhea in combination with syphilis (*Treponema pallidum* infection), chlamydia, human immunodeficiency virus, or hepatitis B virus. Patients with gonorrhea may, therefore, need treatment for more than one pathogen.]

1. **Genitourinary tract infections:** Symptoms of gonococcal infection are more acute and easier to diagnose in males. The patient typically presents with a yellow, purulent urethral discharge and painful urination. In females, infection occurs in the endocervix and extends to the urethra and vagina. A greenish-yellow cervical discharge is most common, often accompanied by intermenstrual bleeding. The disease may progress to the uterus, causing salpingitis (inflammation of the fallopian tubes), pelvic inflammatory disease (PID), and fibrosis. Infertility occurs in approximately twenty percent of women with gonococcal salpingitis, as a result of tubal scarring.

> *N. gonorrhoeae* is a common cause of pelvic inflammatory disease in females.

2. **Rectal infections,** prevalent in male homosexuals, are characterized by constipation, painful defecation, and purulent discharge.

3. **Pharyngitis** is contracted by oral-genital contact. Infected individuals may show a purulent exudate, and the condition may mimic a mild viral or a streptococcal sore throat (see p. 81).

4. **Ophthalmia neonatorum** is an infection of the conjunctival sac that is acquired by a newborn during passage through the birth canal of a mother infected with gonococcus (Figure 11.5). If untreated, acute conjunctivitis may lead to blindness. Treatment is with erythromycin because the antibiotic also eradicates *Chlamydia trachomatis*, if present. [Note: Gonococcal conjunctivitis can also occur in adults.]

5. **Disseminated infection:** Most strains of gonococci have a limited ability to multiply in the bloodstream. Therefore, bacteremia with gonococci is rare. [Note: In contrast, meningococci multiply rapidly in blood (see p. 104).] However, some strains do invade the bloodstream, and may result in a disseminated infection in which the organism can cause fever, a painful, purulent arthritis, and small pustules on the skin that are scattered and single on an erythematous base, and which may develop necrosis. [Note: Gonococcal infection is the most common cause of septic arthritis in sexually active adults.] Disseminated infections are seen in both men and women; however they are more common in women, particularly during pregnancy and menses. All patients treated for disseminated infection should also receive a seven day course of doxycycline to eliminate concurrent infection with *Chlamydia*. Figure 11.6 compares the incidence of some of the common sexually transmitted diseases (STDs). (A summary of organisms causing the most common STDs is presented in Figure 33.2 on p. 368.)

## D. Laboratory identification

In the male, the finding of numerous neutrophils containing gram-negative diplococci in a smear of urethral exudate permits a provisional diagnosis of gonococcal infection, and indicates that the individual should be treated. In contrast, a positive culture is needed to diagnose gonococcal infection in the female, or at other sites in the male. If disseminated gonococcal infection is suspected, appropriate cultures should be set up as indicated, for example, of skin lesions, joint fluid, and blood.

1. **Growth conditions for cell culture:** *N. gonorrhoeae* grows best under aerobic conditions, and most strains require enhanced $CO_2$. *N. gonorrhoeae* ferments glucose but not maltose, lactose, or sucrose. [Note: *N. meningitidis* does ferment maltose (see p. 107).] All members of the genus are oxidase-positive. [Note: The oxidase test (see p. 25) is used to identify neisseriae, but

**Figure 11.4**
Human fallopian tube tissue twenty hours after infection with *Neisseria gonorrhoeae*.

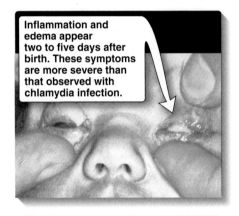

**Figure 11.5**
Gonococcal ophthalmia neonatorum.

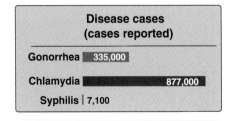

**Figure 11.6**
Incidence of sexually transmitted diseases in the United States (2003).

**Figure 11.7**
Left: Mixed growth on plain chocolate agar. Right: Pure culture on Thayer-Martin chocolate agar medium.

does not distinguish between gonococci, meningococci, and non-pathogenic neisseriae.]

2. **Selective media:** Gonococci, like pneumococci, are very sensitive to heating or drying. Cultures must be plated promptly or, if this is not possible, transport media must be used to extend the viability of the organism to be cultured. Thayer-Martin medium (chocolate agar supplemented with several antibiotics that suppress the growth of nonpathogenic neisseriae and other normal and abnormal flora) is typically used to isolate gonococci (Figure 11.7). The use of this medium is important for cultures that are typically obtained from sites such as the genitourinary tract or rectum, where there is normally an abundance of flora. On nonselective media, the normal flora overgrows the gonococci.

> Culture of *N. gonorrhoeae* on Thayer-Martin agar remains the "gold standard" for diagnosis.

### E. Treatment and prevention

More than twenty percent of current isolates of *N. gonorrhoeae* are resistant to penicillin, tetracycline, cefoxitin, and/or spectinomycin. Penicillin-resistant organisms are called PPNG—penicillinase-producing *N. gonorrhoeae*. These strains contain plasmids that carry the gene for β-lactamase of the TEM type (encoded in a transposable element), such as is seen in *Escherichia coli* and *Haemophilas influenzae*. The frequency of PPNG in the United States is now sufficiently high that penicillin is no longer recommended for treatment of gonorrhea. However, most organisms still respond to treatment with third-generation cephalosporins; for example, a single intramuscular dose of ceftriaxone is recommended therapy for uncomplicated gonococcal infections of the urethra, endocervix, or rectum. Intramuscular spectinomycin is indicated in patients who are allergic to cephalosporins.

> Many patients with gonorrhea have coexisting chlamydial infections. Therefore, doxycycline, a tetracycline effective against chlamydia, is often included as part of the treatment regimen for gonorrhea.

## III. NEISSERIA MENINGITIDIS

*N. meningitidis* is one of the most frequent causes of meningitis. Infection with *N. meningitidis* can also take the form of a fulminant meningococcemia, with intravascular coagulation, circulatory collapse, and potentially fatal shock, but without meningitis. In each case, symptoms can occur with extremely rapid onset and great intensity. Outbreaks of meningitis, most common in winter and early spring, are favored by close contact between individuals; for example, in schools, institutions, and military barracks. Severe epidemics also occur periodically in developing nations, for example, in sub-Saharan Africa and Latin America.

> *N. meningitidis* tends to strike young, previously well individuals and can progress over a matter of hours to death.

## A. Structure

Like *N. gonorrhoeae*, *N. meningitidis* is a nonmotile, gram-negative diplococcus, shaped like a kidney bean, which always appears in pairs (Figure 11.8). It is also piliated; the pili allow attachment of the organism to the nasopharyngeal mucosa where it is harbored both in carriers and in those with meningococcal disease. When meningococcus is isolated from blood or spinal fluid, it is invariably encapsulated. The meningococcal polysaccharide capsule is antiphagocytic and, therefore, the most important virulence factor. [Note: Antibodies to the capsule carbohydrate are bactericidal.]

1. **Serogroups:** The LOS capsule is antigenically diverse, which allows the identification of at least fourteen capsular polysaccharide types, called serogroups (Figure 11.9). Most infections are caused by serogroups A, B, C, W, and Y, although approximately ninety percent of cases of meningococcal disease are caused by serogroups A, B, and C. Serogroup A is usually responsible for massive epidemics in developing countries. In the United States, *N. meningitidis* serogroup B is the predominant cause of disease and mortality, followed by group C. Organisms that do not have a capsule are called "ungrouped."

2. **Serotypes:** A second classification system called serotyping (serotypes 1, 2,....20) is also a serologic classification (see Figure 11.9) that is based on the properties of the outer membrane proteins (OMPs, see p. 102) and LOS. There is no predicable relationship between serogroups and serotypes.

## B. Epidemiology

Transmission occurs through inhalation of respiratory droplets from a carrier or a patient in the early stages of the disease. In addition to contact with a carrier, risk factors include recent viral or mycoplasma upper respiratory tract infection, active or passive smoking, and complement deficiency. In susceptible persons, pathogenic strains may invade the bloodstream and cause systemic illness after an incubation period of two to ten days. The incidence of meningococcal disease in the United States is highest among infants younger than one year (Figure 11.10). Humans are the only natural host.

**Figure 11.8**
Smear of purulent cerebrospinal fluid showing *Neisseria meningitidis*.

| EPIDEMIOLOGIC CLASSIFICATION | ANTIGENIC DETERMINANT |
|---|---|
| Serogroups (>13) | Polysaccharide capsule |
| Serotypes (>20) | Outer membrane proteins and lipo-oligosaccharides |

**Figure 11.9**
Antigenic determinants of *Neisseria meningitidis*.

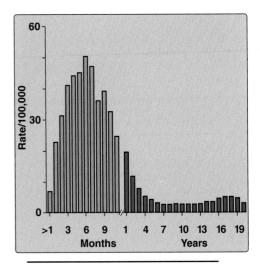

**Figure 11.10**
Incidence of meningococcal infection according to age.

## C. Pathogenesis

Antiphagocytic properties of the meningococcal capsule aid in the maintenance of infection. LOS, released during autolysis and bacterial cell division, is responsible for many of the toxic effects found in disseminated meningococcal disease. As noted on p. 102, gonococci and meningococci make an IgA protease that cleaves $IgA_1$ and, thus, helps the pathogens to evade immunoglobulins of this subclass. [Note: Nonpathogenic neisseriae do not make this protease.]

## D. Clinical significance

*N. meningitidis* initially colonizes the nasopharynx, resulting in a largely asymptomatic meningococcal pharyngitis. In young children and other susceptible individuals, the organism can cause disseminated disease by spreading through the blood, leading to meningitis and/or fulminating septicemia. *N. meningitidis* is currently a leading cause of meningitis.

1. **Meningitis:** The epithelial lining of the nasopharynx normally serves as a barrier to bacteria. Therefore, most persons colonized by *N. meningitides* remain well. As a rare event, meningococci penetrate this barrier and enter the bloodstream where they rapidly multiply (meningococcemia). In patients with fulminating septicemia, meningococci can be detected in blood smears—an unusual occurrence. If not severe, the patient may have only a fever and other nonspecific symptoms. However, the organism can seed from the blood to other sites, for example, crossing the blood-brain barrier and infecting the meninges. There they multiply and induce an acute inflammatory response, accompanied by an influx of polymorphonuclear leukocytes, resulting in a purulent meningitis. Joint symptoms and a petechial rash are also commonly observed in meningococcal infections (Figure 11.11). Within several hours the initial fever and malaise can evolve into severe headache, a rigid neck, vomiting, and sensitivity to bright lights—symptoms characteristic of meningitis. Coma can occur within a few hours. A summary of the major organisms causing meningitis is shown in Figure 33.5, p. 376.

**Figure 11.11**
Petechial rash and neck extension characteristic of meningococcal meningitis.

> The gold standard for diagnosis of systemic meningococcal infection is the isolation of *N. meningitidis* from a usually sterile body fluid, such as blood or cerebrospinal fluid (CSF). In performing a Gram stain on CSF, the clinical sample is centrifuged to concentrate the organisms, because $10^5$ to $10^6$ bacteria per ml are required for this test.

2. **Septicemia:** Meningococci can cause a life-threatening septicemia in an apparently healthy individual in less than twelve hours. Up to thirty percent of patients with meningitis go on to fulminant septicemia. In this condition, the clinical presentation is one of severe

septicemia and shock, for which the bacterial endotoxin (LOS, see p. 105) is largely responsible. Acute, fulminating meningococcal septicemia seen mainly in very young children (the Waterhouse-Friderichsen syndrome). It is characterized by large, purple, blotchy skin hemorrhages, vomiting and diarrhea, circulatory collapse, necrosis of the adrenals, and death within ten to twelve hours.

## E. Laboratory identification

Under the light microscope, *N. meningitidis* obtained from CSF and skin lesion aspirates appear as gram-negative diplococci, often in association with polymorphonuclear leukocytes. Carriers can be detected by culturing swabs from the nasopharyngeal region.

1. **Culture conditions:** Meningococci are cultured on chocolate agar with increased $CO_2$. The sample must be plated promptly or, if this is not possible, transport medium must be used to extend the viability of the organism to be cultured. Unlike gonococci, meningococci are usually cultured from CSF or blood, which are normally sterile; therefore a selective medium is not required, and plain chocolate agar is sufficient. [Note: Thayer-Martin medium (see p. 104) is required for samples obtained from a skin lesion or nasopharyngeal swab, to eliminate contaminating organisms.]

2. **Additional tests:** All *Neisseria* species are oxidase-positive. To differentiate between species, sugar fermentation tests are used (Figure 11.12). *N. meningitidis* ferments both glucose and maltose, whereas *N. gonorrhoeae* ferments only glucose. In bacterial meningitis, the CSF shows increased pressure, elevated protein, decreased glucose (partly resulting from its consumption as a bacterial nutrient), and many neutrophils. The presence of an infecting organism or of antigenic capsular substance confirms the diagnosis.

## F. Treatment and prevention

Bacterial meningitis is a medical emergency. Accordingly, antibiotic treatment cannot await a definitive bacteriologic diagnosis. High fever, headache, and a rash typical of meningococcal infection are treated immediately in an effort to prevent fulminant septicemia in which the mortality rate is high. In the past, meningitis was treated with penicillin G or ampicillin (both of which can pass the inflamed

| | GLUCOSE FERMENTATION | MALTOSE FERMENTATION | PLASMIDS | VACCINE AVAILABLE | POLY-SACCHARIDE CAPSULE | β-LACTAMASE PRODUCTION | OXIDASE |
|---|---|---|---|---|---|---|---|
| *Neisseria gonorrhoeae* | + | − | Common | − | − | Common | + |
| *Neisseria meningitidis* | + | + | Rare | Serogroups A, C, W-135, Y | + | None | + |

**Figure 11.12**
Differential bacteriologic features of *Neisseria gonorrhoeae* and *Neisseria meningitidis*.

blood-brain barrier) in large intravenous doses pending the result of cultures. Most infectious disease specialists now prefer to use cefotaxime or ceftriaxone). Prompt treatment reduces mortality to about ten percent.

> Prompt action is important in treating meningitis. Delays in the administration of antibiotics are likely to have an adverse effect on the outcome of therapy.

1. **Diagnosis:** Gram stains on CSF can be performed immediately, and latex agglutination tests with serogroup-specific anticapsular antibody can be used to obtain rapid presumptive identification of serogroup-specific meningococci in CSF.

2. **Vaccines:** A conjugate meningococcal vaccine (MCV4) was approved in the United States in 2005 for use in adolescents and adults 11 to 55 years of age, and has replaced the quadrivalent polysaccharide vaccine. MCV4 is a tetravalent vaccine that contains capsular polysaccharides from serogroups A, C, W-135, and Y conjugated to diphtheria toxoid. The conjugated vaccine elicits a T cell-dependent memory process that increases the effectiveness of the vaccine, resulting in an improved primary response to the vaccine and a strong response on subsequent exposure to the pathogen. Figure 11.13 summarizes vaccines and serogroups.

3. **Prophylaxis:** Rifampin is usually used to treat family members of an infected individual; the drug is effective in eliminating the carrier state. Other drugs used for prophylaxis include oral ciprofloxacin and intramuscular ceftriaxone.

Figure 11.14 summarizes the diseases caused by *Neisseria* species.

| SEROGROUP CLASSIFICATION | COMMENT |
|---|---|
| A | Usually responsible for massive epidemics in developing countries. |
| B | Does not elicit an effective immune response. |
| B, C | Responsible for most endemic meningitis in the United States. |
| A, C, W-135, Y | Effective capsular vaccine is available. |

**Figure 11.13**
Characteristics of the common serogroups of *Neisseria meningitidis*.

## IV. MORAXELLA

Members of the genus *Moraxella* are nonmotile, gram-negative coccobacilli that are generally found in pairs. *Moraxella* are aerobic, oxidase-positive, fastidious organisms that do not ferment carbohydrates. The most important pathogen in the genus is *Moraxella* (formerly, *Branhamella*) *catarrhalis*. This organism can cause infections of the respiratory system, middle ear, eye, CNS, and joints.

## V. ACINETOBACTER

Members of the genus *Acinetobacter* are nonmotile coccobacilli that are frequently confused with neisseriae in gram-stained samples. Generally encapsulated, oxidase-negative, and obligately aerobic, they do not ferment carbohydrates. They are important nosocomial (hospital-acquired) pathogens.

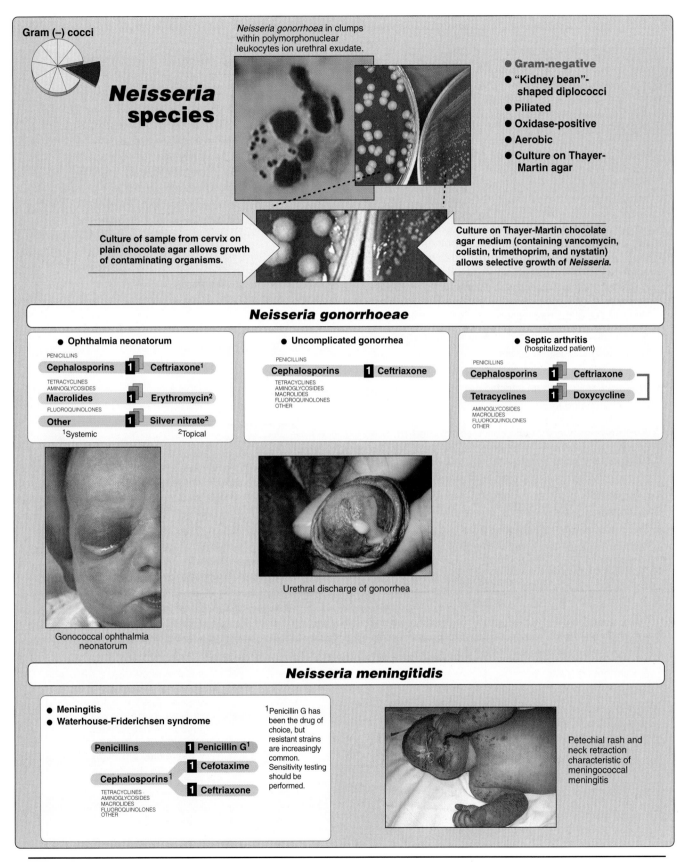

**Figure 11.14**
Summary of neisseria diseases.

## Study Questions

Choose the ONE best answer

11.1 A 14-month-old presented to his family physician with fever, vomiting, and lethargy of 24 hours duration. There was no neck stiffness or photophobia, but a non-blanching rash was found on the boy's chest. The boy's tonsils were inflamed. The child was diagnosed with upper respiratory viral infection and transported to the hospital. That evening, the child became increasingly irritable and drowsy. He was started on parenteral fluids and ceftriaxone. Several hours later, the patient developed seizures. The boy was transferred to the pediatric intensive care unit, where he developed unreactive pupils and central nonresponsive hypothermia. Later that next day, he showed no recordable brainstem activity. The child died two days after admission. Group B meningococcal infection was diagnosed by rapid antigen screen and confirmed on blood culture. The most likely source of the meningococcal infection was:

A. activation of endogenous Neisseria meningitidis.

B. close contact with a carrier.

C. contaminated fomites.

D. close contact with an infected pet.

E. contaminated food.

> Correct answer = B. Transmission occurs through inhalation of respiratory droplets from close contact with a carrier or a patient in the early stages of the disease.

11.2 A gram-negative diplococcus was isolated from a chocolate agar culture of a cerebrospinal fluid sample. Which one of the following tests or observations would be most informative in identifying the organism as N. meningitidis?

A. Appearance of colonies

B. Growth on Thayer-Martin medium

C. Direct oxidase test on spinal fluid

D. Growth in air

E. Positive oxidase test and ability of culture isolate to ferment glucose and maltose

> Correct answer = E. A gram-negative diplococcus may be identified definitively on the basis of positive oxidase test and ability to ferment both glucose and maltose. Growth on Thayer-Martin medium is a nonspecific result because this medium allows growth of neisseriae and several other species. Biochemical determinations are rarely conducted directly on spinal fluid specimens because of the presence of interfering substances which affect the accuracy of the tests. Growth in air only eliminates obligate anaerobes.

11.3 Which one of the following is characteristic of N. meningitidis but not N. gonorrhoeae?

A. Ferments glucose

B. Contains a polysaccharide capsule

C. Is oxidase-positive

D. Most isolates show resistance to penicillin

E. No effective vaccines are available

"This bacteria devours human bank accounts"

> Correct answer = B. N. meningitidis contains a polysaccharide capsule, whereas N. gonorrhoeae does not. N. meningitidis ferments both glucose and maltose, but N. gonorrhoeae metabolizes only glucose. Most isolates of N. meningitidis remain sensitive to penicillin, although resistance is increasing. Effective vaccines exist for N. meningitidis serogroups A, C, W-135, and Y, but not for N. gonorrhoeae.

# Gastrointestinal Gram-negative Rods

# 12

## I. OVERVIEW

All of the organisms covered in this chapter are routinely found in the gastrointestinal (GI) tract of humans or other animals. Many also have alternative habitats in soil or water. All are relatively hardy, but are sensitive to drying, and all grow well in the presence of oxygen, being true facultative anaerobes. They contain lipopolysaccharide (LPS), which is both antigenic and a potential virulence factor (endotoxin). These gram-negative rods belong to diverse taxonomic groups. They constitute only a fraction of the total microbial flora of the GI tract (most bowel organisms are either gram-positive or gram-negative anaerobes). Different enteric gram-negative rods cause diseases in the GI tract, outside the GI tract, or in both locations. For example, diseases caused by members of the genera *Escherichia, Salmonella, Yersinia,* and *Campylobacter* can be both gastrointestinal and extraintestinal, those caused by members of the genera *Shigella, Helicobacter*, and *Vibrio* are primarily gastrointestinal, and those caused by members of the genera *Enterobacter, Klebsiella, Serratia*, and *Proteus* are primarily extraintestinal. Fecal contamination is frequently important in the transmission of those organisms that cause GI diseases. Gram-negative rods discussed in this chapter are listed in Figure 12.1.

## II. ESCHERICHIA COLI

*E. coli* is part of the normal flora of the colon in humans and other animals, but can be pathogenic both within and outside of the GI tract. [Note: The differences in the degree of virulence of different *E. coli* strains are caused by the individual plasmid and integrated prophage repertoire associated with each strain.] *E. coli* has fimbriae or pili that are frequently important for adherence to host mucosal surfaces, and different strains of the organism may be motile or nonmotile. Most strains can ferment lactose (that is, they are Lac$^+$) in contrast to the major intestinal pathogens, *Salmonella* (see p. 115) and *Shigella* (see p. 119), which cannot ferment lactose (that is, they are Lac$^-$). *E. coli* produces both acid and gas during fermentation of carbohydrates.

**Figure 12.1**
Classification of enteric gram-negative rods (figure continues on the next page). See p. 331 for summaries of these organisms.

**Figure 12.1** (continued)
Classification of enteric gram-negative rods. **S** See p. 331 for summaries of these organisms.

**Figure 12.2**
Electron micrograph of *Escherichia coli* showing virulence factors.

## A. Structure and physiology

*E. coli* shares many properties with the other Enterobacteriaceae. They are all true facultative anaerobes (see p. 23). They all ferment glucose, and can generate energy by reducing nitrates to nitrites. They all lack cytochrome oxidase (that is, they are oxidase-negative). Typing strains is based on differences in three structural antigens: O, H, and K (Figure 12.2). The O antigens (somatic or cell wall antigens) are found on the polysaccharide portion of the LPS. These antigens are heat-stable, and may be shared among different Enterobacteriaceae genera. O antigens are commonly used to serologically type many of the enteric gram-negative rods. The H antigens are associated with flagella; therefore, only flagellated (motile) Enterobacteriaceae such as *E. coli* have H antigen. The K antigens are most often associated with the capsule or, less commonly, with the fimbriae. Among *E. coli* species, there are many serologically distinct O, H, and K antigens, and specific serotypes are associated with particular diseases. For example, a serotype of *E. coli* possessing O157 and H7 (designated O157:H7) causes a severe form of hemorrhagic colitis (see p. 113).

## B. Clinical significance: intestinal disease

Transmission of intestinal disease is commonly by the fecal/oral route, with contaminated food and water serving as vehicles for transmission. At least five types of intestinal infections that differ in pathogenic mechanisms have been identified (Figure 12.3). Enterotoxigenic (ETEC), enteropathogenic (EPEC), enterohemorrhagic (EHEC), enteroinvasive (EIEC), and enteroaggregative (EAEC) *E. coli* all are basically the same organism, differing only by the acquisition of specific pathogenic traits.

> Enterohemorrhagic *E. coli* infection should be suspected in all patients with acute bloody diarrhea, particularly if associated with abdominal tenderness and absence of fever.

1. **Enterotoxigenic *E. coli* (ETEC):** ETEC are a common cause of traveler's diarrhea. Transmission occurs through food and water contaminated with human waste, or by person-to-person contact. ETEC colonize the small intestine (pili facilitate the binding of the organism to the intestinal mucosa). In a process mediated by enterotoxins (see p. 51), ETECs cause prolonged hypersecretion of chloride ions and water by the intestinal mucosal cells, while inhibiting the reabsorption of sodium. The gut becomes full of fluid, resulting in significant watery diarrhea that continues over a period of several days. Enterotoxins include a heat-stable toxin (ST) that works by causing an elevation in cellular cyclic guanosine monophosphate (cGMP) levels, whereas a heat-labile toxin (LT) causes elevated cyclic adenosine monophosphate (cAMP) (Figure 12.4). [Note: LT is essentially identical to cholera toxin (see p. 121).]

| STRAIN | ABBREVIATION | SYNDROME | THERAPY[1] |
|--------|--------------|----------|------------|
| Enterotoxigenic E. coli | ETEC | Watery diarrhea | Antibiotics may be useful.[2] |
| Enteropathogenic E. coli | EPEC | Watery diarrhea of long duration, mostly in infants, often in developing countries | Antibiotics may be useful.[2] |
| Enterohemorrhagic E. coli | EHEC | Bloody diarrhea; Hemorrhagic colitis and hemolytic uremic syndrome (HUS) | Avoid antibiotics because of the possible risk of potentiating HUS. |
| Enteroinvasive E. coli | EIEC | Bloody diarrhea | Rehydration and correction of electrolyte abnormalities. |
| Enteroadherent E. coli | EAEC | Persistent watery diarrhea in children and patients infected with HIV | Rehydration and correction of electrolyte abnormalities. |

**Figure 12.3**
Characteristics of intestinal infections caused by *E. coli*. Fluoroquinolones are commonly used in adults for traveler's diarrhea, but are not recommended for children. [1]Rehydration and correction of electrolyte abnormalities are essential for all diarrhea illnesses. [2]Rifaximin is approved for the treatment of diarrhea caused by noninvasive strains of *Escherichia coli* in patients 12 years of age and older. Rifaximin is a nonabsorable, gastrointestinal-selective, oral antibiotic.

2. **Enteropathogenic *E. coli* (EPEC):** EPEC are an important cause of diarrhea in infants, especially in locations with poor sanitation. The newborn becomes infected during birth, or *in utero*. The EPEC attach to mucosal cells in the small intestine, causing destruction of microvilli and development of characteristic lesions. Watery diarrhea results, which on rare occasions may become chronic. Shiga-like toxins are responsible for this destruction (see p. 120).

3. **Enterohemorrhagic *E. coli* (EHEC):** EHEC bind to cells in the large intestine, where they produce an exotoxin (verotoxin, or Shiga-like toxin), causing a severe form of copious, bloody diarrhea (hemorrhagic colitis) in the absence of mucosal invasion or inflammation. Serotype O157:H7 is the most common strain of *E. coli* that produces verotoxin. This strain is also associated with outbreaks of a potentially life-threatening, acute renal failure (hemolytic uremic syndrome, HUS) characterized by fever, acute renal failure, microangiopathic hemolytic anemia and thrombocytopenia in children younger than age five to ten years. The primary reservoir of EHEC is cattle. Therefore, the possibility of infection can be greatly decreased by thoroughly cooking ground beef and pasteurizing milk.

4. **Other *E. coli* infections:** Enteroinvasive *E. coli* (EIEC) cause a dysentery-like syndrome with fever and bloody stools. Enteroadherent *E. coli* (EAEC) also cause traveler's diarrhea and persistent diarrhea of young children.

**C. Clinical significance: extraintestinal disease**

The source of infection for extraintestinal disease is frequently the patient's own flora, in which the individual's own *E. coli* is non-

**Figure 12.4**
The action of *Escherichia coli* LT (heat-labile toxin). [Note: ST (heat-stable toxin) activates guanylate cyclase, causing production of cGMP that also causes secretion.]

pathogenic in the intestine. However, it causes disease in that individual when the organism is found, for example, in the bladder or bloodstream (normally sterile sites).

1. **Urinary tract infections (UTI):** *E. coli* is the most common cause of UTI, including cystitis and pyelonephritis. Women are particularly at risk for infection. Uncomplicated cystitis (the most commonly encountered UTI) is caused by uropathogenic strains of *E. coli*, characterized by P fimbriae (an adherence factor) and, frequently, hemolysin, colicin V, and resistance to the bactericidal activity of serum complement. Complicated UTI (pyelonephritis) occurs in settings of obstructed urinary flow, which may be caused by nonuropathogenic strains.

2. **Neonatal meningitis:** *E. coli* is a major cause of this disease occurring within the first month of life. The K1 (capsular) antigen is particularly associated with such infections.

3. **Nosocomial (hospital-acquired) infections:** These include sepsis/bacteremia, endotoxic shock, and pneumonia.

> The most common causes of neonatal meningitis:
> ● Group B streptococcus ● *E. coli* ● *Listeria*
>
> The most common causes of neonatal sepsis with or without meningitis:
> ● Group B streptococcus ● *E. coli*

## D. Laboratory identification

1. **Intestinal disease:** Because *E. coli* is normally part of the intestinal flora, detection in stool cultures of disease-causing strains is generally difficult. EIEC strains often do not ferment lactose, and may be detected on media such as MacConkey agar (see p. 24). EHEC, unlike most other strains of *E. coli*, ferment sorbitol slowly if at all, and may be detected on MacConkey sorbitol agar.

2. **Extraintestinal disease:** Isolation of *E. coli* from normally sterile body sites (for example, the bladder or CSF) is diagnostically significant. Specimens may be cultured on MacConkey agar. Strains of *E. coli* can be further characterized on the basis of serologic tests.

## E. Treatment and prevention

Intestinal disease can best be prevented by care in selection, preparation, and consumption of food and water. Maintenance of fluid and electrolyte balance is of primary importance in treatment. Antibiotics may shorten duration of symptoms; however, resistance is widespread. Extraintestinal diseases require antibiotic treatment (Figure 12.5). Antibiotic sensitivity testing of isolates is necessary to determine the appropriate choice of drugs.

**Figure 12.5**
Summary of *Escherichia* species.

## III. SALMONELLA

Members of the genus *Salmonella* can cause a variety of diseases, including gastroenteritis and enteric (typhoid) fever. S*almonella* classification has undergone numerous revisions; currently, all strains are grouped in a single species: *S. enterica*, which has approximately 2500 different serotypes, or serovars including the clinically significant serotypes *typhimurium* and *typhi*. Most strains of *Salmonella* are Lac⁻ and produce acid and gas during fermentation of glucose. They also produce $H_2S$ from sulfur-containing amino acids.

### A. Epidemiology

*Salmonella* are widely distributed in nature. Serotype *typhi* is the exclusively human pathogen, whereas other strains are associated with animals and foods (for example, eggs and poultry). Fecal/oral transmission occurs, and may involve chronic carriers. Pet turtles, which may be contaminated by their feed, have also been implicated as sources of infection. Young children and the elderly are particularly susceptible to *Salmonella* infection. Individuals in crowded institutions may also sustain *Salmonella* epidemics.

**Figure 12.6**
Mechanism of salmonella infection causing enteric fever.

**B. Pathogenesis**

*Salmonella* invade epithelial cells of the small intestine. Disease may remain localized or become systemic, sometimes with disseminated foci. The organisms are facultative, intracellular parasites that survive in phagocytic cells (Figure 12.6).

**C. Clinical significance**

*Salmonella* infection can cause both intestinal and extraintestinal diseases (for example, typhoidal salmonella).

1. **Gastroenteritis:** This localized disease (also called salmonellosis) is caused primarily by serotypes *enteriditis* and *typhimurium* (non-typhoidal salmonella). It is characterized by nausea, vomiting, and diarrhea (usually nonbloody), which develop generally within 48 hours of ingesting contaminated food or water. Fever and abdominal cramping are common. In uncompromised patients, disease is generally self-limiting (48 to 72 hours), although convalescent carriage of organisms may persist for a month or more.

> More than 95 percent of cases of salmonella infection are foodborne; salmonellosis accounts for approximately 30 percent of deaths resulting from foodborne illnesses in the United States.

2. **Enteric (typhoid) fever:** This is a severe, life-threatening systemic illness, characterized by fever and, frequently, abdominal symptoms. It is caused primarily by serotype typhi (typhoidal salmonella). Nonspecific symptoms may include chills, sweats, headache, anorexia, weakness, sore throat, cough, myalgia, and either diarrhea or constipation. About thirty percent of patients have a faint maculopapular rash on the trunk (rose spots). The incubation period varies from 5 to 21 days. Untreated, mortality is approximately fifteen percent; among survivors, the symptoms generally resolve in three to four weeks. Timely and appropriate antibiotic therapy reduces mortality to less than one percent, and speeds resolution of fever. Complications can include intestinal hemorrhage and, rarely, focal infections and endocarditis. A small percentage of patients become chronic carriers. [Note: Infected gallbladders are the main source of chronic carriage.] Typhoid fever remains a global health problem. In the United States, however, typhoid fever has become less prevalent, and is now primarily a disease of travelers and immigrants.

3. **Other sites of Salmonella infection:** Sustained bacteremia is often associated with vascular *Salmonella* infections that occur when bacteria seed atherosclerotic plaque. *Salmonella* can also cause abdominal infections (often of the hepatobiliary tract and spleen), osteomyelitis, septic arthritis, and, rarely, infections of other tissues or organs. Chronic carriage may, rarely, develop.

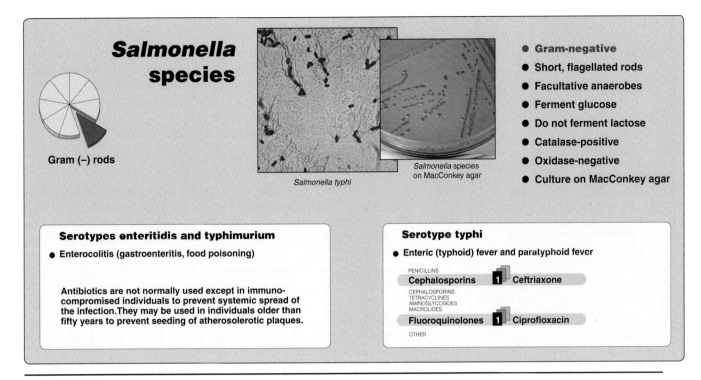

**Figure 12.7**
Summary of salmonella disease.

## D. Laboratory identification

In patients with diarrhea, *Salmonella* can typically be isolated from stools on MacConkey agar or moderately selective media (Figure 12.7). For patients with enteric fever, appropriate specimens include blood, bone marrow, urine, stool, and tissue from typical rose spots.

## E. Treatment and prevention

For gastroenteritis in uncompromised hosts, antibiotic therapy is often not needed, and may prolong the convalescent carrier state. For enteric fever, appropriate antibiotics include β-lactams and fluoroquinolones (see Figure 12.7). Prevention of salmonella infection is accomplished by proper sewage disposal, correct handling of food, and good personal hygiene.

# IV. CAMPYLOBACTER

Members of the genus *Campylobacter* are curved, spiral, or S-shaped organisms that microscopically resemble vibrios (Figure 12.8). A single, polar flagellum provides the organism with its characteristic darting motility. Somatic, flagellar, and capsular antigens all contribute to the numerous serotypes. Most *Campylobacter* are microaerophilic (that is, they require oxygen, but at lower concentrations than that found in air). Members of this genus use a respiratory pathway and do not ferment carbohydrates. *Campylobacter* infect the intestine, and can cause ulcerative, inflammatory lesions in the jejunum, ileum, or colon. Bacteremia may occur.

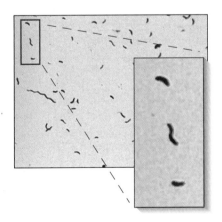

**Figure 12.8**
Micrograph showing the S-shaped cells of *Campylobacter jejuni*.

**ONSET: 1 TO 6 HOURS**

*Bacillus cereus*

*Staphylococcus aureus*

**ONSET: 8 TO 16 HOURS**

*Clostridium perfringens*
*Bacillus cereus*[1]

**ONSET: >16 HOURS**

*Campylobacter jejuni*

*Clostridium botulinum*

*Escherichia coli*
*Salmonella* species
*Shigella* species

[1]Illness caused by diarrheal enterotoxin, rather than preformed enterotoxin)

*Reverse type* = Illness commonly caused by toxin in food; viable bacteria may or may not be present in food.

**Figure 12.9**
Characteristics of common forms of bacterial food poisoning.

## A. Epidemiology

*Campylobacter* are widely distributed in nature as commensals of many different vertebrate species, including mammals and fowl, both wild and domestic. These serve as reservoirs of infection. *Campylobacter* is transmitted to humans primarily via the fecal/oral route—through direct contact, exposure to contaminated meat (especially poultry), or contaminated water supplies.

## B. Pathogenesis and clinical significance

*Campylobacter* may cause both intestinal and extraintestinal disease. [Note: Characteristics of some common forms of bacterial food poisoning are shown in Figure 12.9.] *C. jejuni* typically causes an acute enteritis in otherwise healthy individuals following a one-to-seven day incubation. The disease lasts days to several weeks, and, generally, is self-limiting. Symptoms may be both systemic (fever, headache, myalgia) and intestinal (abdominal cramping and diarrhea, which may or may not be bloody). *C. jejuni* is a cause of both traveler's diarrhea and pseudoappendicitis (symptoms simulating appendicitis without inflammation of the appendix). Bacteremia (often transient) may occur, most often in infants and the elderly. Sustained bacteremia usually reflects host compromise. Complications include septic abortion, reactive arthritis, and Guillain-Barré syndrome.

 Campylobacter is currently the leading cause of food-borne disease in the United States.

## C. Laboratory identification

*Campylobacter* can be isolated from feces using special selective media and microaerophilic conditions. Because of their small size, these organisms are not retained by bacteriologic filters that hold back most other bacteria. Thus, filtration of the fecal suspension may enhance recovery rate. Presumptive diagnosis can be made on the basis of finding curved organisms with rapid, darting motility in a wet mount of feces.

## D. Treatment and prevention

Diarrhea should be treated symptomatically with fluid and electrolyte replacement. For patients with more severe symptoms (for example, high fever, bloody diarrhea, worsening illness, or illness of more than a week's duration), antibiotics should be administered. For *C. jejuni*, ciprofloxacin is the drug of choice; other antibiotics are also effective (Figure 12.10). For *C. fetus*, ampicillin or third-generation cephalosporins are effective. Thorough cooking of potentially contaminated foods (for example, poultry) and pasteurization of milk and milk products is essential to prevention of campylobacteriosis. Also, surfaces used to prepare raw meat or poultry should be disinfected before using them for uncooked food, such as salads.

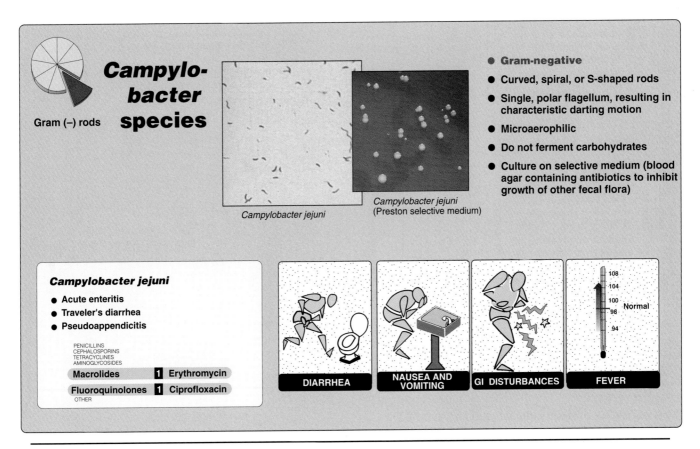

**Figure 12.10**
Summary of campylobacter disease.

# V. SHIGELLA

*Shigella* species cause shigellosis (bacillary dysentery)—a human intestinal disease that occurs most commonly among young children. Shigellae are nonmotile, unencapsulated, and Lac⁻. Most strains do not produce gas in a mixed acid fermentation of glucose.

## A. Epidemiology

Shigellae are typically spread from person to person, with contaminated stools serving as a major source of organisms. Flies and contaminated food or water can also transmit the disease. Shigellosis has a low infectious dose (fewer than 200 viable organisms are sufficient to cause disease). Hence, secondary cases within a household are common, particularly under conditions of crowding or poor sanitation. The forty serotypes of shigella are organized into four groups (A, B, C, and D) based on the serologic relatedness of their polysaccharide O antigens. Group D (*S. sonnei*) is the serogroup found most commonly in the United States.

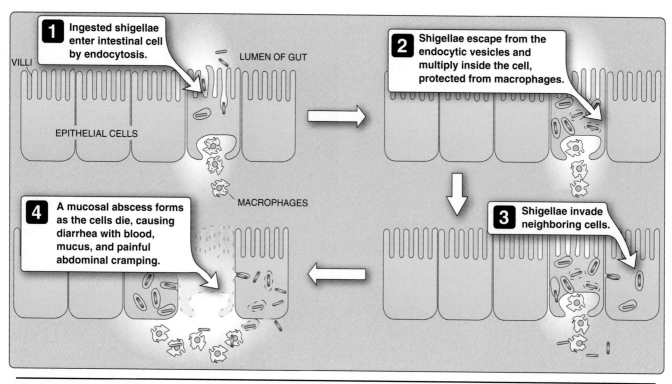

**Figure 12.11**
Mechanism of shigella infection causing diarrhea.

### B. Pathogenesis and clinical significance

Shigellae invade and destroy the mucosa of the large intestine. Infection rarely penetrates to deeper layers of the intestine, and does not lead to shigella bacteremia (Figure 12.11). An exotoxin (Shiga toxin) with enterotoxic and cytotoxic properties has been isolated from these organisms, and its toxicity may play a secondary role in development of intestinal lesions. Shigellae cause classic bacillary dysentery, characterized by diarrhea with blood, mucus, and painful abdominal cramping. The disease is generally most severe in the very young and elderly, and among malnourished individuals, in whom shigellosis may lead to severe dehydration and sometimes death. Among uncompromised populations, untreated dysentery commonly resolves in a week, but may persist longer.

### C. Laboratory identification

During acute illness, organisms can be cultured from stools using differential, selective Hektoen agar or other media specific for intestinal pathogens.

### D. Treatment and prevention

Antibiotics (for example, ciprofloxacin or azithromycin) can reduce the duration of illness and the period of shedding organisms, but usage is controversial because of widespread antibiotic resistance (Figure 12.12). Protection of the water and food supply, and per-

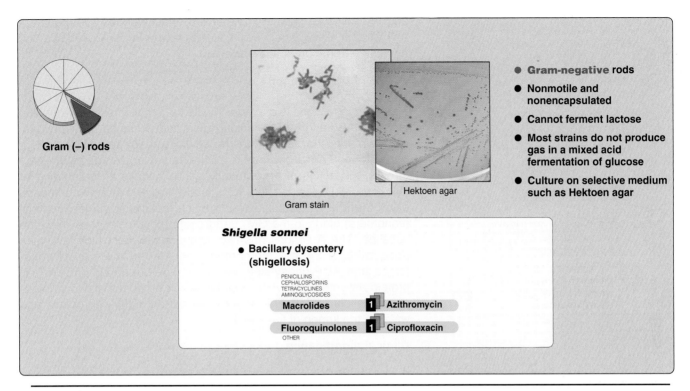

**Figure 12.12**
Summary of shigella disease.

sonal hygiene are crucial for preventing shigella infections. Vaccine development is currently in progress.

## VI. VIBRIOS

Members of the genus *Vibrio* are short, curved, rod-shaped organisms. *Vibrios* are closely related to the family Enterobacteriaceae. They are rapidly motile by means of a single polar flagellum. [Note: This contrasts with the peritrichous flagella (distributed all over the surface) of the motile Enterobacteriaceae.] O and H antigens are both present, but only O antigens are useful in distinguishing strains of vibrios that cause epidemics. Vibrios are facultative anaerobes. The growth of many *Vibrio* strains either requires or is stimulated by NaCl. Pathogenic vibrios include: 1) *V. cholerae*, serogroup O1 strains that are associated with epidemic cholera; 2) non-O1 *V. cholerae* and related strains that cause sporadic cases of choleralike and other illnesses; and 3) *V. parahaemolyticus* and other halophilic vibrios, which cause gastroenteritis and extraintestinal infections.

### A. Epidemiology

*V. cholerae* is transmitted by contaminated water and food. There are no known animal reservoirs, or animal or arthropod vectors. Among humans, long-term carriage is considered uncommon. There are two biotypes (subdivisions) of the species, *V. cholerae*: classic and El Tor. In contrast to the classic strain, the El Tor strain is distinguished by the production of hemolysins, higher carriage rates, and the ability to survive in water for longer periods. Outbreaks of both strains have been associated with raw or undercooked seafood harvested from contaminated waters.

## B. Pathogenesis

Following ingestion, *V. cholerae* infects the small intestine. Adhesion factor(s) are important for colonization and virulence. Achlorhydria, or treatments that lessen gastric acidity, greatly reduce the infectious dose. The organism is noninvasive, and causes disease through the action of an enterotoxin that initiates an outpouring of fluid (Figure 12.13). Cholera toxin is a multimeric protein composed of an A and a B subunit. The B subunit (consisting of five identical monomers) binds to the $GM_1$ ganglioside receptor of cells lining the intestine. The A subunit has two components: A2, which facilitates penetration of the cell membrane, and A1, an ADP-ribosyl transferase that ADP-ribosylates the membrane-bound $G_s$ protein.[1] $G_s$ protein activates adenylate cyclase, which produces elevated levels of intracellular cAMP. This, in turn, causes an outflowing of ions and water to the lumen of the intestine.

## C. Clinical significance

Full-blown cholera is characterized by massive loss of fluid and electrolytes from the body. After an incubation period ranging from hours to a few days, profuse watery diarrhea (rice-water stools) begins. Untreated, death from severe dehydration causing hypovolemic shock may occur in hours to days, and the death rate may exceed fifty percent. Appropriate treatment reduces the death rate to less than one percent. [Note: Non-O1 *V. cholerae* and other non-halophilic vibrios cause sporadic cases of cholera indistinguishable from that caused by *V. cholerae*, serotype O1. They also cause milder illness, comparable to that caused by enterotoxigenic *E. coli*.]

> Patients with suspected cholera need to be treated prior to laboratory confirmation, because death by dehydration can occur within hours.

## D. Laboratory identification

*V. cholerae* grows on standard media such as blood and MacConkey agars. Thiosulfate–citrate–bile salts–sucrose (TCBS) medium can enhance isolation. The organism is oxidase-positive, but further biochemical testing is necessary for specific identification of *V. cholerae*.

## E. Treatment and prevention

Replacement of fluids and electrolytes is crucial in preventing shock, and does not require bacteriologic diagnosis. Antibiotics (doxycycline is the drug of choice) can shorten the duration of diarrhea and excretion of the organism (Figure 12.14). Prevention relies primarily

**Figure 12.13**
Action of cholera toxin.

 [1]See p. 93 in ***Lippincott's Illustrated Reviews: Biochemistry*** (3rd ed.) for a discussion of the mechanism of action of $G_s$ proteins.

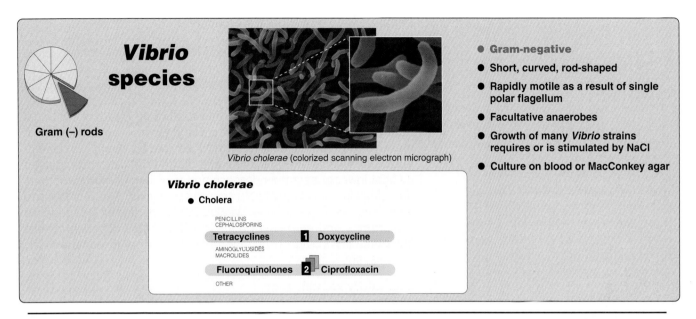

**Figure 12.14**
Summary of *Vibro* disease.

on public health measures that reduce fecal contamination of water supplies and food. Adequate cooking of foods can minimize transmission.

### F. Vibrio parahaemolyticus and other halophilic, noncholera vibrios

These organisms are characterized by a requirement for higher-than-usual concentrations of NaCl, and their ability to grow in ten percent NaCl. They are common in coastal sea waters. *V. parahaemolyticus* is associated with outbreaks of gastrointestinal illness that result from ingestion of contaminated and inadequately cooked seafood, especially shellfish and crustaceans. The disease is self-limiting, and antibiotics do not alter the course of infection. Neither human carriers nor other mammalian reservoirs have been identified. Other halophilic, noncholera vibrios are associated with soft tissue infections and septicemia resulting either from contact of wounds with contaminated sea water or from ingestion of contaminated seafood. For soft tissue infections, prompt administration of antibiotics, such as tetracycline or cefotaxime, is important, and surgical drainage/debridement may be required. Bacteremia is associated with high mortality, especially when caused by *V. vulnificus*.

## VII. YERSINIA

The genus *Yersinia* includes three species of medical importance: *Y. enterocolitica* and *Y. pseudotuberculosis*, both potential pathogens of the GI tract that are discussed in this chapter, and *Y. pestis*, the etiologic agent of bubonic plague, which is discussed in Chapter 13 (see p. 144). *Y. enterocolitica* and *Y. pseudotuberculosis* are both motile when grown at 25°C but not at 37°C. Multiple serotypes of both strains exist, and the V and W antigens are virulence factors. In contrast to most pathogenic Enterobacteriaceae, these strains of *Yersinia* grow well at room temperature as well as at 37°C. Most strains are Lac⁻.

## A. Pathogenesis and clinical significance

Infection occurs via ingestion of food that has become contaminated through contact with colonized domestic animals, abattoirs, or raw meat (especially pork). *Y. enterocolitica* is a relatively uncommon cause of enterocolitis in the United States, and *Y. pseudotuberculosis* is even rarer. Infection results in ulcerative lesions in the terminal ileum, necrotic lesions in Peyer patches, and enlargement of mesenteric lymph nodes. Enterocolitis caused by *Yersinia* is characterized by fever, abdominal pain, and diarrhea. When accompanied by right lower quadrant tenderness and leukocytosis, the symptoms are clinically indistinguishable from appendicitis. Symptoms commonly resolve in one to three weeks. Sequelae may include reactive polyarthritis and erythema nodosum. Other, less common clinical presentations include exudative pharyngitis and, in compromised patients, septicemia.

## B. Laboratory identification

*Yersinia* can be cultured from appropriate specimens on MacConkey or cefsulodin-irgasan-novobiocin (CIN, a medium selective for *Yersinia*) agars. Identification is based on biochemical screening. In the absence of a positive culture, serologic tests for anti-*Yersinia* antibodies may assist in diagnosis.

## C. Treatment and prevention

Reducing infections and outbreaks rests on measures to limit potential contamination of meat, ensuring its proper handling and preparation. Antibiotic therapy (for example, with ciprofloxacin or trimethoprim-sulfamethoxazole) is essential for systemic disease (sepsis), but is of questionable value for self-limited diseases such as enterocolitis (Figure 12.15).

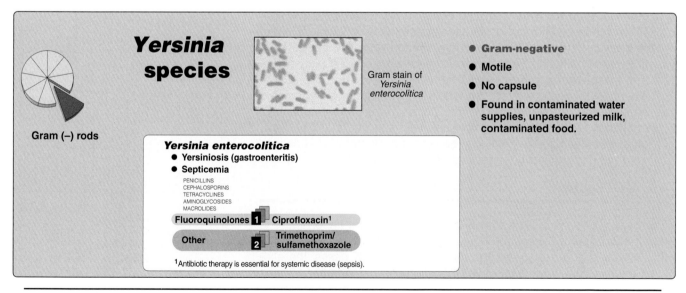

**Figure 12.15**
Summary of *Yersinia enterocolitica* disease.

## VIII. HELICOBACTER

Members of the genus *Helicobacter* are curved or spiral organisms (see Figure 12.17). They have a rapid, corkscrew motility resulting from multiple polar flagella. *H. pylori*, the species of human significance, is microaerophilic, and produces urease. It causes acute gastritis and duodenal and gastric ulcers. *H. pylori* (and several other *Helicobacter* species) are unusual in their ability to colonize the stomach, where low pH normally protects against bacterial infection. *H. pylori* infections are relatively common and worldwide in distribution.

### A. Pathogenesis

Transmission of *H. pylori* is thought to be from person to person; the organism has not been isolated from food or water. Untreated, infections tend to be chronic, even lifelong. *H. pylori* colonizes gastric mucosal (epithelial) cells in the stomach, and metaplastic gastric epithelium in the duodenum or esophagus, but does not colonize the rest of the intestinal epithelium. The organism survives in the mucous layer that coats the epithelium, and causes chronic inflammation of the mucosa (Figure 12.16). Although the organism is non-invasive, it recruits and activates inflammatory cells. Urease released by *H. pylori* produces ammonia ions that neutralize stomach acid in the vicinity of the organism, favoring bacterial multiplication. Ammonia may also both cause injury and potentiate the effects of a cytotoxin produced by *H. pylori*.

**Figure 12.16**
*Helicobacter pylori* infection, resulting in ulceration of the stomach.

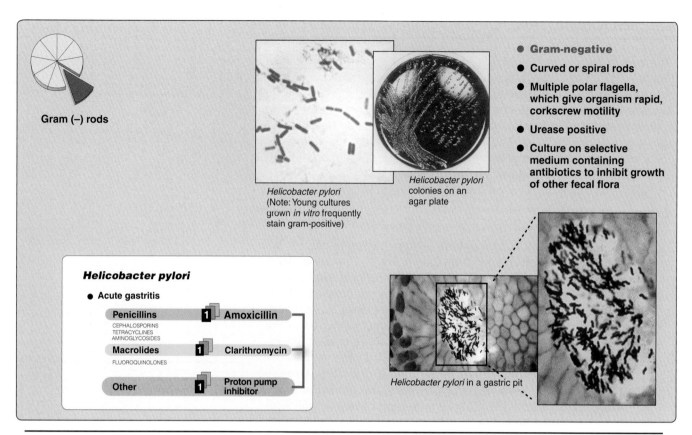

Gram (–) rods

*Helicobacter pylori*
(Note: Young cultures
grown *in vitro* frequently
stain gram-positive)

*Helicobacter pylori*
colonies on an
agar plate

● **Gram-negative**
● Curved or spiral rods
● Multiple polar flagella, which give organism rapid, corkscrew motility
● Urease positive
● Culture on selective medium containing antibiotics to inhibit growth of other fecal flora

*Helicobacter pylori* in a gastric pit

*Helicobacter pylori*

● Acute gastritis

| Penicillins | 1 | Amoxicillin |
CEPHALOSPORINS
TETRACYCLINES
AMINOGLYCOSIDES

| Macrolides | 1 | Clarithromycin |
FLUOROQUINOLONES

| Other | 1 | Proton pump inhibitor |

**Figure 12.17**
Summary of helicobacter disease.

## B. Clinical significance

Initial infection with *H. pylori* causes acute gastritis, sometimes with diarrhea that lasts about one week. The infection usually becomes chronic, with diffuse, superficial gastritis that may be associated with epigastric discomfort. Both duodenal ulcers and gastric ulcers are closely correlated with infection by *H. pylori*. [Note: *H. pylori* infection is found in more than 95 percent of duodenal ulcer patients and in nearly all patients with gastric ulcers who do not use aspirin or other nonsteroidal antiinflammatory drugs, both risk factors for gastric ulcers.] *H. pylori* infection appears to be a risk factor for development of gastric carcinoma and gastric B-cell lymphoma [mucosa-associated lymphoid tumors (MALTomas)].

## C. Laboratory identification

Noninvasive diagnostic tests include serologic tests (ELISA for serum antibodies to *H. pylori*, see p. 28) and breath tests for urease. [Note: Breath tests involve administering radioactively labeled urea by mouth. If *H. pylori* are present in the patient's stomach, the urease produced by the organism will split the urea to $CO_2$ (radioactively labeled and exhaled) and $NH_3$.] Invasive tests involve gastric biopsy specimens obtained by endoscopy. *H. pylori* can be detected in such specimens histologically, by culture, or by a test for urease.

## D. Treatment and prevention

Elimination of *H. pylori* requires combination therapy with two or more antibiotics. Although *H. pylori* is innately sensitive to many antibiotics, resistance readily develops. A typical regimen includes amoxicillin plus clarithromycin plus a proton pump inhibitor, such as omeprazole (Figure 12.17).

# IX. OTHER ENTEROBACTERIACEAE

Other genera of Enterobacteriaceae, such as Klebsiella, Enterobacter, *Proteus*, and *Serratia*, which can be found as normal inhabitants of the large intestine, include organisms that are primarily opportunistic and often nosocomial pathogens. Widespread antibiotic resistance among these organisms necessitates sensitivity testing to determine the appropriate antibiotic treatment.

## A. Enterobacter

*Enterobacter* species are motile and Lac⁺. They rarely cause primary disease in humans, but frequently colonize hospitalized patients, especially in association with antibiotic treatment, indwelling catheters, or invasive procedures. These organisms may infect burns, wounds, and the respiratory (causing pneumonia), or urinary tracts.

## B. Klebsiella

Klebsiellae are large, nonmotile bacilli that possess a luxurious capsule (see Figure 12.17). They are Lac⁺. *K. pneumoniae* and *K. oxytoca* cause necrotizing lobar pneumonia in individuals compromised by alcoholism, diabetes, or chronic obstructive pulmonary disease. *K. pneumoniae* also causes urinary tract infections and bacteremia, particularly in hospitalized patients.

## C. Serratia

*Serratia* are motile and ferment lactose slowly, if at all. The species of *Serratia* that most frequently causes human infection is *S. marcescens*. *Serratia* can cause extraintestinal infections such as those of the lower respiratory and urinary tracts, especially among hospitalized patients.

## D. Proteus, Providencia, and Morganella

Members of these genera are agents of urinary tract and other extraintestinal infections. *Proteus* species are relatively common causes of uncomplicated as well as nosocomial UTIs. Other extraintestinal infections, such as wound infections, pneumonias, and septicemias, are associated with compromised patients. *Proteus* organisms produce urease, which catalyzes the hydrolysis of urea to ammonia. The resulting alkaline environment promotes the precipitation of struvite stones containing insoluble phosphates of magnesium and phosphate.

**Figure 12.18**
Micrograph showing rod-shaped *Klebsiella pneumoniae* cells.

## Study Questions

**Choose the ONE correct answer**

12.1 A Lac⁺, glucose-fermenting, gram-negative rod isolated from a previously healthy child with bloody diarrhea is most likely to be

A. *Shigella sonnei.*

B. *Pseudomonas aeruginosa.*

C. *Escherichia coli.*

D. *Salmonella enterica.*

E. *Helicobacter pylori.*

> Correct answer = C. *E. coli* is Lac⁺, and enteroin-
> vasive strains characteristically cause a dysen-
> terylike syndrome. Shigella characteristically
> causes bloody diarrhea (dysentery) but is Lac⁻. *P.
> aeruginosa* characteristically causes infections in
> compromised hosts, and is Lac⁻. Salmonella is
> also Lac⁻. *H. pylori* causes gastritis.

12.2 An elderly man, hospitalized and recovering from cardiac bypass surgery, develops pneumonia. Sputum
culture reveals a gram-negative rod that produces a
green pigment but does not ferment carbohydrates.
The most likely organism is

A. *Klebsiella pneumoniae.*

B. *Serratia* species.

C. *Proteus* species.

D. *Enterobacter* species.

E. *Pseudomonas aeruginosa.*

> Correct answer = E. All five organisms are oppor-
> tunists capable of causing pneumonia in compro-
> mised patients. However, the first four are
> members of the family Enterobacteriaceae and,
> by definition, can ferment carbohydrates. In addi-
> tion, none of the organisms is known to produce a
> green pigment, although serratia may produce a
> red pigment. *P. aeruginosa* is an obligate aerobe
> that uses respiratory pathways exclusively.
> Production of green pyocyanin pigment regularly
> occurs.

12.3 An elderly, alcoholic male develops severe, necrotizing lobar pneumonia. The organism is Lac⁺ and produces a luxuriant capsule. The most likely agent is

A. *Klebsiella pneumoniae.*

B. *Serratia* species.

C. *Yersinia pseudotuberculosis.*

D. *Pseudomonas aeruginosa.*

E. *Campylobacter fetus.*

> Correct answer = A. The combination of necrotiz-
> ing pneumonia and an alcoholic patient suggests
> *K. pneumoniae*, and the laboratory data (Lac⁺
> and a luxuriant capsule) are consistent. Serratia
> can cause pneumonia in compromised patients;
> necrosis is not a characteristic feature, the organ-
> ism ferments lactose slowly if at all, and does not
> have a luxuriant capsule. *Y. pseudotuberculosis*
> is Lac⁻, and rarely causes pneumonia. *Pseudo-
> monas aeruginosa* can cause pneumonia in com-
> promised patients, but does not ferment lactose.
> *C. fetus* typically causes bacteremia and dissemi-
> nated infections.

"I'm sorry, it's salmonella"

# Other Gram-negative Rods

# 13

## I. OVERVIEW

Although not part of a closely related family, the organisms covered in this chapter do share two significant features of structure and physiology. First, they all have a gram-negative cell envelope and, therefore, contain lipopolysaccharide (LPS), which is a virulence factor. Second, they grow in the presence of oxygen and, therefore, cause infections at sites where oxygen tension is high (for example, in the lungs, and other vital tissues). It is helpful to consider these organisms as follows: 1) those that are primarily or exclusively pathogens of the human respiratory tract (*Haemophilus, Bordetella,* and *Legionella*), 2) one genus that includes an extremely successful opportunistic pathogen (*Pseudomonas*), and 3) those that are primarily pathogens of animals (that is, zoonotic organisms such as *Brucella, Francisella, and Pasteurella,* for which humans are accidental hosts). Although *Yersinia pestis* is a member of the family Enterobacteriaceae (covered in Chapter 12), it is included in this chapter because it is a nongastrointestinal, gram-negative rod. *Bartonella*, another unusual gram-negative rod that is responsible for trench fever and catscratch disease, is also described here. The organisms covered in this chapter are listed in Figure 13.1.

## II. HAEMOPHILUS

Cells of *Haemophilus influenzae*—the major human pathogen of this genus—are pleomorphic, ranging from coccobacilli to long, slender filaments. *H. influenzae* may produce a capsule (six capsular types have been distinguished) or may be unencapsulated (Figure 13.2). The capsule is an important virulence factor. Serious, invasive *H. influenzae* disease is associated particularly with capsular type b (Hib), which is composed of polyribose phosphate. Hib is especially important as a pathogen of young children, although it can cause disease in individuals of all age groups. Nontypeable (unencapsulated) strains may also cause serious disease, and are a significant cause of pneumonia among the elderly and individuals with chronic lung disease.

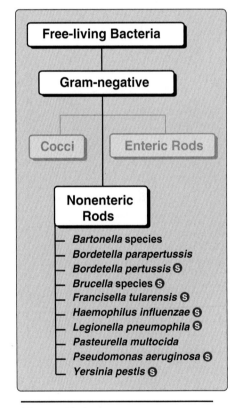

**Free-living Bacteria**

**Gram-negative**

Cocci        Enteric Rods

**Nonenteric Rods**

— *Bartonella* species
— *Bordetella parapertussis*
— *Bordetella pertussis* Ⓢ
— *Brucella* species Ⓢ
— *Francisella tularensis* Ⓢ
— *Haemophilus influenzae* Ⓢ
— *Legionella pneumophila* Ⓢ
— *Pasteurella multocida*
— *Pseudomonas aeruginosa* Ⓢ
— *Yersinia pestis* Ⓢ

**Figure 13.1**
Classification of other gram-negative rods. Ⓢ See p. 331 for summaries of these organisms.

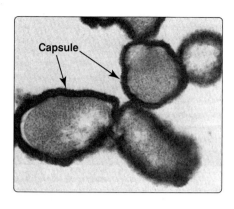

**Figure 13.2**
*Haemphilus influenzae* (electron micrograph) showing thick capsule.

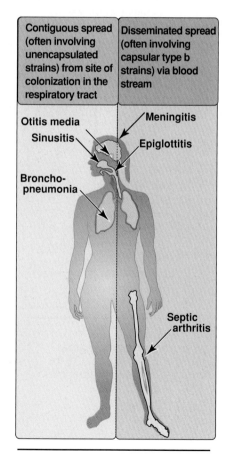

**Figure 13.3**
Infections caused by *Haemophilus influenzae*.

## A. Epidemiology

*H. influenzae* is a normal component of the upper respiratory tract flora in humans, and may also colonize the conjunctiva and genital tract. Humans are the only natural hosts, and colonization begins shortly after birth, with unencapsulated strains and capsular type b being carried most frequently. *H. influenzae* illnesses are usually sporadic in occurrence.

## B. Pathogenesis

*H. influenzae* is transmitted by respiratory droplets. IgA protease produced by the organism degrades secretory IgA, facilitating colonization of the upper respiratory tract mucosa. From this site, *H. influenzae* can enter the bloodstream and disseminate to distant sites. Diseases caused by *H. influenzae*, therefore, fall into two categories (Figure 13.3). First, disorders such as otitis media, sinusitis, epiglottitis, and bronchopneumonia result from contiguous spread of the organism from its site of colonization in the respiratory tract. Second, disorders such as meningitis, septic arthritis, and cellulitis result from invasion of the bloodstream, followed by localization of *H. influenzae* in these and other areas of the body.

## C. Clinical significance

*H. influenzae* has been a leading cause of bacterial meningitis, primarily in infants and very young children, frequently in conjunction with an episode of otitis media. A vaccine against *H. influenzae* type b, administered to infants, has dramatically decreased the frequency of such infections (Figure 13.4). Clinically, *H. influenzae* meningitis is indistinguishable from other purulent meningitides, and may be gradual in onset or fulminant (sudden onset with great severity).

> Mortality from meningitis is high in untreated patients, but appropriate therapy reduces mortality to about five percent. Survivors may be left with permanent neurologic sequelae.

## D. Laboratory identification

A definitive diagnosis generally requires identification of the organism; for example, by culture on chocolate agar. Isolation from normally sterile sites and fluids such as blood, cerebrospinal fluid (CSF), or synovial fluid, is significant, whereas isolation from pharyngeal cultures is inconclusive. Rapid diagnosis is crucial because of the potentially fulminant course of type b infections. In cases of meningitis, Gram staining of CSF commonly reveals pleomorphic, gram-negative coccobacilli (Figure 13.5). Type b capsule may be demonstrated directly in CSF, either by the capsular swelling (quellung) reaction (see p. 27) or by immunofluorescent staining (see p. 29). Capsular antigen may be detected in CSF or other body fluids using immunologic tests, such as latex agglutination, countercurrent immunoelectrophoresis, and radioimmune assay.

## E. Treatment

When invasive *H. influenzae* is suspected, a suitable antibiotic (for example, a third-generation cephalosporin such as ceftriaxone or cefotaxime) should be started as soon as appropriate specimens have been taken for culture (see Figure 13.5). Antibiotic sensitivity testing is necessary because of emergence of strains resistant to antibiotics commonly used to treat *H. influenzae* (for example, strains with β-lactamase-mediated ampicillin resistance). Sinusitis, otitis media, and other upper respiratory tract infections are treated with trimethoprim-sulfamethoxazole or ampicillin plus clavulanate.

## F. Prevention

Active immunization against Hib is effective in preventing invasive disease, and also reduces respiratory carriage of Hib (see Figure 13.4). The current vaccine, generally given to children younger than two, consists of Hib polyribose phosphate (PRP) capsular carbohydrate conjugated to a carrier protein (see p. 35). Rifampin is given prophylactically to individuals in close contact with a patient infected with *H. influenzae*—particularly those patients with invasive disease (for example, *H. influenzae* meningitis).

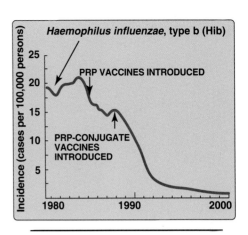

**Figure 13.4**
Incidence of *Haemophilus influenzae* type b meningitis in a pediatric population in the United States.

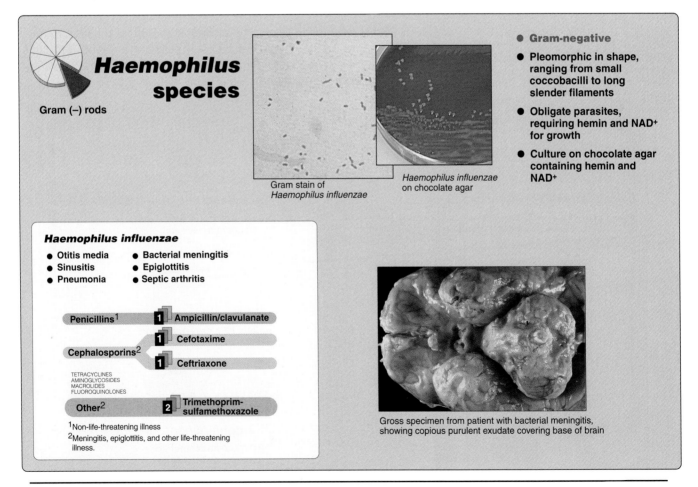

**Figure 13.5**
Summary of haemophilus  isease

## III. BORDETELLA

*Bordetella pertussis* and *B. parapertussis* are the human pathogens of this genus. The former causes the disease pertussis (also known as whooping cough), and the latter causes a mild pertussis-like illness. Whooping cough is a highly contagious disease and a significant cause of morbidity and mortality worldwide (51 million cases and 600,000 deaths each year). Members of the genus *Bordetella* are aerobic. They are small, encapsulated coccobacilli that grow singly or in pairs. They can be serotyped on the basis of cell-surface molecules termed "agglutinogens."

### A. Epidemiology

The major mode of transmission of *Bordetella* is via droplets spread by coughing, but the organism survives only briefly outside the human respiratory tract. The incidence of whooping cough among different age-groups can vary substantially, depending on whether active immunization of young children is widespread in the community. In the absence of an immunization program, disease is most common among young children (ages one to five).

### B. Pathogenesis

*B. pertussis* binds to ciliated epithelium in the upper respiratory tract (see Figure 13.9). There, the bacteria produce a variety of toxins and other virulence factors that interfere with ciliary activity, eventually causing death of these cells (Figure 13.6).

**Figure 13.6**
Toxins produced by *Bordetella pertussis*.

## C. Clinical significance

The incubation period for pertussis generally ranges from one to three weeks (Figure 13.7). The disease can be divided into two phases: catarrhal and paroxysmal.

1. **Catarrhal phase:** This phase begins with relatively nonspecific symptoms such as rhinorrhea, mild conjunctival infection (hyperemia, or bloodshot), malaise, and/or mild fever, and then progresses to include a dry, nonproductive cough.

2. **Paroxysmal phase:** With worsening of the cough, the paroxysmal phase begins. The term whooping cough derives from the paroxysms of coughing followed by a "whoop" as the patient inspires rapidly. Large amounts of mucus may be produced. Paroxysms may cause cyanosis and/or end with vomiting. [Note: Whooping may not occur in all patients.] Pertussis typically causes leukocytosis that can be quite striking as the total white blood cell count sometimes exceeds 50,000 cells/μL (normal range = 4500–11,000 white blood cells/μL), with a striking predominance of lymphocytes. Following the paroxysmal phase, convalescence requires at least an additional three to four weeks. During this period, secondary complications such as infections (for example, otitis media and pneumonia) and CNS dysfunction (for example, encephalopathy or seizures) may occur. Disease is generally most severe in infants.

## D. Laboratory identification

Presumptive diagnosis may be made on clinical grounds once the paroxysmal phase of classic pertussis begins. Pertussis may be suspected in an individual who has onset of catarrhal symptoms within one to three weeks of exposure to a diagnosed case of pertussis. Culture of *B. pertussis* from the nasopharynx of a symptomatic patient supports the diagnosis. The organism produces pinpoint colonies in three to six days on selective agar medium, for example, one that contains blood and charcoal, which serves to absorb and/or neutralize inhibitory substances, and is supplemented with antibiotics to inhibit growth of normal flora. More rapid diagno-

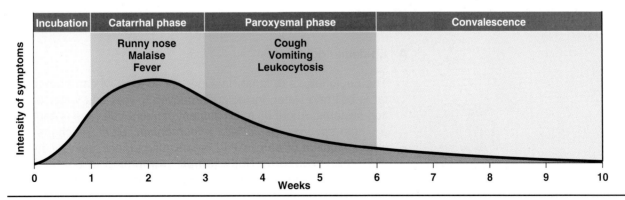

**Figure 13.7**
Clinical presentation of *Bordetella pertussis* disease.

**Figure 13.8**
A. Reported case of pertussis.
B. Incidence of pertussis by age group, United States (2000).

sis may be accomplished using a direct fluorescent antibody (DFA) test to detect *B. pertussis* in smears of nasopharyngeal specimens. Serologic tests for antibodies to *B. pertussis* are primarily useful for epidemiologic surveys.

### E. Treatment

Erythromycin is the drug of choice for infections with *B. pertussis*, both as chemotherapy (where it reduces both the duration and severity of disease), and as chemoprophylaxis for household contacts (see Figure 13.9). For erythromycin treatment failures, trimethoprim-sulfamethoxazole is an alternative choice.

> Patients are most contagious during the catarrhal stage and during the first two weeks after onset of coughing. Treatment of the infected individuals during this period limits the spread of infection among household contacts.

### F. Prevention

Pertussis vaccine is available that has had a significant effect on lowering the incidence of whooping cough. It contains proteins purified from *B. pertussis*, and is formulated in combination with diphtheria and tetanus toxoids (see p. 38). To protect infants who are at greatest risk of life-threatening *B. pertussis* disease, immunization is generally initiated when the infant is two months old. The availability of an effective vaccine led to a dramatic decrease in the incidence of the disease in the United States (Figure 13.8).

## IV. LEGIONELLA

Legionellaceae are facultative intracellular parasites that cause primarily respiratory tract infections. In nature, *Legionella* cells are unencapsulated, relatively slender rods; however, in clinical material, they appear coccobacillary in shape (see Figure 13.11). Members of the Legionellaceae family are aerobic and fastidious, with a particular requirement for L-cysteine.

### A. Epidemiology

The Legionellaceae family includes 34 species whose normal habitat is soil and water, including in cooling towers and water distribution systems. About 85 to 90 percent of human disease is caused by a single species, *Legionella pneumophila*. Most infections result from inhalation of aerosolized organisms but, occasionally, may follow other exposures (for example, swimming in contaminated water). Both sporadic cases and localized outbreaks may occur. One famous outbreak occurred in 1976 during a convention of American Legion members (hence the name, *Legionella*). The

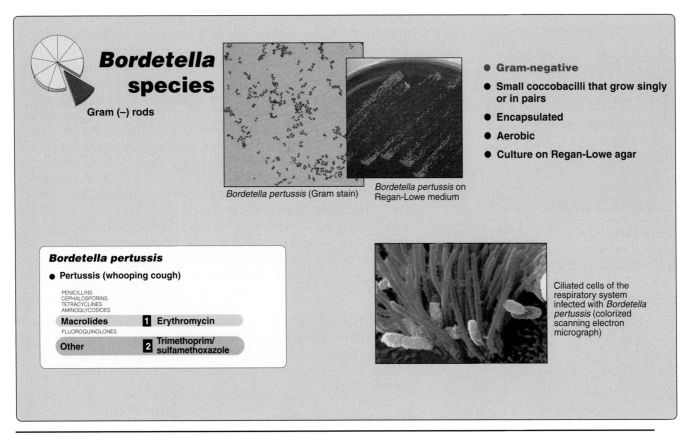

*Bordetella species*

Gram (–) rods

*Bordetella pertussis* (Gram stain)

*Bordetella pertussis* on Regan-Lowe medium

- Gram-negative
- Small coccobacilli that grow singly or in pairs
- Encapsulated
- Aerobic
- Culture on Regan-Lowe agar

**Bordetella pertussis**

- Pertussis (whooping cough)

PENICILLINS
CEPHALOSPORINS
TETRACYCLINES
AMINOGLYCOSIDES

Macrolides        **1** Erythromycin

FLUOROQUINOLONES

Other             **2** Trimethoprim/ sulfamethoxazole

Ciliated cells of the respiratory system infected with *Bordetella pertussis* (colorized scanning electron micrograph)

**Figure 13.9**
Summary of bordetella disease.

organism is chlorine tolerant and thus survives water treatment procedures.

## B. Pathogenesis

The organism gains entry to the upper respiratory tract by aspiration of water containing the organism, or by inhalation of a contaminated aerosol. Failure to clear the organisms permits them to reach the lungs. Alveolar macrophages in the lung bed normally constitute an important line of defense for clearing invading organisms. Although the macrophages do phagocytose *L. pneumophila*, the resulting phagosome fails to fuse with a lysosome. Instead, the organisms multiply within the protected environment of the phagosome until the cell ruptures, releasing a new crop of bacteria.

## C. Clinical significance

Legionellaceae primarily cause respiratory tract infections. There are two distinctly different presentations: Legionnaires' disease and Pontiac fever. The factors that determine which presentation will occur are not understood, although the condition of the host likely plays a role.

**Figure 13.10**
Common pathogens causing community-acquired pneumonia.

1. **Legionnaires' disease (LD):** This is an atypical, acute lobar pneumonia with multisystem symptoms. It may occur sporadically or in outbreaks (for example, nosocomial outbreaks have occurred). LD typically develops in only one to five percent of individuals exposed to a common source. Legionellae are estimated to cause one to five percent of the cases of community-acquired pneumonias in adults (Figure 13.10). The case fatality rate for LD ranges from five to thirty percent, a high rate that may reflect the fact that many LD patients have additional contributing factors, such as pulmonary or immunocompromise. Symptoms develop after an incubation period ranging from two to ten days. Early symptoms may be relatively nonspecific: fever, malaise, myalgia, anorexia, and/or headache. The severity and range of symptoms associated with LD vary substantially. A cough that is only slightly productive then appears, sometimes with respiratory compromise. Diarrhea (watery rather than bloody stools) occurs in 25 to 50 percent of cases. Nausea, vomiting, and neurologic symptoms may also occur.

2. **Pontiac fever:** This is an influenza-like illness that characteristically infects otherwise healthy individuals. The attack rate among those exposed to a common source is typically ninety percent or more. Recovery is usually complete within one week. No specific therapy is required.

### D. Laboratory identification

LD cannot be diagnosed unambiguously on the basis of clinical presentation or radiologic appearance of lungs. Although the organism can be Gram stained, the Gimenez stain is more useful for visualization. The definitive method of diagnosis involves the culturing of *Legionella* from respiratory secretions, using buffered (pH 6.9) charcoal yeast extract (Figure 13.11) enriched with L-cysteine, iron, and α-ketoglutarate. Visible colonies form in three to five days. A urinary antigen test using an enzyme immunoassay is available and has several advantages over culture. For example, the test positivity can persist for days even during administration of antibiotic therapy making it useful in patients who receive empiric anti-Legionella therapy. Further, the results of the urinary antigen test can be available within hours, whereas culture results require three to five days.

 When Legionnaires disease is suspected, both a urinary antigen test and legionella culture of a respiratory specimen should be ordered.

### E. Treatment

Macrolides, such as erythromycin or azithromycin, are the drugs of choice for Legionnaires disease. Fluoroquinolones are also effective (Figure 13.11). Pontiac fever is usually treated symptomatically, without antibiotics.

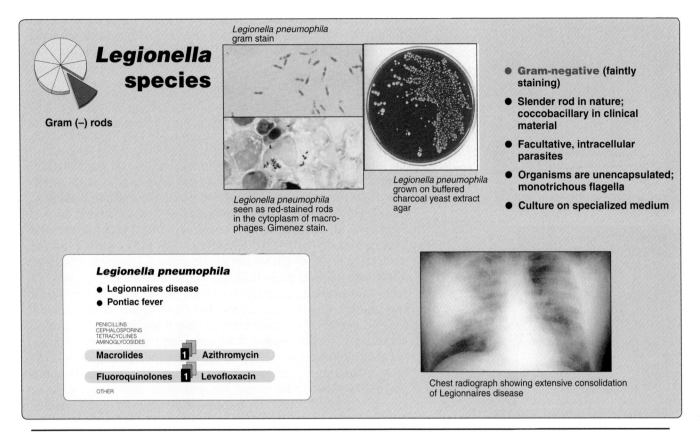

**Legionella species**

Gram (–) rods

*Legionella pneumophila* gram stain

*Legionella pneumophila* seen as red-stained rods in the cytoplasm of macrophages. Gimenez stain.

*Legionella pneumophila* grown on buffered charcoal yeast extract agar

- **Gram-negative (faintly staining)**
- Slender rod in nature; coccobacillary in clinical material
- Facultative, intracellular parasites
- Organisms are unencapsulated; monotrichous flagella
- Culture on specialized medium

**Legionella pneumophila**
- Legionnaires disease
- Pontiac fever

PENICILLINS
CEPHALOSPORINS
TETRACYCLINES
AMINOGLYCOSIDES

Macrolides — 1 — Azithromycin

Fluoroquinolones — 1 — Levofloxacin

OTHER

Chest radiograph showing extensive consolidation of Legionnaires disease

**Figure 13.11**
Summary of legionella disease.

# V. PSEUDOMONAS

*Pseudomonas aeruginosa*, the primary human pathogen in the genus *Pseudomonas*, is widely distributed in nature (it is found in soil, water, plants, and animals). Although it may colonize healthy humans without causing disease, it is also a significant opportunistic pathogen and a major cause of nosocomial (hospital-acquired) infections. *P. aeruginosa* is regularly a cause of nosocomial pneumonia, nosocomial urinary tract infections, surgical site infections, infections of severe burns, and infections of patients undergoing either chemotherapy for neoplastic disease or antibiotic therapy. *P. aeruginosa* is motile (it has polar flagella), encapsulated, and obligately aerobic (it oxidizes but does not ferment carbohydrates). Nutritional requirements are minimal, and the organism can grow on a wide variety of organic substrates. In fact, *P. aeruginosa* can even grow in laboratory water baths, hot tubs, wet IV tubing, and other water-containing vessels. This explains why the organism is responsible for so many nosocomial infections.

## A. Pathogenesis

*P. aeruginosa* disease begins with attachment to and colonization of host tissue. Pili on the bacteria mediate adherence, and a glycocalyx capsule reduces the effectiveness of normal clearance mechanisms. Host tissue damage facilitates adherence and colonization. *P. aeruginosa* produces numerous toxins and extracellular products that promote local invasion and dissemination of the organism.

### B. Clinical significance

*P. aeruginosa* causes both localized and systemic illness. Virtually any tissue or organ system may be affected. Individuals most at risk include those with impaired immune defenses.

1. **Localized infections:** These may occur in the eye (keratitis and endophthalmitis, following trauma), ear (external otitis or swimmer's ear; invasive and necrotizing otitis externa, particularly in elderly diabetic patients or trauma patients), skin (wound sepsis, Figure 13.12, pustular rashes occurring in epidemics associated with use of contaminated whirlpools, hot tubs, and swimming pools), urinary tract (particularly in hospitalized patients who have been subjected to catheterization, instrumentation, surgery, or renal transplantation), respiratory tract (pneumonia in individuals with chronic lung disease, congestive heart failure, or cystic fibrosis, and particularly in patients who have been intubated or are on ventilators), gastrointestinal tract (infections range from relatively mild diarrheal illness in children to severe, necrotizing enterocolitis in infants and neutropenic cancer patients), and the central nervous system (CNS; meningitis and brain abscesses, particularly in association with trauma, surgery, or tumors of the head or neck). Localized infections have the potential to lead to disseminated infection. [Note: The organism has a propensity to invade blood vessel walls.]

2. **Systemic infections:** Infections reflecting systemic spread of the organism include bacteremia (most common in patients whose immune system has been compromised), secondary pneumonia, bone and joint infections (in IV drug users and patients with urinary tract or pelvic infections), endocarditis (in IV drug users and patients with prosthetic heart valves), CNS (mainly when the meninges are breached), and skin/soft tissue infections.

> *P. aeruginosa* is feared because it can cause severe hospital-acquired infections, especially in immunocompromised hosts; it is often antibiotic resistant, complicating the choice of therapy.

### C. Laboratory identification

*P. aeruginosa* can be isolated by plating on a variety of media, both nonselective (for example, blood agar) and moderately selective (for example, MacConkey agar, Figure 13.13). Identification is based on the results of a battery of biochemical and other diagnostic tests. Serologic typing is used in the investigation of clusters of cases, which may stem from exposure to a common source. [Note: A clue to its presence is a characteristic fruity odor, both in the laboratory and at the bedside.]

**1** A 16-year-old wrestler presented with an auricular hematoma.

**2** One day after surgery to repair cartilage, infection with *Pseudomonas aeruginosa* developed.

**3** Appearance of ear three months after completion of gentamicin therapy.

**Figure 13.12**
*Pseudomonas* infection of the pinna of the ear.

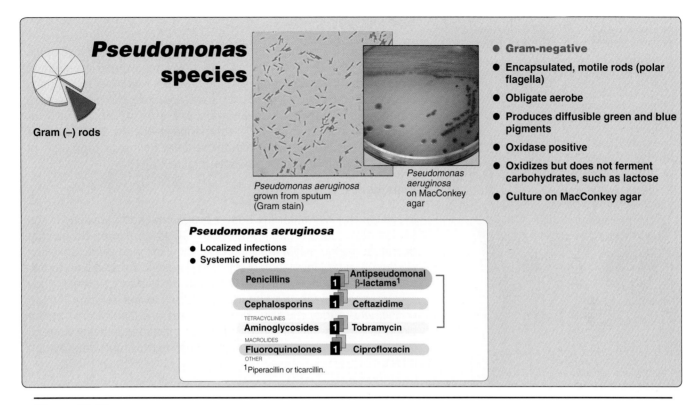

**Figure 13.13**
Summary of pseudomonas disease.

## D. Treatment and Prevention

Specific therapy varies with the clinical presentation and the antibiotic sensitivity pattern of the isolate. It is difficult to find antibiotics effective against *P. aeruginosa*, because of its rapid development of resistance mutations and its own innate mechanisms of antibiotic resistance. Pseudomonas infections typically occur in patients with impaired defenses. Therefore, aggressive antimicrobial therapy (often a combination of two bactericidal antibiotics, such as an aminoglycoside, an antipseudomonal β-lactam, or a quinolone) is generally required (see Figure 13.13).

## VI. BRUCELLA

Members of the genus *Brucella* are primarily pathogens of animals (domestic and feral). Thus, brucellosis (undulant fever) is a zoonosis (a disease of animals that may be transmitted to humans under natural conditions). Different species of *Brucella* are each associated with particular animal species; for example, *B. abortus* (cattle), *B. melitensis* (goats and sheep), *B. suis* (swine), *B. canis* (dogs), and *B. ovis* (sheep). All but *B. ovis* are known to cause disease in humans. The brucellae are aerobic, facultative, intracellular parasites that can survive and multiply within host phagocytes. Cells of the genus *Brucella* are unencapsulated, small coccobacilli arranged singly or in pairs (see Figure 13.15). Lipopolysaccharide is the major virulence factor, as well as the major cell wall antigen.

**Figure 13.14**
Transmission of *Brucella*.

## A. Epidemiology

Brucellosis is a chronic, lifelong infection in animals. Organisms localize in reproductive organs (male and female), and are shed in large numbers in milk, urine, and the placenta and other tissues discharged during delivery or spontaneous abortion. The primary manifestations of infection in animals are sterility and abortion. Transmission to humans characteristically occurs as a result of either direct contact with infected animal tissue or ingestion of unpasteurized milk or milk products (Figure 13.14).

## B. Pathogenesis

Brucellae typically enter the body through cuts and abrasions in the skin or through the gastrointestinal (GI) tract. [Note: Drugs that decrease gastric acidity may increase the likelihood of transmission via the GI route.] Inhalation of infected aerosols can also lead to disease among abattoir workers. Once the organisms gain entry, they are transported via the lymphatic system to the regional lymph nodes, where they multiply. The organisms are then carried by the blood to organs that are involved in the reticuloendothelial system, including the liver, spleen, kidneys, bone marrow, and other lymph nodes.

## C. Clinical significance

The incubation period for *Brucella* infections ranges from five days to several months, but typically lasts several weeks. Symptoms are nonspecific and flulike (malaise, fever, sweats, anorexia, GI symptoms, headache, and back pains), and may also include depression. Their onset may be abrupt or insidious. Objective clinical findings are often few and mild, in contrast to the patient's subjective evaluation. Untreated, patients may develop an undulating pattern of fever (temperatures repeatedly rise then fall, hence the name "undulant fever" is the traditional name for brucellosis). Subclinical infections occur. Manifestations of brucellosis may involve any of a variety of organ systems, including the GI tract, and the skeletal, neurologic, cardiovascular, and pulmonary systems.

> In industrialized countries, brucellosis is largely an occupational disease, occurring in ranchers, dairy farmers, abattoir workers, and veterinarians.

## D. Laboratory identification

Although the nonspecific symptoms may not point to a diagnosis of brucellosis, a detailed history is often crucial, including the patient's occupation, exposure to animals, travel to countries where brucella infection is prevalent, or ingestion of potentially contaminated foods. The organism can be cultured from blood and other body fluids or from tissue specimens. Multiple blood specimens should be cultured. For plated materials, colonies may appear in four to five days; however, longer times are required for blood cultures, and these are routinely examined for up to one month before being declared negative.

**Brucella species**

Gram (–) rods

*Brucella melitensis* (Gram stain)

*Brucella* species on sheep blood agar

- Gram-negative
- Small coccobacilli, arranged singly or in pairs
- Unencapsulated
- Aerobic
- Intracellular parasites
- Culture on blood agar

**Brucella species**
- Brucellosis (undulant fever)

PENICILLINS
CEPHALOSPORINS
**Tetracyclines** 1 **Doxycycline**
**Aminoglycosides** 1 **Gentamicin**[1]
MACROLIDES
FLUOROQUINOLONES
OTHER
                    [1]Or streptomycin

FEVER | DIAPHORESIS | ANOREXIA | GI DISTURBANCES

**Figure 13.15**
Summary of brucella disease.

## E. Treatment

Combination therapy involving doxycycline and gentamicin (or streptomycin) is generally recommended for brucellosis (Figure 13.15). Prolonged treatment (for example, six weeks) is generally necessary to prevent relapse and reduce the incidence of complications.

## VII. FRANCISELLA TULARENSIS

*Francisella tularensis* is primarily a pathogen of animals. Thus, tularemia (also known as rabbit fever and deerfly fever) is a zoonosis. The cells are small, pleomorphic coccobacilli that possess a lipid-rich capsule, which, although nontoxic, may be a virulence factor (Figure 13.16). Members of the genus *Francisella* are facultative intracellular parasites that can survive and multiply within host macrophages, as well as in other types of cells. The organisms are strict aerobes.

### A. Epidemiology

The host range of *F. tularensis* is broad, and includes wild and domestic mammals, birds, and house pets. A number of biting or blood-sucking arthropods (for example, ticks, lice, and mites) can serve as vectors. Infection of humans occurs as a result of contact with infected animal tissues or the bite of an infected arthropod. Within particular geographic regions, specific vertebrates and invertebrate vectors are associated with transmission. For example, in

**Figure 13.16**
Electron micrograph showing the pleomorphic cells of *Francisella tularenis*.

the United States, the major (but not exclusive) endemic tularemic area encompasses Arkansas, Missouri, and Oklahoma. Incidence is most common in the summer months, a fact that reflects the arthropod transmission of the disease. During the winter months, a smaller peak incidence occurs, which reflects exposure of hunters to infected animal carcasses. Infection is also more common in males, because they have a greater exposure risk. Tularemia is an occupational risk for veterinarians, hunters, and trappers (see Figure 13.18), domestic livestock workers, and meat handlers. Recreational activities that increase exposure to ticks and biting flies also increase the risk of acquiring tularemia.

### B. Pathogenesis

In cases involving cutaneous inoculation, the organism multiplies locally for three to five days. It typically produces a papule that ulcerates after several days and may persist for weeks or longer. Organisms spread from the local lesion to the regional lymph nodes, which become large and tender, and may suppurate. From the lymph nodes, the organisms spread via the lymphatic system to various organs and tissues, including skin (Figure 13.17), lungs, liver, spleen, kidneys, and CNS.

**Figure 13.17**
Thumb with skin ulcer of tularemia.

> *F. tularensis* is one of the most infectious pathogenic bacteria known, requiring inoculation or inhalation of as few as ten organisms to cause disease. It is considered to be a dangerous potential biologic weapon because of its extreme infectivity, ease of dissemination, and substantial capacity to cause illness and death.

### C. Clinical significance

Tularemia varies in severity from mild to fulminant and fatal. Clinical presentation, infectious dose, and length of the incubation period depend on the virulence of the organism, portal of entry, and host immunity. Onset of symptoms is usually abrupt. The most common symptoms are flulike (chills, fever, headache, malaise, anorexia, and fatigue), although respiratory and gastrointestinal symptoms may also occur.

1. **Ulceroglandular tularemia:** The most common presentation of tularemia is ulceroglandular. Ulcers may result from contact with contaminated animal products (typically on the hands and/or forearms), or from insect bites (commonly on the trunk and/or lower extremities). Multiple lesions may occur. The location of affected lymph nodes also reflects the type of exposure. Lymphadenopathy is characteristic.

2. **Other forms of tularemia:** Tularemia characterized by lymphadenopathy without evidence of ulceration is known as glandular tularemia. In these cases, the ulcer may have been minimal

or have healed prior to the patient's having sought medical attention. In oculoglandular tularemia, the organism gains entry through the conjunctiva, which becomes inflamed. In pharyngeal tularemia, the organism gains entry through the pharynx, and causes a severe sore throat. In pneumonic tularemia, the prominent feature of initial presentation is pulmonary. The pneumonia may be primary, a result of inhalation of infectious aerosols, or secondary, a result of hematogenous dissemination of the organisms from a primary site elsewhere in the body to the lungs. Systemic illness without lymphadenopathy or ulcerations is called "typhoid tularemia."

## D. Laboratory identification

Clinical presentation and history consistent with possible exposure is of primary importance in diagnosis. Results of routine laboratory tests are not specific to tularemia. The organism may be cultured from ulcer scrapings, lymph node biopsies, gastric washings, and sputum, but rarely from blood. *F. tularensis* is nutritionally fastidious and requires a sulfhydryl source such as cysteine. The organism is highly infectious, and laboratories must take special precautions when culturing specimens to avoid laboratory transmission. For this reason, the laboratory should be notified when there is suspicion of tularemia.

## E. Treatment

The drug of choice for treatment of the forms of tularemia discussed above is streptomycin or, as an alternate, gentamicin (Figure 13.18).

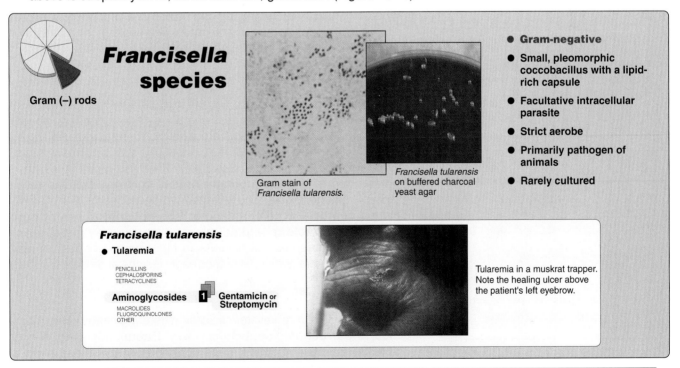

Gram (–) rods

**Francisella species**

Gram stain of *Francisella tularensis.*

*Francisella tularensis* on buffered charcoal yeast agar

- **Gram-negative**
- **Small, pleomorphic coccobacillus with a lipid-rich capsule**
- **Facultative intracellular parasite**
- **Strict aerobe**
- **Primarily pathogen of animals**
- **Rarely cultured**

***Francisella tularensis***
- Tularemia

PENICILLINS
CEPHALOSPORINS
TETRACYCLINES

**Aminoglycosides** 1 **Gentamicin** or **Streptomycin**

MACROLIDES
FLUOROQUINOLONES
OTHER

Tularemia in a muskrat trapper. Note the healing ulcer above the patient's left eyebrow.

**Figure 13.18**
Summary of francisella species.

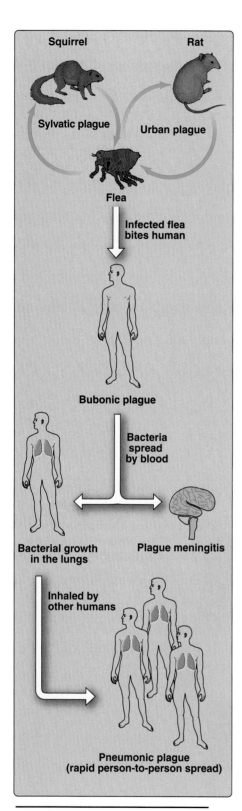

**Figure 13.19**
Epidemiology and pathology of plague.

# VIII. YERSINIA PESTIS

The genus *Yersinia* is a member of the family Enterobacteriaceae, which is presented in Chapter 12. The most clinically notorious member of this genus is *Yersinia pestis*, which causes plague, rather than enteric disease and, therefore, is being discussed separately from the rest of the family. In common with other yersiniae, *Y. pestis* is a small rod that stains bipolarly (see Figure 13.21). It produces V and W antigens, which are virulence factors, as are its endotoxin and antiphagocytic capsule.

## A. Epidemiology

Plague is predominantly a zoonosis with worldwide distribution. In the United States, the Southwest has been a primary focus of *Y. pestis* infection, although the distribution of human cases has been expanding into the Northwest and south-central states. The organism can infect a variety of mammals. For example, rats are common reservoirs in urban areas of some countries (urban plague). However, in the United States, plague is predominantly found in the wild, where prairie dogs and ground squirrels are the most important reservoirs (sylvatic plague). Household pets, particularly cats allowed to roam in plague-enzootic areas, may also become infected. Plague is characteristically transmitted by fleas, which serve to maintain the infection within the animal reservoir. Humans are generally accidental and dead-end hosts. Plague can also be transmitted by ingestion of contaminated animal tissue or via the respiratory route (pneumonic plague). [Note: The latter occurs either when organisms reach the lung and establish a secondary pneumonia, or following exposure to respiratory secretions from a patient or animal with plague pneumonia (Figure 13.19).]

## B. Pathogenesis

Organisms are carried by the lymphatic system from the site of inoculation to regional lymph nodes, where they are ingested by phagocytes. However, the organisms are resistant to intracellular killing by phagocytes and instead may multiply within these cells. Furthermore, the bacteria released from lysed phagocytes have synthesized a new envelope antigen that confers increased resistance to phagocytosis. The affected lymph nodes display hemorrhagic necrosis accompanied by high concentrations of both polymorphonuclear leukocytes and extracellular bacteria. Hematogenous spread of bacteria to other organs or tissues may occur, resulting in additional hemorrhagic lesions at these sites.

## C. Clinical significance

Plague may present several clinically different pictures. Most common is the bubonic/septicemic form. Pneumonic plague may develop during epidemics. Less common presentations include plague meningitis (typically a secondary focus resulting from hematogenous spread of the organisms), cutaneous plague, and pharyngitis (the latter two generally acquired by handling or ingesting contaminated animal tissue).

1. **Bubonic (septicemic) plague:** The infectious cycle begins when a flea ingests a blood meal from an animal that is infected and bacteremic. *Y. pestis* produces a coagulase that causes the blood to clot in the flea's foregut. The organism multiplies in this environment. When the flea next attempts to feed, it regurgitates these bacteria from its foregut into the new animal's skin. The incubation period (from flea bite to development of symptoms) is generally two to eight days. Onset of nonspecific symptoms, such as high fever, chills, headache, myalgia, and weakness that proceeds to prostration, is characteristically sudden. Within a short time, a characteristic, painful bubo develops (Figure 13.20). Buboes (pronounced swellings comprised of one or more infected nodes and surrounding edema that led to the term "bubonic plague") are typically located in the groin, but may also occur in axillae or on the neck. As the disease proceeds, blood pressure generally drops, potentially leading to septic shock and death. Mortality of untreated bubonic plague generally exceeds fifty percent, with untreated and highly contagious pneumonic plague being invariably fatal unless rapidly treated. Other manifestations associated with bubonic plague include pustules or vesicles containing leukocytes and *Y. pestis*. Purpura and necrosis of extremities may occur during systemic disease. [Note: Ingestion of contaminated meat or exposure to airborne bacilli can result in primary lesions in the pharynx. These produce a severe tonsillitis and cervical buboes.] Septicemic plague is a variation in which the patient is overwhelmed by massive bacteremia before the characteristic buboes develop.

**Figure 13.20**
Bubo characteristic of infections due to *Yersinia pestis*.

2. **Pneumonic plague:** If plague bacilli reach the lungs, they cause purulent pneumonia that, if untreated, is rapidly fatal. It is also highly contagious, and the organisms cause pneumonic plague directly when inhaled.

3. **Plague meningitis:** This results from hematogenous dissemination of organisms to the meninges. It may occur following inadequately treated bubonic plague or, like septicemic plague, may occur without, or prior to, development of a bubo. Organisms can be demonstrated in the CSF.

## D. Laboratory identification

Diagnosis of *Y. pestis* infection may be made on the basis of clinical presentation. Laboratory identification can be initiated by a gram-stained smear, and culture of an aspirate from a bubo (or from CSF or sputum in the case of meningitis or pneumonic presentations). The organism grows on both MacConkey and blood agars, although colonies grow somewhat more slowly than those of other Enterobacteriaceae.

## E. Treatment and prevention

Streptomycin is the drug of choice; gentamicin and doxycycline are acceptable alternatives (Figure 13.21). For plague meningitis, chloramphenicol offers good penetration into the CSF. Because of the

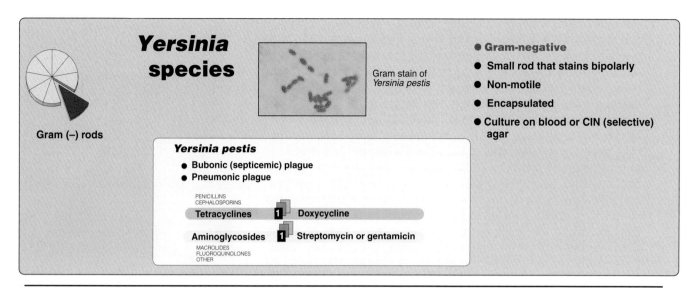

**Figure 13.21**
Summary of *Yersina pestis* disease.

potential for overwhelming septicemia, rapid institution of antibiotic therapy is crucial. Supportive therapy is essential for patients with signs of shock. A formalin-killed vaccine is available for those at high risk of acquiring plague. For individuals in enzootic areas, efforts to minimize exposure to rodents and fleas is important. Sick or dead rodents should never be touched with bare hands.

## IX. BARTONELLA

Members of the genus *Bartonella* (formerly, *Rochalimaea*), facultative, intracellular parasites, can be cultivated on special media in the laboratory. Three species have been implicated in human diseases.

### A. Bartonella quintana

*Bartonella quintana* causes trench fever, an often mild, relapsing fever with maculopapular rash. The organism has a reservoir in humans, and its vector is the human body louse. The disease is, therefore, associated with humans living in poor sanitary conditions. Specific diagnosis can be aided by culture of clinical materials and serologic tests. Broad-spectrum antibiotics are effective in the treatment of the disease (Figure 13.22).

### B. Bartonella henselae

*B. henselae* was recently shown to be associated with most cases of catscratch disease, a syndrome that has been familiar to physicians for decades, but whose etiology had been elusive. The illness is characterized by small abscesses at the site of a cat (less commonly other pets) scratch or bite. This is followed by fever and localized lymphadenopathy. *B. henselae* is also responsible for several other types of infections, such as bacillary angiomatosis—a disease of small blood vessels of the skin and visceral organs—seen primar-

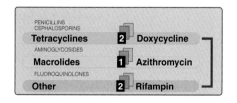

**Figure 13.22**
Antimicrobial agents useful in empiric therapy of infections caused by *Bartonella* species.

ily in immunocompromised patients, such as those with AIDS. *B. henselae* infections are successfully treated with rifampin in combination with doxycycline (see Figure 13.22).

# X. PASTEURELLA

Members of the genus *Pasteurella* primarily colonize mammals and birds, both domestic and feral. Therefore, pasteurella infections are considered zoonoses. The major human pathogen in this genus is *Pasteurella multocida*, which can cause either disease or asymptomatic infections. Pasteurellae are coccobacilli or rods that often exhibit bipolar staining; some strains are encapsulated (Figure 13.23). Virulence factors include the organism's capsule and endotoxin. Pasteurellae are aerobes/facultative anaerobes.

## A. Epidemiology

The majority of pasteurella infections in humans are soft tissue infections that follow an animal bite or cat scratch. A smaller fraction of human pasteurella infections occur either following a non-bite animal exposure, or in the absence of any known animal exposure. The source of pasteurellae in the latter infections is suspected to be nasopharyngeal colonization of the patient.

## B. Clinical significance

*P. multocida* infection should be suspected in cases of acute, painful cellulitis that develop within 24 hours of an animal bite or cat scratch, or an infected animal licking an open wound. Soft tissue infections are characterized by the rapid onset of acute local inflammation within hours of the bite or scratch. Lesions often begin to drain within one to two days. Manifestations of *P. multocida* infection include lymphangitis, lymphadenitis, fever, and local complications such as osteomyelitis or arthritis, which can result in extended disability.

## C. Laboratory identification

Laboratory diagnosis (essential in non–bite/scratch-associated cases) can be accomplished by culturing the organism on blood agar, and performing appropriate biochemical tests.

## D. Treatment

For soft tissue infections, wounds should be cleansed, irrigated, and debrided. Deep-seated infections require surgical drainage and prolonged antibiotic treatment. Penicillin is the drug of choice (Figure 13.24). Fatal infections are uncommon and usually reflect underlying compromise.

**Figure 13.23**
*Pasteurella multocida*. A. Culture on blood agar showing small, translucent nonhemolytic colonies. B. Blood smear, Wright stain. (Note bipolar staining.)

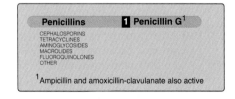

| Penicillins | **1** Penicillin G[1] |
|---|---|
| CEPHALOSPORINS | |
| TETRACYCLINES | |
| AMINOGLYCOSIDES | |
| MACROLIDES | |
| FLUOROQUINOLONES | |
| OTHER | |

[1] Ampicillin and amoxicillin-clavulanate also active

**Figure 13.24**
Antimicrobial agents useful in empiric therapy of infections caused by *Pasteurella multocida*.

## Study Questions

**Choose the ONE correct answer**

13.1 Which of the following is true of *Haemophilus influenzae*?

    A. Invasive infections are most commonly associated with encapsulated strains.

    B. Most invasive infections occur in infants during the neonatal period.

    C. Most human infections are acquired from domestic pets.

    D. The organism can be readily cultured on sheep blood agar in an environment of elevated $CO_2$.

    E. Older adults are rarely at risk for infection with this organism because they typically have a high level of immunity.

> Correct answer = A. The capsule is antiphagocytic, and facilitates hematogenous dissemination of *H. influenzae*. Although *H. influenzae* is an important pathogen of infants and young children, passive transfer of maternal IgG may afford neonates protection. Immunity begins to wane in the elderly, increasing the risk of infection for this population. Humans are the only natural host for *H. influenzae*. *H. influenzae* requires both hemin (X factor) and NAD (V factor), which are not available in sheep blood agar. Heating the blood lyses the erythrocytes, releasing both X and V factors, and simultaneously inactivating an NAD-inactivating enzyme present in blood. Media made with such heated blood is termed chocolate agar. The organism does prefer elevated $CO_2$.

13.2 For which of the following organisms is there no known animal reservoir?

    A. *Francisella tularensis*

    B. *Pasteurella multocida*

    C. *Bordetella pertussis*

    D. *Brucella melitensis*

    E. *Yersinia pestis*

> Correct answer = C. *F. tularensis* has a broad host range, including wild and domestic mammals, birds, and house pets. *P. multocida* primarily colonizes mammals and birds, both domestic and feral. *B. melitensis* primarily infects sheep and goats. *Y. pestis* infects a variety of mammals.

13.3 Which of the following statements about *Bordetella pertussis* infection is true?

    A. Infection causes a leukocytosis characterized primarily by a marked elevation in polymorphonuclear leukocytes.

    B. Isolation of the organism from clinical specimens is greatest during the early stages of illness.

    C. Clinical diagnosis of whooping cough can usually be made within a few days of onset of initial symptoms.

    D. Children who receive a full series of immunizations with the pertussis vaccine generally develop solid, lifelong immunity to pertussis.

    E. The organism can be cultured on standard laboratory media, such as sheep blood agar.

> Correct answer = B. *B. pertussis* typically causes a lymphocytic leukocytosis. Initial symptoms of *Bordetella* infection are relatively nonspecific (rhinorrhea, etc.). The characteristic paroxysmal coughing begins somewhat later. Maintenance of solid immunity depends on repeated exposure to the organism, either through natural causes or by administration of booster shots. Growth of *Bordetella* requires a medium containing a substance such as charcoal to absorb or neutralize inhibitory substances, and also antibiotics that inhibit the growth of normal flora.

*"I'm sorry, it's an ear infection"*

# Clostridia and Other Anaerobic Rods

# 14

## I. OVERVIEW

The organisms discussed in this chapter are all obligate anaerobes; that is, they are microorganisms that obtain energy exclusively by fermentation because they cannot use molecular oxygen (aerobic metabolism) for the production of energy. They are also, in varying degrees, damaged by free oxygen, which limits the conditions under which these organisms can colonize the human body or cause disease. The obligate anaerobic genus, *Clostridium*, consists of gram-positive, spore-forming rods that are associated with soft tissue and skin infections (for example, cellulitis and fasciitis), and antibiotic-associated colitis and diarrhea. These organisms also synthesize some of the most potent exotoxins known. For example, the toxins of specific clostridial species cause botulism, tetanus, gas gangrene, and pseudomembranous colitis. A number of anaerobic, gram-negative rods, such as *Bacteroides* and related genera, are frequently involved in visceral and other abscesses, although these are generally polymicrobic (mixed) infections in which some facultative bacteria are also involved. The organisms discussed in this chapter are listed in Figure 14.1.

## II. CLOSTRIDIA

Clostridia are the anaerobic gram-positive rods of greatest clinical importance. [Note: Other clinically important gram-positive rods are aerobic.] Clinically significant species of *Clostridium* include *C. perfringens*, which causes histotoxic (tissue destructive) infections (myonecrosis) and food poisoning; *C. difficile*, which causes pseudomembranous colitis associated with antibiotic use; *C. tetani*, which causes tetanus ("lockjaw"); and *C. botulinum*, which causes botulism.

### A. General features of clostridia

Clostridia are large, gram-positive, blunt-ended rods. They form endospores; the position of the developing spore within the vegetative cell is useful in identifying the species (see Figure 14.10). Most species are motile.

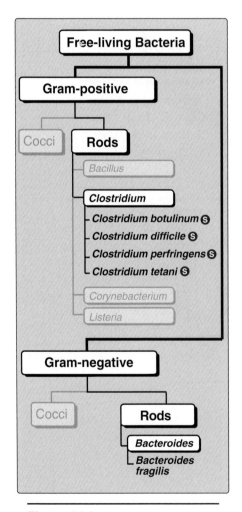

**Figure 14.1**
Classification of organisms in this chapter. ⓢ See p. 331 for summaries of these organisms.

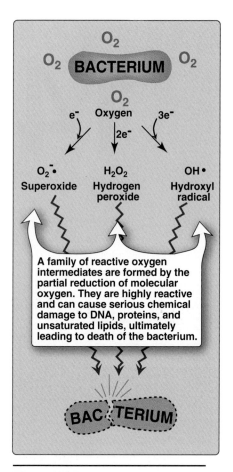

**Figure 14.2**
Toxic effects of reactive oxygen
intermediates on anaerobic bacteria.

1. **Physiology:** Clostridia cannot use free oxygen as the terminal electron acceptor in energy production as do aerobic organisms (see p. 23). Instead, they use a variety of small organic molecules such as pyruvate as the final electron acceptors in the generation of energy. In the vegetative state, clostridia are also variably inhibited or damaged by $O_2$ (Figure 14.2). [Note: The reasons for this damage are not entirely clear. One explanation is that these organisms produce oxygen radicals and peroxides and that some of them cannot detoxify these reactive molecules because they lack enzymes such as peroxidases, catalase, or superoxide dismutase.] Clostridia grow on enriched media in the presence of a reducing agent such as cysteine or thioglycollate (to maintain a low oxidation-reduction potential) or in an $O_2$-free, gaseous atmosphere provided by an air-evacuated glove box, sealed jar, or other device.

2. **Epidemiology:** Clostridia, part of the intestinal flora in humans and other mammals, and are found in soil, sewage, and aquatic settings, particularly those with high organic content. A number of clostridial species produce destructive and invasive infections when introduced into tissues; for example, by a break in the skin resulting from surgery or trauma. Their presence in infectious processes is opportunistic and often derives from the patient's normal flora. Endospore formation facilitates their persistent survival in the environment.

> Spores are resistant to chemical disinfectants, and may withstand ultraviolet irradiation or boiling temperatures for some time, although not standard autoclaving conditions (121°C for fifteen minutes at increased pressure).

### B. Clostridium perfringens

*C. perfringens* is a large, rod-shaped, nonmotile, gram-positive, encapsulated bacillus. It is ubiquitous in nature, with its vegetative form as part of the normal flora of the vagina and gastrointestinal (GI) tract. Its spores are found in soil. [Note: Spores are rarely seen in the body or following *in vitro* cultivation.] When introduced into tissue, however, *C. perfringens* can cause anaerobic cellulitis, and myonecrosis (gas gangrene). Some strains of *C. perfringens* also cause a common form of food poisoning.

1. **Pathogenesis:** *C. perfringens* secretes a variety of exotoxins, enterotoxins, and hydrolytic enzymes that facilitate the disease process (Figure 14.3).

   a. **Exotoxins:** *C. perfringens* elaborates at least twelve exotoxins, designated by Greek letters. The most important of these, and the one that seems to be required for virulence in tissue, is alpha toxin. Alpha toxin is a lecithinase (phospholipase C) that degrades lecithin in mammalian cell membranes, causing lysis of endothelial cells, as well as erythrocytes, leukocytes, and platelets. Other *C. perfringens* exotoxins have hemolytic or other cytotoxic and necrotic effects, either locally or when dispersed in the bloodstream. *C. perfringens* strains are grouped, A through E on the basis of their spectrum of exotoxins. Type A strains, which produce both alpha toxin and enterotoxin, are responsible for most human clostridial infections.

b. **Enterotoxin:** *C. perfringens* enterotoxin, a small, heat-labile protein, acts in the lower portion of the small intestine. The molecule binds to receptors on the epithelial cell surface and alters the cell membrane, disrupting ion transport (primarily in the ileum) and leading to loss of fluid and intracellular proteins. Interestingly, enterotoxin-producing strains are unusually heat resistant, the spores remaining viable for longer than an hour at 100°C, enhancing their threat as food-borne pathogens.

c. **Degradative enzymes:** *C. perfringens* is a metabolically vigorous organism that produces a variety of hydrolytic enzymes, including proteases, DNases, hyaluronidase, and collagenases, which liquefy tissue and promote the spread of infection.

## 2. Clinical significance

The disease processes initiated by *C. perfringens* result from a combination of infection with the production of exotoxins and/or enterotoxins and degradative enzymes.

a. **Myonecrosis (gas gangrene):** Clostridial spores are introduced into tissue, for example, by contamination with infected soil, or by endogenous transfer from the intestinal tract. Severe and open wounds, such as compound fractures and other ischemia-producing injuries (for example, car accidents), are a prime predisposing condition. Alpha toxin and other exotoxins are secreted and extensive cell killing ensues. Production of enzymes that break down ground substance facilitates the spread of infection. Fermentation of tissue carbohydrates yields gas, and an accumulation of gas bubbles in the subcutaneous spaces produces a crinkling sensation on palpation (crepitation); hence, the name gas gangrene (Figure 14.4).

> The majority of infections resulting in necrosis of muscle are due to *Clostridium* species (gas gangrene) and group A streptococcus.

The exudates are copious and foul smelling. As the disease progresses, increased capillary permeability leads to the exotoxins being carried by the circulation from damaged tissue to other organs, resulting in systemic effects such as shock, renal failure, and intravascular hemolysis. Untreated clostridial myonecrosis is uniformly fatal within days of the initiation of gangrene.

**Figure 14.3**
Toxins and degradative enzymes produced by *Clostridium perfringens*. ET = enterotoxin.

Gas gangrene of 5 cm superficial laceration across the left antecubital fossa (depression in front of the elbow) on presentation 3 days after injury.

Following surgical debridement.

**Figure 14.4**
Gas gangrene of arm.

b. **Anaerobic cellulitis:** This is a clostridial infection of connective tissue in which the spread of bacterial growth along fascial planes (fasciitis) does not involve invasion of muscle tissue. Necrotizing processes play a more limited role, but surgical intervention is generally unsuccessful unless it is carried out very promptly and aggressively, because of the rapid spread of infection.

c. **Food poisoning:** *C. perfringens* is a common cause of food poisoning in the United States. Typically, the onset of nausea, abdominal cramps, and diarrhea occurs eight to eighteen hours after eating contaminated food. Fever is absent and vomiting rare. The attack is usually self-limited, with recovery within one to two days. The occurrence of clinical symptoms requires a large inoculum of $10^8$ organisms or greater. Therefore, a typical episode of clostridial enterotoxin food poisoning involves cooking that fails to inactivate spores, followed by holding the food for several hours under conditions that allow bacterial germination and several cycles of growth.

d. **Enteritis necroticans:** Outbreaks of a necrotizing bowel disease with high mortality (greater than fifty percent) caused by *C. perfringens* have been sporadically reported.

e. **Clostridial endometritis:** This condition is a grave complication of incomplete abortion, or the use of inadequately sterilized instruments. Gangrenous infection of uterine tissue is followed by toxemia and bacteremia.

3. **Laboratory identification:** Diagnosis of clostridial myonecrosis or cellulitis rests largely on clinical impression. The presence of clostridia in clinical materials may be adventitious (that is, an accidental contamination). With Gram stain, however, specimens from diseased tissue usually show vegetative clostridial forms (large, gram-positive rods), accompanied by other bacteria and cellular debris. When cultured anaerobically on blood agar, *C. perfringens* grows rapidly, producing colonies with a unique double zone of hemolysis (Figure 14.5). In food poisoning, the organism can be sought in suspected food and patient's feces.

> Increasing pain at the site of prior injury or surgery, together with signs of systemic toxicity and gas in the soft tissue, support the diagnosis of gas gangrene

4. **Treatment and prevention:** The key to both prevention and treatment of gas gangrene is immediate and thorough removal of foreign material and devitalized tissue, and exposure of the wound to $O_2$. Hyperbaric oxygen chambers increase the tissue $O_2$ tension in the affected part and probably inhibit the pathologic pro-

cess. If debridement is unable to control the progression of the gangrene, amputation, when anatomically possible, is still mandatory in gangrene. Supplementary to this is the administration of antibiotics in high dose. *C. perfringens* is sensitive to penicillin and several common inhibitors of prokaryotic protein synthesis (see Figure 14.10).

>  Clostridial infections usually involve a mixture of species; therefore, the use of broad-spectrum antibiotics is appropriate.

### C. Clostridium botulinum

*C. botulinum* causes botulism, which occurs in several clinical forms. Botulism is caused by the action of a neurotoxin that is one of the most potent poisons known. It causes a flaccid paralysis. Contact with the organism itself is not required; hence, the disease can be a pure intoxication.

1. **Epidemiology:** *C. botulinum* is found worldwide in soil and aquatic sediments, and the spores frequently contaminate vegetables and meat or fish. Under appropriate conditions, including a strictly anaerobic environment at neutral or alkaline pH, the organism germinates and toxin is produced during vegetative growth. Because the toxin is often elaborated in food, outbreaks frequently occur in families or other eating groups.

2. **Pathogenesis:** There are several types of botulinum toxin, designated A through G, but human disease is almost always caused by types A, B, or E. The botulinum serotypes and tetanus toxin constitute a homologous set of proteins whose neurotoxicity arises from proteolytic cleavage of specific synaptic vesicle peptides, causing subsequent failure of neurotransmission. In contrast to tetanus toxin, which causes constant contraction (spasms, see p. 154), botulinum toxins affect peripheral cholinergic synapses by blocking the neuromuscular junction and inhibiting release of the neurotransmitter, acetylcholine, preventing contraction and causing flaccid paralysis (Figure 14.6).

3. **Clinical significance:**

   a. **Classic botulism** is a food poisoning in which a patient first begins to experience difficulties in focusing vision, swallowing, and other cranial nerve functions, 12 to 36 hours after ingesting toxin-containing food but not necessarily viable organisms. There is no fever or sign of sepsis. A progressive paralysis of striated muscle groups develops, and mortality is about fifteen percent; the patient usually succumbing to respiratory paralysis. Recovery is protracted, lasting several weeks.

**Figure 14.5**
*Clostridium perfringens.* A. Colonies on blood agar showing double zone of hemolysis. B. Photomicrograph of Gram stain.

**Figure 14.6**
Mechanism of botulinum toxin.  AcCoA = acetyl CoA.

**b. Infant botulism:** The most common form of botulism in the United States today is infant botulism or a cause of floppy baby syndrome (see Figure 14.10). *C. botulinum* colonizes the large bowel of infants 3 to 24 weeks of age; the toxin produced is slowly absorbed. Constipation, feeding problems, lethargy, and poor muscle tone are common early signs. Certain formula supplements, such as honey contaminated with *C. botulinum* spores, may transmit the organism. The condition is possibly a cause of sudden infant death syndrome, but recovery is the usual outcome, following symptomatic treatment that may be prolonged.

**c. Wound botulism:** A rare form of botulism occurs when a wound becomes contaminated with the organism, and toxin is absorbed from that site.

4. **Laboratory identification:** The organism can be cultured and identified by standard anaerobic methods (see p. 23). Toxin is also identifiable in serum, stool, and food.

5. **Treatment and prevention:** Antitoxin, which neutralizes unbound botulinum toxin, should be administered as soon as possible in suspected botulinal intoxication. A trivalent (A, B, E) horse anti-serum is available from the Centers for Disease Control (CDC). Supportive measures, including mechanical ventilation, may be required. In wound botulism, the infection can be treated with penicillin or other antibiotics to which the organism is sensitive. The toxin is inactivated at boiling temperatures, although killing of botulinal spores requires moist heat under pressure (autoclaving). [Note: Even the most severe cases of botulism do not result in immunity.]

### D  Clostridium tetani

The introduction of *C. tetani* spores into even small wounds via contaminated soil is probably a common occurrence. But a combination of the extreme $O_2$ sensitivity of vegetative *C. tetani* and widespread immunization against its exotoxin, make the resulting disease, tetanus, rare in developed countries. In the United States, the disease is seen most often in older individuals who have not received their immunization boosters regularly, and whose immunity has therefore waned.

> Growth of *C. tetani* is completely local, but it produces a powerful neurotoxin that is transported to the central nervous system, where it causes spastic paralysis.

1. **Epidemiology:** *C. tetani* spores are common in barnyard, garden, and other soils. The most typical focus of infection in tetanus is a puncture wound caused, for example, by a splinter. Introduced foreign bodies or small areas of cell killing create a nidus of devitalized material in which tetanus spores can germinate and grow. Special circumstances may also lead to infection, for example, after severe burns or surgery. Illicit drugs often contain spores that are introduced by injection.

2. **Pathogenesis:** Tetanus toxin, called tetanospasmin, is an extremely potent toxin. It is transported from an infected locus by retrograde neuronal flow or blood. A plasmid-coded exotoxin of a single antigenic type; it is produced as a single polypeptide that is cleaved to generate the mature toxin of two chains held together by a disulfide bond. The heavy fragment (B) mediates binding to neurons and cell penetration of the light fragment (A). The A fragment blocks neurotransmitter release at inhibitory synapses, and thus causes severe,

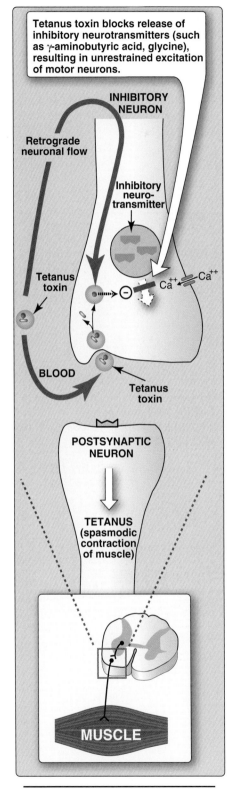

**Figure 14.7**
Mechanism of tetanus toxin.

prolonged muscle spasms (Figure 14.7). The A fragment has been shown to be a protease; it cleaves a small synaptic vesicle protein (synaptobrevin) and abolishes the flow of inhibitory neurotransmitters.

3. **Clinical significance:** Tetanus has an incubation period varying from four days to several weeks. A shorter period is usually associated with more severe disease and wounds closer to the brain. Tetanus presents as a spastic paralysis, in which muscle spasms often first involve the site of infection. In the early stages of the disease, the jaw muscles are affected, so that the mouth cannot open (trismus, or "lockjaw"). Gradually, other voluntary muscles become involved (see Figure 14.10), and any external stimulus (for example, noise or bright light) precipitates a painful spasm, and sometimes convulsions. Death, which occurs in fifteen to sixty percent of cases, is usually the result of paralysis of chest muscles leading to respiratory failure.

4. **Laboratory identification:** Because treatment must be initiated immediately, the diagnosis of tetanus is based largely on clinical findings. The focus of infection is often a trivial wound that may be difficult to locate. *C. tetani* has a characteristic morphology, with a long, slender rod and round, terminal spore (racquet-shaped bacillus, Figure 14.8), and characteristic swarming growth on anaerobic blood agar.

**Figure 14.8**
Photomicrograph of *Clostridium tetani* showing terminal spores.

5. **Treatment:** Prompt administration of antitoxin to neutralize any toxin not yet bound to neurons is the first order of treatment. Treatment with human hyperimmune globulin (tetanus immune globulin) is preferred but, in countries where it is not available, horse antitoxin is used. The organism is sensitive to penicillin, and this drug can be used to eradicate the infection, together with debridement of necrotic tissue at the entry wound.

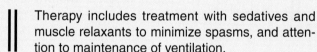

Therapy includes treatment with sedatives and muscle relaxants to minimize spasms, and attention to maintenance of ventilation.

6. **Prevention:** Active immunization with tetanus toxoid (formalin-inactivated toxin) prevents tetanus. It is usually administered to children as a triple vaccine with diphtheria toxoid and pertussis antigens (DPT). Recent studies have confirmed that circulating antibody levels gradually decline, and that many older individuals lose protection. Therefore, booster immunizations with a preparation of diphtheria and tetanus toxoids given every ten years throughout life are recommended. Tetanus immunoglobulin can be used to give immediate passive immunity to injury victims with no history of immunization. Active immunization should also be started. Antitoxin and toxoid, administered in different areas of the body, can be given simultaneously.

## E. Clostridium difficile

Diarrhea, a common complication of antimicrobial drug treatment, can range from loose stools to life-threatening pseudomembranous colitis (PMC, see Figure 14.10). *C. difficile* is estimated to be responsible for about one forth of antibiotic-associated diarrheas (AAD) in hospitalized patients and almost all cases of PMC. After its introduction to a site, the environment—dust, bedding, toilets—becomes persistently contaminated with spores, and new residents are easily colonized. They are then at higher risk for developing the adverse intestinal effect of antibiotic treatments.

1. **Pathogenesis:** *C. difficile* is a minor component of the normal flora of the large intestine. When antimicrobial treatment suppresses more predominant species in this community, *C. difficile* proliferates. Pathogenic strains produce two toxic polypeptides, designated A and B. Toxin A is an enterotoxin that causes excessive fluid secretion, but also stimulates an inflammatory response, and has some cytopathic effect in tissue culture. Toxin B is a cytotoxin; in tissue culture, it disrupts protein synthesis and causes disorganization of the cytoskeleton.

2. **Clinical significance:** Virtually all antimicrobial drugs have been reported as predisposing to clostridial AAD and colitis (Figure 14.9). The three drugs most commonly implicated are clindamycin, ampicillin, and the cephalosporins. The severity of disease varies widely from mild diarrhea through varying degrees of inflammation of the large intestine to a fulminant PMC. The pseudomembranous exudate, composed of mucus, fibrin, inflammatory cells and cell debris overlying an ulcerated epithelium, is best demonstrated by endoscopy.

> Pseudomembranous colitis often begins some time after cessation of drug treatment, or may reoccur after what should be adequate therapy.

3. **Laboratory identification:** *C. difficile* can be cultured from stools and identified by routine anaerobic procedures; however, the more rapid and useful tests are directed at demonstrating toxin production in stool extracts. Recently developed enzyme immunoassays (ELISA, see p. 28) for exotoxins A and B have largely replaced earlier immunologic or tissue culture cytotoxicity assays.

4. **Treatment:** Discontinuance of the predisposing drug and fluid replacement usually lead to resolution of the symptoms. Relapses, however, are common. Oral administration of metronidazole or vancomycin is usually added (see Figure 14.10).

## III. ANAEROBIC GRAM-NEGATIVE RODS

Anaerobic gram-negative rods are normally the most common organisms in the oral cavity (particularly the gingiva), female genital tract, and lower GI tract, where they outnumber *E. coli* 1000:1. They are, therefore,

**Frequently associated**

**Ampicillin**
**Amoxicillin**
**Cephalosporins**
**Clindamycin**

**Occassionally associated**

**Penicillins other than ampicillin**
**Sulfonamides**
**Erythromycin**
**Trimethoprim**
**Quinolones**

**Rarely or never associated**

**Parenteral aminoglycoside**
**Tetracyclines**
**Chloramphenicol**
**Metronidazole**
**Vancomycin**

**Figure 14.9**
The potential of antimicrobial drugs to induce *Clostridium difficile* diarrhea and colitis.

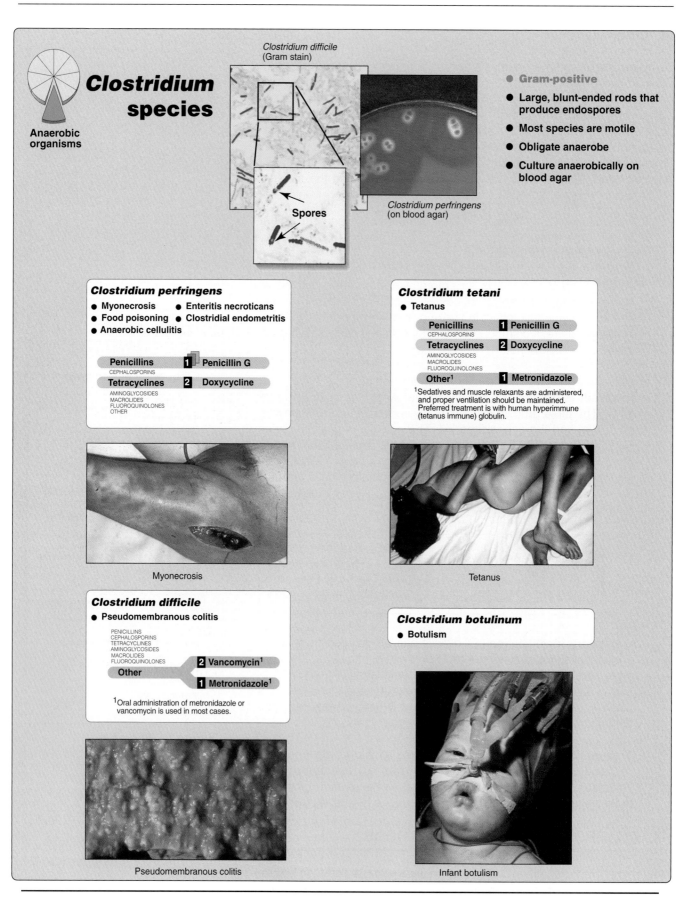

**Figure 14.10**
Summary of clostridial disease.

frequently recovered from infections in various parts of the body; for example, gram-negative anaerobic rods are recovered in about ten percent of bacteremias. Gram-negative rods generally constitute the majority of organisms associated with anaerobic abscesses. Organisms in this group may breach the host epithelial barrier and establish infection in any body tissue. This usually occurs because of trauma, an incident such as a ruptured appendix, or because of compromised immune status. A localized abscess is the most common lesion, and the infectious process often involves two or more species of organisms. For example, various facultative organisms help lower the $pO_2$, thus providing the anaerobic environment required by the coinfecting gram-negative rods (Figure 14.11).

## A. Bacteroides

Members of the genus *Bacteroides* are the predominant anaerobes found in the human colon. They are part of the normal flora, and only cause disease when they gain access to tissues or the blood during bowel penetration (for example, during surgery or trauma). They are, however, the most common cause of serious infections by anaerobic organisms. Bacteroides are slender rods or coccobacilli. Their polysaccharide capsule is an important virulence factor, conveying resistance to phagocytosis.

1. **Epidemiology:** *Bacteroides* are transmitted from the colon to the blood or peritoneum following abdominal trauma. Therefore the source of infection is endogenous (it is not transmitted from person to person).

2. **Pathology and clinical significance:** The major disease-causing *Bacteroides* species is *B. fragilis*. When released from the colon into the blood, *B. fragilis* multiplies rapidly, causing bacteremia. If it is introduced into the abdominal cavity, *B. fragilis* causes peritonitis, and/or abdominal abscesses.

3. **Laboratory identification:** Exudates from mixed anaerobic lesions are often copious and noticeably foul smelling. A Gram stain of such exudates shows numerous faint, slender, gram-negative rods, usually in mixed flora. The organisms are easily obscured by debris and polymorphonuclear leukocytes. *B. fragilis* can be cultured on blood agar under anaerobic conditions. Gas chromatography can be used to identify the characteristic short-chain fatty acids produced by the organism, and biochemical tests can determine its sugar fermentation pattern.

4. **Treatment and prevention:** Drug resistance is common among the *Bacteroides*. Metronidazole is the antibiotic of choice for *B. fragilis* infections (Figure 14.12). Alternative choices include ampicillin-sulbactam, imipenem-cilastin, ticarcillin-clavulanate, cefoxitin, or clindamycin. Aminoglycosides are, of course, ineffective against anaerobes (see p. 44). Surgical drainage of any abscess is essential to ensure penetration of drugs. To prevent *Bacteroides* contamination of a surgical wound, a perioperative antibiotic, such as cefoxitin, can be administered.

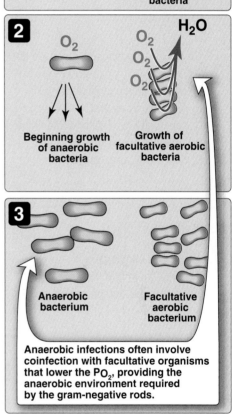

**Figure 14.11**
Anaerobic organisms growth is facilitated by facultative aerobic bacteria.

**Figure 14.12**
Some antimicrobial agents useful in treating infections due to *Bacteroides fragilis*.

## Study Questions

**Choose the ONE correct answer**

14.1 The most common form of infection caused by *Clostridium botulinum* in this country is

    A. infant botulism.

    B. wound infection.

    C. food poisoning.

    D.  primary septicemia.

    E. anaerobic cellulitis.

Correct answer = A. Presently the most common form of botulism in the United States occurs in infants. Malignant food poisoning (C) was the first described form of infection and is probably the best known; a wound focus is rare (B). *C. botulinum* is noninvasive and causes neither septicemia (D) nor cellulitis (E).

14.2 *Clostridium perfringens* infections are commonly associated with

    A. contamination of wounds.

    B. antibiotic treatment.

    C. consumption of water contaminated with sewage.

    D. immunosuppression.

    E. preexisting lung disease.

Correct answer = A. Contamination of wounds is the most common route of infection by this organism. However, the symptoms of gastroenteritis associated with some strains of *C. perfringens* are usually caused by contamination of food.

14.3 Specific antitoxin is an important part of treatment in

    A. gas gangrene.

    B. tetanus.

    C. enteritis necroticans.

    D. pseudomembranous colitis.

    E. bacteroides and prevotella infections.

Correct answer = B. Tetanus antitoxin is an essential reagent in wound prophylaxis and the treatment of clinical disease. It neutralizes only that toxin that has not bound the neuronal receptors. In the case of gas gangrene (A), numerous clinical studies have shown no advantage in the use of antitoxin preparations; presumably the same would be true for enteritis necroticans and pseudomembranous colitis (C and D). Possible toxins among the gram-negative anaerobes are poorly described, and no therapeutic antisera are available (E).

14.4 A predisposing factor in pseudomembranous colitis (PMC) is

    A. clindamycin treatment.

    B.  neonatal age.

    C. diet high in dairy products.

    D. cholecystitis.

    E. older age (older than sixty years of age).

Correct answer = A. Antibiotic or antineoplastic treatment is often complicated by gastrointestinal disturbances, including PMC. Certain drugs, including clindamycin, are more likely to cause this complication.

*"I've decided to leave well enough alone."*

# Spirochetes

15

## I. OVERVIEW

Spirochetes are long, slender, motile, flexible, undulating, gram-negative bacilli that have a characteristic corkscrew or helical shape. Depending on the species, they can be aerobic, anaerobic, or facultatively anaerobic. Some species can be grown in laboratory culture (either cell-free culture or tissue culture), whereas others cannot. Some species are free-living, and some are part of the normal flora of humans and animals. Spirochetes that are important human pathogens are confined to three genera (Figure 15.1): *Treponema* (*T. pallidum* causes syphilis), *Borrelia* (*B. burgdorferi* causes Lyme disease, *B. recurrentis* causes relapsing fever), and *Leptospira* (*L. interrogans* causes leptospirosis).

## II. STRUCTURAL FEATURES OF SPIROCHETES

Spirochetes have a unique structure that is responsible for motility. As illustrated in Figure 15.2, the spirochete cell has a central protoplasmic cylinder bounded by a plasma membrane and a typical gram-negative cell wall. Unlike other bacilli, this cylinder is enveloped by an outer sheath composed of glycosaminoglycans.[1] Between the cell wall and the outer sheath are located multiple periplasmic flagella that do not protrude from the cell but are oriented axially. Bundles of these endo-flagella (axial filaments) span the entire length of the cell and are anchored at both ends. Although the mechanics are not totally clear, it is likely that these axial periplasmic flagella rotate like the external flag-ella of other motile bacteria, propelling the cell in a corkscrew-like manner. Spirochetes can move through highly viscous solutions with little impediment, and it is theorized that this kind of motion is responsible for the ability of spirochete pathogens to penetrate and invade host tissue, just as a corkscrew penetrates cork.

## III. TREPONEMA PALLIDUM

Syphilis is primarily a sexually transmitted disease caused by the spiro-chete *T. pallidum*. Starting with a small lesion (chancre), several pro-gressive stages of the disease can span a period of thirty years or

**Figure 15.1**
Classification of Spirochetes.
Ⓢ See p. 331 for summaries of these organisms.

**Figure 15.2**
Spirochete morphology.

[1]See p.155 in *Lippincott's Illustrated Reviews: Biochemistry* (3rd ed.) for a discussion of glycosaminoglycans.

**Figure 15.3**
Dark-field microscopy of
*Treponema pallidum.*

more, often ending in syphilitic dementia or cardiovascular damage. The causative organism of syphilis is extremely fastidious and fragile. It cannot be cultured routinely in the laboratory, and is sensitive to disinfectants, heat, and drying. *T. pallidum* is so thin that it cannot be observed by conventional light microscopy, but requires immunofluorescent or dark-field techniques (Figure 15.3). The outer surface of the spirochete is sparse in proteins, and the organism is only weakly antigenic. *T. pallidum* appears to produce neither endotoxins nor exotoxins, although it does secrete hyaluronidase, an enzyme that disrupts ground substance, and probably facilitates dissemination of the organism.

## A. Pathogenesis

Transmission of *T. pallidum* is almost always by sexual contact or transplacentally (congenital syphilis). This is understandable because the organism is so sensitive to environmental factors that survival outside of the host for more than a few minutes is highly unlikely. The organism enters the body through a break in the skin, or by penetrating mucous membranes, such as those of the genitalia.

## B. Clinical significance

1. **Syphilis:** Syphilis occurs in three stages (Figure 15.4). The first symptom of primary stage syphilis is a hard genital or oral ulcer (chancre) that develops at the site of inoculation. The average period between infection and the appearance of the chancre is about three weeks, but varies with the number of infecting organisms. This primary lesion heals spontaneously, but the organism continues to spread throughout the body via the lymph and blood. An asymptomatic period ensues, lasting as long as 24 weeks, followed by the secondary stage. This stage is characterized by the

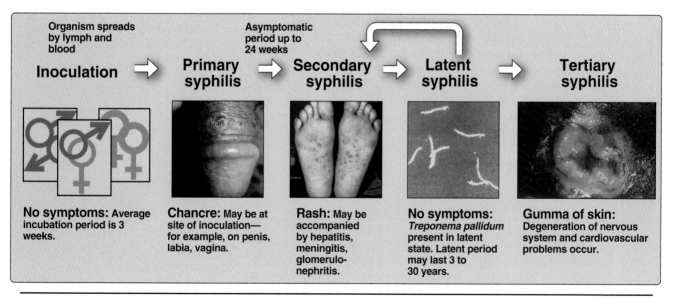

**Figure 15.4**
Clinical stages of untreated syphilis.

appearance of a red, maculopapular rash on almost any part of the body, including the palms of the hands and soles of the feet. Also present are pale, moist, flat papules seen primarily in the anogenital region (where they are called condylomata lata), armpits, and mouth. Both primary and secondary lesions teem with *T. pallidum* and are extremely infectious. The secondary stage may be accompanied by systemic involvement, causing hepatitis, meningitis, nephritis, or chorioretinitis. Upon healing of the secondary lesions, the disease enters a latent period that can last for many years. In approximately forty percent of infected individuals, the disease progresses to a tertiary stage, characterized by degeneration of the nervous system, cardiovascular lesions such as aneurysms, and granulomatous lesions (gummas) in the liver, skin, and bones.

> The chancre represents an initial local infection, but syphilis quickly becomes a systemic disease with widespread dissemination of the spirochete.

2. **Congenital syphilis:** *T. pallidum* can be transmitted through the placenta to a fetus after the first ten to fifteen weeks of pregnancy. Infection can cause death and spontaneous abortion of the fetus or cause it to be stillborn. Infected infants who live develop a condition similar to secondary syphilis, including a variety of central nervous system (CNS) and structural abnormalities. Treatment of the pregnant mother with appropriate antibiotics prevents congenital syphilis.

3. **Other treponemal infections:** Three geographically localized treponemal diseases closely mimic syphilis. They include bejel (found in hot, arid areas of Africa, Southeast Asia, and the Middle East), yaws (found in humid, tropical countries, Figure 15.5), and pinta (found in South and Central America, Mexico, and the Phillipines). Unlike syphilis, direct skin contact, crowded living conditions, and poor hygiene contribute to the spread of these diseases. Sexual contact is usually not the mode of transmission, and congenital infections occur rarely if at all. All three diseases are curable with penicillin.

**Figure 15.5**
Yaws: early stage.

## C. Laboratory identification

Although treponemal spirochetes from primary and secondary lesions can be detected microscopically using immunofluorescent stain or dark-field illumination (see Figure 15.3), syphilis is usually diagnosed serologically. Infection with *T. pallidum* elicits two kinds of antibodies: 1) antitreponemal antibodies that are specific to the treponemal surface proteins; and 2) nontreponemal antibodies (reagin), that are directed against normal phospholipid components—such as cardiolipin[2]—of mammalian membranes. Serologic tests using both kinds of antibodies are available. Antitreponemal antibody tests are more specific than reagin-based tests, but remain positive during and after successful treatment and, are,

[2]See p. 200 in *Lippincott's Illustrated Reviews: Biochemistry* (3rd ed.) for a discussion of the structure of cardiolipin.

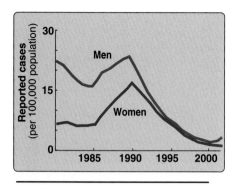

**Figure 15.6**
Incidence of primary and secondary syphilis.

therefore, not useful for monitoring therapy. Cardiolipin-based tests are less specific and liable to give more false-positives. [Note: Non-specific tests are therefore confirmed by a specific test (usually fluorescent treponemal antibody, FTA).] They are, nevertheless, useful in screening and for monitoring therapy because tests for reagin become negative about one year after successful treatment.

### D. Treatment and prevention

One single treatment with penicillin is curative for primary and secondary syphilis; no antibiotic resistance has been reported. In cases of patient sensitivity to penicillin, alternate therapy with erythromycin or tetracyclines may also be effective (see Figure 15.7). In spite of an inexpensive and highly effective cure, there are still over 8000 new cases of syphilis in the United States each year (Figure 15.6). There is no vaccine against *T. pallidum*; prevention depends on safe sexual practices. [Note: More than one sexually transmitted disease (STD) can be passed on at the same time. Therefore, when any STD has been diagnosed, the possibility of the infected individual also having syphilis should be considered.]

## IV. BORRELIA BURGDORFERI

Members of the genus *Borrelia* are relatively large spirochetes that, like *Treponema*, have endoflagella that make them highly motile (see Figure 15.12). *Borrelia* species are unusual among bacteria in that they have linear rather than circular plasmid and chromosomal DNA. Like *T. pallidum*, *Borrelia* do not appear to produce endotoxins or exotoxins.

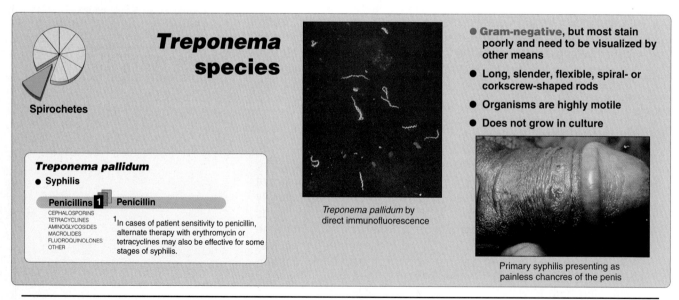

**Figure 15.7**
Summary of *Treponema* species.

## A. Pathogenesis

Lyme disease is caused by the spirochete *B. burgdorferi*, which is transmitted by the bite of a small tick of the genus *Ixodes* (Figure 15.8). [Note: The tick must be attached for at least 24 hours before there is transmission of bacteria.] Mice and other small rodents serve as primary reservoirs for the spirochete, but deer and other mammals serve as hosts for the ticks. Lyme disease is currently the most common arthropod-transmitted disease in the United States, averaging at least 10,000 cases per year.

## B. Clinical significance

The first stage of Lyme disease begins 3 to 32 days after a tick bite, when a characteristic red, circular lesion with a clear center (erythema chronicum migrans) appears at the site of the bite (Figure 15.9). Flulike symptoms often accompany the erythema. The organism spreads via the lymph or blood to musculoskeletal sites, skin, CNS, heart, and other tissues and organs. Weeks to months after the onset, the second stage of the disease begins, with symptoms such as arthritis, arthralgia, cardiac complications, and neurologic complications such as meningitis. Months to years later, the third stage begins with the appearance of chronic arthritis and, in a small number of patients, progressive CNS disease. Lyme disease is rarely fatal, but can result in a poor quality of life if untreated. IgM antibodies, which are directed against flagellar antigens, appear early after the onset of the disease, whereas IgG antibodies appear later. These antibodies offer protective immunity to reinfection, but the immunity is lost if the disease is treated early and successfully. Although caused by different spirochetes, the general similarities in the progression of Lyme disease and syphilis are striking.

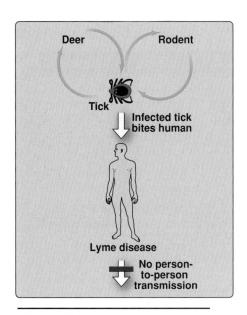

**Figure 15.8**
Transmission of Lyme disease.

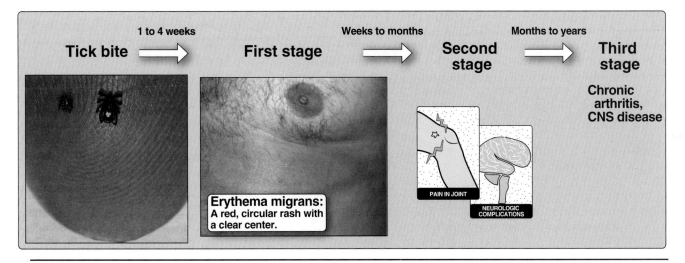

**Figure 15.9**
Clinical stages of untreated Lyme disease.

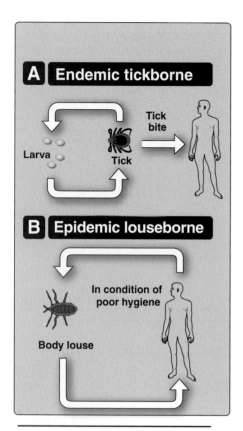

**Figure 15.10**
Endemic (for example, Lyme disease) versus epidemic relapsing fever by *Borrelia recurrentis*.

## C. Laboratory identification

Unlike *T. pallidum*, *B. burgdorferi* can be cultured, but the procedure is difficult, and takes six to eight weeks. Serologic tests have been used to diagnose Lyme disease, but the number of false-positives can outnumber the true-positives. Such tests should be used only as confirmation of a strong clinical suspicion. The most definitive test today is the polymerase chain reaction assay, which is rapid, sensitive, and specific (see p. 30).

## D. Treatment and prevention

Amoxicillin and doxycycline are useful treatments in the early stages of the disease (see Figure 15.12). If arthritic symptoms have already appeared, longer courses of antibiotics are used. Prevention of infection also includes use of insect repellents, and wearing clothing that sufficiently protects the body from tick bites.

# V. BORRELIA RECURRENTIS

*B. recurrentis* is a large, culturable spirochete. The organism is responsible for the disease relapsing fever, which is characterized by several cycles of apparent recovery, each followed by a relapse. A most striking property of *B. recurrentis* is its ability to change its surface protein antigens. This ability accounts for the relapsing nature of the disease because with each relapse a new antigenic variant arises.

## A. Pathogenesis

A distinction is often made between endemic and epidemic relapsing fever. An endemic disease such as Lyme disease, which occurs in most areas of the world, is tickborne (*B. burgdorferi* is passed from the mother tick to her progeny), whereas an epidemic disease such as epidemic relapsing fever, is transmitted from human to human by body lice (Figure 15.10). Fatalities from the endemic disease are rare; however, during epidemics in crowded, unsanitary, louse-infested environments, fatalities can be as high as thirty percent if untreated.

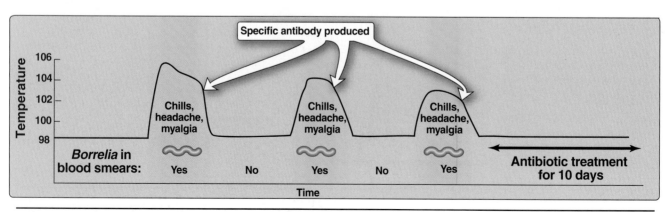

**Figure 15.11**
Clinical stages of relapsing fever.

## B. Clinical significance

The first symptoms of relapsing fever appear three to ten days after exposure to an infected arthropod (Figure 15.11). These symptoms include an abrupt onset of high fever, accompanied by severe headache, muscle pain, and general malaise. During this febrile period, which lasts three to five days, abundant spirochetes are present in the blood. The fever abates along with the number of spirochetes. Apparent recovery is experienced for a period of four to ten days, but is followed by a recurrence of the initial symptoms. There may be as many as ten such recurrences, generally with decreasing severity. In fatal cases, the spirochete invades many organs of the body (heart, spleen, liver, kidney), with death generally due to myocarditis.

## C. Diagnosis and treatment

Diagnosis is usually based on the appearance of Giemsa- or Wright-stainable, loosely coiled spirochetes in the blood during the febrile stage of the disease. Tetracyclines, erythromycin, and penicillin have proven effective treatments (Figure 15.12). However, the relapsing nature of the disease makes it difficult to distinguish spontaneous remissions from response to therapy. No vaccines are available, and prevention is best accomplished by protecting against lice.

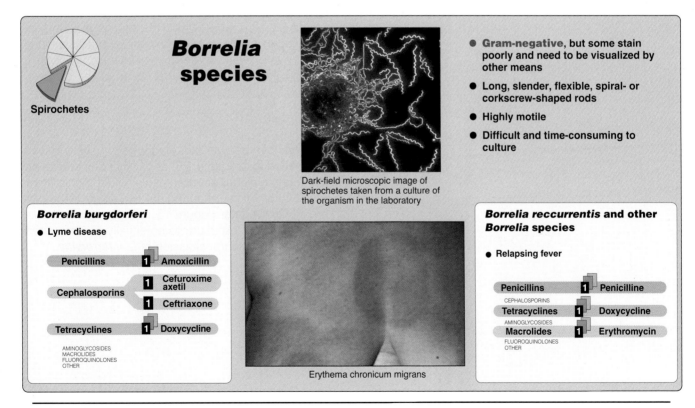

**Figure 15.12**
Summary of *Borrelia* species.

**Figure 15.13**
A. Dark-field micrograph of *Leptospira interrogans*. B. Electron micrograph of one end of a negatively stained *Leptospira interrogans* showing the axial fibril.

# VI. LEPTOSPIRA INTERROGANS

*L. interrogans* infection causes the disease leptospirosis. The organism is a slender (lepto = slender), tightly coiled, culturable spirochete with a single, thin, axial filament, and hooked ends (Figure 15.13). Many serogroups and serotypes (serovars) are recognized and specific to distinct geographic locales. *L. interrogans* is sensitive to drying and a broad range of disinfectants; it can, however, survive for weeks in slightly alkaline water.

## A. Epidemiology and pathogenesis

Leptospirosis is essentially an animal disease that is coincidentally transmitted to humans—primarily by water or food contaminated with animal urine. Entrance to the body can also occur via small skin abrasions or the conjunctiva. Although leptospirosis occurs worldwide (under various local names, such as infectious jaundice, marsh fever, Weil disease, and swineherd's disease), the incidence of the disease today in developed countries is very low; less than 100 cases of clinically significant *L. interrogans* infections are reported annually in the United States.

## B. Clinical significance

Fever occurs one to two weeks after infection, at which time spirochetes appear in the blood. These symptoms decrease after about one week. However, in cases of biphasic disease (that is, the disease having two stages), spirochetes reappear, accompanied by invasion of the liver, kidneys, and CNS. This results in jaundice, hemorrhage, tissue necrosis, and/or aseptic meningitis. This second stage of the disease, which lasts three or more weeks, involves a rise in circulating IgM antibodies. In severe cases of the disease, mortality can be as high as ten percent.

## C. Diagnosis and treatment

Although *L. interrogans* can be cultured, diagnosis is usually based on serologic agglutination tests (see p. 28) and visual demonstration of the spirochetes in urine, blood, or cerebrospinal fluid. Penicillin or doxycycline is useful if administered during the first stage of the disease, but both are ineffective later (Figure 15.14). No vaccine is currently available. Prevention of exposure to potentially contaminated water and food helps control the transmission of *L. interrogans*.

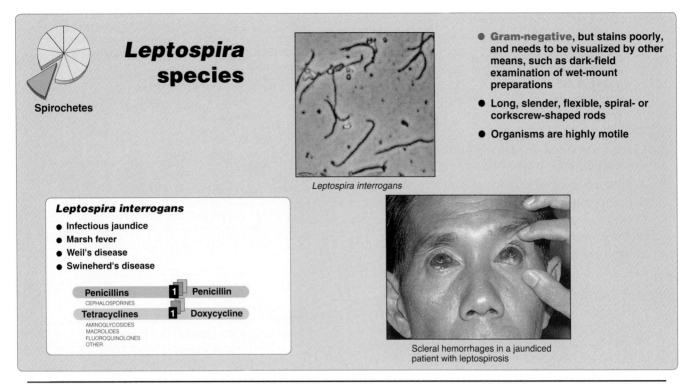

**Leptospira species**

Spirochetes

Leptospira interrogans

- **Gram-negative**, but stains poorly, and needs to be visualized by other means, such as dark-field examination of wet-mount preparations
- Long, slender, flexible, spiral- or corkscrew-shaped rods
- Organisms are highly motile

**Leptospira interrogans**
- Infectious jaundice
- Marsh fever
- Weil's disease
- Swineherd's disease

| Penicillins | 1 | Penicillin |
| CEPHALOSPORINES | | |
| Tetracyclines | 1 | Doxycycline |
| AMINOGLYCOSIDES | | |
| MACROLIDES | | |
| FLUOROQUINOLONES | | |
| OTHER | | |

Scleral hemorrhages in a jaundiced patient with leptospirosis

**Figure 15.14**
Summary of *Leptospira* species.


## Study Questions

**Choose the ONE correct answer**

15.1 The probable cause for the relapsing nature of relapsing fever caused by *Borrelia recurrentis* is

    A. the sequential appearance of new antibiotic resistant variants.

    B. periodic spore dormancy and activation.

    C. successive appearance of antigenic variants.

    D. periodic hormonal fluctuations in the host.

    E. organisms that survive and propagate after spirochete-induced fever.

Correct answer = C. Any of these mechanisms are conceivable with various degrees of plausibility. The weight of evidence, however, favors the mechanism whereby new antigenic variants arise that elude, for a period, the host's immune defenses, to then be replaced by another variant.

15.2 Which of the following spirochete-caused diseases is transmitted by an arthropod?

    A. Leptospirosis

    B. Pinta

    C. Relapsing fever

    D. Yaws

    E. Syphilis

Correct answer = C. *B. recurrentis*, the cause of relapsing fever, is borne by ticks. Pinta, yaws, and syphilis are transmitted by direct human-to-human contact, whereas leptospirosis is transmitted via water contaminated with animal urine.

15.3 A distinctive feature of spirochetes is the presence of

    A. fimbriae.

    B. endoflagella.

    C. helically arranged pili.

    D. nucleosomes.

    E. variable surface antigens.

> Correct answer = B. The endoflagella are thought to be responsible for the corkscrew motion of spirochetes. The other structural features are not specific to spirochetes.

15.4 Syphilis and Lyme disease are strikingly similar in which of the following aspects?

    A. Their modes of transmission are similar.

    B. Both diseases display three similar, distinct phases.

    C. Both causative agents share many antigenic markers.

    D. The diseases show cross-immunity.

    E. Both causative agents can be cultured.

> Correct answer = B. Syphilis, like Lyme disease, has three distinct phases. The other listed properties are either irrelevant or false. Unlike *T. pallidum*, *B. burgdorferi* can be cultured, but the procedure is difficult and takes six to eight weeks.

15.5 A 22-year-old male presents to his physician, complaining of a two-week history of a sore on his penis. Physical examination shows a firm, raised, red, nontender chancre midway between the base and glans. Which of the following is the most appropriate course of action for the physician?

    A. Test a serum sample for antibodies to herpes simplex virus.

    B. Swab the chancre and culture on Thayer-Martin agar.

    C. Swab the chancre and perform a Gram stain.

    D. Perform a dark-field examination on a swab of the active lesion.

    E. Swab the chancre and culture on blood agar.

> Correct answer = D. The patient most likely has primary syphilis rather than herpes simplex virus because the penile chancre is not tender. Herpes lesions are typically very painful. *Treponema pallidum*, the etiologic agent of syphilis, cannot be readily cultured in the routine clinical microbiology laboratory. Treponemal spirochetes from primary and secondary lesions can be detected microscopically using immunofluorescent stain or dark-field illumination. However, syphilis is usually diagnosed serologically by detection of: 1) antitreponemal antibodies that are specific to the treponemal surface proteins, and 2) nontreponemal antibodies (reagin), that are directed against normal phospholipid components.

"I'm not saying it's contagious, however. . . ."

# Mycoplasma

16

## I. OVERVIEW

Mycoplasmas are small, prokaryotic organisms with no peptidoglycan cell walls. Instead, they are enclosed in a single, trilaminar plasma membrane. Because of their extremely small size, mycoplasmas frequently pass through bacteriologic filters. The many *Mycoplasma* species are widely distributed in nature, and include several commensals commonly found in the mouth and genitourinary tract of humans and other mammals. For these reasons, mycoplasmas are often recovered as contaminants or adventitious flora from biologic materials, including clinical samples. Three *Mycoplasma* species are definitively associated with human disease, namely *Mycoplasma pneumoniae*, which is the cause of a primary atypical pneumonia, and *Mycoplasma hominis* and *Ureaplasma urealyticum*, which are associated with a variety of genitourinary diseases, such as urethritis, pelvic inflammatory disease, and intrapartum infections (Figure 16.1). Lacking cell walls, mycoplasmas are insensitive to antibiotics that inhibit cell division by preventing cell wall synthesis (such as penicillin, see p. 42). However, they are susceptible to other inhibitors of prokaryotic metabolism.

## II. GENERAL FEATURES OF MYCOPLASMAS

Lacking cell walls, mycoplasmas are enclosed instead by a membrane composed of a lipid bilayer (Figure 16.2). They are, therefore, plastic and pleomorphic, and thus cannot be classified as either cocci or rods. Mycoplasmas are also the smallest of known free-living, self-replicating prokaryotic cells. Their double-stranded DNA genomes often measure less than $10^9$ daltons. [Note: This may approach the minimum DNA coding capacity required for the free-living state.]

### A. Physiology

Mycoplasmas have limited biosynthetic capabilities, and require a variety of small, organic molecules for growth. Unlike other prokaryotes, mycoplasmas contain sterols in their cell membranes.

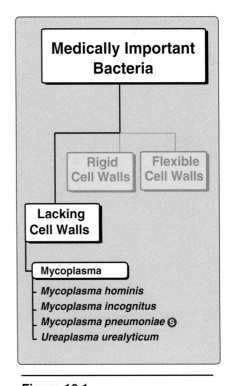

**Figure 16.1**
Classification of Mycoplasma.
Ⓢ See p. 331 for a summary of this organism.

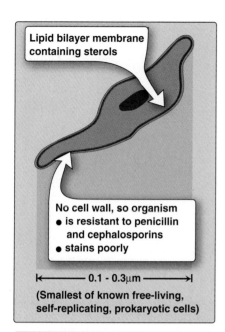

**Figure 16.2**
Structural features of *Mycoplasma*.

Because most mycoplasma species cannot synthesize the sterol ring, they require an external source of cholesterol from serum or a similar medium supplement. Given appropriate supplementation, they can be grown in cell-free media. The medically important species of mycoplasmas are facultative anaerobes (see p. 23), although some genus members are strict anaerobes.

### B. Colony production

Mycoplasmas produce minute colonies on specialized agar after several days of incubation. These are best visualized under 30 to 100x magnification. The central portion of the colony penetrates the agar while the periphery spreads over the adjacent surface, in some cases giving the colony a characteristic "fried egg" appearance (see Figure 16.5).

## III. MYCOPLASMA PNEUMONIAE

*M. pneumoniae* is transmitted by respiratory droplets, and causes a lower respiratory tract infection (primary atypical pneumonia, so named because the signs and symptoms are unlike typical lobar pneumonia). The organism accounts for approximately twenty percent of pneumonia cases, as well as causing milder infections such as bronchitis, pharyngitis, and nonpurulent otitis media. Infections occur worldwide and year-round, with increased incidence in late fall and winter. Cases are usually sporadic, although occasional epidemics among individuals in close contact are reported in both civilian settings (for example, schools and prisons) and among military populations. The highest incidence of clinical disease is seen in older children and young adults (six to twenty years of age).

### A. Pathogenesis

*M. pneumoniae* possesses a membrane-associated protein, P1, which functions as a cytoadhesin. It is concentrated in a specialized organelle, visible under electron microscopy, which binds sialic acid-rich glycolipids found on certain host cell membranes. Among susceptible cell types are ciliated bronchial epithelial cells. The organisms grow closely attached to the host cell luminal surface and inhibit ciliary action. Eventually patches of affected mucosa desquamate, and an inflammatory response develops in bronchial and adjacent tissues involving lymphocytes and other mononuclear cells. The clinical disease is thus largely an expression of host-specific immune response rather than damage created by the organism itself. In infected individuals, organisms are shed in saliva for several days before onset of clinical illness. Reinfection is common, and symptoms are more severe in older children and young adults who have previously encountered the organism.

## B. Clinical significance

Primary atypical pneumonia (lower respiratory tract disease) is the best known form of *M. pneumoniae* infection. However, this disease accounts for a minority of the infectious episodes with this organism, upper respiratory tract and ear infection being much more frequent. Primary atypical pneumonia clinically resembles pneumonia caused by a number of viruses and bacteria, such as *Chlamydia* species. Onset is usually gradual, beginning with nonspecific symptoms such as unrelenting headache, accompanied by fever, chills, and malaise. After two to four days, a dry or scantily productive cough develops. Earache is sometimes an accompanying complaint. Chest radiographs reveal a patchy, diffuse bronchopneumonia involving one or more lobes (Figure 16.3). The infiltration is usually more extensive than physical examination might suggest. Patients often remain ambulatory throughout the illness (hence, "walking pneumonia"). In the absence of preexisting compromise (immunodeficiency, emphysema), the disease remits after three to ten days without specific treatment. X-ray abnormalities resolve more slowly in two weeks to two months. Complications are rare, but include CNS disturbances, a rash (erythema multiform), and mild, hemolytic anemia (the latter associated with production of cold agglutinins, see below).

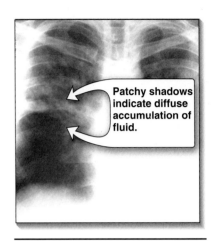

Patchy shadows indicate diffuse accumulation of fluid.

**Figure 16.3**
Radiograph of lung of an individual with *M. pneumoniae*–induced primary atypical pneumonia.

Onset of infection caused by *M. pneumoniae* is gradual, and usually manifested by headache, malaise, and low grade fever. The patient may complain of significant illness despite minimal abnormalities on physical examination.

## C. Immunity

Infection with *M. pneumoniae* elicits both local and systemic immune responses. Only one *M. pneumoniae* serotype has been described. Serum antibody to outer membrane glycolipids and to the P1 adhesin can be demonstrated, with antibody peaking two to four weeks after infection, and gradually disappearing over the following year. An IgM antibody, the cold agglutinin, is produced by approximately sixty percent of infected patients. [Note: This antibody's name derives from the fact that it reacts with the human erythrocyte antigen I, reversibly agglutinating I$^+$ red blood cells at temperatures of 0° to 4°C, but not at 37°C.]

## D. Laboratory identification

Direct microscopic examination of clinical material for *M. pneumoniae* is of limited value. Sputum is scanty and nonpurulent, and the pathogen stains poorly or not at all using standard bacteriologic stains. Sputum samples or throat swabs can be cultured on special media; however, isolation of the organism usually requires eight to fifteen days and, therefore, cannot aid in early treatment decisions.

Serologic tests are the most widely used procedures for establishing a diagnosis of primary atypical pneumonia. Specific antibody is commonly detected by complement fixation using an extract of mycoplasmal glycolipids. A diagnosis is established by a fourfold rise in titer between acute and convalescent samples. Because symptoms of illness develop slowly, the initial serum sample may be positive.

### E. Treatment

*M. pneumoniae* is sensitive to doxycycline or azithromycin (see Figure 16.5). When given early, either antibiotic shortens the course of disease, although symptoms may be eliminated only gradually with such treatment. The organisms, however, may persist in the convalescent upper respiratory tract for weeks.

> Because there is no rapid way to make the diagnosis of *M. pneumoniae* pneumonia, treatment begins with empiric therapy—most often with macrolide antibiotics—for atypical pneumonia.

## IV. GENITAL MYCOPLASMAS

*Mycoplasma hominis* and *Ureaplasma urealyticum* are common inhabitants of the genitourinary tract, particularly in sexually active adults. Because colonization rates in some populations are in excess of fifty percent, it is difficult to establish an unequivocal causal role in various disease states with which the organisms are associated. Both agents can be cultured. They grow more rapidly than *M. pneumoniae*, and can be distinguished by their carbon utilization patterns; *M. hominis* degrades arginine, *U. urealyticum* hydrolyses urea. [Note: *Ureaplasma* is sometimes referred to as a "T-strain" of mycoplasma because it produces tiny colonies not visible to the naked eye.] The major clinical condition associated with *M. hominis* is postpartum or postabortal fever (Figure 16.4). The organism has been isolated from blood cultures in up to ten percent of women so affected. It is also recovered locally in cases of pelvic inflammatory disease, although sometimes in mixed culture. A number of serotypes of *M. hominis* have been described. It is important to note that *M. hominis* isolates are uniformly resistant to erythromycin, in contrast to other mycoplasmas. Tetracycline is effective for specific treatment. *U. urealyticum* is a common cause of **urethritis** when neither gonococcus nor chlamydia can be demonstrated, particularly in men. In women, the organism has been isolated from cases of endometritis and from vaginal secretions of women who undergo premature labor or deliver low-birth-weight babies. The infants are often colonized, and *U. urealyticum* has been isolated from the infant's lower respiratory tract and central nervous system both with and without evidence of inflammatory response.

**Figure 16.4**
A. Diseases caused by *M. hominis* and *U. urealyticum.* B. The antibiotic used to treat these infections.

## V.  OTHER MYCOPLASMAS

Several other species of mycoplasma can be recovered from human sources, for which no pathogenic role is established to date. One such organism, AIDS-associated mycoplasma, or *M. incognitus*, has been isolated in high frequency from patients with that disease, in which the organism may play a role, possibly as a secondary invader.

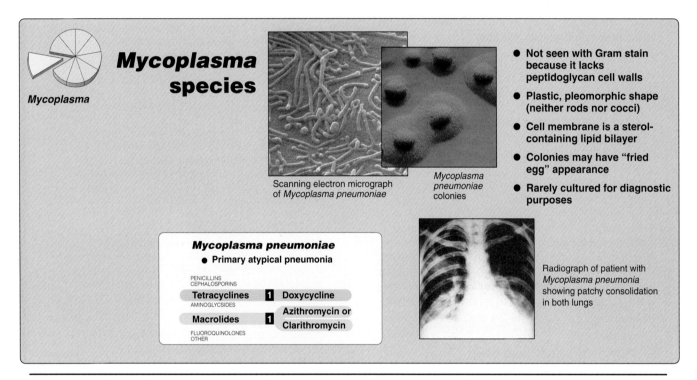

*Mycoplasma*

# *Mycoplasma species*

Scanning electron micrograph of *Mycoplasma pneumoniae*

*Mycoplasma pneumoniae* colonies

- Not seen with Gram stain because it lacks peptidoglycan cell walls
- Plastic, pleomorphic shape (neither rods nor cocci)
- Cell membrane is a sterol-containing lipid bilayer
- Colonies may have "fried egg" appearance
- Rarely cultured for diagnostic purposes

### *Mycoplasma pneumoniae*
- Primary atypical pneumonia

PENICILLINS
CEPHALOSPORINS
**Tetracyclines** 1 Doxycycline
AMINOGLYCSIDES
**Macrolides** 1 Azithromycin or Clarithromycin
FLUOROQUINOLONES
OTHER

Radiograph of patient with *Mycoplasma pneumonia* showing patchy consolidation in both lungs

**Figure 16.5**
Summary of mycoplasma disease.

## Study Questions

Choose the ONE correct answer

16.3 Postpartum fever due to *Mycoplasma hominis* is treated with:

    A. tetracycline.

    B. erythromycin.

    C. penicillin G.

    D.  a second-generation cephalosporin.

    E. vancomycin.

Correct answer = A. Mycoplasmas are small, prokaryotic organisms with no peptidoglycan cell walls. Thus inhibitors of cell wall synthesis, such as penicillins, cephalosporins, and vancomycin are not effective. *M. hominis* isolates, in contrast to other mycoplasmas, are uniformly resistant to erythromycin. Tetracycline is effective for specific treatment.

16.2 A distinguishing feature of human mycoplasma species is that they:

A. stain well with Giemsa, but not by Gram stain.

B. contain no bacterial peptidoglycan.

C. are not immunogenic because they mimic host cell membrane components.

D. cannot be cultivated *in vitro*.

E. are dependent on host sources of ATP.

> Correct answer = B. The distinguishing feature of mycoplasmas is their complete lack of a cell wall.

16.3 Which of the following is most characteristic of *Mycoplasma pneumoniae* infection?

A. Infection results in a fever of sudden onset accompanied by a productive cough.

B. Infection most commonly occurs in the upper respiratory tract.

C. Infection is definitively diagnosed by direct microscopic examination of sputum.

D. Reinfection is rare and less severe than primary infection.

E. Infection causes extensive scarring and calcification of affected lung tissue.

> Correct answer = B. Primary atypical pneumonia is the best known form of *M. pneumoniae* infection. However, upper respiratory tract and ear infection are much more frequent. Atypical pneumonia is characterized by a gradual onset and a scantily productive cough. Direct microscopic examination of clinical material for *M. pneumoniae* is of limited value. Sputum is scanty and nonpurulent, and the pathogen stains poorly or not at all using standard bacteriologic stains. Reinfection causes more severe lesions and a more extensive chronic inflammatory response. Recovery is slow, but without residual damage.

16.4 A 30-year-old woman complained of unrelenting headache, accompanied by fever, chills, and malaise. After two to four days, a dry cough developed. Chest X-rays reveal a patchy, diffuse bronchopneumonia involving both lobes. Her white cell count was not elevated. Which of the following is the most likely diagnosis?

A. Legionellosis

B. Infection with parainfluenza virus

C. Infection with *Streptococcus pneumoniae*

D. Infection with *Haemophilus influenzae*

E. Infection with *Mycoplasma pneumoniae*

> Correct answer = E. The description suggests primary atypical pneumonia caused by *Myoplasma pneumoniae*. Patients often remain ambulatory throughout the illness, hence the name "walking pneumonia." In the absence of preexisting compromise (immunodeficiency, emphysema, etc.), the disease remits after three to ten days without specific treatment. X-ray abnormalities resolve more slowly in two weeks to two months.

*"This will buy you four months."*

# Chlamydiae

# 17

## I. OVERVIEW

*Chlamydia* is a genus of small bacteria that are obligate intracellular parasites, depending on the host cell for energy in the forms of adenosine triphosphate (ATP) and nicotinamide adenine dinucleotide ($NAD^+$). They grow in cytoplasmic vacuoles in a limited number of host cell types. The genus is divided into three species: *Chlamydia trachomatis*, *Chlamydia psittaci*, and *Chlamydia pneumoniae*. *C. trachomatis* infections cause diseases of the genitourinary tract and the eye, including many cases of nongonococcal urethritis and ocular infections such as trachoma. *C. psittaci* and *C. pneumoniae* infect various levels of the respiratory tract. For example, *C. psittaci* causes psittacosis, and *C. pneumoniae* causes atypical pneumonia. Figure 17.1 summarizes the clinically significant chlamydiae.

## II. GENERAL FEATURES OF CHLAMYDIAE

Chlamydiae are small, round-to-ovoid organisms that vary in size during the different stages of their replicative cycle (Figure 17.2). The chlamydial cell envelope consists of two lipid bilayers with associated cell wall material that resembles a gram-negative envelope. However, it contains no peptidoglycan, and muramic acid is not present. The chlamydial DNA genome is less than $10^9$ daltons in size, making it among the smallest found in prokaryotic cells. Chlamydiae possess ribosomes and synthesize their own proteins and, therefore, are sensitive to antibiotics that inhibit this process, such as tetracyclines and macrolides (see pp. 43–44).

### A. Physiology

Chlamydiae are energy parasites; hence, their requirement for growth in living cells. They are unable to synthesize their own pools of ATP or regenerate $NAD^+$ by oxidation. With these high-energy molecules exogenously supplied, chlamydiae produce $CO_2$ from compounds such as glucose, pyruvate, or glutamate and carry out the usual bacterial metabolic activities.

### B. Pathogenesis

Chlamydiae have a unique life cycle, with morphologically distinct infectious and reproductive forms (Figure 17.3). The extracellular infectious form, the elementary body, is a tiny, condensed, apparently inert structure that can survive extracellular cell-to-cell pas-

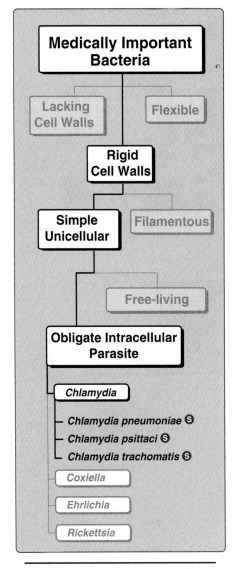

**Figure 17 .1**
Classification of *Chlamydia*.
⑤ See p. 331 for summaries of these organisms.

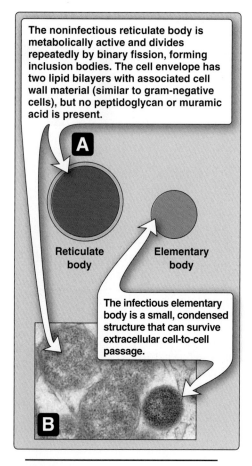

The noninfectious reticulate body is metabolically active and divides repeatedly by binary fission, forming inclusion bodies. The cell envelope has two lipid bilayers with associated cell wall material (similar to gram-negative cells), but no peptidoglycan or muramic acid is present.

**A**

Reticulate body

Elementary body

The infectious elementary body is a small, condensed structure that can survive extracellular cell-to-cell passage.

**B**

**Figure 17.2**
Structural features of *Chlamydia*.
A. Schematic drawing. B. Electron micrograph.

sage and initiate an infection. The elementary body is taken up by phagocytosis into susceptible host cells, a process facilitated by proteins in the chlamydial cell envelope that function as adhesins, directing attachment to glycolipid or glycopolysaccharide receptors on the host cell membrane. Once inside the cell, the elementary body prevents fusion of the phagosome and lysosome, protecting itself from enzymatic destruction. The particle reorganizes over the next eight hours into a larger, noninfectious reticulate body, which becomes metabolically active and divides repeatedly by binary fission within the cytoplasm of the host cell. As the reticulate body divides, it fills the endosome with its progeny, forming an inclusion body. After 48 hours, multiplication ceases and reticulate bodies condense to become new infectious elementary bodies. The elementary bodies are then released from the cell by cytolysis, ending in host cell death.

### C. Laboratory identification

1. **Useful stains:** Chlamydiae are not stained using the Gram stain, but can be visualized under light microscopy by stains that preserve the host cell architecture. Direct immunofluorescence is also a common and useful procedure. In *C. trachomatis* only, a matrix of glycogenlike material accumulates in the inclusions, which can be shown by staining with iodine. Other species do not give this reaction.

2. **Chlamydial antigens:** Although DNA homology among chlamydial species is less than thirty percent, they share lipopolysaccharide antigens that delineate the genus. In addition, there is a class of abundant outer membrane proteins that have species or subspecies specificity and elicit protective antibody. Antigenic classification in this genus is usually done by immunofluorescence, using monoclonal antibodies.

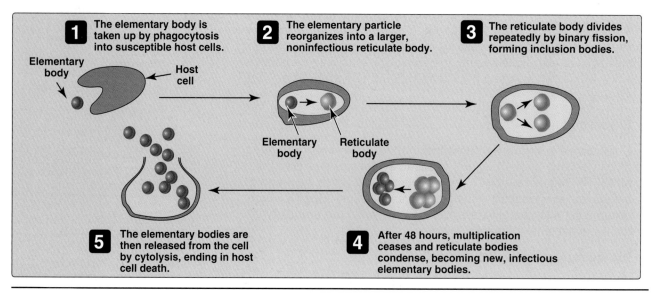

1  The elementary body is taken up by phagocytosis into susceptible host cells.

Elementary body

Host cell

2  The elementary particle reorganizes into a larger, noninfectious reticulate body.

Elementary body     Reticulate body

3  The reticulate body divides repeatedly by binary fission, forming inclusion bodies.

5  The elementary bodies are then released from the cell by cytolysis, ending in host cell death.

4  After 48 hours, multiplication ceases and reticulate bodies condense, becoming new, infectious elementary bodies.

**Figure 17.3**
Reproduction cycle of *Chlamydia*.

## III. CHLAMYDIA TRACHOMATIS

*C. trachomatis* is divided into a number of serotypes, which correlate with the clinical syndrome they cause (Figure 17.4). For example, *C. trachomatis*, the major causal agent of the syndrome, non-gonococcal urethritis (NGU), is currently the most common sexually transmitted bacterial disease in the United States. *C. trachomatis* can also cause eye infections, with symptoms ranging from irritation to blindness. **Trachoma**, which is an ancient disease, was well described in Egyptian writings around 3800 B.C. It remains widely prevalent in developing areas of the world.

### A. Clinical significance

*C. trachomatis* causes a range of genitourinary and eye infections.

1. **Nongonococcal urethritis (NGU):** Annually, more than four million urogenital *C. trachomatis* infections occur in the United States in young, sexually active individuals of all socioeconomic groups. In males, the urethra is the principal locus of infection. Females may present with cervicitis and/or urethritis (see p. 182). Infections are often asymptomatic, although communicable. [Note: Among women, the asymptomatic rate is higher than fifty percent.] Whether locally symptomatic or not, contiguous spread of infection may involve the epididymis in men and fallopian tubes and adjacent tissues in women (pelvic inflammatory disease). Chlamydial NGU is symptomatically similar to infections caused by *Neisseria gonorrhoeae* (see p. 102), although the average incubation time is longer (two to three weeks), and the discharge tends to be more mucoid and contains fewer pus cells. In addition, the two infections often occur simultaneously or sequentially. Therefore, patients suspected of chlamydial infection should be treated for neisserial infection as well. NGU is caused by serotypes D–K of *C. trachomatis* (see Figure 17.4). These serotypes also cause eye infections, for example, in infants born to genitally infected women (Figure 17.5).

| Species and serotype | Disease |
|---|---|
| ***C. trachomatis***<br>A, B, C | ● Trachoma |
| D – K | ● Cervicitis<br>● Endometritis<br>● Epididymitis<br>● Inclusion conjunctivitis of the newborn (ICN) or adult<br>● Infant pneumonia syndrome<br>● Nongonococcal urethritis<br>● Proctitis<br>● Salpingitis |
| $L_1, L_2, L_3$ | ● Lymphogranuloma venereum (LGV) |
| ***C. psittaci***<br>Many | ● Pneumonia (psittacosis) |
| ***C. pneumoniae***<br>One | Acute respiratory diseases, including:<br>● Bronchitis<br>● Pharyngitis<br>● Pneumonia<br>● Sinusitis |

**Figure 17.4**
Correlation between chlamydial species/serotypes and disease.

> Infection with *C. trachomatis* confers little protection against reinfection, which commonly occurs. Repeated or chronic episodes may lead to sterility in both sexes and to ectopic pregnancies.

2. **Lymphogranuloma venereum (LGV):** *C. trachomatis* serotypes $L_1$, $L_2$, and $L_3$ cause LGV, a more invasive sexually transmitted disease (see p. 182). It is uncommon in the United States, but endemic in Asia, Africa, and South America. LGV is characterized by transient papules on the external genitalia, followed in one to two months by painful swelling of inguinal and perirectal lymph nodes. Adenopathy (swelling of the lymph nodes) is often accompanied by mild constitutional symptoms. The inguinal ligament often forms a cleft known as the "groove sign" between masses of inguinal lymph nodes. The affected lymph nodes suppurate, and

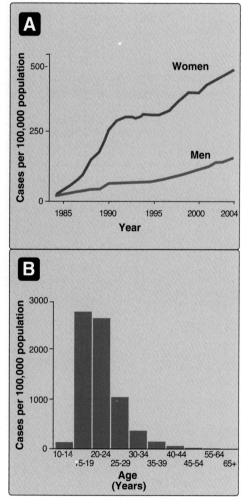

**Figure 17.5**
Neonatal conjunctivitis due to chlamydial infection.

**Figure 17.6**
Prevalence of chlamydial infection.
A. by sex; B. Among females according to age.

chronic inflammation and fibrosis lead to extensive ulceration and blockage of regional lymphatic drainage. (See pp. 367–371 for a summary of sexually transmitted diseases.)

3. **Trachoma:** *C. trachomatis*, serotypes A, B, $B_a$, and C cause a chronic keratoconjunctivitis that often results in blindness (see p. 182). Trachoma is transmitted by personal contact, for example, by eye to eye via droplets, by contaminated surfaces touched by hands and conveyed to the eye, or by flies. Because of persistent or repeated infection over several years, the inflammatory response with attendant scarring leads to permanent opacities of the cornea, and distortion of eyelids.

4. **Neonatal conjunctivitis and other infections:** Over fifty percent of infants born to women infected with *C. trachomatis*, serotypes D–K (see Figure 17.4) will contract symptomatic infection on passage through the birth canal. The most common presentation is inclusion conjunctivitis of the newborn (ICN, see Figure 17.5). This acute, purulent conjunctivitis [named for the inclusion bodies (see p. 178) seen in infected conjunctival epithelial cells] usually heals without permanent damage to the eye. Approximately one of ten infected infants will present with or develop an interstitial pneumonitis, which if left untreated may last several weeks.

5. **Inclusion conjunctivitis in adults:** Individuals of any age may develop transient purulent conjunctivitis caused by *C. trachomatis* serotypes D–K (see Figure 17.4). Such individuals are often found to be genitally infected as well.

### B. Laboratory identification

*C. trachomatis* can be demonstrated in clinical material by several direct procedures, and by culturing in human cell lines. Samples, particularly from urethra and cervix in genitourinary infection and conjunctivae in ocular disease, should be obtained by cleaning away overlying exudate, and gently scraping to exfoliate infected epithelial cells.

1. **Direct tests:** Microscopic examination using direct fluorescent antibody staining reveals characteristic cellular cytoplasmic inclusions. *C. trachomatis* infections can be detected with high sensitivity and specificity using DNA-amplification performed on urine specimens. This permits cost-effective screening of large numbers of individuals without the need for access to a medical clinic and a pelvic examination. For example, Figure 17.6 shows the high prevalence of infection among young females.

2. **Culturing methods:** *C. trachomatis* can be cultivated by tissue culture several human cell lines. In the standard procedure using McCoy cells, addition to the culture medium of a eukaryotic metabolic inhibitor such as cycloheximide enhances growth of the parasite. The presence of chlamydial inclusions can be demonstrated after two to seven days of incubation.

3. **Detection of serotypes:** Serotypes of *C. trachomatis* can be determined by immunofluorescence staining with monoclonal antibodies. However, the procedure is not widely used because it adds

little to clinical impressions. Serologic testing for specific antibodies is similarly not helpful except in suspected lymphogranuloma venereum, in which a single high-titer response is diagnostic.

## C. Treatment and prevention

Chlamydiae are sensitive to a number of broad-spectrum antibacterials. Azithromycin and tetracycline are currently the drugs of choice. Resistant strains have not been reported in the clinical setting. Erythromycin should be used in small children and pregnant women because of the effects of tetracyclines on calcification (see Figure 17.8). [Note: These drugs are also effective in the simultaneous treatment of gonococcal infections that may accompany chlamydial infections.] A topical ocular preparation containing erythromycin provides moderately effective prophylaxis in newborns. Detection—a particular problem in asymptomatic individuals—followed by specific treatment is the key means of control.

## IV. CHLAMYDIA PSITTACI

Psittacosis, or more broadly, ornithosis, denotes a zoonotic disease that is transmitted to humans by inhalation of dust contaminated with respiratory secretions or feces of infected birds. The human disease usually targets the lower respiratory tract (Figure 17.7). There is an acute onset of fever, hacking dry cough, and flulike symptoms. Bilateral patchy pulmonary infiltrates are observed. Enlargement of liver and spleen is a frequent accompanying feature. Frank hepatitis, encephalitis, or myocarditis sometimes ensues. The severity of illness ranges from essentially asymptomatic infection to, rarely, a fatal outcome, usually for older patients. A wide variety of bird species, including psittacines (the parrot family), carry *C. psittaci*, often latently, and contact with either diseased or healthy birds is an important item in formulating the differential diagnosis. A specific diagnosis can be made by showing a four-fold rise in antibody titer with either complement fixation (see p. 274) or indirect immunofluorescence tests (see p. 28). The organism can be grown in tissue culture from sputum and other clinical materials; however, this is not routinely attempted. Some strains are highly contagious and impose a considerable laboratory risk. If given early in the disease, doxycycline or erythromycin is effective in eradicating symptoms, but the organisms sometimes persist well into convalescence, because the drugs are bacteriostatic, not bactericidal (see p. 31).

## V. CHLAMYDIA PNEUMONIAE

*C. pneumoniae* is a respiratory pathogen causing pharyngitis, sometimes followed by laryngitis, bronchitis, or interstitial pneumonia. It is a significant cause of community-acquired respiratory infection, occurring worldwide and without seasonal incidence. Epidemic outbreaks have been reported. About fifty percent of adults in the United States have antibodies to *C. pneumoniae*. Nevertheless, reinfection is known to occur. Several recent studies have linked *C. pneumoniae* antigens (or higher antibody titers to the organism) with atherosclerotic processes and asthma. However, a role for the organism in these diseases has not been established. Neither serologic tests nor recovery by culturing is routinely available. The organism is sensitive to doxycycline and erythromycin.

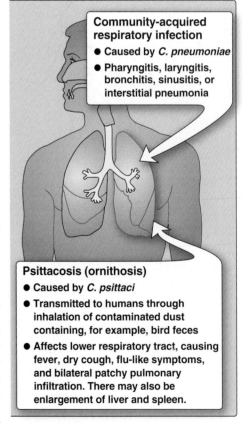

**Community-acquired respiratory infection**
- Caused by *C. pneumoniae*
- Pharyngitis, laryngitis, bronchitis, sinusitis, or interstitial pneumonia

**Psittacosis (ornithosis)**
- Caused by *C. psittaci*
- Transmitted to humans through inhalation of contaminated dust containing, for example, bird feces
- Affects lower respiratory tract, causing fever, dry cough, flu-like symptoms, and bilateral patchy pulmonary infiltration. There may also be enlargement of liver and spleen.

**Figure 17.7**
Diseases caused by *C. psittaci* and *C. pneumoniae*.

# *Chlamydia* species

*Chlamydia trachomatis* inclusion bodies

Inclusion body

- Not routinely stained with Gram stain
- Small, round-to-ovoid organisms
- Envelope consists of two lipid bilayers
- Obligate intracellular parasites, the organisms replicate in endocytic vacuoles, creating characteristic cytoplasmic inclusion bodies

### *Chlamydia pneumoniae*
- Community-acquired respiratory infection

### *Chlamydia psittaci*
- Psittacosis (ornithosis)

### *Chlamydia trachomatis*
- Nongonococcal urethritis
- Trachoma
- Inclusion conjunctivitis of the newborn
- Lymphogranuloma venereum

PENICILLINS
CEPHALOSPORINS
**Tetracyclines**    **1 Doxycycline**
AMINOGLYCOSIDES
**Macrolides**    **1 Azithromycin[1]**
FLUOROQUINOLONES    **1 Erythromycin[1]**
OTHER

[1] Erythromycin should be substituted for doxycycline in small children and pregnant women because of the effects of tetracyclines on calcification of bones and teeth.

No-gonococcal urethritis

Trachoma

Lymphogranuloma venerium

Respiratory infections

Inclusion conjunctivitis of the newborn

Chlamydial cervicitis

**Figure 17.8**
Summary of *Chlamydia* disease.

## Study Questions

**Choose the ONE correct answer**

17.1 Which one of the following is characteristic of chlamydiae?

A. Reticulate bodies are infectious, extracellular form of the organism.

B. Most genital tract infections are asymptomatic and undiagnosed and untreated.

C. Sensitive to β-lactam antibiotics.

D. Stain gram positive.

E. Inclusion bodies are formed from division of elementary bodies.

Correct answer = B. The extracellular infectious form is called the elementary body, not the reticulate body. Once inside the cell, the elementary body reorganizes into a larger, noninfectious reticulate body, which becomes metabolically active and divides repeatedly by binary fission within the cytoplasm of the host cell, forming an inclusion body. Chlamydiae are not stained using the Gram stain. The chlamydial cell envelope contains no peptidoglycan, thus β-lactam antibiotics have no effect on cell growth.

17.2 A feature of *Chlamydia* that is unique to this genus is

A. the requirement of an obligate intracellular habitat.

B. its replicative cycle is distinguished by two morphologic forms that develop in cytoplasmic vacuoles.

C. the lack of muramic acid in its cell envelope.

D. its use of host coenzymes of energy metabolism.

E. all of the above.

Correct answer = B. Extracellularly, chlamydiae exist as small, dense elementary bodies that are highly infective but metabolically inert. In host cell cytoplasmic vacuoles, they develop into larger, metabolically active reticulate bodies that divide, and the progeny finally mature into elementary bodies that are released. Rickettsiae are also obligately intracellular (A) and use certain host energy coenzymes (D). Certain other unrelated species appear to require living host cells for growth. Mycoplasmas, having no peptidoglycan, lack muramic acid (C).

17.3 All of the following are true statements about *Chlamydia trachomatis* EXCEPT which one?

A. It infects several types of epithelial cells.

B. It has a reservoir in domestic fowl.

C. It has a number of serotypes (about fifteen) that correlate with the syndrome produced on infection.

D. It presently causes the most common sexually transmitted disease in the United States.

E. It can be detected by direct immunofluorescence on clinical material.

Correct answer = B. All other items are correct. Whereas other *Chlamydia* species are principally parasites of birds, *C. trachomatis* is a strictly human pathogen.

Questions 17.4 to 17.6:

Match the appropriate bacterium from the following list with the case presented below:

A. *Chlamydia pneumoniae*

B. *Chlamydia psittaci*

C. *Haemophilus influenzae*

D. *Legionella pneumophila*

E. *Mycoplasma pneumoniae*

G. *Streptococcus pneumoniae*

17.4 A 35-year-old, small animal veterinarian presents with severe headache, myalgia, and splenomegaly in addition to pulmonary findings. A scanty sputum was obtained, containing a few mixed bacteria and scattered mononuclear cells on routine Gram staining.

Correct answer = B. The veterinarian probably has psittacosis, which is transmitted to humans by inhalation of dust contaminated with respiratory secretions from infected birds.

**17.5** *Chlamydia trachomatis* and *Chlamydia pneumoniae* share all of the following properties and characteristics EXCEPT

 A. infective stage is the elementary body

 B. growth in cell culture

 C. susceptibility to doxycycline

 D. reproduction by binary fission within the host cell lysosome

 E. implication in inclusion conjunctivitis and interstitial pneumonia of the newborn

Correct answer = E. Newborn infants may be infected with *Chlamydia trachomatis* by the mother, and ten to twenty percent develop a respiratory tract infection that occurs two to twenty weeks after birth and culminates in pneumonia. *Chlamydia pneumoniae* causes an atypical pneumonia in young persons, but not neonates.

**17.6** A 22-year-old man complains of a urethral discharge and urethral itching. The discharge is noted to be whitish in color, but the result of the Gram stain is negative; however, leukocytes are present. The patient is told that he has nongonococcal urethritis and is given a prescription for doxycycline. All of the following statements are correct EXCEPT

 A. the organism that is most likely causing his symptoms is *Chlamydia trachomatis*

 B. his sexual partner should also be examined and treated; his partner may be an asymptomatic carrier, causing the patient to become reinfected

 C. the selected antibiotic is appropriate for this case

 D. the organism that is most likely causing this disease is an extracellular pathogen

 E. the organism that is most likely causing this disease can cause serious complications, including death, in women

Correct answer = D. *Chlamydia trachomatis* is the most common cause of nongonoccocal urethritis. The organism is spread by sexual contact, and it may exist asyptomatically in women. Untreated carriers may continue to reinfect their partners. The organism is also capable of causing serious harm to women, including salpingitis and pelvic inflammatory disease, which can lead to infertility, ectopic pregnancy, and death. Tetracycline and other antibiotics (for example, erythromycin, doxycycline) that can penetrate into eukaryotic cells are appropriate treatments, because this organism is metabolically active only inside cells.

"Ah, Mr. Bromley. Nice to put a face on a disease."

# Mycobacteria and Actinomycetes

# 18

## I. OVERVIEW

Mycobacteria are slender rods with lipid-rich cell walls that are resistant to penetration by chemical dyes, such as those used in the Gram stain. They stain poorly but, once stained, cannot be easily decolorized by treatment with acidified organic solvents. Hence, they are termed "acid-fast" (see p. 22). Mycobacterial infections are intracellular, and generally result in the formation of slow-growing granulomatous lesions that are responsible for major tissue destruction. For example, *Mycobacterium tuberculosis* causes tuberculosis, the principal chronic bacterial disease in humans, and a leading cause worldwide of death from infection. This organism has increasingly become a cause for special concern in immunocompromised patients. Members of the genus *Mycobacterium* also cause leprosy, as well as several tuberculosis-like human infections. This genus belongs to the order of organisms (Actinomycetales) that also includes the genera *Actinomyces* and *Nocardia*. These organisms all cause granulomatous lesions with various clinical presentations. Mycobacteria and other clinically significant Actinomycetales discussed in this chapter are listed in Figure 18.1.

## II. MYCOBACTERIA

Mycobacteria are long, slender rods that are nonmotile and do not form spores (Figure 18.2). Mycobacterial cell walls are unusual in that they are approximately sixty percent lipid, including a unique class of very long-chain (75 to 90 carbons), β-hydroxylated fatty acids (mycolic acids). These complex with a variety of polysaccharides and peptides, creating a waxy cell surface that makes mycobacteria strongly hydrophobic, and accounts for their acid-fast staining characteristic. Their unusual cell walls make mycobacteria impervious to many chemical disinfectants, and convey resistance to the corrosive action of strong acids or alkalis. Use is made of this fact in decontaminating clinical specimens such as sputum, where nonmycobacterial organisms are digested by such treatments. Mycobacteria are also resistant to drying, but not to heat or ultraviolet irradiation. Mycobacteria are strictly aerobic. Most species grow slowly with generation times of 8 to 24 hours, in part because their hydrophobic surface promotes clumped growth.

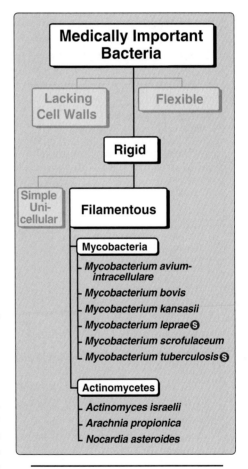

**Figure 18.1**
Classification of *Mycobacteria* and *Actinomycetes*.
Ⓢ See p. 331 for summaries of these organisms.

**Figure 18.2**
*Mycobacterium tuberculosis.*
A. Acid-fast stain of sputum from a patient with tuberculosis. B. Typical growth pattern showing "cording" (that is, growing in strings).

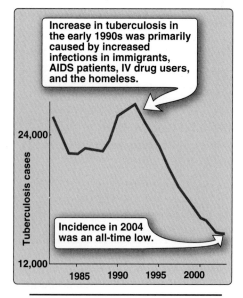

**Figure 18.3**
Incidence of new cases of tuberculosis (United States).

## A. Mycobacterium tuberculosis

It is currently estimated that about one third of the world's population is infected with *M. tuberculosis* (tubercle bacillus), with thirty million people having active disease. The incidence of tuberculosis in the United States has declined for many years and is now at a historic low (Figure 18.3). In contrast to the decline of tuberculosis in the West, the incidence of the disease in some Asian and sub-Saharan African nations has dramatically increased. In some of these nations, nearly fifty percent of the HIV-infected population is co-infected with *M. tuberculosis.*

1. **Epidemiology:** Patients with active pulmonary tuberculosis shed large numbers of organisms by coughing, creating aerosol droplet nuclei. Because of resistance to dessication, the organisms can remain viable in the environment for a long time. The principal mode of contagion is person-to-person transmission by inhalation of the aerosol, and repeated or prolonged contact is usually required for transmission of infection. However, a single infected person can pass the organism to numerous people in an exposed group, such as a family, classroom, or hospital ward.

2. **Pathogenicity:** After being inhaled, mycobacteria reach the alveoli, where they multiply in the pulmonary epithelium or macrophages. Within two to four weeks, many bacilli are destroyed by the immune system, but some survive and are spread by the blood to extrapulmonary sites. The virulence of *M. tuberculosis* rests with its ability to survive and grow within host cells (Figure 18.4). The organism produces no demonstrable toxins; however, when engulfed by macrophages, bacterial sulfolipids inhibit the fusion of phagocytic vesicles with lysosomes.

> The ability of *M. tuberculosis* to grow even in immunologically activated macrophages and to remain viable within the host for decades, are unique characteristics of tuberculosis.

3. **Immunity:** *M. tuberculosis* stimulates both a humoral and a cell-mediated immune response. Although circulating antibodies appear, they do not convey resistance to the organism. Instead, cellular immunity (CD4+ T cells) and the accompanying delayed hypersensitivity directed against a number of bacterial protein antigens, develop in the course of infection, and contribute to both the pathology of and immunity to the disease.

4. **Clinical significance:** Primary tuberculosis occurs in a person who has had no previous contact with the organism. For the majority of cases (about 95 percent), the infection becomes arrested, and most people are unaware of this initial encounter. The only evidence of tuberculosis may be a positive tuberculin test (see p. 189). A chest radiograph sometimes shows the initial pulmonary nodule (a healing tubercle, see below), and some fibrosis—the

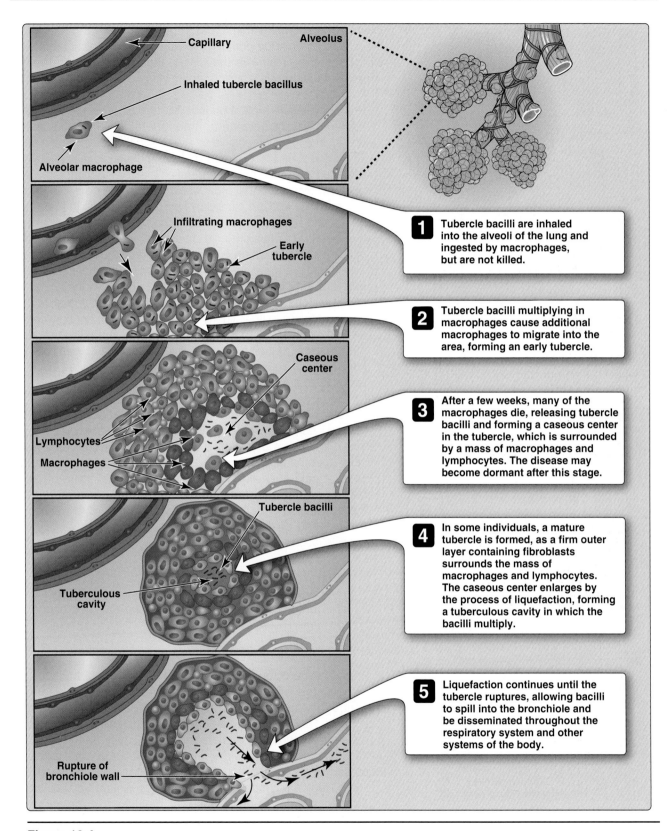

**Figure 18.4**
Progression of active tuberculosis infection.

Fibrosis

**Figure 18.5**
A chest radiograph showing some
fibrosis—the classic Ghon complex.

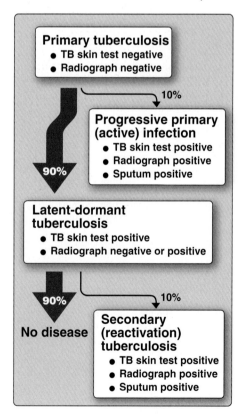

**Primary tuberculosis**
• TB skin test negative
• Radiograph negative

10%

90%

**Progressive primary
(active) infection**
• TB skin test positive
• Radiograph positive
• Sputum positive

**Latent-dormant
tuberculosis**
• TB skin test positive
• Radiograph negative or positive

90%                    10%

**No disease**

**Secondary
(reactivation)
tuberculosis**
• TB skin test positive
• Radiograph positive
• Sputum positive

**Figure 18.6**
Stages in the pathogenesis of
tuberculosis.

classic Ghon complex (Figure 18.5). Approximately ten percent of
those with an arrested primary infection develop clinical tuberculosis at some later time in their lives. Figure 18.4 illustrates the
course of tuberculosis infection progressing to clinical disease.

a. **Primary disease—initial phase:** Primary tuberculosis is usually
acquired via the respiratory tract; therefore, the initial lesion
occurs in a small bronchiole or alveolus in the midlung periphery.
The organisms are engulfed by local mononuclear phagocytes,
and their presence initiates an inflammatory reaction. However,
because tubercle bacilli grow well in phagocytic cells, the bacteria proliferate and are carried by lymphatic drainage to the lymph
nodes and beyond to set up additional foci. This initial phase of
the infection is usually mild or asymptomatic, and results in
exudative lesions where fluid and polymorphonuclear leukocytes
accumulate around the bacilli. A specific immune response
develops after about one month, and this changes the character
of the lesions. Cell-mediated immunity to *M. tuberculosis* and
hypersensitivity to its antigens (tuberculoproteins) not only confer
an enhanced ability to localize the infection and curb growth of
the organism, but also cause a greater capacity to damage the
host. Macrophages, activated by specific T lymphocytes, begin to
accumulate and destroy the bacilli.

b. **Primary disease—tubercle formation:** The productive (granulomatous) lesion that develops is known as a tubercle (see Figure
18.4). It consists of a central area of large, multinucleate giant
cells (macrophage syncytia) containing tubercle bacilli, a mid-
zone of pale epithelioid cells, and a peripheral collar of fibroblasts and mononuclear cells. Tissue damage is produced by
the destruction of both bacilli and phagocytes, which results in
the release of degradative enzymes and reactive oxygen
species, such as superoxide radicals.

> The center of the tubercule develops a charac-
> teristic expanding, caseous (cheesy) necrosis
> (see Figure 18.4).

c. **Primary tuberculosis follows one of two courses:** If the lesion
arrests, the tubercle undergoes fibrosis and calcification,
although viable but nonproliferating organisms may persist
(Figure 18.6). Alternatively, if the lesion breaks down, the
caseous material is discharged, and a cavity is created that
can facilitate spread of the infection. The organisms are dispersed by the lymph and the bloodstream, and can seed the
lungs, regional lymph nodes, or various distant tissues, such
as liver, spleen, kidneys, bone, or meninges. In progressive
disease, one or more of the resulting tubercles may expand,
leading to destruction of tissue and clinical illness; for example,
chronic pneumonitis, tuberculous osteomyelitis, or tuberculous
meningitis. In the extreme instance, active tubercles develop
throughout the body, a serious condition known as miliary (disseminated) tuberculosis.

**Figure 18.7**
Mantoux skin test for tuberculosis. [Note: For some people, determination of a positive reaction may be interpreted more stringently (see Figure 18.8).]

   **d. Reactivation of tuberculosis:** This is usually caused by *M. tuberculosis* that has survived in a dormant primary tubercle lesion (see Figure 18.6). Any of the preexisting tubercles may be involved, but pulmonary sites are most common, particularly the lung apices where high oxygen tension favors mycobacterial growth. Bacterial populations in such lesions often become quite large and many organisms are shed (for example, in sputum). The patient again becomes capable of exposing others to the disease. Reactivation is apparently caused by an impairment in immune status, often associated with malnutrition, alcoholism, advanced age, or severe stress. Immunosuppressive medication or diseases such as diabetes and, particularly, AIDS, are common preconditions.

5. **Tuberculin reaction:** The tuberculin reaction test is a manifestation of delayed hypersensitivity to protein antigens of *M. tuberculosis*. Whereas such tests can be used to document contact with the tubercle bacillus, they do not confirm that the patient currently has active disease. In the Mantoux test, purified protein derivative (PPD) is prepared from culture filtrates of the organism, and biologically standardized. Activity is expressed in tuberculin units (TU). In the routine procedure (Mantoux test), a measured amount of PPD is injected intradermally in the forearm (Figure 18.7). It is read 48 to 72 hours later for the presence and size of an area of induration (hardening) at the site of injection, which must be observed for the test to be positive (Figure 18.8). A positive reaction usually develops four to six weeks after initial contact with the organism. It remains positive for life, although it may wane after some years, or in the presence of immunosuppression by medications or disease.

**An induration of >5 mm is interpreted as positive in the following populations:**

- Persons who have had contact with infectious individuals
- Persons with an abnormal chest radiograph
- HIV-infected and other immuno-suppressed persons

**An induration of >10 mm is interpreted as positive in the following populations:**

- Foreign-born persons from high-prevalence countries
- Residents of prisons, nursing homes, and other institutions
- Healthcare workers
- Persons with other medical risk factors

**An induration of >15 mm is interpreted as positive in the following populations:**

- Persons with no risk factors

**Figure 18.8**
Interpretations of the Mantoux skin test for tuberculosis.

**6. Laboratory identification:** Diagnosis of active pulmonary tuberculosis includes demonstration of clinical symptoms and abnormal chest radiographs, and confirmation by isolation of *M. tuberculosis* from relevant clinical material.

a. **Identification of *M. tuberculosis* in clinical specimens:** A microscopic search for acid-fast bacilli using techniques such as the Ziehl-Neelsen stain is the most rapid test for mycobacteria. However, *M. tuberculosis* cannot be reliably distinguished on morphologic grounds from other occasional pathogens in the genus, from some saprophytic mycobacterial species that may contaminate glassware and reagents in the laboratory, or from those mycobacteria that may be part of the normal flora. Therefore, a definitive identification of *M. tuberculosis* can only be obtained by culturing the organism, or by using one of the newer molecular methods described below. Although two to eight weeks are required to culture the tubercle bacillus because of its slow growth on laboratory media, such cultures can detect small numbers of organisms in the original sample. Figure 18.9 shows a culture of *M. tuberculosis*.

**Figure 18.9**
*Mycobacterium tuberculosis* colonies grown on Lowenstein-Jensen medium.

> Isolation of the organism is essential for determining its antibiotic sensitivity in addition to confirming the specific identity of the bacillus by growth and biochemical characteristics.

b. **Nucleic acid amplification:** Molecular techniques are increasingly important in the diagnosis of tuberculosis because they have the potential to shorten the time required to detect and identify *M. tuberculosis* in clinical specimens. For example, the amplified *M. tuberculosis* direct test use enzymes that rapidly make copies of *M. tuberculosis* 16S ribosomal RNA, which can be detected using genetic probes. The sensitivity of the test ranges from 75 to 100 percent, with a specificity of 95 to 100 percent (see p. 19), and it is used for patients whose clinical smears are positive for acid-fast bacilli and for which cultures are in progress. A second technique, the polymerase chain reaction (PCR), amplifies a small portion of a predetermined target region of the *M. tuberculosis* DNA. Using human sputum, commercial PCR kits can confirm the diagnosis of tuberculosis within eight hours, with a sensitivity and specificity that rival culture techniques. In addition, PCR analysis facilitates DNA fingerprinting of specific strains, allowing studies of the progress of epidemics.

**7. Treatment:** Several chemotherapeutic agents are effective against *M. tuberculosis*. Because strains of the organism resistant to a particular agent emerge during treatment, multiple drug therapy is employed to delay or prevent emergence. Isoniazid, rifampin, ethambutol, streptomycin, and pyrazinamide are the principal or "first-line" drugs because of their efficacy and acceptable degree of toxicity (see Figure 18.14).

a. **Drug resistance:** Mutants resistant to each of these agents have been isolated even prior to drug treatment. Therefore, the standard procedure is to begin treatment with two or more drugs to prevent outgrowth of resistant strains. Sensitivity tests, administered as soon as sufficient cultured organisms are available, are an important guide to modifying treatment. In most parts of the United States, eight to fourteen percent of *M. tuberculosis* strains are resistant to one or more of the primary drugs when initially isolated from new cases of tuberculosis. The higher incidence of multiple-drug-resistant strains (MDR-TB) in some locations and patient populations (for example, prisons) is obviously a cause for great concern.

b. **Course of treatment:** Clinical tuberculosis requires a long course of treatment because of the characteristics of the organisms and the lesions they produce. For example, as intracellular pathogens, the bacilli are shielded from drugs that do not penetrate host cells, and large cavities with avascular centers are penetrated by drugs with difficulty. Further, in chronic or arrested tubercles, the organisms are nonproliferating and, therefore, not susceptible to many antimicrobial agents. Until recently, twelve to eighteen months of drug administration was thought to be required for a clinical cure. In recent years, short courses of six months, beginning with a daily dose of a combination of drugs and later by twice weekly doses have been successful in curing uncomplicated tuberculosis (Figure 18.10).

> If the drugs are effective in the pulmonary form of tuberculosis, sputum acid-fast bacteria smears become negative, and the patient becomes non-infectious in two to three weeks.

c. **Directly observed therapy:** Patient compliance is often low when multiple drug schedules last for six months or longer. One successful strategy for achieving better treatment completion rates is "directly observed therapy," in which patients take their medication while being supervised and observed. Some healthcare providers have embraced the concept of directly observed therapy; others regard the strategy as expensive and intrusive, suitable only for individuals who have a history of noncompliance.

8. **Prevention:** Public health measures such as tuberculin tests, chest radiographs, case registries, and contact tracing have done much to control tuberculosis at the population level. However, these measures were relaxed in the late 1980s, resulting in an increasing incidence of disease (see Figure 18.3).

a. **Latent TB chemotherapy:** For individuals who are tuberculin-positive but asymptomatic, chemotherapy is indicated in sev-

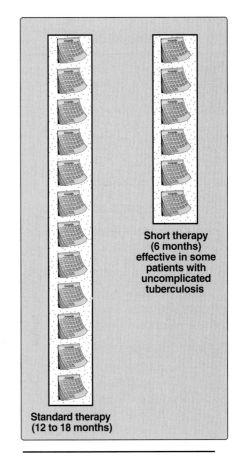

**Short therapy (6 months) effective in some patients with uncomplicated tuberculosis**

**Standard therapy (12 to 18 months)**

**Figure 18.10**
Duration of treatment for tuberculosis.

In the United States, BCG vaccine is recommended only for tuberculin-negative individuals under sustained heavy risk of infection.

**Figure 18.11**
Bacille Calmette-Guérin (BCG) vaccine is used throughout the world, but seldom in the United States.

eral situations, usually with the single antibiotic, isoniazid. For example, people in whom a recent skin test conversion is documented, or tuberculin-positive patients who need immuno-suppressive therapy for another illness, can be protected from active tuberculosis by this treatment.

b. **Vaccines:** A vaccine against tuberculosis has been available since early in the twentieth century. It is produced from Bacille Calmette-Guérin (BCG), an attenuated strain of *M. bovis*. When injected intradermally, it can confer tuberculin hypersensitivity and an enhanced ability to activate macrophages that kill the pathogen. This vaccine is about eighty percent protective against serious forms of tuberculosis, such as meningitis in children, and has been used in mass immunization campaigns by the World Health Organization and in several European countries. However, recommendations by public health officials in the United States are that vaccination be considered only for tuberculin-negative individuals under sustained heavy risk of infection, such as special groups of health-care workers or those at high risk in areas where multiple-drug-resistant TB is common (Figure 18.11).

## B. Mycobacterium leprae

Leprosy (specified by the United States Public Health Service as Hansen disease) is rare in this country, but a small number of cases, both imported and domestically acquired, are reported each year. Worldwide, it is a much larger problem, with an estimated ten to twelve million cases.

1. **Pathogenicity:** *M. leprae* is transmitted from human to human through prolonged contact; for example, between exudates of a leprosy patient's skin lesions and the abraded skin of another individual.

> The infectivity of *M. leprae* is low and the incubation period protracted, so that clinical disease may develop years or even decades after initial contact with the organism.

2. **Clinical significance:** Leprosy is a chronic granulomatous condition of peripheral nerves and mucocutaneous tissues, particularly the nasal mucosa. It occurs as a continuum between two clinical extremes: tuberculoid and lepromatous leprosy (Figure 18.12). In tuberculoid leprosy, the lesions occur as large maculae (spots) in cooler body tissues such as skin (especially the nose, outer ears, and testicles), and in superficial nerve endings. Neuritis leads to patches of anesthesia in the skin. The lesions are heavily infiltrated by lymphocytes and giant and epithelioid cells, but caseation does not occur. The patient mounts a strong cell-mediated immune response and develops delayed hypersensitivity,

---

**Tuberculoid leprosy**

- The lesions occur as large maculae in cooler body tissues such as skin (especially nose and outer ears), testicles, and superficial nerve endings
- Cell-mediated immune response
- Low infectivity

↓
**Progression of disease**
↓

**Lepromatous leprosy**

- Extensive erythematous macules, papules, or nodules; extensive destruction of skin
- Immunity is severely depressed
- High infectivity

**Figure 18.12**
Classification of leprosy.

which can be shown by skin test with lepromin, a tuberculin-like extract of lepromatous tissue. The course of lepromatous leprosy is slow but progressive (Figure 18.13). Large numbers of organisms are present in the lesions and reticuloendothelial system, and immunity is severely depressed.

3. **Laboratory identification:** *M. leprae* is an acid-fast bacillus. It has not been successfully maintained in artificial culture, but can be grown in the footpads of mice and in the armadillo, which may also be a natural host although playing no role in human disease. Laboratory diagnosis of lepromatous leprosy, where organisms are numerous, involves acid-fast stains of specimens from nasal mucosa or other infected areas. In tuberculoid leprosy, organisms are extremely rare, and diagnosis depends on clinical findings and the histology of biopsy material.

4. **Treatment and prevention:** Several drugs are effective in the treatment of leprosy, including sulfones such as dapsone, rifampin, and clofazamine (see Figure 18.14). Treatment is prolonged, and combined therapy is necessary to ensure the suppression of resistant mutants. The fact that vaccination with BCG (see p. 192) has shown some protective effect in leprosy has encouraged further interest in vaccine development. Thalidomide, an inhibitor of TNF-α, is being distributed under tight restrictions for use as a treatment for erythema nodosum leprosum, a serious and severe skin complication of leprosy.

## III. ACTINOMYCETES

Actinomycetes are a group of filamentous, branching, gram-positive organisms that easily fragment into slender rods (Figure 18.15). Although they superficially resemble fungi on morphologic grounds, they are prokaryotes of bacterial size. They are free-living, mostly soil organisms that are related to corynebacteria and mycobacteria, as well as to the streptomycetes that are sources of important antibiotics.

### A. Actinomyces israelii, Arachnia propionica

*A. israelii* and *A. propionica* are part of the normal oral and intestinal flora in humans. They are strict anaerobes.

1. **Clinical significance:** Actinomycosis is an opportunistic infection, in which a chronic suppurative abscess leads to scarring and disfigurement. The infection is probably initiated by accidental introduction of organisms into the underlying soft tissue during conditions of sufficient anaerobiasis to support their growth. About half of the cases have a cervicofacial location, and are associated with poor dental hygiene and/or tooth extraction. Other cases involve the lung and chest wall, cecum, appendix, abdominal wall, and pelvic organs. The lesion (mycetoma) begins as a hard, red, relatively nontender swelling that develops slowly, becomes filled with liquid, and ruptures to the surface, discharging quantities of pus. It also spreads laterally, draining pus through several sinus tracts.

**Figure 18.13**
A. Leprosy in a 13-year-old Hawaiian boy in 1931. B. Same boy two years later. [Note: This patient had the misfortune of contracting leprosy before the era of effective antibiotics.]

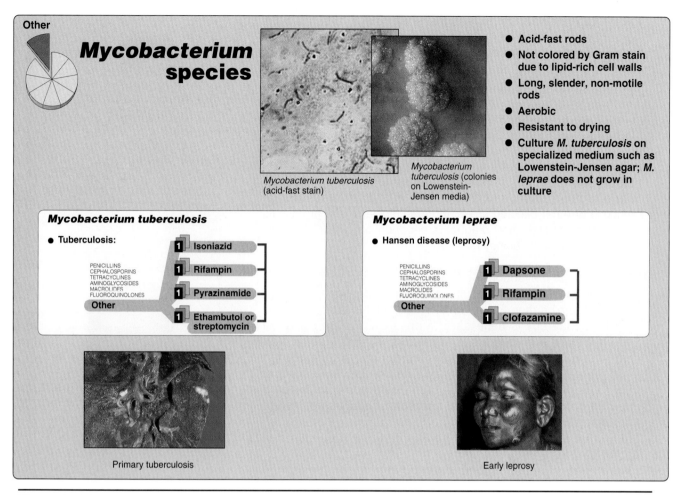

**Figure 18.14**
Summary of mycobacterium disease.

**Figure 18.15**
Actinomycetoma of the foot using a Brown-Brenn stain. Actinomycetoma is a chronic, granulomatous infection of the skin and subcutaneous tissue caused by *Actinomycetes*.

**2. Laboratory identification:** The most typical and diagnostic finding in actinomycosis is the presence of "sulfur granules" in the draining pus. These are small, firm, usually yellowish particles, which in fact do not contain sulfur. When examined under the microscope, these appear as microcolonies composed of filaments of the organism embedded in an amorphous, eosinophilic material thought to be antigen-antibody complexes. The organism can be grown anaerobically on enriched media such as thioglycollate broth or blood agar. Growth is slow, often requiring ten to fourteen days for visible colonies.

**3. Treatment:** Penicillin G is the treatment of choice for actinomycosis, although a number of antibiotics (clindamycin, erythromycin, and tetracycline) have been shown to have clinical effect. Treatment must be sustained for weeks to months, and may be accompanied by surgical debridement and/or drainage. No significant resistance to penicillin G has been reported. [Note: Good oral hygiene is an important preventive measure.]

## B. Nocardia asteroides, Nocardia brasiliensis

Nocardiae are aerobic soil organisms. Infections of humans and domestic animals are opportunistic and not transmissible from person to person. Instead, nocardiae are inhaled or acquired by contamination of skin wounds.

**Figure 18.16**
*Nocardia*

1. **Clinical significance:** The most common presentation of human **nocardiosis** is a pneumonia of rather chronic course with abscesses, extensive necrosis, and cavity formation. The organisms may metastasize, with the brain and kidneys the most common secondary locations. Common predisposing conditions are immunosuppression associated with lymphoma or other malignancy or with drugs. In the United States, *N. asteroides* is the more common organism.

2. **Laboratory identification:** Nocardiae are gram-positive, but irregularly staining, branched filaments (Figure 18.16). They are usually numerous in clinical material, and do not form sulphur granules. They stain weakly acid-fast after decolorization with one percent sulfuric acid alcohol, but fully decolorize with the routine Ziehl-Neelsen procedure. Nocardiae are strictly aerobic. They grow slowly on a variety of simple media (such as fungal media without antibiotics) and on standard blood agar.

3. **Treatment:** The sulfonamides such as sulfamethoxazole, with or without trimethoprim, are the drugs of choice for treating nocardiosis.. The nocardiae are relatively resistant to penicillin. Surgical drainage of the lesions is important, and prolonged therapy may be required to eliminate the infection.

## Study Questions

**Choose the ONE correct answer**

18.1 Which one of the following is characteristic of mycobacteria?

    A. They contain mycolic acids.

    B. They are resistant to inactivation by heat.

    C. They grow extracellularly.

    D. They are anaerobic.

    E. They are spore-forming.

Correct choice = A. Mycobacteria are unique in that their cell wall contains high concentrations of mycolic acids. Mycobacteria are not particularly heat resistant, as witness their susceptibility to pasteurization. They are aerobic, intracellular organisms that do not form spores.

18.2 An acid-fast smear on a patient's sputum is positive. The tuberculin test, however, is negative. A more definitive diagnosis could be obtained by

   A. paying attention to the patient's history.

   B. a more extensive physical examination.

   C. a chest radiograph.

   D. repeat of the sputum smear.

   E. laboratory culture and speciation.

Correct answer = E. Laboratory culture and speciation would best resolve the question, although any of the procedures listed might yield helpful information. The possibility of anergy could be investigated by skin-testing for delayed hypersensitivity to unrelated antigens, but the patient might be anergic and still be infected with a mycobacterium other than *M. tuberculosis* (MOTT).

18.3 Which of the following statements regarding *Actinomyces* and *Nocardia* is true?

   A. Both organisms have branching growth but are prokaryotes.

   B. Neither stains with Gram stain

   C. *Nocardia* infections are endogenous, and often initiated by trauma.

   D. *Actinomyces* usually causes infections in systemically compromised patients.

   E. Neither is sensitive to anti-bacterial drugs.

Correct answer = B. Both species appear as gram-positive, filamentous rods or branching forms on Gram staining. *Actinomyces* are often seen in association with amorphous material from "sulfur granules" in such smears. *Nocardia* is weakly acid-fast, in addition to being gram-positive. *Actinomyces* infections are endogenous, and often initiated by trauma. *Nocardia* usually causes infections in systemically compromised patients.

18.4 The treatment of tuberculosis

   A. is initiated with a single "first-line" drug.

   B. is initiated after the results of sensitivity testing is available.

   C. is most effective in patients with chronic or arrested tubercles.

   D. may last two to three weeks.

   E. should be directly observed in individuals who have a history of noncompliance.

Correct answer = E. The standard procedure is to begin treatment with two or more drugs to prevent outgrowth of resistant strains. Sensitivity tests are an important guide to modifying treatment, but sensitivity data are not required to initiate therapy. In chronic or arrested tubercles, the organisms are nonproliferating, and therefore are not susceptible to many antimicrobial agents. Therapy may last from six to eighteen months.

18.5 Virulence in mycobacteria is most strongly correlated with:

   A. mycotoxin production.

   B. slow growth.

   C. composition of the cell envelope.

   D. small size of cells.

   E. dependence on oxygen for growth.

Correct answer = C: Several cell wall components promote the intracellular growth of the organisms, and their dissemination in the infected host.)

"It's O.K, I'm past the contagious stage."

# Rickettsiae

19

## I. OVERVIEW

The group of organisms known as rickettsiae (family Rickettsiaceae) consists of three genera: *Rickettsia*, *Ehrlichia*, and *Coxiella* (Figure 19.1), which have a number of features in common. For example: 1) They grow only inside living host cells. [Note: Many pathogenic bacteria grow well inside particular cell types, but do not require this environment for multiplication; rickettsiae, like chlamydiae, are obligately intracellular parasites.] 2) Most rickettsial infections are transmitted by infected arthropods—lice, ticks, fleas, and/or mites. 3) Rickettsial diseases, such as typhus, spotted fevers, human ehrlichiosis, and Q fever, are generalized infections, with rash sometimes being a prominent feature. Mortality rates of these diseases are variable, but may be high in the absence of appropriate treatment.

## II. RICKETTSIA

Rickettsia have the structural features of typical prokaryotic cells. They are small, rodlike or coccobacillary shaped (Figure 19.2), and have a typical double-layered, gram-negative cell wall. However, they stain poorly, and because of their usual occurrence inside host cells are best visualized under the light microscope with one of the polychrome stains, such as Giemsa or Macchiavello.

### A. Physiology

The obligate requirement for an intracellular environment for rickettsial replication is not fully understood, but its plasma membrane is leaky and, therefore, easily permeable to host cell nutrients and coenzymes. Rickettsia contain a number of antigens that convey both group and species specificity.

### B. Pathogenesis

*Rickettsia* are transmitted to humans by arthropods such as fleas, ticks, mites, or lice. Depending on the rickettsial species, rodents, humans, or arthropods can serve as reservoirs of infectious organisms. *Rickettsia* species have an affinity for endothelial cells located throughout the circulatory system. Following a bite by an infected arthropod, the organisms are taken into cells by a process similar to phagocytosis. The organisms multiply in both the nucleus and cytoplasm of host cells. They appear to mobilize host cell actin fibrils

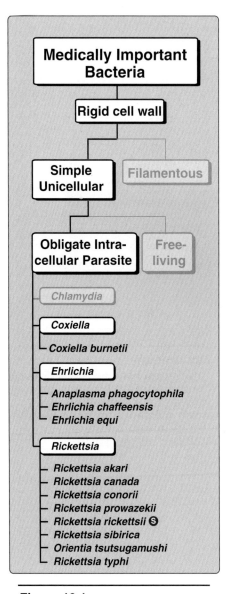

**Figure 19.1**
Classification of *Rickettsiae*.
Ⓢ See p. 331 for a summary of this organism.

**Figure 19.2**
Electron micrograph of *Rickettsia prowazekii* in experimentally infected tick tissue.

**Figure 19.3**
Child's right hand and wrist displaying the characteristic spotted rash with raised or palpable pur pura, which is pathognomonic of vasiculitis (the fundamental lesion of Rocky Mountain spotted fever).

that facilitate their exit into adjacent cells in a manner similar to that of the genus *Listeria* (see p. 97). Ultimately host cells are killed, and rickettsia spread throughout the body via the bloodstream or lymphatics Focal thrombi are formed in various organs including the skin (Figure 19.3), and a variety of small hemorrhages and hemodynamic disturbances create the symptoms of illness.

## C. Clinical significance

1. **Rocky Mountain spotted fever**, a potentially lethal but usually curable tickborne disease, and is the most common rickettsial infection in the United States. The disease is caused by *Rickettsia rickettsii*. Human infection is initiated by the bite of an infected wood or dog tick. Ticks can transmit the organism transovarially to their progeny and, thereby, the organism can be maintained without mammalian hosts in specific geographic regions for many years. Currently in the United States, such infected tick populations are prevalent in south-central states and along the mid-Atlantic coast. The disease usually occurs with highest frequency during the warmer months when tick activity is greatest. Symptoms begin to develop an average of seven days after infection. The disease is characterized by high fever and malaise, followed by a prominent rash that is initially macular but may become petechial or frankly hemorrhagic (Figure 19.3). The rash typically begins on the extremities, involving the palms and soles, and develops rapidly to cover the body. In untreated cases, vascular disturbances and myocardial or renal failure may ensue. Two-thirds of cases of Rocky Mountain spotted fever occur in children younger than fifteen years, with the peak incidence occurring between the ages of five and nine years.

> A potential diagnostic problem occurs in those infected patients (approximately ten percent) in whom a rash does not occur. These cases of "spotless" Rocky Mountain spotted fever may be severe and end fatally.

2. **Other spotted fevers:** Tickborne spotted fevers similar to Rocky Mountain spotted fever are found in several regions of the world. They vary in severity, and are caused by organisms such as *R. conorii*, *R. canada*, and *R. sibirica*. A clinically different disease, rickettsialpox, is caused by *R. akari*. It has been reported in the United States and Japan. The vector for *R. akari* is a mite, and its reservoir is the common house mouse or similar small rodents. Rickettsialpox is characterized by scattered papulovesicles that are preceded by an eschar at the site of the mite bite, and with mild constitutional symptoms of a few days' duration. Figure 19.4 illustrates the spotted fevers caused by rickettsial organisms.

3. **Louseborne (epidemic) typhus** is caused by *Rickettsia prowazekii*. [Note: Epidemic typhus is a different disease from salmonella-induced typhoid fever (see p. 86). Both were originally thought to be variations of the same disease, which was called "typhus" after

the Greek word meaning "stupor". When the two diseases were determined to be caused by different organisms, the salmonella-induced disease was named "typhoid," meaning "typhuslike."] *R. prowazekii* is transmitted from person to person by an infected human body louse that excretes organisms in its feces. The introduction of the pathogen from lice feces into a bite wound is facilitated by scratching the louse bites. Infected lice are themselves eventually killed by the infecting bacterium. Thus, this disease is not maintained in the louse population, but rather lice serve as vectors, transmitting the organism between humans.

a. **Typhus epidemics:** Typhus occurs most typically in large epidemics under conditions of displacement of people, crowding, and poor sanitation. Currently a major focus of such outbreaks is found in northeast Africa. The epidemic form of typhus has not occurred in the United States since early in the twentieth century. Clinical symptoms of typhus develop an average of eight days after infection and include high fever, chills, severe headache, and often a considerable degree of prostration and stupor. Rash may be observed. The disease lasts two weeks or longer, and tends to be more severe in older individuals. Complications of epidemic typhus may include central nervous system (CNS) dysfunction and myocarditis.

b. **Brill-Zinsser disease (recrudescent typhus):** This is a usually milder form of typhus that occurs in persons who previously recovered from primary infections (ten to forty years earlier). Latent infection is thought to be maintained in the reticuloendothelial system, and probably serves as a reservoir for the organism in interepidemic periods.

4. **Other forms of typhuslike fever:** Murine (endemic) typhus, caused by *R. typhi*, is a clinically similar, but usually milder disease than that caused by *R. prowazekii*. Human infections are initiated by the bites of infected rat fleas, and a worldwide reservoir for *R. typhi* exists in urban rodents. Murine typhus was endemic in rat-infested areas, particularly in the southeastern United States and in the Gulf of Mexico region. However, with improving rodent control, it has become rare in this country. [Note: The cat flea, which also resides on skunks, opossums, and raccoons, is still a significant vector of murine typhus in the United States.] *Orientia tsutsugamushi* (formerly, *R. tsutsugamushi*), the cause of scrub typhus, occurs in Asia and the South Pacific. The disease is transmitted by mite larvae (chiggers) from a reservoir in common rodents.

## D. Laboratory identification

A variety of serologic procedures have been developed, most of which rely on the demonstration of a rickettsia-specific antibody response during the course of infection. Suspensions or soluble extracts of rickettsiae are used to demonstrate group- and species-specific antibodies by indirect immunofluorescence. Alternatively, although not widely available, infected cells can be detected by immunofluorescence or histochemical procedures on some clinical samples, such as punch biopsies from areas of rash.

**ROCKY MOUNTAIN SPOTTED FEVER**
- *R. rickettsii*
- Maintained in wood and dog tick populations
- Causes high fever, malaise, and a prominent rash
- Complications (if untreated): Vascular disturbances Myocardial failure Renal failure

**RICKETTSIALPOX**
- *R. akari*
- Caused by the bite of a mite that has a small rodent reservoir
- Eschar (thick crust) at site of bite, and papulovesicular rash

**Figure 19.4**
Spotted fevers caused by *Rickettsia*.

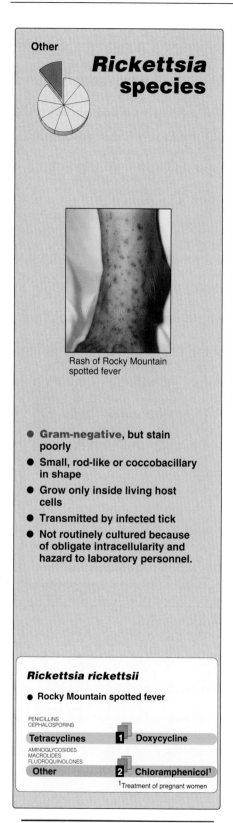

**Other**

## *Rickettsia* species

Rash of Rocky Mountain spotted fever

- **Gram-negative, but stain poorly**
- **Small, rod-like or coccobacillary in shape**
- **Grow only inside living host cells**
- **Transmitted by infected tick**
- **Not routinely cultured because of obligate intracellularity and hazard to laboratory personnel.**

*Rickettsia rickettsii*

- **Rocky Mountain spotted fever**

PENICILLINS
CEPHALOSPORINS

**Tetracyclines**    **1** Doxycycline

AMINOGLYCOSIDES
MACROLIDES
FLUOROQUINOLONES

**Other**    **2** Chloramphenicol[1]

[1]Treatment of pregnant women

**Figure 19.5**
Summary of *Richettsia* disease.

### E. Treatment

Doxycycline is the drug of choice for the treatment of Rocky Mountain spotted fever in both adults and children, except for pregnant women who should be treated with chloramphenicol (Figure 19.5). The risk of dental staining with doxycycline is minimal if a short course is administered. The decision to treat must be made on clinical grounds, together with a history or suspicion of contact with an appropriate arthropod vector, before the seroconversion data are available.

> Early therapy for Rocky Mountain spotted fever is important, because delay beyond the fifth day of illness is associated with an increased mortality rate. (Mortality is extremely rare if treatment is begun by the fourth day of illness.)

### F. Prevention of infection

Prevention depends on vector control; for example, delousing, rodent-proofing buildings, or clearing brush in tick- or mite-infested areas as appropriate. Personal protection should include wearing clothes that cover exposed skin, use of tick repellents, and frequent inspection of the body and removal of attached ticks. It is of interest that infected ticks do not transmit the infection until several hours of feeding have elapsed.

Prophylactic therapy with doxycycline or another tetracycline is not recommended following tick exposure because less than one percent in endemic areas are infected with *R. rickettsii*. Patients who report tick bites should seek treatment if any systemic symptoms, especially fever and headache, occur in the following 14 days. Vaccines are not currently licensed for use in the United States.

## III. EHRLICHIA

*Ehrlichia* resembles *Rickettsia* in appearance and behavior; however, these organisms parasitize leukocytes and grow in cytoplasmic vacuoles, creating characteristic inclusions called morulae. Human infection by *Ehrlichia* was not recognized in the United States until recently, although there were known pathogens of this group in some animals (for example, horses and dogs).

### A. Clinical significance

Currently, two tickborne forms of ehrlichiosis are known: human monocytic ehrlichiosis (HME) caused by *E. chaffeensis,* and human granulocytic anaplasmosis (HGA) caused by the organism *Anaplasma phagocytophilum*, which is closely related to *E. equi* (Figure 19.6). The major clinical features of ehrlichiosis are acute fever, myalgia, and a moderate to severe leucopenia and thrombocytopenia. Rash is seldom seen for HME; deaths from HGA and HME have occurred. HME has been confirmed in some thirty states in the southeastern and south-central United States, and has been most commonly associated with bites of the Lone Star tick. HGA has been associated with the bites of deer and dog ticks.

### B. Laboratory identification

Antibody assays and a polymerase chain reaction method have been diagnostically useful in investigative laboratories. Occasionally the characteristic morulae can be seen in peripheral blood smears during acute illness.

### C. Treatment

The treatment of choice is doxycycline.

## IV. COXIELLA

*Coxiella burnetii*, the causal agent of Q fever, is found worldwide (the "Q" stands for "query" because the cause of the fever was unknown for many years). It has several features that distinguish it from other rickettsiae. For example: 1) It grows in cytoplasmic vacuoles and seems to be stimulated by the low pH of a phagolysosome, being resistant to the host degradative enzymes within that structure. 2) It is extremely resistant to heat and drying, and can persist outside its host for long periods. 3) It causes disease in livestock such as cattle and in other mammals, but it does not seem to be transmitted to humans by arthropods. Although the organism has been reported to be recovered from ticks, human infection usually occurs following inhalation of infected dust in barnyards, slaughterhouses, and such—a transmission route made possible because of the ability of *C. burnetii* to withstand drying. [Note: *C. burnetii* has also been known to enter the body via other mucous membranes, abrasions, and the gastrointestinal tract through consumption of milk from infected animals.]

### A. Clinical significance

*C. burnetii* reproduces in the respiratory tract and then (in the absence of treatment) is disseminated to other organs. Clinical illness takes several forms. Classic Q fever is an interstitial pneumonitis (not unlike some viral or mycoplasmal illnesses) that may be complicated by hepatitis, myocarditis, or encephalitis. *C. burnetii* should also be considered as a potential causative agent in culture-negative endocarditis. Infections are usually self-limiting but, in rare instances—especially endocarditis—can become chronic.

### B. Laboratory identification

Serologic assays are the principal means of specific diagnosis, and serologic surveys indicate that inapparent infections are common.

### C. Treatment and prevention

Doxycycline is the drug of choice for treatment. A vaccine has been reported to be of limited use in occupationally exposed individuals, but it is not readily available in the United States.

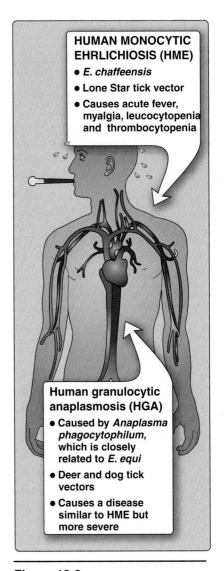

**HUMAN MONOCYTIC EHRLICHIOSIS (HME)**
- *E. chaffeensis*
- Lone Star tick vector
- Causes acute fever, myalgia, leucocytopenia and thrombocytopenia

**Human granulocytic anaplasmosis (HGA)**
- Caused by *Anaplasma phagocytophilum*, which is closely related to *E. equi*
- Deer and dog tick vectors
- Causes a disease similar to HME but more severe

**Figure 19.6**
Diseases caused by *Ehrlichia*.

## Study Questions

**Choose the ONE correct answer**

19.1 Rickettsiae

    A. grow only extracellularly.

    B. have eukaryotic-type cell organization.

    C. cause contagious infections because they are disseminated by respiratory droplets.

    D. are clinically sensitive to penicillin.

    E. generally invade the endothelial lining of capillaries, causing small hemorrhages.

> Correct answer = E. Most rickettsiae cause rashes resulting from damage of the vascular system. They are obligate intracellular, prokaryotic parasites (A and B). With the exception of coxiella, which is transmitted by inhalation of infected dust, rickettsiae are transmitted by bite of an arthropod. They are sensitive to tetracyclines, but not to penicillin.

19.2 The vector of Rocky Mountain spotted fever is the:

    A. human body louse.

    B. rat flea.

    C. deer tick.

    D. dog tick.

    E. mosquito.

> Correct answer = D.

19.3 Ehrlichiosis and Rocky Mountain spotted fever have all but which of the following clinical features in common?

    A. Both involve parasitized blood cells.

    B. Both are acute fevers.

    C. Both are transmitted by the same vector.

    D. Both can be treated by doxycycline.

    E. Both are caused by members of the family Rickettsiaceae.

> Correct answer = A. *Ehrlichia* parasitizes leukocytes, whereas *R. rickettsii* invades capillary linings, causing the "spotted" rash of RMSF.

19.4 Coxiella burnetii

    A. cannot survive outside its host.

    B. has no reservoir other than humans.

    C. causes a pneumonitis called Q fever.

    D. causes symptomatic disease only in the lower respiratory tract.

    E. is found only in the United States.

> Correct answer = C. Whereas lower respiratory tract disease is most characteristic, the organism fairly frequently causes hepatitis, myocarditis or endocarditis, and other visceral infections. It is resistant to drying and heat, and infects a variety of animals (including ticks, but they play no role in human disease). Its distribution is worldwide.

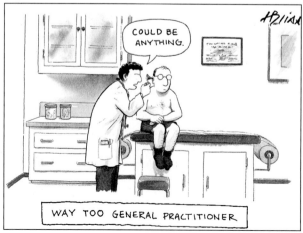

# Fungi

# 20

## I. OVERVIEW

Fungi are a diverse group of saprophytic (derives nourishment from dead organic matter) and parasitic eukaryotic organisms. Although formerly considered to be plants, they are now generally assigned their own kingdom, Mycota. Virtually all organisms are subject to fungal infection. Of some 100,000 fungal species, only about 100 have pathogenic potential for humans; of these, only a few species account for most clinically important fungal infections (Figure 20.1). Human fungal diseases (mycoses) are classified by the location on or in the body where the infection occurs. They are called cutaneous when limited to the epidermis, subcutaneous when the infection penetrates significantly beneath the skin, and systemic when the infection is deep within the body or disseminated to internal organs. Systemic mycoses can be further divided into those that are caused by true pathogenic fungi capable of infecting healthy individuals, and those that are opportunistic, infecting primarily those individuals who have predisposing conditions such as immunodeficiency or debilitating diseases (for example, diabetes, leukemia, and Hodgkin and other lymphomas). Fungi produce and secrete a variety of unusual metabolic products, some of which, when ingested, are highly toxic to animals, including humans. Thus, fungi can cause poisonings as well as infections. Lastly, fungal spores are important as human allergenic agents.

## II. CHARACTERISTICS OF MAJOR FUNGAL GROUPS

Fungi can be distinguished from other infectious organisms such as bacteria or viruses because they are eukaryotes (that is, they have a membrane-enclosed nucleus). Their characteristic structures, habitats, and modes of growth and reproduction are used to distinguish between different groups of fungi.

### Pathogenic Fungi

**TRUE PATHOGENS**

**Cutaneous infective agents**
- *Epidermophyton* species
- *Microsporum* species
- *Trichophyton* species

**Subcutaneous infective agents**
- *Actinomadura madurae*
- *Cladosporium*
- *Madurella grisea*
- *Phialophora*
- *Sporothrix schenckii*

**Systemic infective agents**
- *Blastomyces dermatitidis*
- *Coccidioides immitis*
- *Histoplasma capsulatum*
- *Paracoccidioides brasiliensis*

**OPPORTUNISTIC PATHOGENS**
(continued on next page)

**Figure 20.1**
Classification of pathogenic fungi (figure continues on next page).

**Pathogenic fungi**
(continued)

**OPPORTUNISTIC PATHOGENS**

— *Absidia corymbifera*
— *Aspergillus fumigatus*
— *Candida albicans*
— *Cryptococcus neoformans*
— *Pneumocystis jiroveci*
— *Rhizomucor pusillus*
— *Rhizopus oryzae (R. arrhizus)*

**Figure 20.1 (continued)**
Classification of pathogenic fungi.

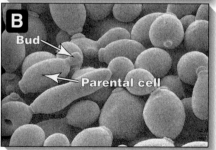

**Figure 20.2**
A. Filamentous (mold-like) fungi
(light micrograph). B. Budding
yeast-like fungi (scanning electron
micrograph).

## A. Cell wall and membrane components

The fungal cell wall and cell membrane are fundamentally different from those of bacteria and other eukaryotes. Fungal cell walls are composed largely of chitin, a polymer of N-acetylglucosamine,[1] rather than peptidoglycan—a characteristic component of bacterial cell walls. Fungi are, therefore, unaffected by antibiotics (for example, penicillin) that inhibit peptidoglycan synthesis. The fungal membrane contains ergosterol, rather than the cholesterol found in mammalian membranes. These chemical characteristics are useful in targeting chemotherapeutic agents against fungal infections. Many such agents interfere with fungal membrane synthesis or function. For example, amphotericin B and nystatin bind to ergosterol present in cell membranes of fungal cells. There they form pores that disrupt membrane function, resulting in cell death. Imidazole antifungal drugs (clotrimazole, ketoconazole, miconazole) and triazole antifungal agents (fluconazole and itraconazole) interact with C-14 $\alpha$-demethylase to block demethylation of lanosterol to ergosterol. Ergosterol is a vital component of the cell membrane of fungi, and disruption of its biosynthesis results in cell death.

## B. Habitat and nutrition

All fungi are heterotrophs; that is, they require some preformed organic carbon source for growth. Fungi do not ingest food particles as do organisms such as protozoa (see p. 217), but depend upon transport of soluble nutrients across their cell membranes. To obtain these soluble nutrients, fungi secrete degradative enzymes (for example, cellulases, proteases, nucleases) into their immediate environment. It is this ability that enables fungi to live saprophytically on organic waste. Therefore, the natural habitat of almost all fungi is soil or water containing decaying organic matter. [Note: Some fungi can be parasitic on living organisms. However, these parasitic infections usually originate from the individual's contact with fungus-infested soil, an exception being *Candida*, which is part of the normal human mucosal flora (see p. 7).]

## C. Modes of fungal growth

Most fungi exist in one of two basic morphologic forms (that is, either as filamentous mold or unicellular yeast). However, some fungi are dimorphic (that is, they switch between these two forms in response to environmental conditions).

1. **Filamentous (mold like) fungi:** The vegetative body, or thallus, of mold-like fungi is typically a mass of threads with many branches (Figure 20.2A). This mass is called a mycelium, which grows by branching and tip elongation. The threads (hyphae) are actually tubular cells that, in some fungi, are partitioned into segments (septate); whereas, in other fungi, the hyphae are uninterrupted by crosswalls (nonseptate). Even in septate fungi, however, the septae are perforated so that the cytoplasm of the hyphae is continuous. When hyphal filaments become densely packed, the

[1]See p. 158 in *Lippincott's Illustrated Reviews: Biochemistry* (3rd ed.) for a discussion of N-acetylglucosamine.

mycelium may have the appearance of a cohesive tissue. An example of this is the body of a mushroom.

2. **Yeast-like fungi:** These fungi exist as populations of single, unconnected, spheroid cells, not unlike many bacteria, although they are some ten times larger than a typical bacterial cell (Figure 20.2B). Yeast-like fungi generally reproduce by budding.

> Some fungal species, especially those that cause systemic mycoses, are dimorphic, being usually yeast-like in one environment and mold-like in another. Examples of conditions that affect the choice of morphology are temperature and carbon dioxide levels.

## D. Sporulation

Sporulation is the principal means by which fungi reproduce and spread through the environment. Fungal spores are metabolically dormant, protected cells, released by the mycelium in enormous numbers. They can be borne by air or water to new sites, where they germinate and establish colonies. Spores can be generated either asexually or sexually (Figure 20.3).

**Figure 20.3**
Examples of: A. Asexual sporulation. B. Sexual sporulation. Both spores are *Aspergillus nidulans*.

1. **Asexual sporulation:** Asexual spores (conidia) are formed by mitosis in or on specialized hyphae (conidiophores, Figure 20.3A). The color of a typical fungal colony seen on bread, fruit, or culture plate is caused by the conidia, which can number tens of millions per cm$^3$ of surface. Because they are easily detached from their underlying mycelial mats, conidia can become airborne and, therefore, are a major source of fungal infection (see p. 209).

2. **Sexual sporulation:** This process is initiated when a haploid nucleus from each of two compatible strains of the same species fuse to form a transient diploid (Figure 20.3B). The products of meiosis of this transient diploid become sexual spores (ascospores). Compared to asexual sporulation, sexual sporulation is relatively rare among human fungal pathogens. Spores, especially sexual spores, often have a characteristic shape and surface ornamentation pattern that may serve as the primary or only means of species identification.

### E. Laboratory identification

Most fungi can be propagated on any nutrient agar surface. The standard medium is Sabouraud dextrose agar, which, because of its low pH (5.0), inhibits bacterial growth while allowing fungal colonies to form (Figure 20.4). Various antibacterial antibiotics can also be added to the medium to further inhibit bacterial colony formation. Cultures can be started from spores or hyphal fragments. Clinical samples may be pus, blood, spinal fluid, sputum, tissue biopsies, or skin scrapings. Identification is usually based on the microscopic morphology of conidial structures. Serologic tests and immunofluorescent techniques are also useful in identification of fungi from clinical isolates.

**Figure 20.4**
Colonies of *Nocardia asteroides* grown on Sabouraud dextrose agar.

## III. CUTANEOUS MYCOSES

Also called dermatophytoses, these common diseases are caused by a group of related fungi, the dermatophytes. Dermatophytes fall into three genera, each with many species: *Trichophyton*, *Epidermophyton*, and *Microsporum*.

### A. Epidemiology

The causative organisms of the dermatophytoses are often distinguished according to their natural habitats: anthropophilic (residing on human skin), zoophilic (residing on the skin of domestic and farm animals), or geophilic (residing in the soil). Most human infections are by anthropophilic and zoophilic organisms. Transmission from human to human or animal to human is by infected skin scales.

### B. Pathology

A defining characteristic of the dermatophytes is the ability to use keratin as a source of nutrition. This ability allows them to infect keratinized tissues and structures, such as skin, hair, and nails. There is some specificity, however. Whereas all three genera attack the skin, *Microsporum* does not infect nails and *Epidermophyton* does not infect hair. None invade underlying, nonkeratinized tissue.

## C. Clinical significance

Dermatophytoses are characterized by itching, scaling skin patches that can become inflamed and weeping. Specific diseases are usually identified according to affected tissue (for example, scalp, pubic area, or feet), but a given disease can be caused by any one of several organisms, and some organisms can cause more than one disease depending, for example, on the site of infection or condition of the skin. The following are the most commonly encountered dermatophytoses.

1. **Tinea pedis (athlete's foot):** Organisms most often isolated from infected tissue are *Trichophyton rubrum*, *Trichophyton mentagrophytes*, and *Epidermophyton floccosum*. The infected tissue is initially between the toes, but can spread to the nails, which become yellow and brittle. Skin fissures can lead to secondary bacterial infections, with consequent lymph node inflammation (Figure 20.5A).

2. **Tinea corporis (ringworm):** Organisms most often isolated are *E. floccosum* and several species of *Trichophyton* and *Microsporum*. Lesions appear as advancing annular rings with scaly centers (Figure 20.5B). The periphery of the ring, which is the site of active fungal growth, is usually inflamed and vesiculated. Although any site on the body can be affected, lesions most often occur on nonhairy areas of the trunk.

3. **Tinea capitis (scalp ringworm):** Several species of *Trichophyton* and *Microsporum* have been isolated from scalp ringworm lesions, the predominant infecting species depending on the geographic location of the patient. In the United States, for example, the predominant infecting species is *Trichophyton tonsurans*. Disease manifestations range from small, scaling patches, to involvement of the entire scalp with extensive hair loss (Figure 20.5C). The hair shafts can become invaded by *Microsporum* hyphae, as manifested by their green fluorescence in long-wave ultraviolet light (Wood lamp).

4. **Tinea cruris ("jock itch"):** Causative organisms are *E. floccosum* and *T. rubrum*. Disease manifestations are similar to ringworm, except that lesions occur in the moist groin area, where they can spread from the upper thighs to the genitals (Figure 20.5D).

5. **Tinea unguium (onychomycosis):** The causative organism is most often *T. rubrum*. The nails are thickened, discolored, and brittle. Treatment must be continued for three to four months until all infected portions of the nail grow out and are trimmed off (Figure 20.5E).

**Figure 20.5**
Cutaneous mycoses.

**Figure 20.6**
Subcutaneous mycoses.
A. Sporotrichosis. The forearm of a
gardener exhibiting the cutaneous-
lymphatic form of sporotrichosis.
B. Chromomycosis. Multiple
plaques on the lower leg.
C. Mycetoma of the arm.

## D. Treatment

Removal of infected skin, followed by topical application of antifungal antibiotics such as miconazole or clotrimazole, is the first course of treatment. Refractory infections usually respond well to oral griseofulvin and itraconazole. Infections of the hair and nails usually require systemic (oral) therapy. Terbinafine is the drug of choice for onychomycosis.

## IV. SUBCUTANEOUS MYCOSES

Subcutaneous mycoses are fungal infections of the dermis, subcutaneous tissue, and bone. Causative organisms reside in the soil and decaying or live vegetation.

### A. Epidemiology

Subcutaneous fungal infections are almost always acquired through traumatic lacerations or puncture wounds. Sporotrichosis, for example, is often acquired from the prick of a thorn. As expected, these infections are more common in individuals who have frequent contact with soil and vegetation and wear little protective clothing.

> The subcutaneous mycoses are not transmissible from human to human under ordinary conditions.

### B. Clinical Significance

With the rare exception of sporotrichosis, which shows a broad geographic distribution in the United States, the common subcutaneous mycoses discussed below are confined to tropical and subtropical regions.

1. **Sporotrichosis:** This infection, characterized by a granulomatous ulcer at the puncture site, may produce secondary lesions along the draining lymphatics (Figure 20.6A). The causative organism, *Sporothrix schenckii*, is a dimorphic fungus that exhibits the yeast form in infected tissue (see Figure 20.7) and the mycelial form upon laboratory culture. In most patients, the disease is self-limiting, but may persist in a chronic form. Oral itraconazole is the drug of choice.

2. **Chromomycosis (also called chromoblastomycosis):** This infection is characterized by warty nodules that spread slowly along the lymphatics and develop crusty abscesses (Figure 20.6B). Pathogens causing this mycosis include several species of pigmented soil fungi, for example, *Phialophora* and *Cladosporium*, and the infection is most commonly seen in the tropics. Treatment is difficult. Surgical removal of small lesions is effective, but must

be performed cautiously and with wide margins to prevent dissemination. More advanced stages of the disease are treated with itraconazole and terbinafine.

3. **Mycetoma (Madura foot):** Mycetoma appears as a localized abscess, usually on the feet, that discharges pus, serum, and blood through sinuses (in this usage, sinus means "abnormal channel"). The infection can spread to the underlying bone and results in crippling deformities (Figure 20.6C). The pathogenic agents are various soil fungi or actinomycetes (see p. 163), depending on the climate of the geographic area. Most common are *Madurella grisea* and *Actinomadura madurae*. Mycetomas appear similar to the lesions of chromomycosis, but the defining characteristic of mycetoma is the presence of colored grains, composed of compacted hyphae, in the exudate. The color of the grains (black, white, red, or yellow) is characteristic of the causative organism and, therefore, useful in identifying the particular pathogen. There is no effective chemotherapy for fungal mycetoma; the treatment is usually surgical excision.

**Figure 20.7**
Tissue section showing the budding yeast *Sporothrix schenckii.*

## V. SYSTEMIC MYCOSES

The organisms responsible for systemic mycoses fall into two general categories: 1) those that infect normal healthy individuals ("true" pathogens), and 2) those that primarily infect debilitated, and/or immunocompromised individuals ("opportunistic pathogens," see p. 385). In the United States, coccidioidomycosis, histoplasmosis, and blastomycosis are the most common systemic mycotic infections in the immunocompetent host. These infections occur in defined geographic areas where fungal pathogens are found in the soil and can be aerosolized. Clinical manifestations closely resemble those seen in tuberculosis in that asymptomatic primary pulmonary infection is common, whereas chronic pulmonary or disseminated infection is rare. The fungi causing these diseases are uniformly dimorphic, exhibiting the yeast form in infected tissue, and the mycelial form in culture or in their natural environment.

### A. Epidemiology and pathology

Entry into the host is by inhalation of airborne spores, which germinate in the lungs. From the lungs, dissemination can occur to any organ of the body where the fungi can invade and destroy tissue (Figure 20.8).

### B. Clinical significance

In spite of the seemingly grave nature of potentially systemic disease, most cases of coccidioidomycosis, histoplasmosis, and paracoccidioidomycosis in otherwise healthy patients present only mild symptoms and are self-limiting. In immunosuppressed patients, however, the same infections can be life-threatening.

**Figure 20.8**
Systemic mycoses.

1. **Coccidioidomycosis** is caused by *Coccidioides immitis*. Most cases of coccidioidomycosis occur in the arid areas of southwestern United States (Figure 20.9) and Central and South America. In the soil, the fungus generates spores by septation of hyphal filaments (arthrospores). These spores become readily airborne and enter the lungs, where they germinate and develop into large (twenty to forty μm) spherules filled with many endospores. Rupture of the spherule releases the endospores, each of which can form a new spherule. In cases of disseminated disease, lesions occur most often in the bones and the central nervous system (CNS) where they result in meningitis.

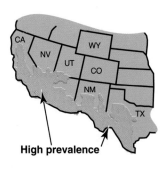

**Figure 20.9**
Geographic prevalence of coccidioidomycosis in the United States.

2. **Histoplasmosis** is caused by *Histoplasma capsulatum*. In the soil, the fungus generates conidia, which, when airborne, enter the lungs and germinate into yeast-like cells. These yeast cells become engulfed by macrophages in which they multiply. Pulmonary infections may be acute but relatively benign and self-limiting, or chronic, progressive, and fatal. Dissemination is rare. Disseminated disease results in invasion of cells of the reticuloendothelial system, which distinguishes this organism as the only fungus to exhibit intracellular parasitism. Definitive diagnosis is by isolation and culture of the organism, which is a slow process taking four to six weeks, or by detection of exoantigen, which can be completed in several days. The disease occurs worldwide, but is most prevalent in central North America, especially the Ohio and Mississippi River Valleys (Figure 20.10). Soils that are laden with bird, chicken, or bat droppings are a rich source of *H. capsulatum* spores. Local epidemics of the disease can occur, in particular, in areas where construction has disturbed bird, chicken, and bat roosts. AIDS patients who live in or travel through endemic areas are especially at risk.

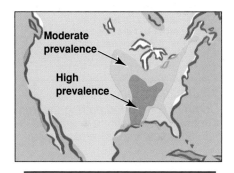

**Figure 20.10**
Endemic areas of histoplasmosis in North America.

> The wide range of clinical manifestations of histoplasmosis makes it a particularly complex disease, often resembling tuberculosis.

3. **Blastomycosis** is caused by *Blastomyces dermatitidis*. Like *Histoplasma,* the fungus produces microconidia, most often in the soil, which become airborne and enter the lungs. There they germinate into thick-walled yeast cells that often appear with buds. Initial pulmonary infections (Figure 20.11) rarely disseminate to other sites; however, when dissemination occurs, secondary sites include skin (seventy percent), bone (thirty percent), and genitourinary tract (twenty percent), where they manifest as ulcerated granulomas. Definitive diagnosis is accomplished by isolation and culture of the organism. Identifiable colonies can be obtained in one to three weeks, but identity can be established more rapidly by subjecting the young mycelial colonies to an exoantigen test. Infections are most common in the South Central and South Eastern United States, and are much more common in adult males than in females or children.

**Figure 20.11**
Chest radiograph showing a diffuse reticulonodular infiltrate of the lungs in a male landscaper. Bronchoalveolar lavage recovered *Blastomyces dermatitidis*.

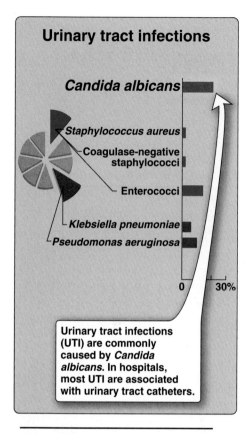

**Urinary tract infections**

*Candida albicans*

*Staphylococcus aureus*

Coagulase-negative
staphylococci

Enterococci

*Klebsiella pneumoniae*

*Pseudomonas aeruginosa*

0          30%

Urinary tract infections
(UTI) are commonly
caused by *Candida
albicans*. In hospitals,
most UTI are associated
with urinary tract catheters.

**Figure 20.12**
Commonly reported pathogens from
urinary tract infections in patients in
adult medical intensive care units.

**Figure 20.13**
*Candida albicans.*

**4. Paracoccidioidomycosis**, also called South American blastomycosis, is caused by *Paracoccidioides brasiliensis*. The clinical presentation is much like that of histoplasmosis and blastomycosis except that the most common secondary site of infection is the mucosa of the mouth and nose, where painful, destructive lesions may develop. Like other dimorphic pathogens, morphologic identification via conidia is slow, but the yeast form observed in infected tissue or exudates has a characteristic ship's steering wheel appearance caused by the presence of multiple buds (see Figure 20.8). The disease is restricted to Central and South America, and over ninety percent of patients with symptomatic disease are mature males. It is speculated that female sex hormones may inhibit formation of the yeast form.

**C. Laboratory identification**

These diseases are not communicable from one person to another. However, laboratory cultures should be handled cautiously, especially those of *C. immitis*, because under culture conditions the fungi revert to the spore-bearing, infectious form. Because these organisms have slow growth rates, morphologic identification of the characteristic conidia can take several weeks. A rapid and simple method for identifying the four systemic pathogens discussed above is the exoantigen test in which cell-free antigens produced by young mycelial colonies (or liquid cultures) are detected by immunodiffusion assay. A rapid and accurate diagnostic method uses nucleic acid probes that detect specific fungal sequences.

**D. Treatment**

Systemic mycoses are usually treated with amphotericin B, sometimes in combination with flucytosine. Ketoconazole, fluconazole, and itraconazole are also used, depending on the stage and site of the disease.

## VI. OPPORTUNISTIC MYCOSES

Opportunistic mycoses afflict debilitated or immunocompromised individuals, and are rare in healthy individuals. The use of immunosuppressive drugs for organ transplantation, widespread use of chemotherapy in cancer treatment, and the high frequency of immunodeficient individuals caused by the AIDS epidemic have resulted in significant expansion of the immunocompromised population, as well as increasing the spectrum of opportunistic fungal pathogens.

Fungal infections represent approximately fifteen percent of all nosocomial infections in intensive care units in the United States, with *Candida* species being the most commonly occurring fungal pathogen (Figure 20.12).

The opportunistic mycoses most commonly encountered today include the following.

A. **Candidiasis** (**candidosis**) is caused by the yeast *Candida albicans*, and other *Candida* species, which are normal body flora found in the skin, mouth, vagina, and intestines. Although considered a yeast, *C. albicans* is dimorphic, and can form a true mycelium (Figure 20.13). Infections occur when competing bacterial flora are eliminated, for example, by antibacterial antibiotics, allowing the yeast to overgrow. *Candida* infections have various manifestations depending on the site. For example, oral candidiasis (thrush) presents as raised, white plaques on the oral mucosa, tongue, or gums (Figure 20.14). The plaques can become confluent and ulcerated and spread to the throat. Most HIV-positive individuals eventually develop oral candidiasis, which often spreads to the esophagus. The latter condition is considered an indicator of full-blown AIDS. Vaginal candidiasis presents as itching and burning pain of the vulva and vagina, accompanied by a thick or thin white discharge. HIV-positive females often experience recurrent vaginal candidiasis. Systemic candidiasis is a potentially life-threatening infection that occurs in debilitated individuals, cancer patients (with neutropenia secondary to chemotherapy), individuals on systemic corticosteroids, and patients treated with broad-spectrum antibiotics. Systemic candidiasis may involve the gastrointestinal tract, kidneys, liver, and spleen. Both oral and vaginal infections are treated topically with nystatin or clotrimazole. Oral systemic antifungal agents such as ketoconazole, fluconazole, and itraconazole are preferred for ease of administration and increased efficacy. Amphotericin B by itself or in combination with flucytosine is used in systemic disease.

B. **Cryptococcosis** is caused by the yeast *Cryptococcus neoformans* (Figure 20.15), which is found worldwide. The organism is especially abundant in soil containing bird (especially pigeon) droppings, although the birds are not infected. The organism has a characteristic thick capsule that surrounds the budding yeast cell, which is observable on a background of India ink. A positive India ink test on cerebral spinal fluid (CSF) can give a quick diagnosis of cryptococcal meningitis, but false negatives are common. The most common form of cryptococcosis is a mild, subclinical lung infection. In immunocompromised patients, the infection often disseminates to the brain and meninges, with fatal consequences. However, about half of patients with cryptococcal meningitis have no obvious immunologic defect.

 In AIDS patients, cryptococcosis, the second most common fungal infection (after candidiasis), is potentially the most serious.

The antifungal drugs used to treat cryptococcosis are amphotericin B and flucytosine, the precise treatment regimen depending on the

**Figure 20.14**
Oral candidiasis (thrush).

**Figure 20.15**
*Cryptococcosis neoformans.*

**Figure 20.16**
*Aspergillus* species.

**Figure 20.17**
Fungus ball.

**Figure 20.18**
*Rhizopus oryzae.*

stage of disease, site of infection, and whether the patient has AIDS. Fluconazole is the drug of choice for prevention of cryptococcal meningitis in AIDS patients.

C. **Aspergillosis** is caused by several species of the genus *Aspergillus*, but primarily by *Aspergillus fumigatus. Aspergillus* is rarely pathogenic in the normal host, but can produce disease in immunosuppressed individuals and patients treated with broad-spectrum antibiotics. The disease has a worldwide distribution. Aspergilli are ubiquitous, growing only as filamentous molds (Figure 20.16) and producing prodigious numbers of conidiospores. They reside in dust and the soil, decomposing organic matter. In fact, hospital outbreaks affecting neutropenic patients (that is, those with decreased neutrophils in their blood) have been traced to dust from neighboring construction work. Aspergillosis manifests itself in several forms, depending in part on the immunologic state of health of the patient.

1. **Acute aspergillus infections:** The most severe, and often fatal, form of aspergillosis is acute invasive infection of the lung, from which the infection can be disseminated to the brain, gastrointestinal tract, and other organs. A less severe, noninvasive lung infection gives rise to a fungus ball (aspergilloma), a mass of hyphal tissue that can form in lung cavities derived from prior diseases, such as tuberculosis (Figure 20.17). Although the lung is the most common primary site of infection, the eye, ear, nasal sinuses, and skin can also be primary sites.

2. **Diagnosis and treatment:** Definitive diagnosis of an aspergillus infection is afforded by detection of hyphal masses, and isolation of the organism from clinical samples. Aspergillus hyphae characteristically form V-shaped branches (septate hyphae that branch at a 45-degree angle, see Figure 20.16) that are distinguished from *Mucor* species, which form right-angle branches. Also, septae are present in aspergillus hyphae but absent from mucor hyphae. In culture, the spore-bearing structures of the aspergilli are unmistakable but, because these organisms are so ubiquitous, external contamination of clinical samples can give false-positives. Treatment of aspergillus infections is typically by amphotericin B and surgical removal of fungal masses or infected tissue. The antifungal drugs miconazole, ketoconazole, and fluconazole have not proved useful, although itraconazole has been used with some effectiveness for *Aspergillus* osteomyelitis.

D. **Mucormycosis** is caused most often by *Rhizopus oryzae* (also called *R. arrhizus,* Figure 20.18) and less often by other members of the Order Mucorales, such as *Absidia corymbifera* and *Rhizomucor pusillus*. Like the aspergilli, these organisms are ubiquitous in nature, and their spores are found in great abundance on rotting fruit and old bread. *Mucor* infections occur worldwide, but are almost entirely restricted to individuals with some underlying predisposing condition, such as burns, leukemias, or acidotic states such as diabetes mellitus. The most common form of the disease, which can be fatal within one week, is rhinocerebral mucormycosis, in which the infection begins in the nasal mucosa or sinuses and progresses to the orbits, palate, and brain. Because the disease is so aggressive, many cases are not diagnosed until after death. Treatment is based on high-dose amphotericin B, but must be accompanied, when possible, by surgical debridement of necrotic tissue, and correction of the underlying predisposing condition. Antifungal drugs other than amphotericin have not proven useful. With early diagnosis and optimal treatment, about half of diabetic patients survive rhinocerebral mucormycosis; however, prognosis is very poor for leukemic patients.

**Figure 20.19**
*Pneumocystis jiroveci.*

**E. Pneumocystis jiroveci** pneumonia is caused by the unicellular eukaryote, *P. jiroveci* (formerly, *P. carinii*). Before the use of immunosuppressive drugs and the onset of the AIDS epidemic, infection with this organism was a rare occurrence. It is one of the most common opportunistic diseases of individuals infected with HIV-1 (see Figure 33.10, p. 388) and almost 100 percent fatal if untreated.

1. **Classification:** Previously, *P. jiroveci* had been considered a protozoan, but recent molecular homology studies of both protein and nucleic acid sequences strongly indicate that *P. jiroveci* is a fungus related to the ascomycetous yeasts. However ergosterol, which is an essential component of most fungal membranes, is lacking in *P. jiroveci*. It has so far not been possible to cultivate *P. jiroveci* in culture, limiting understanding of its life cycle.

2. **Pathology:** The infectious form and the natural reservoir of this organism have not been identified, but they must be ubiquitous in nature because almost 100 percent of children worldwide have antipneumocystis antibodies. The disease is not transmitted from person to person. Instead, development of *P. jiroveci* in immunodeficient patients is thought to be by activation of preexisting dormant cells in the lungs. The encysted forms induce inflammation of alveoli, resulting in production of an exudate that blocks gas exchange. Figure 20.20 shows typical radiographic findings in *Pneumocystis* pneumonia.

**Figure 20.20**
*Pneumocystis* pneumonia.

3. **Diagnosis and treatment:** Because *P. jiroveci* cannot be cultivated, diagnosis is based on microscopic examination of biopsied lung tissue or washings. The most effective therapy is a combination of sulfamethoxazole and trimethoprim, which is also used prophylactically to prevent infection in AIDS patients. Aggressive treatment can spare about half of patients.

> Because the mechanism of action of many antifungal drugs, such as amphotericin, involves interfering with ergosterol synthesis or function, these drugs are useless for ergosterol-lacking fungi.

## Study Questions

**Choose the ONE correct answer**

20.1 A component of the cell membrane of most fungi is

    A. cholesterol.

    B. chitin.

    C. ergosterol.

    D. peptidoglycan.

    E. keratin.

Correct answer = C. Ergosterol in fungi is the functional equivalent of cholesterol in higher organisms. Peptidoglycan is a component of the bacterial cell wall, whereas chitin is a component of the cell wall of fungi. [Note: Chitin also comprises the exoskeletons of insects and crustacea.] Keratin is the major protein of hair and nails.

20.2 A physician visiting a rural Latin American village finds that many mature males but few immature males or females of any age are afflicted by a particular fungal disease. What is likely to be the diagnosis?

    A. Mycetoma

    B. Blastomycosis

    C. Paracoccidioidomycosis

    D. Mucormycosis

    E. Histoplasmosis

Correct answer = C. For some reason, possibly hormonal, this disease favors mature males.

20.3 A fungus that can attack hair is

    A. *Trichophyton*.

    B. *Rhizopus*.

    C. *Microsporum*.

    D. *Sporothrix*.

    E. *Epidermophyton*.

Correct answer = C. All attack skin, but only *Microsporum* attacks hair.

20.4 A farmer in Mississippi presents with a chronic cough. Chest radiograph reveals an opaque mass. Biopsy of the lung shows macrophages with multiple yeast forms. Which one of the following diagnoses is most likely?

    A. Coccidioidomycosis

    B. Histoplasmosis

    C. Blastomycosis

    D. Paracoccidioido-mycosis

    E. Sporotrichosis

Correct answer = B. Histoplasmosis is caused by *Histoplasma capsulatum*. In the soil, the fungus generates conidia, which, when airborne, enter the lungs and germinate into yeast-like cells. These yeast cells become engulfed by macrophages in which they multiply. Pulmonary infections may be acute but relatively benign and self-limiting or chronic, progressive and fatal. Dissemination is rare. The disseminated disease results in invasion of cells of the reticuloendothelial system, which distinguishes this organism as the only fungus to exhibit intracellular parasitism. The disease occurs worldwide, but is most prevalent in central North America, especially the Ohio and Mississippi River Valleys.

*"On the other hand, he never takes a sick day."*

# Protozoa

**21**

## I. OVERVIEW

Protozoa are a diverse group of unicellular, eukaryotic organisms. Many have evolved structural features (organelles) that mimic the organs of multicellular organisms. Reproduction is generally by mitotic binary fission, although in some protozoal species, sexual (meiotic) reproduction with several variations occurs as well. Only a few of the many tens of thousands of protozoan species are pathogenic for humans. Those discussed in this chapter are listed in Figure 21.1. These pathogens are of two general kinds: those that parasitize the intestinal and urogenital tracts, and those that parasitize blood cells and tissues. Protozoal infections are common in developing tropical and subtropical regions where sanitary conditions and control of the vectors of transmission are poor. However, with increased world travel and immigration, protozoal diseases are no longer confined to specific geographic locales. Because they are eukaryotes, protozoa, like fungi, have metabolic processes closer to those of the human host than to prokaryotic bacterial pathogens. Protozoal diseases are thus less easily treated than bacterial infections because many antiprotozoal drugs are toxic to the human host.[1]

## II. CLASSIFICATION OF CLINICALLY IMPORTANT PROTOZOA

Among the pathogenic protozoa, there are important common features that are clinically relevant. For example, many protozoa have both a dormant, immotile cyst stage that permits survival when environmental conditions are hostile, and a motile, actively feeding and reproducing, vegetative (trophozoite) stage. For convenience, protozoa are classified according to mode of locomotion. The clinically relevant protozoa are divided into four groups (Figure 21.2).

### A. Amebas

Amebas move by extending cytoplasmic projections (pseudopodia) outward from the main cell body. A single cell can have several pseudopodia projecting in the same general direction, with the remainder of the cytoplasm flowing into the pseudopodia. Amebas feed by engulfing food particles with their pseudopodia. [Note: Some amebas have flagella as well.]

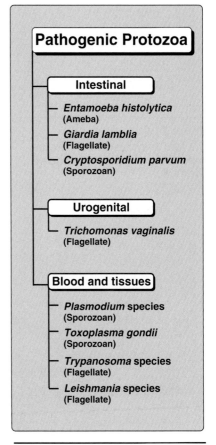

**Pathogenic Protozoa**

**Intestinal**
- *Entamoeba histolytica* (Ameba)
- *Giardia lamblia* (Flagellate)
- *Cryptosporidium parvum* (Sporozoan)

**Urogenital**
- *Trichomonas vaginalis* (Flagellate)

**Blood and tissues**
- *Plasmodium* species (Sporozoan)
- *Toxoplasma gondii* (Sporozoan)
- *Trypanosoma* species (Flagellate)
- *Leishmania* species (Flagellate)

**Figure 21.1**
Clinically relevant protozoa, classified according to site of infection.

[1]See Chapter 36, pp. 413-425 in ***Lippincott's Illustrated Reviews: Pharmacology*** (3rd ed.) for a more in depth discussion of the drugs used for treatment of clinically important protozoa.

**Figure 21.2**
The four major protozoal groups, classified according to mode of locomotion.

### B. Flagellates

Flagellates move by means of two or more whip-like projections (flagella) that rotate and propel the cells through their liquid environment. Some flagellates, for example, the pathogen *Trichomonas vaginalis*, also have undulating membranes that assist in swimming. Flagellates ingest food particles through an oral groove called a cytostome.

### C. Ciliates

Ciliates move by means of many hair-like projections (cilia) arranged in rows that cover the cell surface and beat in synchrony, propelling the cell much like an oar-driven galley. Most ciliates have cytostomes that pass food particles through a cytopharynx and finally into vacuoles where digestion takes place. Although there are some 7000 species of ciliates, only *Balantidium coli* is pathogenic for humans, and the disease, balantidiasis, is rare.

### D. Sporozoa

Sporozoans (also called apicomplexa) are obligate, intracellular parasites. They generally have nonmotile adult forms; however, in some species, male gametes have flagella. An example of a sporozoan is *Plasmodium vivax* (see p. 221), which causes malaria. Sporozoans can have complex life cycles with more than one host. The definitive

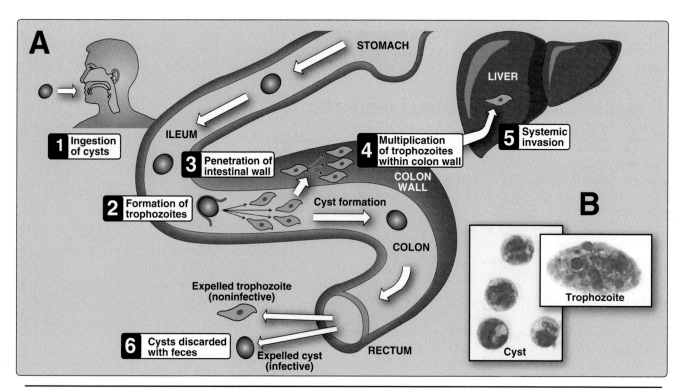

**Figure 21.3**
A. Life cycle of *Entamoeba histolytica*. B. Photomicrographs of tropozoite and cyst forms.

host is that which harbors the sexually reproducing stage, whereas the intermediate host provides the environment in which asexual reproduction occurs.

## III. INTESTINAL PROTOZOAL INFECTIONS

There are three principal protozoal intestinal parasites: the ameba, *Entamoeba histolytica*; the flagellate, *Giardia lamblia*; and several varieties of the sporozoan, *Cryptosporidium*. Each causes dysentery, which, although similar, differ in the site of infection, its severity, and secondary consequences.

### A. Amebic dysentery (*Entamoeba histolytica*)

Ingested cysts from contaminated food or water form trophozoites in the small intestine (Figure 21.3). These pass to the colon, where they feed on intestinal bacteria, and may invade the epithelium, potentially inducing ulceration. The parasite can further spread to the liver and cause abscesses. In the colon, trophozoites form cysts that pass in the feces (amebic cysts are resistant to chlorine concentrations used in most water treatment facilities). Diagnosis is made by examination of fecal samples for motile trophozoites or cysts (Figure 21.4). Serologic test kits are useful when microscopic examination is negative. Liver abscesses should be biopsied from the abscess edge where the active amebas accumulate. Mild cases of luminal amebic dysentery are treated with iodoquinol, paramomycin, or diloxanide furoate. More severe cases, including liver infections, are treated with metronidazole (which also has antibacterial activity) in combination with chloroquine and/or diloxamide furoate or emetine.

**Figure 21.4**
*Entamoeba histolytica* cysts.

### B. Giardiasis (*Giardia lamblia*)

Similar to *E. histolytica*, *Giardia lamblia* has two life-cycle stages: the binucleate trophozoite that has four flagella, and the drug-resistant, four-nucleate cyst. Ingested cysts form trophozoites in the duodenum where they attach to the wall but do not invade (Figure 21.5). *Giardia* infections are often clinically mild, although in some individuals, massive infection may inflame and damage the duodenal mucosa.

Giardiasis is the most commonly diagnosed parasitic intestinal disease in the United States.

Because the *Giardia* parasite preferentially inhabits the duodenum, fecal examination may be negative. A commercial immunologic ELISA test to measure *Giardia* antigen in fecal material has proven useful. Metronidazole is an effective treatment. [Note: *G. lamblia* cysts are resistant to chlorine concentrations used in most water treatment facilities.]

**Figure 21.5**
*Giardia lamblia* trophozoite in stool sample.

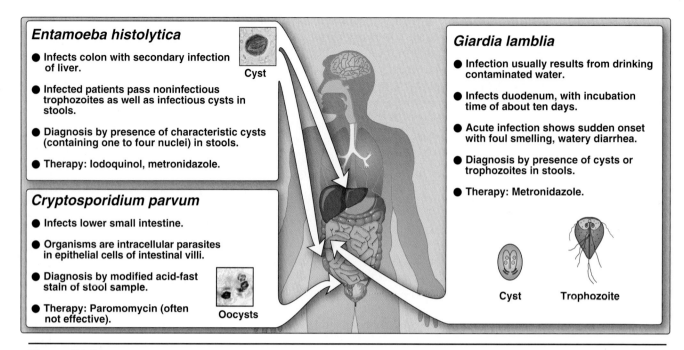

**Entamoeba histolytica**

● Infects colon with secondary infection of liver.

● Infected patients pass noninfectious trophozoites as well as infectious cysts in stools.

● Diagnosis by presence of characteristic cysts (containing one to four nuclei) in stools.

● Therapy: Iodoquinol, metronidazole.

Cyst

**Cryptosporidium parvum**

● Infects lower small intestine.

● Organisms are intracellular parasites in epithelial cells of intestinal villi.

● Diagnosis by modified acid-fast stain of stool sample.

● Therapy: Paromomycin (often not effective).

Oocysts

**Giardia lamblia**

● Infection usually results from drinking contaminated water.

● Infects duodenum, with incubation time of about ten days.

● Acute infection shows sudden onset with foul smelling, watery diarrhea.

● Diagnosis by presence of cysts or trophozoites in stools.

● Therapy: Metronidazole.

Cyst            Trophozoite

**Figure 21.6**
Summary of intestinal protozoal infections.

### C. Cryptosporidiosis (*Cryptosporidium* species)

*Cryptosporidium* is an intracellular parasite that inhabits the epithelial cells of the villi of the lower small intestine. The source of infection is often the feces of domestic animals, and farm run-off has been implicated as a source of *Cryptosporidium* contamination of drinking water. Asymptomatic to mild cases are common, and if the immune system of the patient is normal, the disease usually resolves without therapy. However, in immunocompromised individuals (for example, those with AIDS), infection may be severe and intractable, although paromomycin has provided some improvement. Diagnosis is made by acid-fast staining of the tiny (four to six μm) oocysts in fresh stool samples. A summary of intestinal protozoal infections is shown in Figure 21.6.

## IV. UROGENITAL TRACT INFECTIONS

Trichomoniasis is caused by *T. vaginalis*. Trichomoniasis is the most common protozoal urogenital tract infection of humans. The trichomonads are pear-shaped flagellates, with undulating membranes. Several nonpathogenic species, including *T. tenax* and *T. hominis*, can be found in the human mouth and intestines, respectively. In the living state, these species, which are part of the normal flora, are not easily distinguished morphologically from the pathogenic species, *T. vaginalis*.

### A. Trichomoniasis (*T. vaginalis*)

*T. vaginalis* is responsible for the most common form of human trichomoniasis (Figure 21.7). In females, it causes inflammation of the

**Figure 21.7**
*Trichomonas vaginalis.*

mucosal tissue of the vagina, vulva, and cervix, accompanied by a copious, yellowish, malodorous discharge. Less commonly, it infects the male urethra, prostate, and seminal vesicles, producing a white discharge. The disease is largely sexually transmitted, and both (or all) sexual partners should be treated. The optimum pH for growth of this organism is about 6.0; therefore, *T. vaginalis* does not thrive in the normal, acidic vagina, which has a pH of about 4.0. Abnormal alkalinity of the vagina thus favors acquisition of the disease. Diagnosis is made by detection of motile trophozoites in vaginal or urethral secretions. If the concentration of parasites is too low to be observed directly, laboratory culture can be used to obtain observable organisms. Effective treatment is afforded by metronidazole. Figure 21.8 summarizes urogenital infections caused by *T. vaginalis*.

# V. BLOOD AND TISSUE PROTOZOAL INFECTIONS

The major protozoal diseases that involve the blood and internal organs are malaria (*Plasmodium* species), toxoplasmosis (*Toxoplasma* species), trypanosomiasis (*Trypanosoma* species), and leishmaniasis (*Leishmania* species). *Plasmodium* and *Toxoplasma* are sporozoans (apicomplexa), whereas *Trypanosoma* and *Leishmania* are flagellates, sometimes referred to as hemoflagellates.

## A. Malaria (*Plasmodium falciparum* and other species)

Malaria is an acute infectious disease of the blood, caused by one of four species of the protozoal genus, *Plasmodium*, a sporozoan. *P. falciparum* accounts for some fifteen percent of all malaria cases, and *P. vivax* for eighty percent of malarial cases.

> The plasmodial parasite is transmitted to humans through the bite of a female *Anopheles* mosquito, or by an infected, blood-contaminated, needle.

Sporozoans reproduce asexually in human cells by a process called schizogony, in which multiple nuclear divisions are followed by envelopment of the nuclei by cell walls producing merozoites. These, in turn, become trophozoites. Sexual reproduction occurs in the mosquito, where new spores (sporozoites) are formed.

1. **Pathology and clinical significance:** *Plasmodium* sporozoites are injected into the bloodstream, where they rapidly migrate to the liver. There they form cyst-like structures containing thousands of merozoites. Upon release, the merozoites invade red blood cells, using hemoglobin as a nutrient. Eventually, the infected red cells rupture, releasing merozoites that can invade other erythrocytes. If large numbers of red cells rupture at roughly the same time, a paroxysm (sudden onset) of fever can result from the massive release of toxic substances.

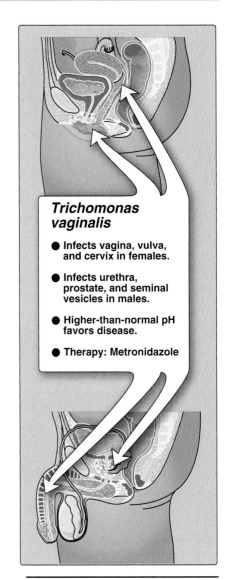

***Trichomonas vaginalis***

● Infects vagina, vulva, and cervix in females.

● Infects urethra, prostate, and seminal vesicles in males.

● Higher-than-normal pH favors disease.

● Therapy: Metronidazole

**Figure 21.8**
Summary of urogenital infection.

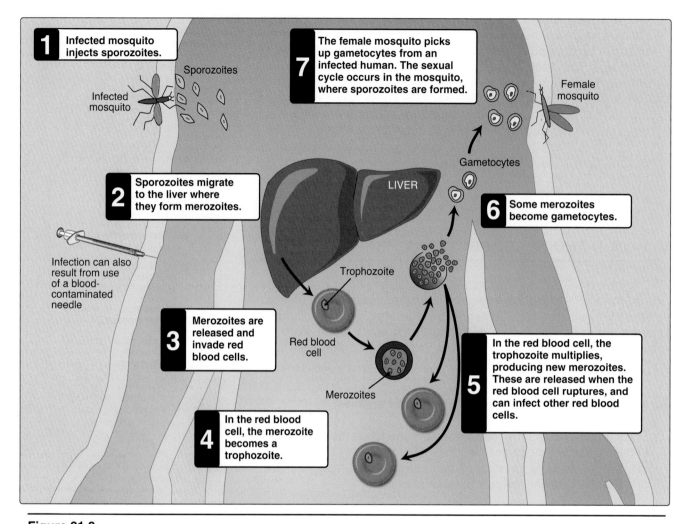

**Figure 21.9**
Life cycle of the malarial parasite, *Plasmodium falciparum*.

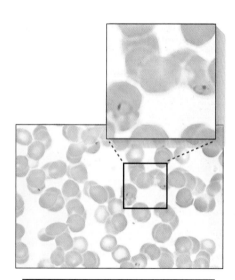

**Figure 21.10**
Ring form of *Plasmodium falciparum* in red blood cell.

*Plasmodium falciparum* is the most dangerous plasmodial species. It can cause a rapidly fulminating disease, characterized by persistent high fever and orthostatic hypotension. Infection can lead to capillary obstruction and death if treatment is not prompt. *P. malariae*, *P. vivax*, and *P. ovale* cause milder forms of the disease, probably because they invade either young or old red cells, but not both. This is in contrast to *P. falciparum*, which invades cells of all ages. Even today, malarial infection is a common and serious disease, causing some 300 million cases per year, with a death rate of about one percent. A summary of the life cycle of *Plasmodium* is shown in Figure 21.9.

2. **Diagnosis and treatment:** Diagnosis depends on detection of the parasite inside red blood cells (Figure 21.10). Thick blood smears stained with Giemsa stain provide the most sensitive visual test. Thin blood smears, in which more detail can be discerned, are used to determine the species involved, which is important in planning a course of therapy. [Note: Serologic tests are usually too slow for diagnosis of acute disease.] Drug treatment depends on the stage of infection. Primaquine is effective against the exo-

erythrocytic forms in the liver and bloodstream and also against the gametocytic form, but inactive against parasites in red blood cells. Therefore, for the erythrocytic form, primaquine is administered in conjunction with a blood schizontocide such as chloroquine, quinine, artemisinin, mefloquine, or pyrimethamine. All species may develop drug resistance. [Note: Patients with glucose 6-phosphate dehydrogenase deficiency develop hemolytic anemia if they are treated with primaquine.[1]]

## B. Toxoplasmosis (*Toxoplasma gondii*)

*Toxoplasma gondii* is a sporozoan, distributed worldwide, that infects all vertebrate species, although the definitive host is the cat. Humans can become infected by the accidental ingestion of oocysts present in cat feces, by eating raw or undercooked meat, congenitally from an infected mother, or from a blood transfusion.

1. **Pathology and clinical significance:** There are two kinds of *Toxoplasma* trophozoites found in human infections: rapidly growing tachyzoites (tachy = rapid) that are seen in body fluids in early, acute infections, and slowly growing bradyzoites (brady = slow) that are contained in cysts in muscle and brain tissue and in the eye. Tachyzoites directly destroy cells, particularly parenchymal and reticuloendothelial cells, whereas bradyzoites released from ruptured tissue cysts cause local inflammation with blockage of blood vessels and necrosis. Infections of normal human hosts are common and usually asymptomatic. However, they can be very severe in immunocompromised individuals, who may also suffer recrudescence (relapse) of the infection. Congenital infections can also be severe, resulting in stillbirths, brain lesions, and hydrocephaly, and they are a major cause of blindness in newborns.

2. **Diagnosis and treatment:** The initial diagnostic approach involves detection of parasites in tissue specimens, but this may often be inconclusive. With the recent availability of commercial diagnostic kits, serologic tests to identify toxoplasma are now routinely used. These include tests for *Toxoplasma*-specific IgG and IgM. The treatment of choice for this infection is the antifolate drug pyrimethamine, given in combination with sulfadiazine.

## C. Trypanosomiasis (various trypanosome species)

Trypanosomiasis refers to two chronic, eventually fatal, diseases (African sleeping sickness and American trypanosomiasis) caused by several trypanosome species. Some of the differences between these diseases and the available chemotherapeutic agents are summarized in Figure 21.11.

1. **Pathology and clinical significance:** African sleeping sickness is caused by the closely related flagellates, *Trypanosoma brucei gambiense* or *Trypanosoma brucei rhodesiense* (Figure 21.12). These parasites are injected into humans by the bite of the tsetse fly, producing a primary lesion or chancre. The organism then

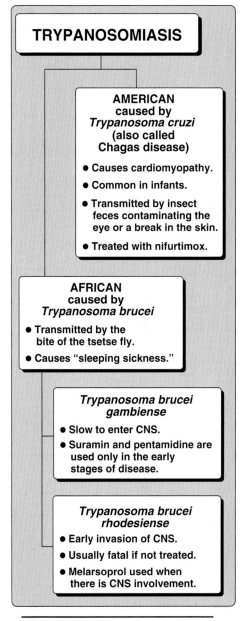

**Figure 21.11**
Summary of trypanosomiasis.

[2]See p. 149 in *Lippincott's Illustrated Reviews: Biochemistry* (3rd ed.) for a discussion of glucose 6-phosphate dehydrogenase deficiency.

spreads to lymphoid tissue and reproduces extracellularly in the blood. Later, the parasite invades the central nervous system (CNS), causing inflammation of the brain and spinal cord, mediated by released toxins. This inflammation produces the characteristic lethargy and, eventually, continuous sleep and death. American trypanosomiasis (Chagas disease), caused by *Trypanosoma cruzi*, occurs in Central and South America. Unlike African forms of the disease, infection is not transmitted by insect bite, but rather by insect feces contaminating the conjunctiva or a break in the skin.

2. **Diagnosis and treatment:** Diagnosis of African trypanosomiasis is made primarily by detection of motile trypanosomes in Giemsa-stained smears of body fluids (for example, blood, cerebrospinal fluid, and lymph node aspirates). Highly specific serologic tests are also available, that are often used for diagnostic confirmation. Early-stage African trypanosomiasis is treated with suramin or pentamidine. Melarsoprol is used in late-stage disease when the CNS is involved. American trypanosomiasis is treated with nifurtimox, but the drug's effectiveness is limited.

D. **Leishmaniasis (various *Leishmania* species)**

Leishmaniasis refers to a group of infections caused by the flagellate protozoa of the genus *Leishmania*. About half a million new cases are reported each year, and it is estimated that 12,000,000 people are currently infected with this parasite. There are three clinical types of leishmaniasis: cutaneous, mucocutaneous, and visceral. The various infective organisms are indistinguishable

**Figure 21.12**
*Trypanosoma brucei.*

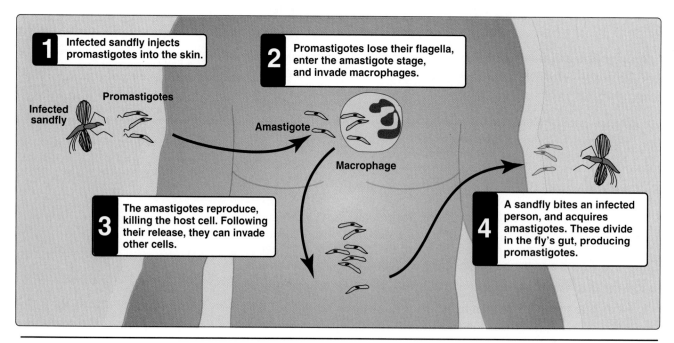

**Figure 21.13**
Life cycle of *Leishmania*.

morphologically, but can be differentiated by biochemical means. Two subgenera are recognized (*L. leishmania* and *L.viannia*), each with several species. Any species has the potential to cause one of three clinical manifestations. The natural reservoir of the parasite varies with geography and species, but is usually wild rodents, dogs, and humans. Transmission to humans is by the bite of a sandfly of the genus *Phlebotomus* or *Lutzomyia*. The life cycle of *Leishmania* is shown in Figure 21.13.

1. **Cutaneous leishmaniasis (local name, oriental sore):** This disease is caused by *Leishmania tropica* in north and west Africa, Iran, and Iraq. The cutaneous form of the disease is characterized by ulcerating single or multiple skin sores (Figure 21.14). Most cases spontaneously heal, but the ulcers leave unsightly scars. In Mexico and Guatemala, the cutaneous form is due to *Leishmania mexicana*, which produces single lesions that rapidly heal.

**Figure 21.14**
Skin ulcer due to leishmaniasis, on the hand of a Central American adult.

2. **Mucocutaneous leishmaniasis (local name, espundia):** This disease is caused by *Leishmania viannia brasiliensis* in Central and South America, especially the Amazon regions. In this form of the disease, the parasite attacks tissue at the mucosal-dermal junctions of the nose and mouth, producing multiple lesions. Extensive spreading into mucosal tissue can obliterate the nasal septum and the buccal cavity, ending in death from secondary infection.

3. **Visceral leishmaniasis (local name, kala-azar):** This disease is caused by *Leishmania donovani* in India, East Africa, and China. In the visceral disease, the parasite initially infects macrophages, which, in turn, migrate to the spleen, liver, and bone marrow, where the parasite rapidly multiplies. The spleen and liver enlarge, and jaundice may develop. Most individuals have only minor symptoms, and the disease may resolve spontaneously. However, in some cases, complications resulting from secondary infection and emaciation result in death.

4. **Diagnosis and treatment:** Diagnosis is made by examination of Giemsa-stained tissue and fluid samples for the nonflagellated form (amastigote), which is the only form of the organism that occurs in humans and other mammals. Cutaneous and mucocutaneous disease can be diagnosed from tissue samples taken from the edges of lesions or lymph node aspirates. Visceral disease is more difficult to diagnose, requiring liver, spleen, or bone marrow biopsy. Serologic tests (for example, indirect fluorescent antibody, see p. 29, and complement fixation, see p. 27) are useful and used by the Centers for Disease Control and Prevention. The treatment of leishmaniasis is difficult because the available drugs have considerable toxicity and high failure rates. Pentavalent antimonials, such as sodium stibogluconate, are the conventional therapy, with pentamidine and amphotericin B as second-line agents.

## Study Questions

**Choose the ONE correct answer**

21.1  The protozoal trophozoite phase is characterized by

A. metabolic dormancy.

B. toxin production.

C. active feeding and reproduction.

D. flagellar locomotion.

E. residence in the intermediate host.

> Correct answer = C. The trophozoite is, generally speaking, the active phase, in contrast to the cyst, which is the dormant phase. In some species, several varieties of trophozoites are recognized, such as the tachyzoites and bradyzoites of *Toxoplasma gondii*.

21.2  The definitive host of a parasite is the host

A. in which asexual reproduction occurs.

B. in which sexual reproduction occurs.

C. that is obligatory for the parasite.

D. that is capable of destroying the parasite.

E. that is the vector organism that transports a parasite from an uninfected to an infected host.

> Correct answer = B. Sexual reproduction occurs in the definitive host, whereas asexual reproduction occurs in the intermediate host. For example, in the case of the malarial *Plasmodium*, the definitive host is the mosquito and the intermediate host is the human. In most cases, both hosts are obligatory for propagation of the parasite.

21.3  *Plasmodium falciparum*, which causes malaria, is an example of

A. an ameboid protozoan.

B. a sporozoan.

C. a flagellate.

D. a ciliate.

E. a schizont.

> Correct answer = B. The sporozoans are also called apicomplexa, because of the presence of a complex of organelles at the cell tip that facilitate penetration of the parasite into host tissue. A schizont is not a taxonomic group but a mass of trophozoites.

21.4  A United States businessman who has recently returned home from Haiti suddenly develops a periodic high fever followed by orthostatic hypotension. What is the likely preliminary diagnosis?

A. Chagas disease

B. Giardiasis

C. Syphilis

D. Malaria

E. Toxoplasmosis

> Correct answer = D. All of the signs point to malaria, especially the periodicity of the fever that results from synchronous rupturing of large numbers of red blood cells.

*"I suppose this is goodbye."*

# Helminths

# 22

## I. OVERVIEW

Helminths are worms, some of which are parasitic to humans. These parasites belong to one of three groups: cestodes (tapeworms), trematodes (flukes), or nematodes (roundworms) (Figure 22.1). Although individual species may have preferred primary sites of infestation—often the intestines where they generally do little damage—these organisms may disseminate to vital organs (for example, the brain, lungs, or liver) where they can cause severe damage. It is estimated that at least seventy percent of the world's population is infected with a parasitic helminth. The mode of transmission to humans varies from species to species, includes ingestion of larvae in raw or undercooked pork, beef, or fish and helminth eggs in feces, by insect bites, or by direct skin penetration. In North America, helminthic diseases are becoming rare, whereas they are endemic in regions of the world where community sanitary conditions are poor and human feces is used as fertilizer.

## II. CESTODES

Cestodes (tapeworms) are ribbon-like, segmented worms that are primarily intestinal parasites. They totally lack a digestive system and do not ingest particulate matter, but instead they absorb soluble nutrients directly through their cuticle. In the small intestine some species (for example, the tapeworm *Diphyllobothrium latum)* can attain enormous lengths of up to fifteen meters. Cestodes cause clinical injury by sequestering the host's nutrients, by excreting toxic waste, and, in massive infestations, by causing mechanical blockage of the intestine. The anterior end of the worm consists of a scolex, a bulbous structure with hooks and suckers that functions to attach the worm to the intestinal wall (Figure 22.2). The body (strobila) is composed of many segments (proglottids), which form continuously in the region just behind the scolex. Each proglottid has a complete set of sexual organs—both male and female—that generate fertilized eggs. The mature, egg-filled proglottids are located at the posterior end of the organism. These can break off the chain and pass out of the body in the stool. Characteristics of infections by the four medically important cestodes are summarized in Figure 22.3. Note that *Taenia solium* has two different disease manifestations, depending on whether transmission is by ingestion of larvae from undercooked pork, or by ingestion of its eggs. In the former case, infestation is limited to the intestines; in the latter case, the eggs develop into larvae that form cysts (cysticerci) in the brain and other tissues.

**Helminths**

**CESTODES (TAPEWORMS)**

- *Diphyllobothrium latum*
  (Broad fish tapeworm)
- *Echinococcus granulosus*
  (Dog tapeworm)
- *Taenia saginata*
  (Beef tapeworm)
- *Taenia solium*
  (Pork tapeworm)

**TREMATODES (FLUKES)**

- *Clonorchis sinensis*
  (Chinese or Oriental liver fluke)
- *Paragonimus westermani*
  (Lung fluke)
- *Schistosoma mansoni*
  (Blood fluke)
- *Schistosoma haematobium*
  (Blood fluke)

**NEMATODES (ROUNDWORMS)**

*Intestinal infections*
- *Ancylostoma duodenale*
- *Necator americanus*
  (Old World and New World hookworms)
- *Ascaris lumbricoides*
  (Giant roundworm)
- *Enterobius vermicularis*
  (Pinworm)
- *Strongyloides stercoralis*
  (Small roundworm)
- *Trichinella spiralis*
- *Trichuris trichiura*
  (Whipworm)

*Tissue infections*
- *Brugia malayi*
- *Dracunculus medinensis*
  (Guinea fire worm**)**
- *Loa loa*
  (Filarial worm, or African eye worm)
- *Onchocerca volvulus*
  (Filarial worm)
- *Toxocara canis*
  (Dog worm)
- *Wuchereria bancrofti*
  (Filarial worm)

**Figure 22.1**
Clinically important helminths.

**Figure 22.2**
The scolex of *Taenia solium* is 1 mm wide and has four suckers.

## III. TREMATODES

Trematodes, commonly called flukes, are small (about 1 cm), flat, leaf-like worms that, depending on the species, infest various organs of the human host (for example, intestinal veins, urinary bladder, liver, or lung). All parasitic trematodes use freshwater snails as an intermediate host.

### A. Hermaphroditic flukes

Developmental events in the life cycle of a typical fluke begin when the adult fluke, which is hermaphroditic, produces eggs in the human (the definitive host). The eggs are then excreted into the environment. The first larval stage (miracidium) develops inside the eggs. These larvae seek out and infect suitable snail species, which are the first intermediate host. In the snail, asexual reproduction occurs, during which several intermediate developmental forms can be distinguished, including sporocyst, redia (an early larval stage) and eventually large numbers of the final larval stage, called cer-

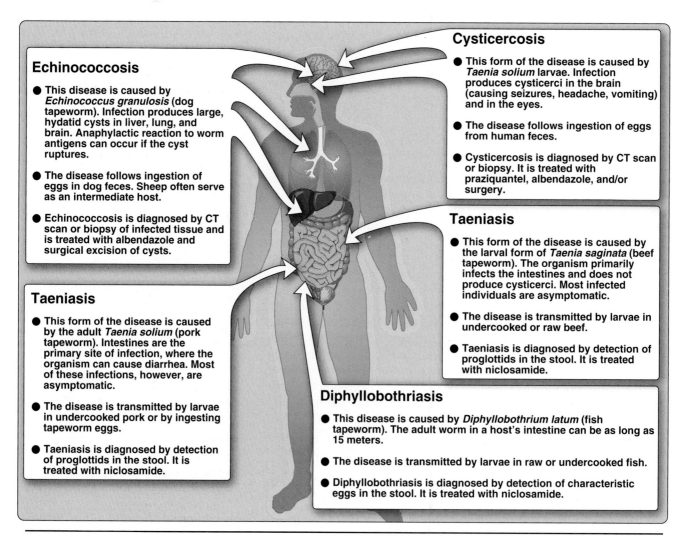

**Echinococcosis**

● This disease is caused by *Echinococcus granulosis* (dog tapeworm). Infection produces large, hydatid cysts in liver, lung, and brain. Anaphylactic reaction to worm antigens can occur if the cyst ruptures.

● The disease follows ingestion of eggs in dog feces. Sheep often serve as an intermediate host.

● Echinococcosis is diagnosed by CT scan or biopsy of infected tissue and is treated with albendazole and surgical excision of cysts.

**Taeniasis**

● This form of the disease is caused by the adult *Taenia solium* (pork tapeworm). Intestines are the primary site of infection, where the organism can cause diarrhea. Most of these infections, however, are asymptomatic.

● The disease is transmitted by larvae in undercooked pork or by ingesting tapeworm eggs.

● Taeniasis is diagnosed by detection of proglottids in the stool. It is treated with niclosamide.

**Cysticercosis**

● This form of the disease is caused by *Taenia solium* larvae. Infection produces cysticerci in the brain (causing seizures, headache, vomiting) and in the eyes.

● The disease follows ingestion of eggs from human feces.

● Cysticercosis is diagnosed by CT scan or biopsy. It is treated with praziquantel, albendazole, and/or surgery.

**Taeniasis**

● This form of the disease is caused by the larval form of *Taenia saginata* (beef tapeworm). The organism primarily infects the intestines and does not produce cysticerci. Most infected individuals are asymptomatic.

● The disease is transmitted by larvae in undercooked or raw beef.

● Taeniasis is diagnosed by detection of proglottids in the stool. It is treated with niclosamide.

**Diphyllobothriasis**

● This disease is caused by *Diphyllobothrium latum* (fish tapeworm). The adult worm in a host's intestine can be as long as 15 meters.

● The disease is transmitted by larvae in raw or undercooked fish.

● Diphyllobothriasis is diagnosed by detection of characteristic eggs in the stool. It is treated with niclosamide.

**Figure 22.3**
Characteristics and therapy for commonly encountered cestode infections.

caria, which leave the snail and seek out a second intermediate host (a fish or crustacean, depending on the species of fluke). In this second intermediate host, the cercaria form cysts called metacercaria that can remain viable indefinitely. Finally, if the infected raw or undercooked fish or crustacean is eaten by a human, the metacercaria excysts, and the fluke invades tissues such as the lung or the liver and begins producing eggs, thus completing the life cycle.

## B. Sexual flukes (schistosomes)

The life cycle of schistosomes is similar to that of hermaphroditic flukes. One difference is that schistosomes have only one intermediate host, the snail. Another difference is that schistosomiasis is not acquired by ingestion of contaminated food, but rather from schistosome cercaria directly penetrating the skin of waders or swimmers in contaminated rivers and lakes. After dissemination and development in the human host, adult schistosomes take up residence in various abdominal veins, depending on the species; they are, therefore, called "blood flukes." Also in contrast to the "typical" hermaphroditic flukes described above, schistosomes have separate, distinctive sexes. A remarkable anatomic feature is the long groove or schist on the ventral surface of the large male in which the smaller female resides and continuously mates with the male (Figure 22.4). This mating takes place in the human liver. Fertilized

**Figure 22.4**
Male schistosome has a long groove in which the smaller female resides and continuously mates with the male.

## Paragonimiasis

● This disease is caused by *Paragonimus westermani* (lung fluke). The organisms move from the gastrointestinal tract to the lung, which is the primary site of damage. Secondary bacterial infections can result in a cough that produces bloody sputum.

● The disease is transmitted by eating raw crab meat.

● Paragonimiasis is diagnosed by identifying eggs in the sputum and stool. It is treated with praziquantel.

## Clonorchiasis

● This disease is caused by *Clonorchis sinensis* (Oriental liver fluke). The primary site of infection is the biliary tract, where the resulting inflammatory response can cause fibrosis and hyperplasia.

● The disease is transmitted by eating raw freshwater fish.

● Clonorchiasis is diagnosed by identifying eggs in the stool. It is treated with praziquantel.

## Schistosomiasis (New World)

● This disease is caused by *Schistosoma mansoni* and *Schistosoma japonicum*. The primary site of infection is the gastrointestinal tract. Damage to the intestinal wall is caused by the host's inflammatory response to eggs deposited at that site. The eggs also secrete proteolytic enzymes that further damage the tissue.

● Clinical presentation includes GI bleeding, diarrhea, and liver damage.

● The disease is transmitted by direct skin penetration.

● This form of schistosomiasis is diagnosed by Identification of characteristic eggs in the stool. It is treated with praziquantel.

## Schistosomiasis (Old World)

● This disease is caused by *Schistosoma haematobium*. The primary sites of infection are veins of the urinary bladder, where the organism's eggs can induce fibrosis, granulomas, and hematuria.

● The disease is transmitted by direct skin penetration.

● This form of schistosomiasis is diagnosed by identifying characteristic eggs in the urine or bladder wall. It is treated with praziquantel.

**Figure 22.5**
Characteristics and therapy for commonly encountered trematode infections.

**Figure 22.6**
Coiled larva of *Trichinella spiralis* in skeletal muscle.

eggs penetrate the human host's vascular walls and enter the intestine or bladder, emerging from the body in feces or urine. In fresh water, the organisms infect snails in which they multiply, producing cercaria (the final, free-swimming larval stage), which are released into the fresh water to complete the cycle. Characteristics of clinically important trematodes are summarized in Figure 22.5.

## IV. NEMATODES

The nematodes (roundworms) are elongated, nonsegmented worms that are tapered at both ends (Figure 22.6). Unlike other helminths, nematodes have a complete digestive system, including a mouth, an intestine that spans most of the body length, and an anus. The body is

### Onchocerciasis (River Blindness)

- This disease is caused by *Onchocerca volvulus*. It is characterized by subcutaneous nodules, pruritic skin rash, and ocular lesions often causing blindness.

- The disease is transmitted by the bite of a blackfly.

- Onchocerciasis is diagnosed by detection of microfilariae in skin biopsy. It is treated with ivermectin and/or surgery.

### Visceral Larva Migrans

- This disease is caused by *Toxocara canis*. It is primarily a disease of young children. The larval form matures in the intestines, then migrates to the liver, brain, and eyes (only the larvae cause disease).

- The disease is transmitted by ingestion of eggs from dog feces.

- Visceral larval migrans is diagnosed by detecting larvae in the tissue. It is treated with mebendazole or thiabendazole.

### Filariasis (Elephantiasis)

- The most frequent organisms causing this disease are *Wuchereria bancrofti* and *Brugia malayi*. These filarial worms block the flow of lymph, causing edematous arms, legs, and scrotum.

- The disease is transmitted by the bite of infected female *Anopheles* and *Culex* mosquitoes.

- Filariasis is diagnosed by detection of microfilariae in blood. It is treated with a combination of diethylcarbamazine and abendazole.

### Loiasis

- This disease is caused by *Loa loa*. The larvae crawl under the skin, leaving characteristic tracks. They can enter the eye where adult worms are visible in the subconjuctival space around the iris.

- The disease is transmitted by deer flies. There is no animal reservoir, and humans are the only definitive host.

- Loiasis is diagnosed by detection of microfilariae in blood. It is treated with diethylcarbamazine.

### Dracunculiasis

- This disease is caused by *Dracunculus medinensis*. Adult worms cause skin inflammation and ulceration. Adult females can be as long as 100 cm; males are much smaller.

- The disease is transmitted by drinking water containing the intermediate host copepods in which the larvae live.

- Dracunculiasis is diagnosed by finding the head of the worm in a skin lesion or larvae that are released from a lesion following contact with water. The disease is treated by removing subcutaneous worms—formerly by winding them on a thin stick, now usually by surgery.

### Trichinosis

- This disease is caused by *Trichinella spiralis*—an intestinal nematode that encysts in the tissue of human and porcine hosts.

- The disease is transmitted by eating undercooked pork.

- Trichinosis is diagnosed by locating coiled encysted larvae in a muscle biopsy. In its early stages, the disease is treated with thiabendazole; no treatment is available for the late stages.

**Figure 22.7**
Characteristics and therapy for commonly encountered nematode infections of tissues other than intestine.

### Enterobiasis (Pinworm Disease)

● This disease is caused by *Enterobius vermicularis*. It is the most common helminthic infection in the United States. Pruritus ani occurs, with white worms visible in the stools or perianal region.

● The disease is transmitted by ingesting the organism's eggs. Humans are the only host.

● Pinworm disease is diagnosed by identifying eggs present around the perianal region. It is treated with mebendazole or pyrantel pamoate.

### Ascariasis (Roundworm Disease)

● This disease is caused by *Ascaris lumbricoides*. It is second only to pinworms as the most prevalent multicellular parasite in the United States. Approximately one-third of the world's population is infected with this worm.

● The disease is transmitted by ingestion of soil containing the organism's eggs. Humans are the sole host. Larva grow in the intestine, causing abdominal symptoms, including intestinal obstruction. Roundworms may pass to the blood and through the lungs.

● Roundworm disease is diagnosed by detection of characteristic eggs in the stool. It is treated with pyrantel pamoate or mebendazole.

### Trichuriasis (Whipworm Disease)

● This disease is caused by *Trichuris trichiura*. The infection is usually asymptomatic; however, abdominal pain, diarrhea, flatulence, and rectal prolapse can occur.

● The disease is transmitted by ingestion of soil containing the organism's eggs.

● Whipworm disease is diagnosed by identifying characteristic eggs in the stool. It is treated with mebendazole.

### Hookworm Disease

● This disease is caused by *Ancylostoma duodenale* (Old World hookworm) and *Necator americanus* (New World hookworm). The worm attaches to the intestinal mucosa, causing anorexia, ulcer-like symptoms, and chronic intestinal blood loss, leading to anemia.

● The disease is transmitted through direct skin penetration by larvae found in soil.

● Hookworm disease is diagnosed by identification of characteristic eggs in the stool. It is treated with pyrantel pamoate or mebendazole.

### Strongyloidiasis (Threadworm Disease)

● This disease is caused by *Strongyloides stercoralis*. It is relatively uncommon compared with infections by other intestinal nematodes. It is a relatively benign disease in healthy individuals, but can progress to fatal outcome in immunocompromised patients.

● The disease is transmitted through direct skin penetration by larvae found in soil.

● Threadworm disease is diagnosed by identifying larvae in the stool. It is treated with thiabendazole or invermectin.

**Figure 22.8**
Characteristics and therapy for commonly encountered intestinal nematode infections.

protected by a tough, noncellular cuticle. Most nematodes have separate, anatomically distinctive sexes. The mode of transmission varies widely, depending on the species and includes direct skin penetration by infectious larvae, ingestion of contaminated soil, eating undercooked pork, and insect bites. The parasites can invade almost any part of the body: liver, kidneys, intestines, subcutaneous tissue, or eyes. Generally, nematodes are categorized by whether they infect the intestine or other tissues (Figures 22.7 and 22.8). Alternatively, they can be divided into those for which the eggs are infectious and those for which the larvae are infectious. The most common nematode infection in the United States is enterobiasis (pinworm disease), which causes anal itching (Figure 22.9) but otherwise does little damage. A more serious disease of worldwide occurrence is ascariasis, caused by *Ascaris lumbricoides* (see Figure 22.8).

**Figure 22.9**
Pinworms leaving the anus of a five-year-old child.

## Study Questions

**Choose the ONE correct answer**

22.1 A patient is diagnosed as having a trematode infection. Lacking a more specific identification of the causative organism, which of the following drugs would most likely be effective?

A. Niclosamide

B. Thiabendazole

C. Praziquantel

D. Diethylcarbamazine

E. Tetracycline

> Correct answer = C. Praziquantel is the drug of choice for most trematode infections.

22.2 Which of the following is the most common helminthic infection in the United States?

A. Schistosomiasis

B. Diphyllothriasis

C. Clonorchiasis

D. Trichinosis

E. Enterobiasis

> Correct answer = E. Enterobiasis is known as pinworm disease.

22.3 Which of the following helminthic diseases is transmitted by the bite of a mosquito?

A. Filariasis

B. Onchocerciasis

C. Taeniasis

D. Schistosomiasis

E. Visceral larval migrans

> Correct answer = A. Mosquitoes ingest filarial embryos (microfilariae) from infected blood. In the insect, the embryos develop into infective filariform larvae that are injected into the human host.

22.4 Which of the following helminthic diseases is transmitted by direct skin penetration by helminth larva?

A. Filariasis

B. Onchocerciasis

C. Dracunculiasis

D. Schistosomiasis

E. Visceral larval migrans

> Correct answer = D. Schistosome cercaria released from snails in fresh water are capable of penetrating human skin.

*"I already diagnosed myself on the Internet. I'm only here for a second opinion."*

# Introduction to the Viruses

# 23

## I. OVERVIEW

A virus is an infectious agent that is minimally constructed of two components: 1) a genome consisting of either ribonucleic acid (RNA) or deoxyribonucleic acid (DNA), but not both, and 2) a protein-containing structure (capsid) designed to protect the genome (Figure 23.1A). Many viruses have additional structural features, for example, an envelope composed of a protein-containing lipid bilayer, whose presence or absence further distinguishes one virus group from another (Figure 23.1B). A complete virus particle combining these structural elements is called a virion. In functional terms, a virion can be envisioned as a delivery system that surrounds a nucleic acid payload. The delivery system is designed to protect the genome and enable the virus to bind to host cells. The payload is the viral genome and may also include enzymes required for the initial steps in viral replication—a process that is obligately intracellular. The pathogenicity of a virus depends on a great variety of structural and functional characteristics. Therefore, even within a closely related group of viruses, different species may produce significantly distinct clinical pathologies.

## II. CHARACTERISTICS USED TO DEFINE VIRUS FAMILIES, GENERA, AND SPECIES

Viruses are divided into related groups, or families, and, sometimes into subfamilies based on: 1) type and structure of the viral nucleic acid, 2) the strategy used in its replication, 3) type of symmetry of the virus capsid (helical versus icosahedral), and 4) presence or absence of a lipid envelope. Within a virus family, differences in additional specific properties, such as host range, serologic reactions, amino acid sequences of

**Figure 23.1**
General structure: A. nonenveloped; B. enveloped viruses.

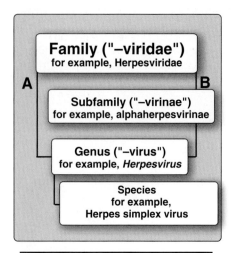

**Figure 23.2**
Classification of viruses: A. No subfamilies present. B. Subfamilies present.

viral proteins, degree of nucleic acid homology, among others, form the basis for division into genera (singular = genus) and species (Figure 23.2). Species of the same virus isolated from different geographic locations may differ from each other in nucleotide sequence. In this case, they are referred to as strains of the same species.

## A. Genome

The type of nucleic acid found in the virus particle is perhaps the most fundamental and straightforward of viral properties. It may be RNA or DNA, either of which may be single-stranded (ss) or double-stranded (ds). The most common forms of viral genomes found in nature are ssRNA and dsDNA. However, both dsRNA and ssDNA genomes are found in viruses of medical significance (Figure 23.3). Single-stranded viral RNA genomes are further subdivided into those of "positive polarity" (that is, of messenger RNA sense, which can therefore be used as a template for protein synthesis), and those of "negative polarity" or are antisense (that is, complementary to messenger RNA sense, which cannot therefore be used directly as a template for protein synthesis). Viruses containing these two types of RNA genomes are commonly referred to as positive-strand and negative-strand RNA viruses, respectively.

## B. Capsid symmetry

The protein shell enclosing the genome is, for most virus families, found in either of two geometric configurations (see Figure 23.3): helical (rod-shaped or coiled) or icosahedral (spherical or symmetric). The capsid is constructed of multiple copies of a single polypeptide type (found in helical capsids) or a small number of different polypeptides (found in icosahedral capsids), requiring only a limited amount of genetic information to code for these structural components.

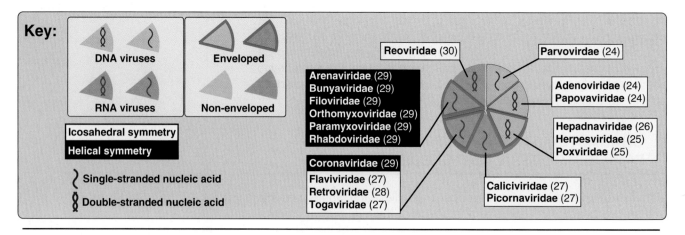

**Figure 23.3**
Viral families classified according to type of genome, capsid symmetry, and presence or absence of an envelope. [Note: Numbers indicate chapters where detailed information is presented]. RNA shown in blue, DNA in red, nucleic acids (either RNA or DNA) in purple, and viral envelope in green.

1. **Helical symmetry:** Capsids with helical symmetry, such as the paramyxoviridae (see p. 312), consist of repeated units of a single polypeptide species that—in association with the viral nucleic acid—self-assemble into a helical cylinder (Figure 23.4). Each polypeptide unit (protomer) is hydrogen-bonded to neighboring protomers. The complex of protomers and nucleic acid is called the nucleocapsid.

 Because the nucleic acid of a virus is surrounded by the capsid, it is protected from environmental damage.

2. **Icosahedral symmetry:** Capsids with icosahedral symmetry are more complex than those with helical symmetry, in that they consist of several different polypeptides grouped into structural subassemblies called capsomers. These, in turn, are hydrogen-bonded to each other to form an icosahedron (Figure 23.5). The nucleic acid genome is located within the empty space created by the rigid, icosahedral structure.

## C. Envelope

An important structural feature used in defining a viral family is the presence or absence of a lipid-containing membrane surrounding the nucleocapsid. This membrane is referred to as the envelope. A virus that is not enveloped is referred to as a naked virus. In enveloped viruses, the nucleocapsid is flexible and coiled within the envelope, resulting in most such viruses appearing to be roughly spherical (Figure 23.6). The envelope is derived from host cell membranes. However, the cellular membrane proteins are replaced by virus-specific proteins, conferring virus-specific antigenicity upon the particle.

 Among viruses of medical importance, there are both naked and enveloped icosahedral viruses, but all the helical viruses of animals are enveloped and contain RNA.

## III. VIRAL REPLICATION: THE ONE-STEP GROWTH CURVE

The one-step growth curve is a representation of the overall change, with time, in the amount of infectious virus in a single cell that has been infected by a single virus particle. In practice, this is determined by following events in a large population of infected cells in which the infection is proceeding as nearly synchronously as can be achieved by manipulating the experimental conditions. Whereas the time scale and yield of progeny virus vary greatly among virus families, the basic features of the infectious cycle are similar for all viruses. The one-step growth curve begins with the eclipse period, which is followed by a period of exponential growth (Figure 23.7).

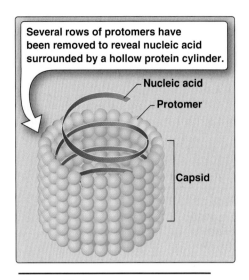

**Figure 23.4**
Nucleocapsid of a helical virus.

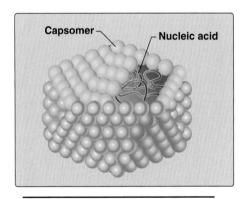

**Figure 23.5**
Structure of a nonenveloped virus showing icosahedral symmetry.

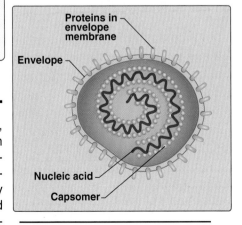

**Figure 23.6**
Structure of an enveloped helical virus.

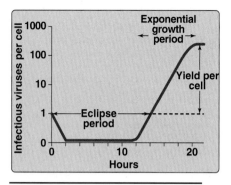

**Figure 23.7**
One-step growth curve of a single cell infected with a single virus particle. Initiation of infection is at zero time.

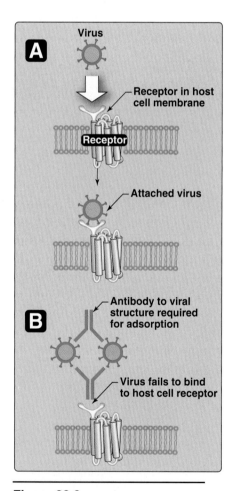

**Figure 23.8**
A. Attachment of virus to receptor on host cell membrane. B. Antibody prevents adsorption of virus.

## A. Eclipse period

Following initial attachment of a virus to the host cell, the ability of that virus to infect other cells disappears. This is the eclipse period, and it represents the time elapsed from initial entry and disassembly of the parental virus to the assembly of the first progeny virion. During this period, active synthesis of virus components is occurring. The eclipse period for most human viruses falls within a range of one to twenty hours.

## B. Exponential growth

The number of progeny virus produced within the infected cell increases exponentially for a period of time, then reaches a plateau, after which no additional increase in virus yield occurs. The maximum yield per cell is characteristic for each virus-cell system, and reflects the balance between the rate at which virus components continue to be synthesized and assembled into virions, and the rate at which the cell loses the synthetic capacity and structural integrity needed to produce new virus particles. This may be from 8 to 72 hours or longer, with yields of 100 to 10,000 virions per cell.

# IV. STEPS IN THE REPLICATION CYCLES OF VIRUSES

The individual steps in the virus replication cycle are presented below in sequence, beginning with virus attachment to the host cell and leading to penetration and uncoating of the viral genome. Gene expression and replication are followed by assembly and release of viral progeny.

## A. Adsorption

The initial attachment of a virus particle to a host cell involves an interaction between specific molecular structures on the virion surface and receptor molecules in the host cell membrane that recognize these viral structures (Figure 23.8A).

1. **Attachment sites on the viral surface:** Some viruses have specialized attachment structures, such as the glycoprotein spikes found in viral envelopes (for example, rhabdoviruses, see p. 310); whereas for others, the unique folding of the capsid proteins forms the attachment sites (for example, picornaviruses, see p 284). In both cases, multiple copies of these molecular attachment structures are distributed around the surface of the virion. [Note: In some cases, the mechanism by which antibodies neutralize viral infectivity is through antibody binding to the viral structures that are required for adsorption (Figure 23.8B).]

2. **Host cell receptor molecules:** The receptor molecules on the host cell membrane are specific for each virus family. Not surprisingly, these receptors have been found to be molecular structures that usually carry out normal cell functions. For example, cellular

membrane receptors for compounds such as growth factors may also inadvertently serve as receptors for a particular virus. Many of the compounds that serve as virus receptors are present only on specifically differentiated cells or are unique for one animal species. Therefore, the presence or absence of host cell receptors is one important determinant of tissue specificity within a susceptible host species, and also for the susceptibility or resistance of a species to a given virus.

> ‖ Information about the three-dimensional structure of virus binding sites is being used to design antiviral drugs that specifically interact with these sites, blocking viral adsorption.

## B. Penetration

Penetration is the passage of the virion from the surface of the cell, across the cell membrane and into the cytoplasm. There are two principal mechanisms by which viruses enter animal cells: receptor-mediated endocytosis and direct membrane fusion.

1. **Receptor-mediated endocytosis:** This is basically the same process by which the cell internalizes compounds such as growth regulatory molecules and serum lipoproteins, except the infecting virus particle is bound to the host cell surface receptor in place of the normal ligand (Figure 23.9). The cell membrane invaginates, enclosing the virion in an endocytotic vesicle (endosome). Release of the virion into the cytoplasm occurs by various routes, depending on the virus but, in general, it is facilitated by one or more viral molecules. In the case of an enveloped virus, its membrane may fuse with the membrane of the endosome, resulting in the release of the nucleocapsid into the cytoplasm.

> ‖ Failure to exit the endosome before fusion with a lysosome generally results in degradation of the virion by lysosomal enzymes. Therefore, not all potentially infectious particles are successful in establishing infection.

2. **Membrane fusion:** Some enveloped viruses (for example, human immunodeficiency virus, see p. 297) enter a host cell by fusion of their envelope with the plasma membrane of the cell (Figure 23.10). One or more of the glycoproteins in the envelope of these viruses promotes the fusion. The end result of this process is that the nucleocapsid is free in the cytoplasm, whereas the viral membrane remains associated with the plasma membrane of the host cell.

**Figure 23.9**
Receptor-mediated endocytosis of virus particle.

**Figure 23.10**
Fusion of viral envelope with membrane of host cell.

## C. Uncoating

"Uncoating" refers to the stepwise process of disassembly of the virion that enables the expression of the viral genes that carry out replication. For enveloped viruses, the penetration process itself is the first step in uncoating. In general, most steps of the uncoating process occur within the cell and depend on cellular enzymes; however in some of the more complex viruses, newly synthesized viral proteins are required to complete the process. The loss of one or more structural components of the virion during uncoating predictably leads to a loss of the ability of that particle to infect other cells, which is the basis for the eclipse period of the growth curve (see Figure 23.7). It is during this phase in the replication cycle that viral gene expression begins.

## D. Mechanisms of DNA virus genome replication

Each virus family differs in significant ways from all others in terms of the details of the macromolecular events comprising the replication cycle. The wide range of viral genome sizes gives rise to great differences in the number of proteins for which the virus can code. In general, the smaller the viral genome, the more the virus must depend on the host cell to provide the functions needed for viral replication. For example, some small DNA viruses, such as polyomavirus (see p. 249), produce only one or two replication-related gene products, which function to divert host cell processes to those of viral replication. Other larger DNA viruses, such as poxvirus (see

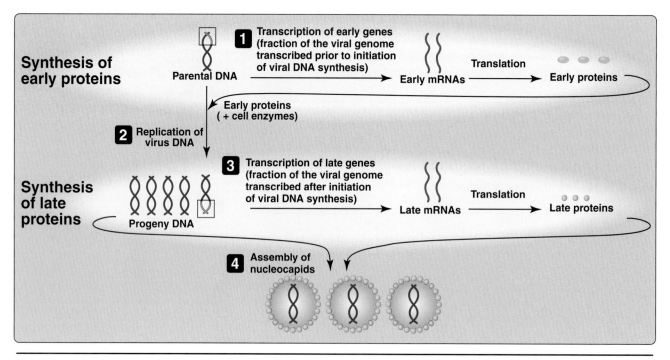

**Figure 23.11**
Replication of DNA viruses.

p. 270), provide virtually all enzymatic and regulatory molecules needed for a complete replication cycle. Figure 23.11 outlines the essential features of gene expression and replication of DNA viruses.

## E. Mechanisms of RNA virus genome replication

Viruses with RNA genomes must overcome two specific problems that arise from the need to replicate the viral genome, and to produce a number of viral proteins in eukaryotic host cells. First, there is no host cell RNA polymerase that can use the viral parental RNA as a template for synthesis of complementary RNA strands. Second, translation of eukaryotic mRNAs begins at only a single initiation site, and they are, therefore, translated into only a single polypeptide. However, RNA viruses, which frequently contain only a single molecule of RNA, must express the genetic information for at least two proteins: an RNA-dependent RNA polymerase and a minimum of one type of capsid protein. Although the replication of each RNA virus family has unique features, the mechanisms evolved to surmount these restrictions can be grouped into four broad patterns (or "types") of replication.

> For both DNA and RNA viruses, the information contained in the viral genome is expressed using the cellular machinery of the host cell.

1. **Type I: RNA viruses with a single-stranded genome (ssRNA) of (+) polarity that replicates via a complementary (–) strand intermediate:** In Type I viral replication, the infecting parental RNA molecule serves both as mRNA and later as a template for synthesis of the complementary (–) strand (Figure 23.12).

   a. **Role of (+) ssRNA as mRNA:** Because the parental RNA genome is of (+), or messenger, polarity, it can be translated directly upon uncoating and associating with cellular ribosomes. The product is usually a single polyprotein from which individual polypeptides, such as RNA-dependent RNA polymerase and various proteins of the virion, are cleaved by a series of proteolytic processing events carried out by a protease domain of the polyprotein (see Figure 23.12).

   b. **Role of (+) ssRNA as the template for complementary (–) strand synthesis:** The viral (+) ssRNA functions early in infection, not only as mRNA for translation of polyproteins but also as a template for virus-encoded RNA-dependent RNA polymerase to synthesize complementary (–) ssRNA (see Figure 23.12). The progeny (–) strands, in turn, serve as templates for synthesis of progeny (+) strands, which can serve as additional mRNAs, amplifying the capacity to produce virion proteins for progeny virus. When a sufficient quantity of capsid proteins has

**Figure 23.12**
Type I virus with a ssRNA genome of (+) polarity replicates via a complementary (–) strand intermediate.

**1** Transcription of (+) strand mRNAs from the parental viral (−) strand RNA template

(−) ssRNA

RNA-dependent RNA polymerase from infecting virus particle

(+) ssRNA          mRNAs          Viral proteins

**2** (+) ssRNA serves as a template for complementary (−) strand (viral genome) synthesis-

RNA-dependent RNA polymerase

(−) ssRNA

Assembly into nucleocapsids

**Figure 23.13**
Type II virus with an ssRNA genome of (−) polarity that replicates via a complementary (+) strand intermediate.

accumulated later in the infection, progeny (+) ssRNAs begin to be assembled into newly formed nucleocapsids.

2. **Type II: Viruses with a ssRNA genome of (−) polarity that replicate via a complementary (+) strand intermediate:** Viral genomes with (−) polarity, such as the (+) strand genomes, also have two functions: 1) to provide information for protein synthesis, and 2) to serve as templates for replication. Unlike (+) strand genomes, however, the (−) strand genomes cannot accomplish these goals without prior construction of a complementary (+) strand intermediate (Figure 23.13).

   a. **Mechanism of replication of viral ssRNA with (−) polarity:** The replication problems for these viruses are two-fold. First, the (−) strand genome cannot be translated and, therefore, the required viral RNA polymerase cannot be synthesized immediately following infection. Second, the host cell has no enzyme capable of transcribing the (−) strand RNA genome into (+) strand RNAs capable of being translated. The solution to these problems is for the infecting virus particle to contain viral RNA-dependent RNA polymerase, and to bring this enzyme into the host cell along with the viral genome. As a consequence, the first synthetic event after infection is transcription of (+) strand mRNAs from the parental viral (−) strand RNA template.

   b. **Mechanisms for multiple viral protein synthesis in Type II viruses:** The synthesis of multiple proteins is achieved in one of two ways among the (−) strand virus families: 1) the viral genome may be a polycistronic molecule, from which transcription produces a number of mRNAs, each specifying a single polypeptide; 2) alternatively, the (−) strand viral genome may be segmented (that is, composed of a number of different RNA molecules, most of which code for a single polypeptide).

   c. **Production of infectious virus particles:** Although the details differ, the flow of information in both segmented and unsegmented genome viruses is basically the same. In the Type II replication scheme, an important control element is the shift from synthesis of (+) strand mRNAs to production of progeny (−) strand RNA molecules that can be packaged in the virions. This shift is not a result of different polymerase, but rather to the sequestering of (+) strand RNA molecules by interaction with one or more of the newly synthesized proteins. This makes the (+) strands available as templates for the synthesis of genomic (−) strands. Further, segmented genome viruses have the additional problem of assuring that all segments are incorporated into the progeny virions. The mechanism by which this occurs is not clear.

3. **Type III: Viruses with a dsRNA genome.** The dsRNA genome is segmented, with each segment coding for one polypeptide (Figure 23.14). However, eukaryotic cells do not have an enzyme

capable of transcribing dsRNA. Type III viral mRNA transcripts are, therefore, produced by virus-coded, RNA-dependent RNA polymerase (transcriptase) located in a subviral core particle. This particle consists of the dsRNA genome and associated virion proteins, including the transcriptase. The mechanism of replication of the dsRNA is unique, in that the (+) RNA transcripts are not only used for translation, but also as templates for complementary (–) strand synthesis, resulting in the formation of dsRNA progeny.

4. **Type IV: Viruses with a genome of ssRNA of (+) polarity that is replicated via a DNA intermediate.** The conversion of a (+) strand RNA to a double-stranded DNA is accomplished by an RNA-dependent DNA polymerase, commonly referred to as a "reverse transcriptase," that is contained in the virion. The resulting dsDNA becomes integrated into the cell genome by the action of a viral "integrase." Viral mRNAs and progeny (+) strand RNA genomes are transcribed from this integrated DNA by the host cell RNA polymerase (Figure 23.15).

## F. Assembly and release of progeny viruses

Assembly of nucleocapsids generally takes place in the host cell compartment where the viral nucleic acid replication occurs (that is, in the cytoplasm for most RNA viruses and in the nucleus for most DNA viruses). For DNA viruses, this requires that capsid proteins be transported from their site of synthesis (cytoplasm) to the nucleus. The various capsid components begin to self-assemble, eventually associating with the nucleic acid to complete the nucleocapsid.

**Figure 23.14**
Type III virus with a dsRNA genome.

**Figure 23.15**
Type IV virus with a ssRNA genome of (+) polarity that replicates via a DNA intermediate.

**1** Virus-specific glycoproteins are synthesized and transported to the host cell membrane.

Host cell membrane

Viral protein

**2** The cytoplasmic domains of membrane proteins bind nucleocapsids.

Nucleocapsid

**3** A nucleocapsid is enveloped by the host cell membrane.

**4** The host cell membrane provides the viral envelope by a process of "budding".

**5** The enveloped virion is released from the host cell.

**Figure 23.16**
Release of enveloped virus from a host cell by the process of "budding."

1. **Naked viruses:** In naked (unenveloped) viruses, the virion is complete at this point. Release of progeny is usually a passive event resulting from the disintegration of the dying cell and, therefore, may be at a relatively late time after infection.

2. **Enveloped viruses:** In enveloped viruses, virus-specific glycoproteins are synthesized and transported to the host cell membrane in the same manner as cellular membrane proteins.[1] When inserted into the membrane, they displace the cellular glycoproteins, resulting in patches on the cell surface that have viral antigenic specificity. The cytoplasmic domains of these proteins associate specifically with one or more additional viral proteins (matrix proteins) to which the nucleocapsids bind. Final maturation then involves envelopment of the nucleocapsid by a process of "budding" (Figure 23.16). A consequence of this mechanism of viral replication is that progeny virus are released continuously while replication is proceeding within the cell and ends when the cell loses its ability to maintain the integrity of the plasma membrane. A second consequence is that with most enveloped viruses, all infectious progeny are extracellular. The exceptions are those viruses that acquire their envelopes by budding through internal cell membranes, such as those of the endoplasmic reticulum or nucleus.

> Viruses containing lipid envelopes are sensitive to damage by harsh environments and, therefore, tend to be transmitted by the respiratory, parenteral, and sexual routes. Nonenveloped viruses are more stable to hostile environmental conditions and often transmitted by the fecal-oral route.

## G. Effects of viral infection on the host cell

The response of a host cell to infection by a virus ranges from: 1) little or no detectable effect; to 2) alteration of the antigenic specificity of the cell surface due to presence of virus glycoproteins; to 3) latent infections that, in some cases, cause cell transformation; or, ultimately, to 4) cell death due to expression of viral genes that shut off essential host cell functions (Figure 23.17).

1. **Viral infections in which no progeny virus are produced:** In this case, the infection is referred to as abortive. An abortive response to infection is commonly caused by: 1) a normal virus infecting cells that are lacking in enzymes, promoters, transcription factors, or other compounds required for complete viral replication, in

[1]See p. 166 in *Lippincott's Illustrated Reviews: Biochemistry* (3rd ed.) for a discussion of the mechanism of insertion of glycoproteins into cell membranes.

which case the cells are referred to as nonpermissive; 2) infection by a defective virus of a cell that normally supports viral replication (that is, by a virus that itself has genetically lost the ability to replicate in that cell type); or 3) death of the cell as a consequence of the infection, before viral replication has been completed.

2. **Viral infections in which the host cell may be altered antigenically but is not killed, although progeny virus are released:** In this case, the host cell is permissive, and the infection is productive (progeny virus are released from the cell), but viral replication and release neither kills the host cell nor interferes with its ability to multiply and carry out differentiated functions. The infection is therefore said to be persistent. The antigenic specificity of the cell surface may be altered as a result of the insertion of viral glycoproteins.

3. **Viral infections that result in a latent viral state in the host cell:** Some viral infections result in the persistence of the viral genome inside a host cell with no production of progeny virus. Such latent viruses can be reactivated months or years in the future, leading to a productive infection. Some latently infected cells contain viral genomes that are stably integrated into a host cell chromosome. This can cause alterations in the host cell surface, cellular metabolic functions, and, significantly, cell growth and replication patterns. Such viruses may induce tumors in animals; in this case, they are said to be tumor viruses, and the cells they infect are transformed.

4. **Viral infections resulting in host cell death and production of progeny virus:** Eliminating host cell competition for synthetic enzymes and precursor molecules increases the efficiency with which virus constituents can be synthesized. Therefore, the typical result of a productive (progeny-yielding) infection by a cytocidal virus is the shut-off of much of the cell's macromolecular syntheses by one or more of the virus gene products, causing the death of the cell. Such an infection is said to be lytic. The mechanism of the shut-off varies among the viral families.

---

In summary, all viruses
- are small
- contain only one species of nucleic acid, either DNA or RNA.
- attach to their host cell with a specific receptor-binding protein;
- requires the assistance of a host cell to reproduce its genomic information.

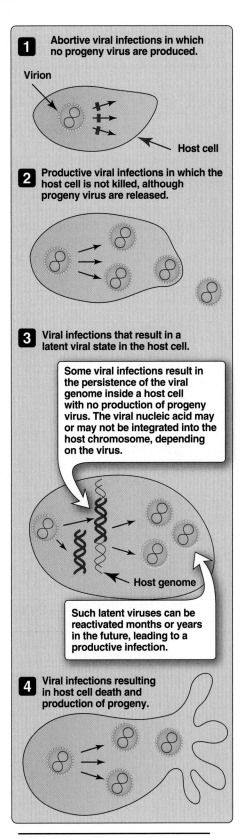

**Figure 23.17**
Effects of viral infection on a host cell.

## Study Questions

**Choose the ONE correct answer**

23.1 The capsid of a virus with helical symmetry is composed of

    A. multiple identical copies of a single polypeptide molecule.

    B. several polypeptides produced by sequential processing of a single large protein molecule.

    C. several different polypeptides encoded by different open reading frames in the viral genome.

    D. several different polypeptides generated by differential splicing of the same RNA transcript.

    E. each of the above occurs and is characteristic of the specific virus family.

> Correct answer = A. B, C, and D each occur in families with icosahedral symmetry, but helical capsids are composed of only one species of polypeptide, encoded by a single gene. In contrast, none of those with icosahedral symmetry have only a single polypeptide species.

23.2 The term "eclipse period" refers to

    A. the period between epidemic outbreaks of diseases that occur in a cyclic pattern.

    B. the period between recurrences of disease in individuals with latent virus infections.

    C. the time between exposure of an individual to a virus and the first appearance of disease.

    D. the time between infection of a susceptible cell by a cytocidal virus and the first appearance of cytopathic effects (CPE).

    E. the time between entry into the cell and disassembly of the parental virus and the appearance of the first progeny virion.

> Correct answer = E. C: This time is referred to as the incubation period. There is no specific term applied to the time periods described by A, B, and D.

23.3 The early genes of DNA viruses code primarily for proteins whose functions are required for

    A. transcription of viral mRNA.

    B. translation of the capsid proteins.

    C. replication of the viral DNA.

    D. final uncoating of the infecting virions.

    E. processing of the mRNA precursors

> Correct answer = C. Depending on the virus family, this may consist of a DNA polymerase and other enzymes directly involved in DNA replication or, alternatively, may be a product that stimulates the cell to produce all of the enzymes and precursors needed for DNA synthesis. A: Transcription for the most part is carried out by cellular RNA polymerase. B: Similarly, translation is done with the cell's translation system. D: The poxviruses do code for proteins that are involved in completion of uncoating, but this is an exception. E: mRNA processing is accomplished by cell enzymes.

*"You caught a virus from your computer and we had to erase your brain. I hope you kept a back-up copy."*

# Nonenveloped DNA Viruses

# 24

## I. OVERVIEW

The DNA viruses discussed in this Papovaviridae, Adenoviridae, and Parvoviridae (Figure 24.1)—share the properties of lacking an envelope and having relatively simple structures and genome organization. However, the diseases commonly associated with these viruses and their mechanisms of pathogenesis are quite different, ranging from upper respiratory infections to tumors.

## II. INTRODUCTION TO THE PAPOVAVIRIDAE

Papovaviruses are nonenveloped (naked), have icosahedral nucleocapsids, and contain supercoiled, double-stranded, circular DNA. However, basic differences in genome complexity and regulation of gene expression led to division of this family into two subfamilies: the Papillomavirinae and the Polyomavirinae. Papovaviruses induce both lytic infections and either benign or malignant tumors, depending on infected cell type.

## III. PAPOVAVIRIDAE: SUBFAMILY PAPILLOMAVIRINAE

All papillomaviruses induce hyperplastic epithelial lesions in their host species. Over 100 types (species) of human papillomaviruses (HPVs) are now recognized, based on differences in their DNA base sequences in certain well-characterized virus genes. HPVs exhibit great tissue and cell specificity, infecting only surface epithelia of skin and mucous membranes. The HPVs within each of these tissue-specific groups have varying potentials for causing malignancies. For example, there are: 1) a small number of virus types that produce lesions having a high risk of progression to malignancy, such as in cervical carcinoma; 2) other virus types produce mucosal lesions that progress to malignancy with lower frequency, causing, for example, anogenital warts (condyloma acuminata, a common sexually transmitted disease) and laryngeal papillomas (the most common benign epithelial tumors of the larynx); and 3) still other virus types that are associated only with benign lesions (for example, common, flat, and plantar warts).

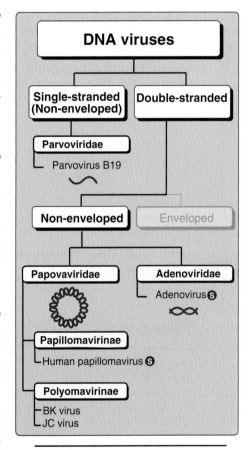

**Figure 24.1**
Classification of Non-enveloped DNA viruses. ⑤ See p. 331 for summaries of these viruses.

⌣ = Single-stranded, linear DNA

∝∝ = Double-stranded, linear DNA

⬭ = Double-stranded, circular DNA

## A. Epidemiology

Transmission of HPV infection requires direct contact with infected individuals (for example, sexual contact) or with contaminated surfaces (fomites), such as communal bathroom floors. HPV can also be transmitted from mother to infant during passage down the birth canal. Because the initial phase, as well as the maintenance of infection, occurs in cells of the basal layer of the skin, access to these cells is presumably via epithelial surface lesions, such as abrasions.

## B. Pathogenesis

The most striking characteristics of HPV multiplication and pathogenesis are its specificity for epithelial cells and its dependence on the differentiation state of the epithelial host cell.

1. **Wart formation:** The development of a typical wart results from cell multiplication and delayed differentiation induced by certain papillomavirus early proteins. In cutaneous tissues, for example, infected cells leave the basal layer and migrate toward the surface of the skin. The virus replication cycle proceeds in parallel with the steps of keratinocyte differentiation, which end with the terminally differentiated cornified layer of the growing wart. An important function of two early viral proteins is the activation of host cells, causing them to divide. This activation involves interaction between these viral proteins and cellular proteins (anti-oncoproteins) that normally function to regulate the cell cycle. Two of these antioncogenic cellular proteins are p53 (cellular growth suppressor protein) and pRb

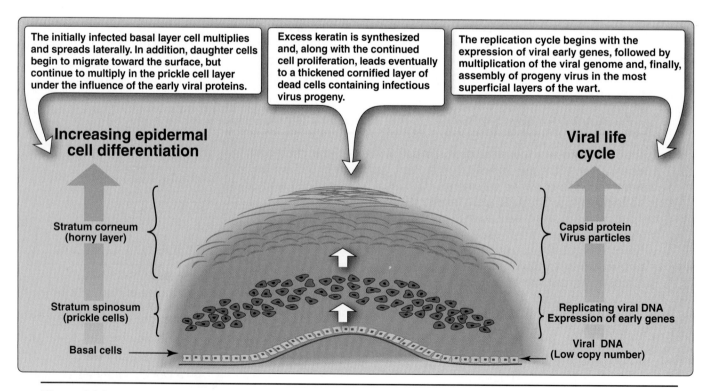

**Figure 24.2**
Relationship between steps in the development of a skin wart and the life cycle of papilloma virus.

(retinoblastoma gene product). The viral genome is maintained in low copy numbers as a plasmid in the nuclei of multiplying basal cells. Expression of only one early gene appears to be required for maintaining this balance between plasmid persistence and basal cell division. (See Figure 24.2 for a summary of papillomavirus replication and wart formation.)

2. **Development of malignancies:** Progression to malignancy occurs primarily in warts located on mucosal surfaces, particularly those of the genital tract, and is associated with a limited number of papillomavirus types. The affinity of binding between virus early proteins and cellular anti-oncoproteins p53 and pRb (which inactivate these cellular regulatory proteins) correlates with a high risk for malignant progression. However, it is clear that this interaction is only the first step in a multistep process involving alterations in expression of other cell oncoproteins and anti-oncoproteins and including, at some point, the non–site-specific integration of part of the viral genome into a host cell chromosome.

## C. Clinical significance

HPVs cause diseases that cover the spectrum from simple warts to malignancies. Warts can occur on any part of the body, including both cutaneous and mucosal surfaces (Figure 24.3). Specific HPV types tend to be associated with specific wart morphology, although a wart's morphologic type is also related to its location (Figure 24.4).

1. **Cutaneous warts:** These warts may be classified as common (fingers and hands), plantar (sole of foot), or flat (arms, face, and knee). Another category of cutaneous lesion occurs in patients with what appears to be an inherited predisposition for multiple warts that do not regress, but instead spread to many body sites (epidermodysplasia verruciformis). Of particular interest is that these lesions frequently give rise to squamous cell carcinomas several years after initial appearance of the original warts, especially in areas of skin exposed to sunlight.

2. **Mucosal infections:** HPV infections of the mucosal surfaces of greatest clinical importance are those of the genital tract. All of these are acquired primarily as sexually transmitted infections. Several types of HPV produce anogenital warts (condyloma acuminata), which are occasionally large but usually benign

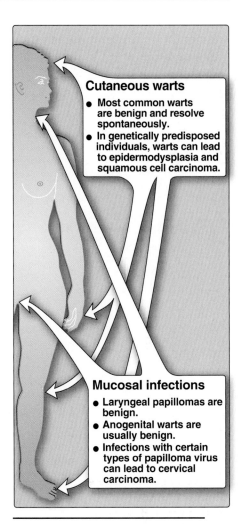

**Cutaneous warts**
- Most common warts are benign and resolve spontaneously.
- In genetically predisposed individuals, warts can lead to epidermodysplasia and squamous cell carcinoma.

**Mucosal infections**
- Laryngeal papillomas are benign.
- Anogenital warts are usually benign.
- Infections with certain types of papilloma virus can lead to cervical carcinoma.

**Figure 24.3**
Location and properties of papilloma infections.

**Figure 24.4**
Warts caused by papilloma virus.

**Figure 24.5**
Treatment of papilloma.

lesions that often regress spontaneously. Infections with other types of HPV do not lead to overt wart formation, but have a high risk of progressing to malignancy. In fact, HPV has been established as the primary cause of cervical cancer in the majority of cases. Other mucosal surfaces are infected by some of these same HPV types, affecting such sites as the respiratory tract, oral cavity, and conjunctiva. Most of these infections result in benign papillomas.

### D. Laboratory identification

Diagnosis of cutaneous warts generally involves no more than visual inspection. The major role of laboratory identification in papillomavirus infections is to: 1) determine whether HPV is present in abnormal tissue recovered by biopsy or cervical swab, and 2) whether the HPV type detected is one considered a high risk for progression to malignancy (the latter applying primarily to infections of the genital tract). The lack of any tissue culture system for recovery of the virus, and the fact that HPV types are defined by molecular criteria, means that typing is done by DNA hybridization reactions, using defined, type-specific nucleic acid probes (see p. 30).

### E. Treatment and prevention

Treatment of warts generally involves surgical removal or destruction of the wart tissue with liquid nitrogen, laser vaporization, or cytotoxic chemicals such as podophyllin or trichloroacetic acid (Figure 24.5). Such treatments remove the wart; however, HPV often remains present in cells of the surrounding tissue, and recurrence rates of fifty percent have been reported. Common warts often regress spontaneously, and removal is not usually warranted unless there is unusual pain caused by the location or for cosmetic reasons. Cidofovir, an inhibitor of DNA synthesis, appears to be effective when applied topically. Interferon, given orally, has been shown to cause regression of laryngeal papillomas; when injected directly into genital warts, it has given positive results in about one half of patients. Because transmission of the infection is by direct inoculation, avoidance of the opportunity for contact with wart tissue is the primary means of prevention. In genital tract warts, all of the procedures for prevention of sexually transmitted diseases are appropriate.

## IV. PAPOVAVIRIDAE: SUBFAMILY POLYOMAVIRINAE

All members of this virus subfamily have the capacity to transform normal cells in culture and to induce tumors in species other than those in which they are normally found in nature.

"Polyoma" means many (poly-) tumor (-oma). However, polyomavirus has not yet been shown to cause tumors in humans.

There are two human polyoma viruses: BK and JC viruses (BKV and JCV). JCV has been associated with progressive multifocal leukoencephalopathy (PML), a rare, fatal, demyelinating disease, that occurs only in patients with impaired immune function (for example those with AIDS). BKV can cause cystitis in this same population.

## A. Epidemiology and pathogenesis

Human polyomaviruses, BKV and JCV, are transmitted by droplets from the upper respiratory tract of infected persons, and possibly through contact with their urine. Infection with these viruses usually occurs in childhood. Specific antibody to one or both human polyomaviruses is present in seventy to eighty percent of the adult population. There is evidence that both BKV and JCV spread from the upper respiratory tract to the kidneys, where they may persist in an inactive state in the tubular epithelium of healthy individuals. Polyomaviruses follow the basic pattern of DNA virus genome replication and gene expression in the nucleus. The enzymes and precursors synthesized in preparation for cellular DNA synthesis are made available for synthesis of viral DNA. This productive cycle leads to viral multiplication and, ultimately, to death of the host cell.

## B. Clinical significance

Immune compromise of various types can be associated with the development of PML, so named because the lesions are restricted to white matter (Figure 24.6). PML, thought to be caused by reactivated JCV that has entered the CNS via the blood, occurs as a complication of a number of lymphoproliferative disorders and chronic diseases that affect immune competence. [Note: In recent years, PML has been seen especially in patients with AIDS.] In PML, JCV carries out a cytocidal infection of the brain, specifically of oligodendrocytes, leading to demyelination resulting from myelinated cells losing their capacity to maintain their myelin sheaths. Early development of impaired speech and mental capacity is rapidly followed by paralysis and sensory abnormalities, with death commonly occurring within three to six months of the initial symptoms. [Note: BKV is also found in the urine (Figure 24.7), but rarely has pathologic consequences except in immunocompromised patients, who may develop hemorrhagic cystitis.]

## C. Laboratory identification

Because most people have antibodies to these viruses, serologic techniques are not generally useful in the diagnosis of acute infections. Identification by DNA hybridization of BKV in the urine or JCV in PML lesions in brain tissue are the most sensitive and specific techniques for diagnosis of these infections.

## D. Treatment and prevention

No successful, specific, antiviral therapy is available. Because JCV and BKV infection is nearly universal and asymptomatic, and PML represents reactivation of "latent" virus, there are presently no viable preventive measures.

**Progressive multifocal leukoencephalopathy**
- Rare, fatal demyelinating disease caused by JCV
- Occurs in immuno-compromised patients

**Hemorrhagic cystitis**
- Caused by BKV
- Most commonly seen in immunocompromised patients

**Figure 24.6**
Location and properties of polyoma-virus infections.

**Figure 24.7**
Electron micrograph of BK virions from the urine of an infected patient.

**Figure 24.8**
A. Electron micrograph of an adenovirus virion with fibers. B. Model of
adenovirus. C. Crystalline aggregate
of adenovirus in the nucleus of a cell.

# V. ADENOVIRIDAE

Adenoviruses are nonenveloped, icosahedral viruses containing double-stranded linear DNA (Figure 24.8). They commonly cause diseases
such as respiratory tract infections, gastroenteritis, and conjunctivitis.
Adenoviruses were first discovered during screenings of throat washings and cultures of adenoids and tonsils, performed in the search for
the common cold virus. They are now recognized as a large group of
related viruses commonly infecting humans, other mammals, and birds.
Over forty serotypes (species) of human adenoviruses are known, and
antibody surveys have shown that most individuals have been infected
by several different types by adulthood.

> Although some human serotypes are highly
> oncogenic in experimental animals, none have
> been associated with human malignancies.

## A. Epidemiology and pathogenesis

The site of the clinical syndrome caused by an adenovirus infection
is generally related to the mode of virus transmission. For example,
most adenoviruses are primarily agents of respiratory disease, which
are transmitted via the respiratory route. However, most adenoviruses also replicate efficiently and asymptomatically in the intestine, and can be isolated from the stool well after respiratory disease
symptoms have ended, as well as from the stools of healthy persons.
Similarly, ocular infections are transmitted by direct inoculation of the
eye by virus-contaminated hands, ophthalmologic instruments, or
bodies of water in which groups of children swim together.

## B. Structure and replication

The adenovirus capsid is composed of hexon capsomers making up
the triangular faces of the icosahedron, with a penton capsomer at
each of the vertices (see Figure 24.8). Replication of adenoviruses
essentially follows the general model for DNA viruses (see p. xxx).
Attachment to a host cell receptor occurs via knobs on the tips of
the viral fibers, which is follow by entry into the cell by receptor-
mediated endocytosis. The viral genome is then progressively
uncoated while it is transported to the nucleus, where all transcription of viral genes, genome replication, and assembly occurs. Two
early viral genes have the same function as the early proteins of the
papovaviruses [that is, inactivating cellular regulatory proteins
(including p53 and pRb) that normally prevent progression through
the cell cycle (see p. xxx)]. However, the considerably larger adenovirus genome encodes a number of additional early proteins,
including a DNA polymerase and others that affect transcription and
replication of the viral genome. The productive cycle kills the host
cell, as cellular DNA, RNA, and protein synthesis are all shut off
during the course of infection. Release of infectious virus from the
cell occurs by slow disintegration of the dying cell.

## C. Clinical significance

Adenoviruses all replicate well in epithelial cells. The observed disease symptoms are related primarily to the killing of these cells; systemic infections are rare. Most adenovirus infections are asymptomatic, but certain types are more commonly associated with disease than others. These diseases can be conveniently grouped into those affecting the: 1) respiratory tract; 2) eye; 3) gastrointestinal (GI) tract, and, less commonly, 4) other tissues, including the urinary tract and heart (Figure 24.9).

1. **Respiratory tract diseases:** The most common manifestation of adenovirus infection of infants and young children is acute febrile pharyngitis, characterized by a cough, sore throat, nasal congestion, and fever. Isolated cases may be indistinguishable from other common viral respiratory infections. Some adenovirus types tend additionally to produce conjunctivitis, in which case the syndrome is referred to as pharyngoconjunctival fever. This entity is more prevalent in school-aged children and occurs both sporadically, and in outbreaks, often within family groups or in groups using the same swimming facility ("swimming pool conjunctivitis"). The syndrome referred to as acute respiratory disease occurs primarily in epidemics among new military recruits. It is thought to reflect the lowered resistance brought on by exposure to new strains, fatigue, and crowded living conditions, promoting efficient spread of the infection. Lastly, the respiratory syndromes described above may progress to true viral pneumonia, which has a mortality rate of about ten percent in infants.

2. **Ocular diseases:** In addition to the conjunctivitis that sometimes accompanies the upper respiratory syndrome described above, a similar follicular conjunctivitis may occur as a separate disease. It is self-limiting and has no permanent sequelae. A more serious infection is epidemic keratoconjunctivitis, which involves the corneal epithelium, and may be followed by corneal opacity lasting several years. The epidemic nature of this disease partly results from transmission via shared towels or ophthalmic solutions, person-to-person contact, or improperly sterilized ophthalmologic instruments.

3. **Gastrointestinal diseases:** Most human adenoviruses multiply in the GI tract and can be found in stools; however, these are generally asymptomatic infections. Two serotypes have been associated specifically with infantile gastroenteritis.

> Adenovirus infections have been estimated to account for five to fifteen percent of all viral diarrheal disease in children.

4. **Less common diseases:** Several adenovirus serotypes have been associated with an acute, self-limited, hemorrhagic cystitis, which occurs primarily in boys. It is characterized by hematuria, and virus

**Ocular infections**
- Follicular conjunctivitis
- Keratoconjunctivitis

**Respiratory infections**
- Acute febrile pharyngitis
- Pharyngoconjunctival fever
- Acute respiratory disease
- Viral pneumonia

**Gastrointestinal infections**
- Infantile gastroenteritis

**Urinary tract infections**
- Hemorrhagic cystitis

**Figure 24.9**
Adenovirus infections.

**Figure 24.10**
Replication of B19 parvovirus.

can usually be recovered from the urine. Similarly, adenovirus infection of heart muscle has recently been shown to be one cause of left ventricular dysfunction in both children and adults. In immunocompromised patients, such as those with AIDS, the common respiratory adenovirus infections have a greater risk of proceeding to serious, often fatal, pneumonia. Other disseminated infections leading to a fatal outcome have been reported in patients with a compromised immune system or those immunosuppressed from drug therapy.

### D. Laboratory identification

Isolation of virus for identification is not done on a routine basis, but may be desirable in cases of epidemic disease or nosocomial outbreak, especially in the nursery. Identification of the adenovirus serotype can be done by neutralization or hemagglutination inhibition using type-specific antisera. They are more commonly detected by direct test of stool specimens by ELISA (see p. xxx).

### E. Treatment and prevention

No antiviral agents are currently available for treating adenovirus infections. Prevention of epidemic respiratory disease by immunization has been used only for protection of the military population. A live, attenuated adenovirus vaccine is used for this purpose that produces a good neutralizing antibody response. The oncogenic capacity of the adenoviruses in experimental animals has inhibited the use of vaccines on a wider scale.

## VI. PARVOVIRIDAE

Parvoviruses are the smallest of the DNA viruses. They are nonenveloped and icosahedral, with single-stranded, linear DNA. A human parvovirus, B19, has been isolated and identified as the cause of transient aplastic crisis in patients with sickle cell disease and implicated in adult acute polyarthritis. This virus is also the cause of the common childhood disease erythema infectiosum, and is associated with fetal death in pregnant women experiencing a primary infection. The parvovirus family is divided into two genera, based on whether their ability to replicate requires coinfection with a helper DNA virus, or if they are capable of independent replication ("autonomous parvoviruses"). Members of the first group are referred to as adenoassociated viruses (AAV), because they are usually found in infected cells in combination with a helper adenovirus.

### A. Epidemiology and pathogenesis

Transmission of parvoviruses is by the respiratory route. A high-titered viremia lasting a few days follows about one week after infection, during which time virus is also present in throat secretions. A specific antibody response occurs rapidly, resulting in suppression of the viremia. Replication of parvoviruses requires a host cell in which DNA synthesis is in progress. Therefore, damage is limited primarily to specific tissues that are mitotically active. [Note: In the case of B19 virus, these are primarily tissues of erythroid origin.] Because of the single-stranded nature of the genome, conversion to a double stranded DNA molecule by a cellular DNA polymerase must occur before production of additional single-stranded viral DNA genomes or viral mRNA transcription can begin. Despite the limited amount of genetic material, two or three capsid proteins and two nonstructural regulatory proteins are produced by a combination of alternative RNA splicing patterns and posttranslational processing. The parvovirus life cycle is summarized in Figure 24.10.

## B. Clinical significance

The single human pathogen in this family is the autonomous parvovirus, B19. The spectrum of illnesses caused by this virus is related to its unique tropism for cycling erythroid progenitor cells. Although B19 was initially isolated from sickle cell disease patients undergoing a transient aplastic crisis, it has since been recognized that chronic, progressive bone marrow suppression results from B19 infection of immunocompromised patients unable to mount an immune response capable of eliminating the virus.

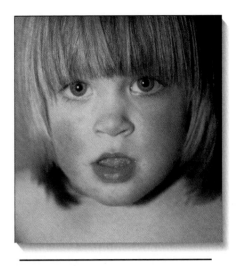

**Figure 24.11**
Typical "slapped cheek" appearance of a child infected with parvovirus B19 ("fifth disease").

1. **Erythema infectiosum:** The observation that thirty to sixty percent of some human populations have antibodies to B19 led eventually to the identification of this virus as the causative agent of the common childhood rash, erythema infectiosum ("fifth disease", Figure 24.11). The characteristic rash ("slapped cheek" appearance) occurs about two weeks after initial exposure, when the virus is no longer detectable. It is apparently immune system–mediated. Another complication accompanying B19 infection is an acute arthritis that usually involves joints symmetrically. This is considerably more frequent in adults than in children, and usually resolves within several weeks.

2. **Birth defects:** Spontaneous abortion rate is elevated in women having a primary infection during the first trimester; primary infection during the second or third trimester is associated with some instances of hydrops fetalis.

## C. Laboratory identification

Laboratory identification of B19 infection is not routinely done. The large amount of virus present during the viremic (usually asymptomatic) phase permits detection of viral proteins by immunologic methods, or of viral DNA by various hybridization techniques. Retrospective diagnosis can be made by any of the usual procedures used to demonstrate a specific antibody response.

## D. Treatment and prevention

No antiviral agent or vaccine is available for treating human B19 infections. Isolation of patients with signs of parvovirus disease is not a useful approach to control because subclinical infections occur and infected individuals shed virus before symptoms appear.

## Study Questions

**Choose the ONE correct answer**

24.1 An important step in the mechanism proposed for oncogenesis by human papillomaviruses is

A. inactivation of a cellular regulatory gene by HPV integration into the coding region of the gene.

B. transactivation of a normally silent cellular oncogene by an HPV early protein.

C. reversal of keratinocyte differentiation caused by continued active replication and production of progeny HPV.

D. specific binding of certain HPV early proteins to cellular anti-oncoproteins.

E. induction of a specific chromosome translocation that results in activation of a cellular oncogene.

Correct answer = D. The early proteins of both adenoviruses and papovaviruses required for immortalization and transformation of normal cells have been shown to bind specifically to cellular proteins p53 and pRb, which are important in maintaining regulation of the mitotic cycle. Interaction with viral proteins is believed to result in loss of their normal functions, as do the mutations that are commonly associated with spontaneously occurring cancers. A, B: Neither gene inactivation by integration nor transcriptional activation by an early protein has been observed. C: Virus replication occurs only in differentiated keratinocytes, but dedifferentiation does not occur. E: Multiple chromosome rearrangements are observed late in progression to malignancy, but none are specific for HPV-transformed cells.

24.2 The characteristic spectrum of diseases caused by autonomous parvoviruses is related to the fact that they

A. integrate into a specific chromosomal site that disrupts an essential gene and leads to death of the cell.

B. require host cells that are actively progressing through the mitotic cycle.

C. infect only terminally differentiated cells.

D. code for an early protein that shuts off cellular protein synthesis.

E. increase the severity of the disease normally caused by their associated helper virus.

Correct answer = B. The diseases caused by the autonomous parvoviruses all result from the effects of killing multiplying cells that are essential for normal functions; for example, B19 specifically infects erythroblasts, leading to anemia in the fetus or in immunodeficient patients. A, C, D: Parvoviruses are not observed to integrate during the replicative cycle, they cannot replicate in terminally differentiated cells, and they do not shut off cell syntheses. E: By definition, the autonomous parvoviruses do not require a helper virus for replication.

24.3 The characteristic rash of erythema infectiosum is due to

A. virion/antibody immune complex formation.

B. bone marrow suppression caused by killing of erythrocyte precursors by B19 infection.

C. damage to the liver.

D. B19 infection of epithelial cells.

E. the inflammatory response to B19 infection of capillary endothelium.

*"Don't think of it as getting a flu shot.
Think of it as installing virus protection software."*

Correct answer = A. The appearance of the rash coincides with production of antibodies to B19, which occurs several days after the peak of viremia. B: Infection in immunodeficient individuals can lead to chronic, progressive depletion of erythrocyte precursors and severe anemia, but not rash. C: The host range of B19 is restricted to erythroid precursors, including those found in the fetal liver. Whereas this may be a factor in causing hydrops fetalis due to B19 infection of a pregnant woman, it is not related to the rash. D and E: Again, B19 is not known to infect other than erythroid precursor cells.

# Enveloped DNA Viruses

# 25

## I. OVERVIEW

Two of the three enveloped DNA virus families—the Herpesviridae and the Poxviridae—are discussed in this chapter. [Note: Hepadnaviridae, the third enveloped DNA virus family, is discussed in Chapter 26.] The Herpesviridae and the Poxviridae are both structurally and genetically more complex than the DNA viruses discussed in Chapter 24. For example, there is less dependence on host cell-supplied functions, with a correspondingly greater number of virus-coded functions involved in viral replication. This latter fact contributes to the greater success in developing antiviral drugs against these viruses (more virus-specific enzymes that can serve as targets for inhibitors, in contrast to viruses that are more host cell function-dependent). Replication of herpesviruses and poxviruses is also independent of the host cell cycle. The herpesvirus family includes important human pathogens (Figure 25.1). The one highly virulent member of the poxvirus family, variola (the cause of smallpox), is the only human pathogen that has been successfully eradicated. This success serves as a model for attempts to control and potentially eradicate other infectious diseases.

## II. HERPESVIRIDAE: STRUCTURE AND REPLICATION

Eight human herpesvirus species are known. All have the ability to enter a latent state following primary infection of their natural host and be reactivated at a later time. However, the exact molecular nature of the latency and the frequency and manifestation of reactivation vary with the species of herpesvirus.

### A. Structure of herpesviruses

Herpesvirus virions consist of an icosahedral capsid enclosed in a lipoprotein envelope (Figure 25.2). Between the envelope and the capsid lies an amorphous proteinaceous material (tegument) that contains virus-coded enzymes and transcription factors essential for initiation of the infectious cycle, although none of these is a polymerase. The genome is a single molecule of linear, double-stranded DNA, encoding from 70 to 200 proteins, depending on the species. Although all members of the family have some genes with homologous functions, there is little nucleotide sequence homology and little antigenic relatedness between species.

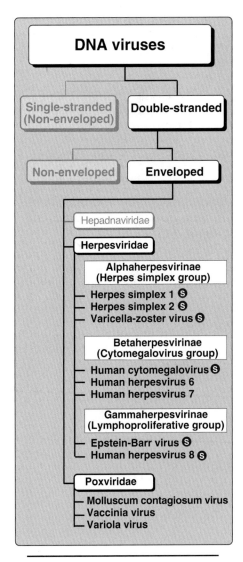

**Figure 25.1**
Classification of enveloped DNA viruses. Ⓢ See p. 331 for summaries of these viruses.

**Figure 25.2**
Structure of herpesvirus.
A. Schematic drawing.
B. Transmission electron micrograph.

## B. Classification of herpesviruses

Herpesviridae cannot readily be differentiated by morphology in the electron microscope—they all have similar appearances. However, Herpesviridae have been divided into three subfamilies, based primarily on biologic characteristics (see Figure 25.1).

1. **Alphaherpesvirinae (herpes simplex virus group):** These viruses have a relatively rapid, cytocidal growth cycle and establish latency in nerve ganglia. Herpes simplex virus types 1 and 2 (HSV-1 and HSV-2) and varicella-zoster virus (VZV) belong to this group. HSV-1 and HSV-2 share significant nucleotide homology and, therefore, share many common features in replication and pathogenesis. VZV has a smaller genome than HSV, but the two viruses have many genes that are homologous.

2. **Betaherpesvirinae (cytomegalovirus group):** These viruses have a relatively slow replication cycle that results in the formation of characteristic, multinucleated, giant host cells. Latency is established in nonneural tissues, primarily lymphoreticular cells and glandular tissues. Human cytomegalovirus (HCMV) and human herpesviruses types 6 and 7 (HHV-6 and HHV-7) are in this group.

3. **Gammaherpesvirinae (lymphoproliferative group):** These viruses replicate in mucosal epithelium, where they also establish latent infections. They induce cell proliferation in lymphoblastoid cells. Epstein-Barr virus (EBV) was previously the only well-characterized human gammaherpesvirus. However, genome analysis of a virus recovered from cells of Kaposi sarcoma revealed it to also be a human member of the gammaherpesvirinae. It has been designated human herpesvirus type 8 (HHV-8).

## C. Replication of the Herpesviruses

Herpesviruses replicate in the nucleus, following the basic pattern of DNA virus replication (see p. 238). Regulation of herpesvirus transcription is referred to as "cascade control," in that expression of a first set of genes is required for expression of a second set, which in turn is required for expression of a third set of genes. [Note: A similar pattern is found in some other DNA virus families in which the genes are referred to as immediate early, delayed early, and late.] The general features of herpesvirus replication are summarized in Figure 25.3.

1. **Virus adsorption and penetration:** Herpesviruses adsorb to host cell receptors that can differ according to the virus species and the tissue type being infected. Viral envelope glycoproteins promote fusion of the envelope with the cell's plasma membrane, depositing the nucleocapsid and tegument proteins in the cytosol. One of the tegument proteins induces a host cell RNase that degrades cellular mRNA, effectively shutting off host cell protein synthesis.

2. **Viral DNA replication and nucleocapsid assembly:** The nucleocapsid is transported to a nuclear pore, through which viral DNA is

released into the nucleus. Another tegument protein is an activator of cellular RNA polymerase that causes the enzyme to initiate transcription of the set of viral immediate early genes, which code for a variety of regulatory functions, including initiation of further gene transcription. Next, delayed early genes are expressed. They code primarily for enzymes that are required for replication of viral DNA, such as viral DNA polymerase, helicase, and thymidine kinase.

> Because these enzymes are virus-specific, they provide excellent targets for antiherpes agents (such as acyclovir), that are relatively nontoxic for the cell.

As is the case with other DNA viruses, late genes code for structural proteins of the virion and proteins involved in assembly and maturation of viral progeny.

3. **Acquisition of the viral envelope:** Newly synthesized envelope proteins accumulate in patches on the nuclear membrane, and nucleocapsids that have been assembled in the nucleus acquire their envelopes by budding through these patches. The completed virus is transported by a vacuole to the surface of the cell. Additional copies of the envelope glycoproteins are also transported to the plasma membrane, which acquires herpesvirus antigenic determinants. These glycoproteins may also cause fusion of neighboring cells, in some cases producing characteristic multinucleated giant cells. The end result of this productive cycle is death of the cell resulting from most cellular synthetic pathways being turned off.

4. **Latency:** All herpesviruses can undergo an alternative infection cycle, entering a quiescent state (latency) from which they subsequently can be reactivated. The cell type in which this occurs is usually not the same cell type in which productive, cytocidal infection occurs. Because the mechanism of latency, the cells in which it is established, the frequency of reactivation, and the nature of the recurrent disease are characteristic for each of the herpesviruses, the topic of latency is discussed in this chapter in the context of the individual virus species.

## III. HERPES SIMPLEX VIRUS, TYPES 1 AND 2

HSV-1 and HSV-2 are the only human herpesviruses that have a significant degree of nucleotide homology (about fifty percent). They therefore share many common features in replication, disease production, and latency.

### A. Epidemiology and pathogenesis

Transmission of both HSV types is by direct contact with virus-containing secretions or with lesions on mucosal or cutaneous surfaces. Primary or recurrent infections in the oropharyngeal region,

**Figure 25.3**
Replication of herpes viruses.

**Figure 25.4**
Herpes simplex gingivostomatitis.

Male

Female

**Figure 25.5**
Genital herpes simplex infections.

caused primarily by HSV-1, are accompanied by virus release into saliva; therefore kissing or saliva-contaminated fingers are major modes of transmission. In genital tract infections, caused primarily by HSV-2, virus is present in genital tract secretions. Consequently, sexual intercourse and infections of newborns during passage through the birth canal are major modes of transmission. Both HSV-1 and HSV-2 multiply in epithelial cells of the mucosal surface onto which they have been inoculated, resulting in production of vesicles or shallow ulcers containing infectious virus. In immunocompetent individuals, epithelial infection remains localized because cytotoxic T lymphocytes recognize the HSV-specific antigens on the surface of infected cells and kill these cells before progeny virus has been produced. A lifelong latent infection is usually established in the regional ganglia as a result of entry of infectious virions into sensory neurons that terminate at the site of the infection.

## B. Clinical significance

A useful generality is that HSV-1 is most commonly found in lesions of the upper body, and HSV-2 is more commonly the cause of genital tract lesions. Either can, however, infect and cause similar lesions at the opposite site.

1. **Primary infections of the upper body:** Many primary HSV infections are subclinical, but the most common symptomatic infections of the upper body are gingivostomatitis in young children (Figure 25.4) and pharyngitis or tonsillitis in adults. The lesions typically consist of vesicles and shallow ulcers, which are often accompanied by systemic symptoms such as fever, malaise, and myalgia. Another clinically important site of infection is the eye, in which keratoconjunctivitis can lead to corneal scarring and eventual blindness. If HSV infection spreads to the central nervous system (CNS) it can cause encephalitis, which, if untreated, has a mortality rate estimated to be seventy percent. Survivors are usually left with neurologic deficits.

> In the United States, HSV-1 infection of the eye is the second most common cause of corneal blindness (after trauma), HSV infections of the CNS account for up to twenty percent of encephalitis viral infections.

2. **Primary infections of the genital tract:** Primary genital tract lesions are similar to those of the oropharynx; however, based on the frequency of antibody in the population, the majority of these infections are asymptomatic. When symptomatic (genital herpes), local symptoms include painful vesiculoulcerative lesions on the vulva, cervix, and vagina, or penis (Figure 25.5). Systemic symptoms of fever, malaise, and myalgia may also be more severe than those that accompany primary oral cavity infections. In pregnant women with a primary genital HSV infection, the risk of infecting

the newborn during birth is estimated to be thirty to forty percent (neonatal herpes). Because such infants have no protective maternal antibody, a disseminated infection, often involving the CNS, results. There is a high mortality rate if untreated, and survivors are likely to have permanent neurologic sequelae. A newborn is also at risk of acquiring infection from an infected mother by transfer on contaminated fingers or in saliva. However, infection *in utero* appears to occur only rarely.

3. **Latency:** In latently infected cells of the ganglia—HSV-1 in trigeminal ganglia and HSV-2 in sacral or lumbar ganglia—from one to thousands of copies of the viral genome are present as nonintegrated, circular molecules of DNA in the nuclei (Figure 25.6). Expression of HSV genes is shut off in latently infected cells.

4. **Reactivation:** Several factors, such as hormonal changes, fever, and physical damage to the neurons, are known to induce reactivation and replication of the latent virus (see Figure 25.6). The newly synthesized virions are transported down the axon to the nerve endings from which the virus is released, infecting the adjoining epithelial cells. Characteristic lesions are thus produced in the same general area as the primary lesions. [Note: Virus replication occurs in only a fraction of the latently infected neurons, and these nerve cells eventually die.] The presence of circulating antibody does not prevent this recurrence, but does limit the spread of virus to surrounding tissue. Sensory nerve symptoms, such as pain and tingling, often precede and accompany the appearance of lesions. In general, the severity of any systemic symptoms is considerably less than that of a primary infection, and many recurrences, in fact, are characterized by shedding of infectious virus in the absence of visible lesions.

   a. **HSV-1:** The frequency of oropharyngeal symptomatic recurrences is variable, ranging from none to several a year. The lesions occur as clusters of vesicles at the border of the lips (herpes labialis or "cold sores", "fever blisters") and heal without scarring in eight to ten days.

   b. **HSV-2:** Reactivation of HSV-2 genital infections can occur with considerably greater frequency (for example, monthly) and is often asymptomatic, but still results in viral shedding. Consequently, sexual partners or newborn infants may be at increased risk of becoming infected resulting from lack of precautions against transmission. The risk of transmission to the newborn is much less than in a primary infection because considerably less virus is shed and there is maternal anti-HSV antibody in the baby. This antibody also lessens the severity of the disease if infection does occur.

**Figure 25.6**
Primary and recurrent herpes simplex infections.

**Figure 25.7**
Mechanism of action of acyclovir.

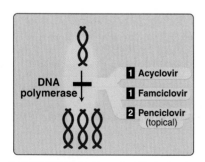

**Figure 25.8**
Drug therapy for herpes simplex
infection.

## C. Laboratory identification

Laboratory identification is not required for diagnosis of characteristic HSV lesions in normal individuals. Identification is important, however, to prevent neonatal infection and HSV encephalitis and keratoconjunctivitis, in which early initiation of therapy is essential but characteristic lesions are not present. Further, for purposes of therapy in the immunocompromised patient, HSV infection must be distinguished from that of VZV (see p. 261). It must also be distinguished from similar exanthems (skin eruptions) caused by other viruses or, in some cases, by bacteria, or noninfectious, allergy-based reactions. Demonstration of HSV by inoculation of human cell tissue culture with a sample of vesicle scraping, fluid, or genital swab is the definitive method for demonstrating infection. Gross cytopathic changes may require several days to appear, but individual infected cells can be detected within 24 hours by use of immunofluorescence (see p. 29) or immunoperoxidase staining with antibodies directed against viral early proteins. Using these same techniques, infected cells can also be demonstrated directly in clinical specimens, although this approach is generally less sensitive than virus isolation in tissue culture. Direct detection of viral DNA by liquid or *in situ* hybridization complements these procedures, and, after amplification of the DNA by the polymerase chain reaction (see p. 30), is considerably more sensitive. For example, in patients with encephalitis, HSV etiology can be confirmed by demonstration of viral DNA in the cerebral spinal fluid (CSF) instead of by brain biopsy.

## D. Treatment

The guanine analog, acycloguanosine (acyclovir), is selectively effective against HSV because it becomes an active inhibitor of DNA synthesis only after initially being phosphorylated by the HSV thymidine kinase (Figure 25.7). The drug of choice for any primary HSV infection, it is especially important in treating herpes encephalitis, neonatal herpes, and disseminated infections in immunocompromised patients. Other drugs effective in treating herpes simplex infection include famciclovir and topical penciclovir (Figure 25.8). Famciclovir is a prodrug that is metabolized to the active penciclovir. It provides more convenient dosing and greater bioavailability than oral acyclovir. Penciclovir is active against HSV-1 and HSV-2, and against VZV. None of these drugs can cure a latent infection, but they can minimize asymptomatic viral shedding, and recurrences of symptoms (Figure 25.9).

## E. Prevention

Prevention of HSV transmission is enhanced by avoidance of contact with potential virus-shedding lesions and by safe sexual practice. Prevention of neonatal HSV infections is of great importance; however, genital infection of the mother is difficult to detect because it is often asymptomatic. When overt genital tract lesions are detected at the time of delivery, cesarean section is usually warranted. Prophylactic therapy of the mother and the newborn with acyclovir can be employed if the presence of HSV is detected just before or at the time of birth; measures to prevent physical transmission following birth are also important. A vaccine is not currently available.

## IV. VARICELLA-ZOSTER VIRUS

VZV has biologic and genetic similarities to HSV, and is classified with HSVs in the Alphaherpesvirinae subfamily. Biologic similarities between VZV and HSV include the fact that latency is established in sensory ganglia and infections are rapidly cytocidal. Primary infections with VZV cause varicella ("chickenpox"), whereas reactivation of the latent virus causes herpes zoster ("shingles").

### A. Epidemiology and pathogenesis

Transmission of VZV is usually via respiratory droplets, which results in initial infection of the respiratory mucosa, followed by spread to regional lymph nodes (Figure 25.10). Progeny virus enter the bloodstream, undergo a second round of multiplication in cells of the liver and spleen, and are disseminated throughout the body by infected mononuclear leukocytes. Endothelial cells of the capillaries and, ultimately, skin epithelial cells become infected, resulting in the characteristic, virus-containing vesicles of chickenpox that appear from 14 to 21 days after exposure. The infected individual is contagious from one to two days before the appearance of the exanthem, implying that viruses reinfect cells of the respiratory mucosa near the end of the incubation period. Contact with vesicular fluid does not appear to be a common mode of transmission.

### B. Clinical significance

In contrast to HSV infections, the primary and recurrent diseases (varicella and zoster) due to VZV are quite distinct. Whereas neither is usually life-threatening in the normal, healthy individual, both can have severe complications in immunocompromised patients.

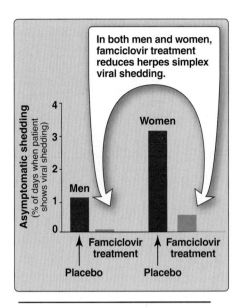

**Figure 25.9**
Chronic suppressive antiviral therapy reduces the frequency of asymptomatic herpes simplex virus shedding.

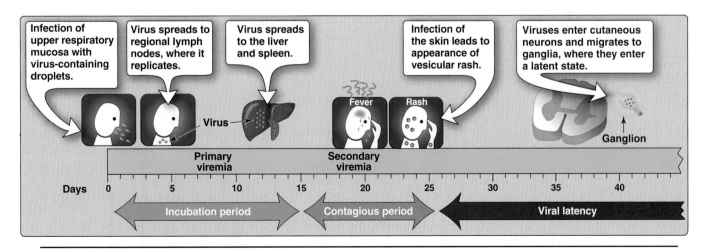

**Figure 25.10**
Time course of varicella (chickenpox) in children. In adults, the disease shows a longer time course and is more severe.

**Figure 25.11**
Appearance of chickenpox with lesions at all stages of development.

1. **Primary infection (varicella, or "chickenpox"):** In a normal, healthy child, the incubation period is most commonly from 14 to 16 days. The first appearance of exanthem is often preceded by one or two days of a prodrome of fever, malaise, headache, and abdominal pain. The exanthem begins on the scalp, face, or trunk as erythematous macules, which evolve into virus-containing vesicles that begin to crust over after about 48 hours (Figure 25.11). Itching is most severe during the early stage of vesicle development. While the first crop of lesions is evolving, new crops appear on the trunk and extremities. In older adults and the immunocompromised, lesions may also appear on mucous membranes, such as in the oropharynx, conjunctivae, and vagina. New lesions continue to appear over a period of up to six or seven days. Healing occurs without scarring.

> Reye syndrome, an acute encephalopathy accompanied by fatty liver, is a complication of VZV and influenza A and B infections of children. A possible relationship exists between the use of aspirin to control the child's pain and fever and the manifestation of Reye syndrome.

Varicella is a more serious disease in healthy adults and immunocompromised patients. Varicella pneumonia is the most common of the serious complications, but fulminant hepatic failure and varicella encephalitis may also result. Primary infection of a pregnant woman may cause her to contract the more severe adult form of varicella, and may affect the fetus or neonate as well. Fetal infection early in pregnancy is uncommon, but can result in multiple developmental anomalies. More commonly, a fetus infected near the time of delivery may exhibit typical varicella at birth or shortly thereafter. The severity of the disease depends on whether the mother has begun to produce anti-VZV IgG by the time of delivery.

2. **Recurrent infection (herpes zoster, or "shingles"):** Due to the disseminated nature of the primary infection, latency is established in multiple sensory ganglia, the trigeminal and dorsal root ganglia being most common. Unlike most of the herpesviruses, asymptomatic virus shedding is a rare event. Herpes zoster results from reactivation of the latent virus, not from new, exogenous exposure. Reactivation occurs in approximately fifteen percent of infected individuals. The most striking feature of herpes zoster is that distribution of the clustered vesicular lesions is dermatomal (affecting the area of skin supplied by cutaneous branches from a single spinal nerve, Figure 25.12).

### C. Laboratory identification

Laboratory diagnosis of uncomplicated varicella or zoster is generally not necessary and not usually done because of the typical clinical appearance and distribution of lesions. However, in the immuno-compromised patient in whom therapy is warranted, it is important to distinguish VZV infection from other similar exanthems. Cell tissue cultures inoculated with a sample of vesicle fluid show gross cytopathic changes in several days; individual infected cells can be detected within 24 hours by use of immunofluorescence or immunoperoxidase staining with antibodies against viral early proteins. More rapid diagnosis can be made by reacting epithelial cells scraped from the base of vesicles with the stains described above, or by doing *in situ* hybridization with VZV-specific DNA probes.

## D. Treatment

Treatment of primary varicella in immunocompromised patients, adults, and neonates is warranted by the severity of the disease (Figure 25.13). Acyclovir has been the drug of choice in such patients, but requires intravenous administration to achieve effective serum levels. Oral acyclovir reduces the time course and acute pain of zoster, but has little or no effect on the subsequent postherpetic neuralgia. Famciclovir and valacyclovir—base analogues similar to acyclovir—have greater activity against VZV.

## E. Prevention

Susceptible individuals (for example, neonates, nonimmune healthy adults, and immunocompromised children who have been exposed to chickenpox or to zoster lesion fluid) can be protected by administration of varicella-zoster immunoglobulin (VZIg). Administration of VZIg has no effect on the occurrence of zoster.

> A live, attenuated vaccine that was approved in 1995 for use in the United States by children one year of age or older is now recommended as one of the routine childhood vaccines. It is also indicated for non-immune adults at risk of being exposed to contagious individuals.

Vesicles erupt on an erythematous base and eventually dry and scab. The vesicles appear in regions supplied by the peripheral sensory nerves arising in latently infected root ganglia.

**Figure 28.12**
Cutaneous manifestations of acute herpes zoster.

## V. HUMAN CYTOMEGALOVIRUS

Human cytomegalovirus (HCMV) is a member of the Betaherpesvirinae subfamily and, as such, differs from HSV and VZV in several ways. Its replication cycle is significantly longer, and infected cells typically are greatly enlarged and multinucleated(hence, "cytomegalo-", Figure 25.14). There is only one recognized human species of HCMV, but there are many distinct strains that can be distinguished by antigenic differences as well as by restriction fragment analysis of their genomes. HCMV is the most common cause of intrauterine infections and congenital abnormalities in the United States. It also represents a serious threat to immunodeficient or immunosuppressed patients.

DNA polymerase

1 Famciclovir
1 Valaciclovir
1 Acyclovir

**Figure 25.13**
Drug therapy for varicella virus.

**Figure 25.14**
Cytomegalovirus infection. Lung section showing typical owl-eye inclusions.

## A. Epidemiology and pathogenesis

Initial infection with HCMV commonly occurs during childhood. Depending on geographic location and socioeconomic group, 35 to 90 percent of the population have antibody against the virus by adulthood.

1. **Transmission:** Infection in children is usually asymptomatic; these children continue to shed virus for months in virtually all body fluids, including tears, urine, and saliva. Transmission is by intimate contact with these fluids, although saliva may be the most common source. In adults, the virus can also be transmitted by: 1) sexual means because it is present in semen and vaginal secretions; 2) organ transplants; and 3) blood transfusions. Similarly, virus is present in breast milk and, thus, neonates can be infected by this route. HCMV can also cross the placenta and infect a fetus *in utero*. Initial replication of the virus in epithelial cells of the respiratory and gastrointestinal (GI) tracts is followed by viremia and infection of all organs of the body. In symptomatic cases, kidney tubule epithelium, liver, and CNS, in addition to the respiratory and GI tracts, are most commonly affected.

2. **Latency and reactivation:** A distinctive feature of HCMV latency is the phenomenon of repeated episodes of asymptomatic virus shedding over prolonged periods. Latency is probably established in monocytes and macrophages, but other cell types, such as those of the kidney, are also involved.

## B. Clinical significance

In healthy individuals, primary HCMV infection is usually inapparent. Whereas most infections occur in childhood, primary infection as an adult may result in a mononucleosis syndrome clinically identical to that caused by Epstein-Barr virus (EBV, see p. 268).

 It is estimated that about eight percent of infectious mononucleosis (IM) cases are caused by HCMV.

Persistent fever, muscle pain, and lymphadenopathy are characteristic IM symptoms, as are elevated levels of abnormal lymphocytes and liver enzymes. The major distinguishing feature of HCMV IM is the absence of heterophile antibodies that characterize IM caused by EBV (see p. 268). Two specific situations have greater clinical significance, namely, congenital infections and infection of immunocompromised patients.

1. **Congenital infections:** HCMV is the most common intrauterine viral infection. However, there is a great disparity in incidence of fetal infection and severity of outcome, depending on whether the mother is experiencing a primary or recurrent infection. In women experiencing their first HCMV infection during pregnancy (who, therefore, have not yet produced antibodies against HCMV), 35 to

50 percent of fetuses will be infected, and ten percent of these will be symptomatic (Figure 25.15). The severity of the symptoms is most pronounced when infection occurs during the first trimester. Referred to as cytomegalic inclusion disease, results caused by the infection range from fetal death to various degrees of damage to liver, spleen, blood-forming organs, and components of the nervous system. The latter is a common cause of hearing loss and mental retardation. Even in infants who are asymptomatic at birth, hearing deficits and ocular damage (for example, chorioretinitis) may appear later and continue to progress during the first few years of life.

> Congenitally and perinatally infected infants may continue to excrete virus for years after birth, serving as an important virus reservoir.

2. **Infections of immunosuppressed and immunodeficient patients:** Immunosuppressed transplant recipients are multiply at risk from: 1) HCMV present in the tissue being transplanted; 2) virus carried in leukocytes in the associated blood transfusions; and 3) reactivation of their own endogenous latent virus. Immune suppression for the transplant can negate any protective advantage of a seropositive recipient. Destruction of GI tract tissue, hepatitis, and pneumonia are common, the latter being a major cause of death in bone marrow transplant recipients. HCMV infection is also associated with decreased survival of solid tissue grafts (heart, liver, kidney). HCMV coinfection of patients with HIV infection occurs frequently, probably because of their similar modes of transmission (see p. 364). As a common opportunistic infection in AIDS patients, invasive HCMV infections—arising from reactivation of latent virus—become increasingly important as CD4+ lymphocyte counts and immune competence decline (see p. 367). Any organ system can be affected; however, pneumonia and blindness caused by HCMV retinitis are especially common. Encephalitis, dementia, esophagitis, enterocolitis, and gastritis are other significant problems. In addition, coinfection with HCMV may accelerate the progression of the pathology of AIDS (Figure 25.16).

## C. Laboratory identification

Because the incidence of HCMV infection in the population is so high, and periodic inapparent recurrent infections occur frequently, simple detection of virus or anti-HCMV antibody is not generally useful. Recovery of virus is not usually done. Serologic diagnosis using ELISA techniques can distinguish primary from recurrent infection by demonstrating IgG seroconversion or the presence of HCMV-specific IgM. The use of purified HCMV antigens produced by recombinant DNA methods has improved the reliability of both IgG and IgM determinations. Direct determination of the presence and amount of viral DNA or proteins in white blood cells is useful as an indicator of invasive disease, whereas extracellular virus in urine or saliva may simply result from asymptomatic recurrence. Any of

**Figure 25.15**
Newborn with congenital cytomegalovirus disease, showing hepatosplenomegaly and rash.

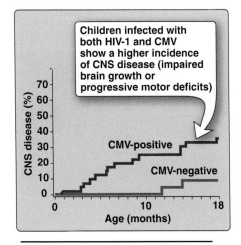

**Figure 25.16**
Incidence of central nervous system (CNS) disease in HIV-1-infected children, with or without cytomegalovirus infection.

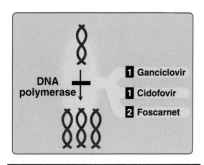

**Figure 25.17**
Drug therapy for cytomegalovirus.

these techniques can be used to screen transplant donors and recipients to determine HCMV status.

### D. Treatment and prevention

Treatment of HCMV infections is indicated primarily in immunocompromised patients (Figure 25.17). Acyclovir is ineffective because HCMV lacks its own thymidine kinase. However, two inhibitors of HCMV DNA polymerase are available: ganciclovir, a guanine analog that is phosphorylated by a virus-coded protein kinase, and cidofovir, a deoxycytidine analog. A third inhibitor of DNA polymerase, unrelated to the two just described, is phosphonoformic acid (foscarnet). Ganciclovir is used for invasive infections of transplant recipients and AIDS patients, but it has considerable toxicity. For retinitis in AIDS patients, toxic adverse effects can be avoided by direct intraocular inoculation. A vaccine for active immunization is not available.

## VI. HUMAN HERPESVIRUS TYPES 6 AND 7

HHV-6 and HHV-7, classified as members of the Betaherpesvirinae, have marked similarities to HCMV in biologic and genome characteristics. Both HHV-6 and HHV-7 are causative agents of roseola infantum (exanthem subitum), although infection with HHV-7 is more frequently asymptomatic.

### A. Epidemiology and pathogenesis

Most infections with HHV-6 and HHV-7 occur during the first three years of life, with overall incidence of antibody approaching ninety percent of the population by age three. Transmission is thought to be via oral secretions because the viruses are replicated in salivary glands and secreted into saliva. HHV-7, in particular, has been recovered frequently from saliva of healthy individuals. These viruses also infect peripheral blood lymphocytes and the cells of various solid organs, including the CNS. HHV-6 infection of lymphoid cells induces a number of significant cell responses, including the synthesis of CD4 glycoprotein, interferon-$\alpha$, tumor necrosis factor-$\alpha$, and interleukin-1-$\beta$. The ability of HHV-6 to induce expression of CD4 in cells not normally expressing it extends the range of cells infectible by HIV. In addition, HHV-6 transactivates transcription of HIV, accelerating the rate of cell death in coinfected cells. Latently infected cells are found among the peripheral blood lymphocyte population.

### B. Clinical significance

HHV-6 infections resulting in disease are most common in infants and individuals who are immunocompromised.

1. **Primary infections:** Symptomatic roseola infantum (exanthem subitum) occurs in roughly one third to one half of infants with a primary HHV-6 infection. It is characterized by a high fever of three to five days, after which a characteristic erythematous macular rash appears on the neck and trunk, resolving after several more days without sequelae (Figure 25.18). HHV-7 infection has been shown to produce an identical clinical picture. Of greater clinical significance is the fact that primary HHV-6 infection of

**Figure 25.18**
Roseola infantum.

infants is the cause of many acute febrile illnesses and febrile seizures in the absence of the characteristic rash (Figure 25.19). In some of these cases, HHV-7 has been shown to be the causative agent; in others, the patient was coinfected with both HHV-6 and HHV-7.

> Over twenty percent of emergency room visits for febrile illness in infants, and one third of febrile seizures are caused by primary infection with HHV-6 and/or HHV-7.

2. **Recurrent infections:** Following immunosuppression for organ transplantation, or immunocompromise related to HIV infection, reactivation of latent HHV-6, frequently together with HCMV, has been associated with sometimes-fatal interstitial pneumonitis, fever, hepatitis, and encephalitis, as well as with transplant rejection. The relationship of HHV-6 to AIDS has not been completely elucidated. However, the fact that: 1) HHV-6 broadens the range of cell types infectible by HIV by inducing CD4; 2) coinfected cells are killed more rapidly; and 3) extensively disseminated HHV-6 infection frequently occurs in terminal AIDS patients, suggests that HHV-6 may be an important factor in accelerating the progression from early HIV infection to terminal AIDS. The most common clinical syndrome associated with HHV-6 in AIDS patients is encephalitis (Figure 25.20).

## C. Laboratory identification

A simple diagnostic test for primary infection with HHV-6 or HHV-7 is not available. PCR amplification has been used to demonstrate HHV-6 DNA in the CSF of patients with neurologic disease and in the serum of patients undergoing posttransplant reactivation of a latent infection.

## D. Treatment and prevention

Because of its genetic relationship to HCMV, HHV-6 is generally inhibited by the same drugs (see p. 266), but extensive clinical trials have not yet been done. In AIDS patients, treatment of the HIV infection appears to reduce the amount of HHV-6 as well. No vaccine is currently available for these viruses.

# VII. HUMAN HERPESVIRUS TYPE 8

HHV-8 infection appears not to occur as frequently as the other human herpesviruses in the normal, healthy population. Yet the virus genome and/or viral proteins have been detected in more than ninety percent of patients with Kaposi sarcoma (KS), but in less than one percent of non-KS tissues. The notable feature of pathogenesis by HHV-8 is the finding that the viral genome encodes a number of cell-derived genes related to growth regulation. These include genes for several cytokines, cytokine receptors, growth factors that promote angiogenesis, and a

**Figure 25.19**
Clinical signs of human herpes virus 6 infection occurring without the characteristic rash.

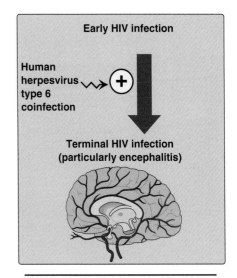

**Figure 25.20**
Coinfection with human herpesvirus type 6 accelerates the progression of HIV symptoms.

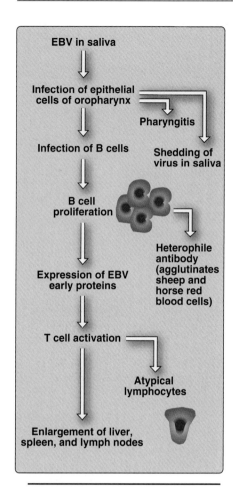

**Figure 25.21**
Pathogenesis of infectious mononucleosis caused by Epstein-Barr
virus.

factor that inhibits apoptosis. The primary method for detection of HHV-8 is by DNA hybridization following PCR amplification.

## VIII. EPSTEIN-BARR VIRUS

EBV is most commonly known as the causative agent of infectious mononucleosis in young adults. Its initial discovery in association with the childhood disease Burkitt lymphoma led to its recognition as the first human virus clearly related to a malignancy. More recently, EBV has been associated with several additional human neoplastic diseases.

### A. Epidemiology and pathogenesis

Most transmission of EBV occurs by intimate contact with saliva that contains virus during both primary infection and in repeated episodes of asymptomatic shedding. The initial site of virus replication appears to be the oropharyngeal epithelium, following which some of the progeny viruses infect B lymphocytes (Figure 25.21). The B-cell receptor for EBV is the complement component C3b receptor (see p. 92). The B-cell infection is an abortive one, in that only a limited number of early proteins are synthesized. The infection also causes the induction of a number of cellular lymphokines, including B-cell growth factors. In contrast to other herpesviruses, the early genes of EBV induce cell multiplication and immortalization, rather than cell death. Thus, infection induces a polyclonal B-cell proliferation and an accompanying nonspecific increase in total IgM, IgG, and IgA. The IgM class contains "heterophile antibodies" that agglutinate sheep and horse red blood cells. These antibodies are the basis for the classic diagnostic test for EBV-associated infectious mononucleosis (see p. 269).

### B. Clinical significance

As stated earlier, primary infection in infancy or childhood is usually asymptomatic, but as high as fifty percent of those infected later in life develop infectious mononucleosis. Although B cells are the primary target of infection as a result of the presence of the EBV receptor molecule, EBV has more recently been found to be associated with a small number of T-cell malignancies as well. In patients who are immunodeficient or immunosuppressed, the lack of cell-mediated immune control increases the likelihood of lymphoproliferative disorders of various kinds. Throughout life, healthy EBV carriers continue to have episodes of asymptomatic virus shedding. The source of this virus is presumably productively infected oropharyngeal cells that acquire the virus from latently infected B cells in which the lytic cycle has been activated.

1. **Infectious mononucleosis (IM):** The manifestations and severity of primary EBV infection vary greatly, but the typical IM syndrome appears after an incubation period of four to seven weeks, and includes pharyngitis, lymphadenopathy, increased levels of liver enzymes in the blood, and fever (Figure 25.22). Headache and malaise often precede and accompany the disease, which may last several weeks. Complete recovery may take much longer.

**2. EBV and malignancies:** Following the initial discovery of EBV in association with Burkitt lymphoma (BL), it has been shown to be associated with a number of other human neoplastic diseases.

    **a. Burkitt lymphoma (BL):** BL was first described in 1958 as a rather unique malignancy of the jaw, found in an unusually high frequency in children in regions of equatorial Africa. Burkitt lymphoma cells all contain one of three characteristic chromosome translocations. The breakpoints of these translocations are such that the c-myc proto-oncogene on chromosome eight is constitutively activated. Malarial infection and HIV infection are known risk factors for development of BL.

    **b. EBV-associated nasopharyngeal carcinoma (NPC):** NPC is one of the most common cancers in southeast Asia, North Africa, and the Eskimo population, but it is less common elsewhere. NPC differs from BL in that there is no characteristic chromosomal alteration, and the cells involved are epithelial in origin. The role of EBV is indicated because all cells of the tumor contain cytoplasmic viral DNA molecules.

**c. EBV infections in immunocompromised and immunosuppressed patients:** In BL and NPC, EBV infection appears to be only one step in a multistep, disease-causing process, and its specific role is still not well defined. In contrast, EBV alone appears to be sufficient for induction of B-cell lymphomas in immunocompromised patients, such as transplant recipients and individuals with AIDS, who cannot control the cell multiplication induced by the early proteins. For example, many AIDS patients develop a B-cell malignancy of some type: BL of the sporadic type occurs with high frequency in earlier stages of AIDS progression, whereas non–BL-type lymphoblastic lymphomas are more characteristic in late-stage AIDS patients. Not all of the HIV-associated BL cases contain the EBV genome. [Note: AIDS patients infected with EBV may exhibit nonmalignant, white-gray lesions on the tongue ("hairy leukoplakia," Figure 25.23).]

## C. Laboratory identification

Atypical lymphocytes (cytotoxic T cells) can be observed in the blood smear of a patient with IM (Figure 25.24). Detection of EBV DNA or RNA by hybridization or of virus antigens using immunohistochemical techniques can be done with cell homogenates or by *in situ* methods for visualization of individual infected cells. The classic test for infectious mononucleosis, the Paul-Bunnell test, is based upon the fact that polyclonal stimulation of B cells by EBV infection results in nonspecific elevation of all immunoglobulins, including heterophile antibodies that specifically agglutinate horse and sheep red blood cells. These heterophile antibodies are diagnostic for EBV-related IM, although they are not present in all cases of EBV IM.

---

**Classic clinical triad of infectious mononucleosis:**

- Fever
- Pharyngitis
- Lymphadenopathy (usually enlargement of anterior and posterior cervical lymph nodes)

Note: Acute infection is often asymptomatic in children, whereas adolescents and young adults show the typical symptoms of infectious mononucleosis.

---

**Transmission:**

- Exposure to oropharyngeal secretions

---

**Clinical manifestations of Epstein-Barr-associated infectious mononucleosis by age-group:**

Key:
- Patients < 35 years old
- Patients > 35 years old

---

**Incidence of Epstein-Barr-associated infectious mononucleosis:**

- Peak incidence occurs between ages of 15 and 19.
- Incidence is 30 times higher in blacks than whites in the United States.
- No difference in incidence between sexes.
- Ninety percent of the general population shows evidence of previous infection with Epstein-Barr virus.

**Figure 25.22**
Characteristics of infectious mononucleosis.

**Figure 25.23**
Hairy leukoplakia caused by Epstein-Barr virus infection.

**Figure 25.24**
Abnormal mononuclear cells commonly seen in infectious mononucleosis.

**D. Treatment and prevention**

Although acyclovir inhibits EBV replication, none of the antiherpes drugs have been effective in modifying the course or severity of IM due to EBV or in preventing development of EBV-related B-cell malignancies. Acyclovir has been successful in treating oral hairy leukoplakia, in which the virus is actively replicating in the epithelial cells of the tongue. No vaccine for prevention of EBV infections is currently available. Some properties of the common herpesvirus infections are summarized in Figure 25.25.

# IX. POXVIRIDAE

Poxviruses are a family of large, genetically complex viruses having no obvious symmetry. Members of this family are widely distributed in nature. The agent of previous medical importance to humans, variola virus, was the cause of smallpox, the first infectious disease to be declared eradicated from the earth. Among the factors that led to this success are: 1) the availability of an effective, attenuated vaccine; 2) variola was antigenically stable and only a single antigenic type existed; 3) the absence of asymptomatic cases or persistent carriers; 4) the absence of an animal reservoir; and 5) the emotional effect of this highly lethal, disfiguring disease helping gain public cooperation in the eradication efforts. Currently, the highly effective poxvirus used to make vaccine is vaccinia virus; it is being used in attempts to construct vectors carrying immunizing genes from other infectious agents. Finally, the poxvirus, molluscum contagiosum virus (MCV), causes small, wartlike tumors (not to be confused with true warts caused by papilloma virus, see p. 245).

**A. Structure and classification of the family**

The genome is a single linear molecule of double-stranded DNA, with a coding capacity for more than 200 polypeptides. The virion contains enzymes that are involved in early steps of replication. The vertebrate poxviruses are related by a common nucleoprotein anti-

| VIRUS | VIRUS SUBFAMILY | CLINICAL MANIFESTATIONS OF PRIMARY INFECTION | CLINICAL MANIFESTATIONS OF RECURRENT INFECTION | SITE OF INITIAL INFECTION | SITE OF LATENCY |
|---|---|---|---|---|---|
| Herpes simplex-1 | α | Keratoconjunctivitis, gingivostomatitis, pharyngitis, tonsilitis | Herpes labialis ("cold sores") | Mucoepithelial | Trigeminal sensory ganglia |
| Herpes simplex-2 | α | Genital herpes; perinatal disseminated disease | Genital herpes | Mucoepithelial | Lumbar or sacral sensory ganglia |
| Varicella-zoster virus | α | Varicella ("chickenpox") | Herpes-Zoster ("shingles") | Mucoepithelial | Dorsal root ganglia |
| Cytomegalo-virus | β | Congenital infection (*in utero*); mononucleosis-like syndrome | Asymptomatic shedding of virus | Monocytes, lymphocytes, and epithelial cells | Monocytes, lymphocytes |
| Epstein-Barr virus | γ | Infectious mononucleosis; Burkitt lymphoma | Asymptomatic shedding of virus | Mucosal epithelium, B lymphocytes | B lymphocytes |

**Figure 25.25**
Properties of common herpesvirus infections.

gen, but are otherwise quite distinct. Humans are the natural host for variola and MCV; however, monkeypox, cowpox, and several other animal poxviruses can also cause human disease.

## B. Replication of the poxviruses

Poxviruses follow the basic replication pattern for DNA viruses (see p. 238)p, with a few notable exceptions. The most striking of these is that the entire replication cycle takes place in the cytoplasm, the virus providing all of the enzymes (including a viral DNA-dependent RNA polymerase) necessary for DNA replication and gene expression. Final maturation by acquisition of a lipoprotein envelope occurs as the virus buds from the cell. The replication cycle is rapid and results in early shut-off of all cell macromolecular syntheses, causing the death of the cell.

## C. Epidemiology and clinical significance

The stages of are illustrated in Figure 25.26. Whereas there is no longer the threat of naturally occurring smallpox, the mutation of one of the animal poxviruses to a form more virulent for humans has continued to be of concern. Human infections with monkeypox are clinically similar to smallpox and, although somewhat less severe, still have a mortality rate of about eleven percent. Such infections have only been observed where the human population comes into close contact with infected monkeys; in its natural state, monkeypox is not readily transmitted among humans. Molluscum contagiosum infection occurs only in humans, causing benign wart-like tumors on various body surfaces. Usually spread by direct contact, it is now recognized as a sexually transmitted disease.

## D. Laboratory identification

The unique cellular localization of poxvirus replication has enabled rapid diagnosis by observation of DNA-containing intracytoplasmic inclusion bodies in cells scraped from skin lesions.

## E. Treatment and prevention

Whereas immunization with vaccinia is no longer done routinely, it is still carried out in certain groups, such as the military and laboratory workers. Although one of the safest vaccines in healthy recipients, individuals with eczema may develop a generalized vaccinia rash covering the surface of the body. Immunocompromised patients are likely to develop progressive vaccinia, which has a high mortality rate. Postvaccinal encephalitis, with a mortality of forty percent, is a second hazard accompanying vaccination.

## F. Smallpox as a biologic weapon

Smallpox is potentially a devastating biologic weapon because it is highly contagious and has a high case fatality rate—more than thirty percentage among unvaccinated persons. In 1972, the United States stopped routine vaccination of civilians against smallpox. As a result, more than forty percent of the population are now vulnerable to smallpox infection, with the percent increasing each year. Stores of vaccine and vaccinia immune globulin are currently inadequate to combat a massive outbreak of the disease.

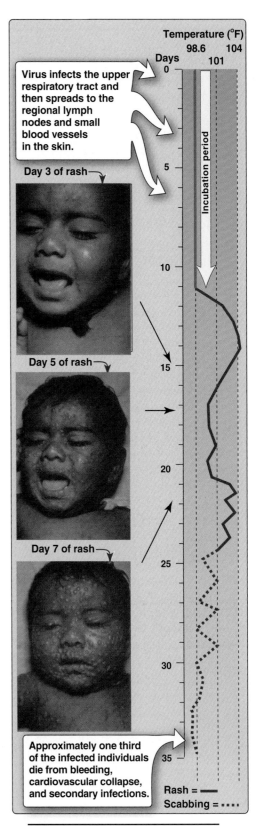

**Figure 25.26**
Time course of smallpox.

# Study Questions

**Choose the ONE correct answer**

25.1 The initial infection with human cytomegalovirus most commonly occurs

　A. during early childhood, by exchange of body fluids.

　B. *in utero*, by transplacental transmission from a latently infected pregnant woman.

　C. by transfer of saliva between young adults.

　D. by sexual intercourse.

　E. as a result of blood transfusion or organ transplantation.

> Correct answer = A. Depending on the population, up to ninety percent have antibody by adulthood. B: The most serious complications of infection are those resulting from transplacental transmission, but this is not the common mode of transmission. C and D: Transmission by kissing or sexual intercourse can occur, but most individuals have already been infected by this age. E: This mode of transmission has serious consequences in antibody-negative recipients, but most recipients had been infected at an earlier age. More common is reactivation of latent HCMV in recipients who have been immuno-suppressed for purposes of transplantation.

25.2 The cellular response typical of infectious mononucleosis caused by Epstein-Barr virus is due to:

　A. stimulation of B-cell proliferation by the EBV early proteins synthesized in the infected cells.

　B. proliferation of cytotoxic T cells responding to EBV antigens expressed on the surface of infected B cells.

　C. a primary humoral immune response to the EBV infection.

　D. macrophages responding to the death of EBV-infected cells.

　E. activation of an oncogene resulting from a chromosome translocation in EBV-infected lymphocytes.

> Correct answer = B. A: Polyclonal stimulation of B cells by EBV infection occurs, and results in appearance of the characteristic "heterophile antibodies," but it is the CTL response that comprises atypical lymphocytosis of IM. C: EBV-specific humoral immune response is not related to lymphocytosis. D: B cells are not killed by infection with EBV. E: Whereas this is the process that results in EBV-associated Burkitt lymphoma, it occurs only years after the initial virus infection.

25.3 Acyclovir is largely ineffective in the treatment of human cytomegalovirus infections because

　A. HCMV exhibits a high rate of mutation in the target enzyme.

　B. HCMV depends upon the host cell's DNA polymerase for replication of its DNA.

　C. HCMV lacks the thymidine kinase required for activation of acyclovir.

　D. The tissues in which HCMV multiplies are largely inaccessible to the drug.

　E. HCMV codes for an enzyme that inactivates the drug.

> Correct answer = C. The specificity of acyclovir derives from the fact that it must be phosphorylated by the HSV or VZV thymidine kinase to be an active inhibitor of viral DNA synthesis. HCMV does not have a corresponding enzyme. A: HCMV develops resistance to those drugs that are effective, such as ganciclovir and cidofovir, after long term therapy, but because their mechanisms of action are different, mutants resistant to one are usually not resistant to the other. B: All herpesviruses code for their own DNA polymerase. D: In those cases where access is a problem for treatment of herpesvirus infections, direct inoculation of the drug has been done. E: Resistance to antiherpesvirus drugs has generally involved mutation of the enzyme interacting with the drug, not inactivation of the drug.

*"You probably came in contact with someone who has an infectious smile."*

# Hepatitis B and Hepatitis D (Delta) Viruses

# 26

## I. OVERVIEW

Hepatitis (inflammation of the liver) can be caused by a variety of organisms and toxins. For example, there are many viral diseases that involve some degree of liver damage as a secondary effect (such as infectious mononucleosis caused by the Epstein-Barr virus, see p. 268). However, the viruses referred to as "hepatitis viruses" are those whose pathogenesis specifically involves replication in and destruction of hepatocytes. This chapter describes the only human hepatitis virus that has a DNA genome, hepatitis B virus (HBV, Figure 26.1). This chapter also discusses the defective agent that sometimes accompanies HBV during infections—the "delta agent," or hepatitis D virus (HDV). With the exception of HBV, hepatitis viruses thus far identified—hepatitis A, C, D, and E viruses—contain RNA and belong to several different families (Figure 26.1), but the acute disease produced by each is similar. (See p. 378 for a summary of hepatitis). Outcome of infection and mode of transmission, however, differ significantly from virus to virus (Figure 26.2). Worldwide, chronic HBV infection affects almost 300 million people, three quarters of whom are in Asia. HBV is a leading cause of chronic hepatitis, cirrhosis, and hepatocellular carcinoma, accounting for one million deaths annually.

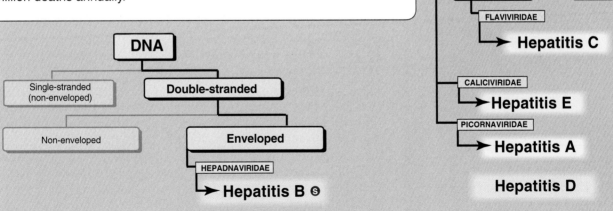

**Figure 26.1**
Classification of major viral agents causing hepatitis. [Note: Hepatitis D is a defective virus and is classified in its own "floating" genus. Hepatitis A, C, and E are discussed in Chapter 27.] ⑤ See p. 331 for a summary of this virus.

**Figure 26.2**
Classification of hepatitis viruses based on mode of transmission.

## II. HEPADNAVIRIDAE

The family Hepadnaviridae (hepatotropic DNA viruses) consists of hepatitis-causing viruses with DNA genomes. Each hepadnavirus has a narrow host range in which it produces both acute and chronic, persistent infections; HBV is the only member of this family that infects humans. Because of highly infectious virus in the blood of both symptomatic and asymptomatic patients, chronically infected individuals poses a serious threat to all healthcare workers, and immunization of such individuals is generally required. A highly effective vaccine produced in genetically engineered yeast cells is available and included among routine childhood immunizations (see p. 39). Biologically, HBV is unique among human disease agents in that replication of the DNA genome proceeds via an RNA intermediate, which, in turn, is "reverse transcribed" by a viral enzyme homologous to the retrovirus reverse transcriptase (see p. 296). However, whereas retroviruses package an RNA genome, Hepadnaviridae package a DNA genome.

### A. Structure and replication of HBV

The HBV virion, historically referred to as the Dane particle, consists of an icosahedral nucleocapsid enclosed in an envelope (Figure 26.3).

1. **Organization of the HBV genome:** The short HBV DNA genome is unusual in that it is a partly single-stranded, partly double-stranded, noncovalently closed, circular DNA molecule (that is, one strand is longer than the other, Figure 26.4). The short "plus" strand, which can vary in length, is only fifty to eighty percent as long as its mate, the "minus" strand. The circular structure of the genome is maintained by base-pairing the strands at one end. A summary of HBV replication is shown in Figure 26.4.

2. **Viral proteins:** The four proteins encoded by viral DNA are: 1) the capsid protein [hepatitis B capsid antigen (HBcAg)]; 2) envelope protein [a glycoprotein referred to as hepatitis B surface antigen (HBsAg)]; 3) multifunctional reverse transcriptase/DNA polymerase, which is complexed with the DNA genome within the capsid; and 4) a nonstructural regulatory protein designated the X protein.

### B. Transmission

Infectious HBV is present in all body fluids of an infected individual. Therefore, blood, semen, saliva, and mother's milk, for example, serve as sources of infection. The titer of infectious virus in the blood of an acutely infected patient can be as high as $10^8$ virus particles per ml, but generally is lower in other body fluids. In areas of high endemicity, for example, Southeast Asia, Africa, and the Middle East, the majority of the population becomes infected at or shortly after birth from a chronically infected mother or from infected siblings. Individuals infected at this young age have a significant chance of becoming chronic carriers (see p. 10), maintaining the high prevalence of virus in the population. In the United States and other western countries, the carrier rate is much lower, and primary infection rarely occurs in newborns.

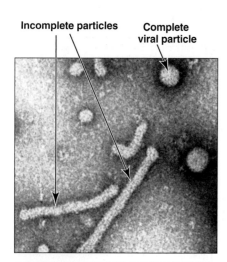

**Figure 26.3**
Electron micrograph of a fraction of serum from a patient with severe hepatitis.

Hepatitis B is primarily a disease of infants in developing nations; however, in Western countries, it is mostly confined to adults who usually contract HBV infection through sexual intercourse or intravenous (IV) drug use.

## C. Pathogenesis

Fully differentiated hepatocytes are the primary cell type infected by HBV. The primary cause of hepatic cell destruction appears to be the cell-mediated immune response. The cells involved are HLA–I-restricted cytotoxic T cells, which react specifically with the fragments of nucleocapsid proteins (HBcAg and HBeAg), expressed on the surface of infected hepatocytes. This response also contributes to control of the infection by eliminating virus-producing cells. Enhanced natural killer cell activity, as well as production of interferon-α, also contribute to limiting the extent of infection. Humoral anti-HBsAg antibody, which is the neutralizing antibody (Ab), does not appear until well into the convalescence period, when it may aid in clearing any remaining circulating free virus. Of greater importance, however, is that this antibody provides protection against reinfection. However, it is this same humoral antibody that is considered the source of extrahepatic damage seen in ten to twenty percent of patients, through the formation and deposition of HBsAg/anti-HBs Ab immune complexes and the consequent activation of complement.

## D. Clinical significance: acute disease

HBV is of medical and public health importance, not only as the cause of acute liver disease but also as the cause of chronic, persistent infections that can result in the eventual death of infected individuals from cirrhosis and liver cancer. Chronically infected people serve as the reservoir of transmissible virus in the population. In most individuals, the primary infection is asymptomatic, and resolves as a result of an effective cell-mediated immune response (Figure 26.5).

1. **Phases in acute HBV infections:** Following infection, HBV has a long but variable incubation period of between 45 and 120 days. Following this period, a pre-icteric (pre-jaundice) phase occurs, lasting several days to a week. This is characterized by mild fever, malaise, anorexia, myalgia, and nausea. The acute, icteric phase then follows and lasts for one to two months. During this phase, dark urine, due to bilirubinuria, and jaundice (a yellowish coloration of mucous membranes, conjunctivae, and skin) are evident. There usually is an enlarged and tender liver as well. In eighty to ninety percent of adults, a convalescent period of several more months is followed by complete recovery (Figure 26.6).

2. **Monitoring the course of acute HBV infection:** Whereas liver-specific enzymes are important clinical determinants of all of the viral hepatitides, HBV infection is unusual in that the quantities of

**Figure 26.4**
Replication of hepatitis B virus.

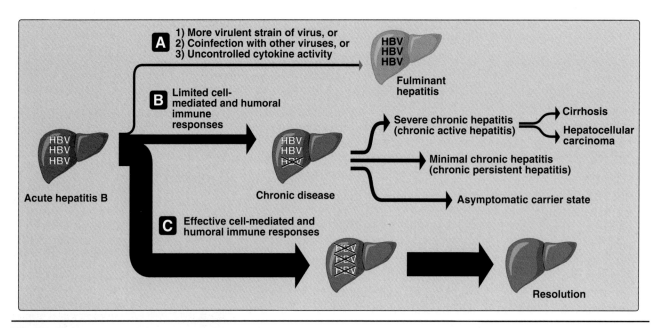

**Figure 26.5**
Clinical outcomes of acute hepatitis B infection.

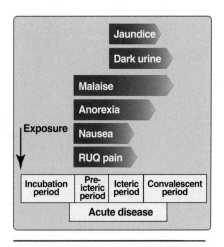

**Figure 26.6**
Symptoms of acute hepatitis B infection. RUQ = right upper quadrant.

virions and virion components in the blood are so great that the time course of their appearance and clearance, along with that of the antibodies directed against them, serve as convenient markers of the stage of the disease and the likely future course (Figure 26.7A).

a. **Appearance of viral antigens:** During the incubation period, HBsAg and HBeAg are the first indicators of HBV infection to appear in the blood. Their presence indicates an active infection, but does not distinguish between acute and chronic infections. Next, viral DNA, viral DNA polymerase, and complete virions become detectable. These continue to increase during the acute disease phase, when a patient's blood has the highest titer of infectious virus.

b. **Appearance of antiviral antibodies:** Antibodies to the HBcAg rise concurrently with liver enzymes in the serum, whereas anti-HBe antibodies and still later, anti-HBs antibodies do not appear until the beginning of convalescence—generally after the respective antigens have disappeared from the blood. In those patients in whom the infection resolves completely, anti-HBc and anti-HBs antibodies remain present for life, providing immunity to reinfection. Continued presence of HBsAg beyond six months and absence of anti-HBs indicates that the infection has become chronic (Figure 26.8).

3. **Fulminant hepatitis:** In one to two percent of acute symptomatic cases, much more extensive necrosis of the liver occurs during the first eight weeks of the acute illness. This is accompanied by high fever, abdominal pain, and eventual renal dysfunction, coma, and seizures. Termed fulminant hepatitis, this condition is fatal in roughly eight percent of cases. Whereas it is not clear why the

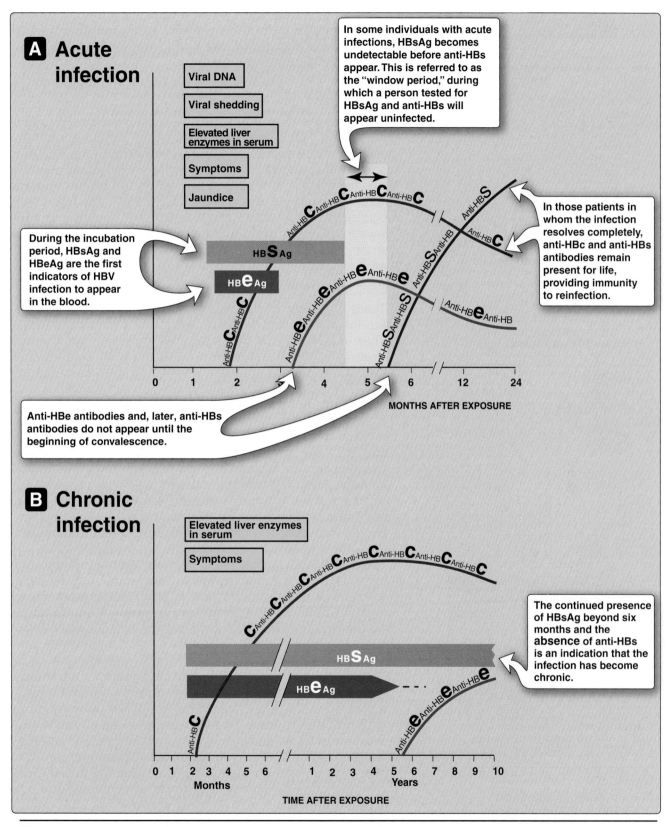

**Figure 26.7**
Typical course of hepatitis B virus infection. A. Acute infection. B. Chronic infection.

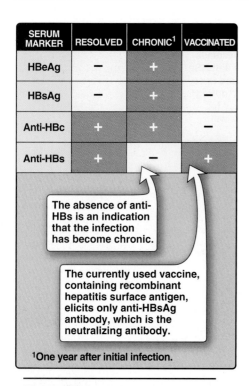

| SERUM MARKER | RESOLVED | CHRONIC[1] | VACCINATED |
|---|---|---|---|
| HBeAg | − | + | − |
| HBsAg | − | + | − |
| Anti-HBc | + | + | − |
| Anti-HBs | + | − | + |

The absence of anti-HBs is an indication that the infection has become chronic.

The currently used vaccine, containing recombinant hepatitis surface antigen, elicits only anti-HBsAg antibody, which is the neutralizing antibody.

[1]One year after initial infection.

**Figure 26.8**
Interpretation of serologic markers of HBV infection.

- 90% Infants born to infected mothers
- 25-50% Infected children five years of age or less
- 5% Infected adults

0  20  40  60  80  100

Percentage of HBV-infected individuals in the United States that progress to chronic disease.

**Figure 26.9**
Effect of patient's age on the tendency of acute HBV infection to progress to chronic disease.

acute disease takes this course, a more highly virulent strain of HBV, coinfection with HDV or another hepatitis virus (for example, HCV), and/or perhaps an uncontrolled immune response by the patient, are thought to play a role.

### E. Clinical significance: chronic disease

In about two thirds of individuals, the primary infection is asymptomatic, even though such patients may later develop symptomatic chronic liver disease, indicating persistence of the virus. Following resolution of the acute disease (or asymptomatic infection), about two to ten percent of adults and over twenty five percent of young children remain chronically infected (Figure 26.9). The high rate of progression to chronic liver disease seen in infants born to HBV-infected mothers is thought to be related to the less competent immune status of newborns. Adults with immune deficiencies also have a considerably higher probability of developing chronic infection than individuals with normal immune systems.

1. **Types of chronic carriers:** The asymptomatic carriers of HBsAg are the most common type of persistently infected individuals. They usually have anti-HBe antibodies and little or no infectious virus in their blood (see Figures 26.7B and 26.8). Later progression of liver damage or recurrence of acute episodes of hepatitis is rare in such patients. Those carriers with minimal chronic hepatitis (formerly, "chronic persistent hepatitis") are asymptomatic most of the time, but have a higher risk of reactivation of disease, and a small fraction do progress to cirrhosis. Severe chronic hepatitis (formerly, "chronic active hepatitis") results in more frequent exacerbations of acute symptoms, including progressive liver damage, potentially leading to cirrhosis and/or hepatocellular carcinoma (see below), chronic fatigue, anorexia, malaise, and anxiety. These symptoms are accompanied by active virus replication and the corresponding presence of HBeAg in the blood. Serum levels of liver enzymes and bilirubin are increased to varying degrees, reflecting the extent of necrosis. The risk of developing cirrhosis is highest in those carriers with more frequent recurrences of acute disease and those in whom HBeAg is not cleared from the blood, indicating continuing virus replication. Overall life expectancy is significantly shorter in those individuals with cirrhosis.

2. **Development of hepatocellular carcinoma (HCC, hepatoma):** HCC is fairly uncommon in the United States, whereas it is ten to a hundred times more frequent in areas of high HBV endemicity. In all populations, males experience a higher rate of chronic HBV infections, a higher rate of progression to cirrhosis, and ultimately a higher rate of HCC, for which the male-to-female ratio is six to one. HCC typically appears many years after the primary HBV infection, and the tumor itself is rather slow growing and only occasionally metastasizes. Clinically, a patient with HCC exhibits weight loss, right upper quadrant pain, fever, and intestinal bleeding. Although there is no doubt that chronic HBV infection greatly increases the risk of HCC, the mechanisms relating HBV and

HCC are not understood. However, by causing continuing liver necrosis accompanied by continuing regeneration of the damaged tissue, chronic HBV infection provides the opportunity for chromosome rearrangements and mutations. The presence of environmental carcinogens could further contribute to the disease process.

> HCC is a major cause of death due to malignancy worldwide, and its distribution parallels HBV incidence (approximately eighty percent of primary HCCs occur in HBV-infected individuals).

## F. Laboratory identification

The purpose of diagnostic laboratory studies of patients with clinical hepatitis is to first, determine which hepatitis virus is the cause of the illness, and second (for HBV), to distinguish acute from chronic infections. The diagnosis of hepatitis is made on clinical grounds, coupled with biochemical tests that evaluate liver damage. Elevations of aminotransferases, bilirubin, and prothrombin time, all contribute to the initial evaluation of hepatitis. ELISA (see p. 28) and other immunologic techniques for detection of viral antigens and antibodies are the primary means to distinguish among HAV, HBV, HCV and HDV. In addition, identification of the presence or absence of specific antiviral antibodies and viral antigens permits differentiating between acute and chronic HBV infections (see Figure 26.7).

## G. Treatment

In the past, treatment for acute hepatitis was largely supportive and not directed toward inhibiting virus replication. Prolonged (months) treatment with interferon-α has succeeded in reducing or eliminating indicators of HBV replication in about one third of patients but, in some of these, recurrence of indications of the infection occurs after discontinuance of the therapy. Antiviral analogs used in HIV therapy (see p. 304) and targeted especially against the reverse transcriptase have been tested and had some success. In clinical trials, lamivudine, an oral nucleoside analog, has been shown to be an effective treatment in patients with previously untreated chronic hepatitis B (Figure 26.10). Treatment with lamivudine for one year was well tolerated. It decreased histologic liver abnormalities and increased the rate of HBeAg seroconversion (defined as the loss of HBeAg in serum, undetectable HBV DNA levels, and the presence of antibodies against HBeAg). Most lamivudine-treated patients had undetectable serum HBV DNA during the one year of treatment, but four months after treatment was stopped, the median HBV DNA level had returned to about fifty percent of the pretreatment value. Initial reports show no greater benefits from combination therapy with interferon plus lamivudine than with lamivudine monotherapy.

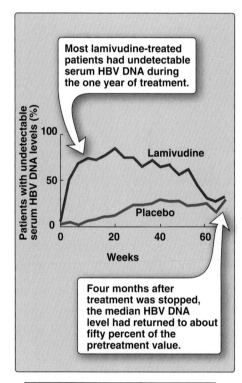

**Figure 26.10**
Effect of lamivudine therapy on the levels of serum HBV DNA (expressed as percentages of patients with undetectable HBV DNA).

**Routine immunization**
- All infants and previously unvaccinated children by the age of 11 years

**Increased risk of hepatitis B**
- People with multiple sexual partners
- Sexual partner or household contacts of HBsAg-positive people
- Homosexually active men
- Users of illicit injection drugs
- Travelers to regions of endemic disease
- People occupationally exposed to blood or body fluids
- Hemodialysis patients
- Patients receiving clotting-factor concentrates

**Figure 26.11**
Candidates for hepatitis B virus immunization.

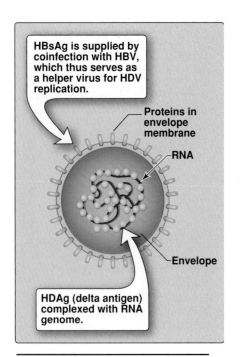

HBsAg is supplied by coinfection with HBV, which thus serves as a helper virus for HDV replication.

Proteins in envelope membrane

RNA

Envelope

HDAg (delta antigen) complexed with RNA genome.

**Figure 26.12**
Structure of hepatitis D virus.

## H. Prevention

The purpose of controlling the spread of HBV infection is to prevent cases of acute hepatitis. An additional goal is to decrease the pool of chronically infected individuals who serve as reservoirs for infectious virus in the population, and who are at greatly increased risk for developing cirrhosis and liver cancer. The availability of a highly effective vaccine has led to a several-pronged approach: 1) protection of those adults who are at risk because of lifestyle or occupation; 2) protection of newborns from infection by transmission from HBV-positive mothers (important because of the high rate of resulting chronic infections, see p. 274); and 3) protection of siblings and other children from infection by chronically infected family members.

1. **Active immunization:** HBsAg is used to prepare vaccines conferring protection because it is antibody to this virion component that neutralizes infectivity. HBV vaccination is now recommended as a routine infant immunization, as is the immunization of adolescents who were not given the vaccine as infants. An unusual feature of the recommended vaccination schedule (see Figure 5.8, p. 39) is to initiate an HBV vaccine series at birth. This is possible because infants have adequate antibody response to neonatal vaccination with the HBV vaccine. Other individuals who are candidates for HBV vaccine are shown in Figure 26.11.

2. **Passive immunization:** Hepatitis B immunoglobulin (HBIG) is prepared from the blood of donors having a high titer of anti-HBs antibody. Immediate administration of HBIG is recommended as the initial step in preventing infection of individuals accidentally exposed to HBV-contaminated blood by needlestick or other means, and of those exposed to infection by sexual contact with an HBV-positive partner. [Note: In such cases, this should be accompanied by a course of active immunization with the hepatitis B vaccine.] It is also strongly recommended that pregnant women should be screened for HBsAg. Infants born to mothers who are HBV-positive are given HBIG plus hepatitis B vaccine at birth, followed by additional doses of vaccine at one and six months.

## III. HEPATITIS D VIRUS (DELTA AGENT)

Hepatitis D virus (HDV) is found in nature only as a coinfection with HBV. It is significant because its presence results in more severe acute disease, with a greater risk of fulminant hepatitis and, in chronically infected patients, a greater risk of cirrhosis and liver cancer.

## A. Structure and replication

HDV does not fall into any known group of animal viruses. It has a circular, single-stranded RNA genome with negative polarity that codes for one protein (delta antigen), with which the genome is complexed in the virion (Figure 26.12). In the infectious particle, the nucleoprotein complex is enclosed within an envelope containing

HBV-coded HBsAg. Thus, HDV requires HBV to serve as a helper virus for infectious HDV production. The HDV RNA genome is replicated and transcribed in the nucleus by cellular enzymes, whose specificity is probably modified by complexing with the delta protein. [Note: This phase of HDV replication is independent of HBV, whose only helper function is to supply HBsAg for the envelope.]

### B. Transmission and pathogenesis

Because HDV exists only in association with HBV, it can be transmitted by the same routes. However, it does not appear to be transmitted sexually as frequently as HBV or HIV. Pathologically, liver damage is essentially the same as in other viral hepatitides, but the presence of HDV usually results in more extensive and severe damage.

### C. Clinical significance

Disease HDV can occur in one of three variations (Figure 26.13). First, simultaneous primary coinfection with both HBV and HDV can cause an acute disease that is similar to that caused by HBV alone, except that, depending on the relative concentrations of the two agents, two successive episodes of acute hepatitis may occur. The risk of fatal fulminant hepatitis caused by the presence of HDV is also considerably higher than with HBV alone. The likelihood of progression to the second variation of HDV disease (chronic coinfection with HBV) is greatly increased as well. In this case, cirrhosis and HCC or death due to liver failure also develop more frequently than with HBV infection alone. The third variation—primary HDV infection of a chronically HBV-infected individual—leads to an episode of severe acute hepatitis after a short incubation period and develops into chronic HDV infection in more than seventy percent of the cases. Again in this situation, the risk of acute hepatitis becoming fulminant is greatly increased, and the persistent infection is often of the severe chronic type (see p. 276).

### D. Laboratory identification

The immunologically based methods used to diagnosis HBV are also applied to HDV. The delta (D) antigen and IgM antibodies to it can be detected in serum. The presence of HDV RNA in serum or liver tissue, as detected by hybridization with or without the use of reverse transcriptase and PCR amplification, is an indicator of active infection.

### E. Treatment and prevention

No specific treatment for HDV infection is available. Because HDV depends on coinfection with HBV, the approaches for preventing HBV infection are also effective in preventing HDV infection. There is no vaccine specifically for HDV. Therefore, those who are chronically infected with HBV can only be protected from HDV infection by limiting chances for exposure. Those who are protected against HBV infection through vaccination will not be affected by HDV.

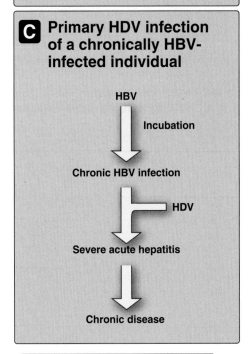

**Figure 26.13**
Consequences of HDV infection.

## Study Questions

**Choose the ONE correct answer**

26.1 Killing of liver cells infected with hepatitis B virus is primarily caused by

   A. shut-off of cellular protein synthesis.

   B. intracytoplasmic accumulation of HBV antigen aggregates.

   C. degradation of cellular mRNA.

   D. attack by cytotoxic T lymphocytes directed against HBV antigens.

   E. virus-induced aberrant chromosome rearrangements and deletions.

Correct answer = D. There is no evidence that HBV infection is cytocidal. Protein synthesis is not shut off, and mRNA is not degraded in infected cells. Accumulation of HBV proteins is not observed, rather they are actively exported. Whereas chromosome damage is observed in cells of primary hepatocellular carcinoma, it is not characteristic of nonmalignant infected liver cells.

26.2 The most common natural mode of transmission of infection with hepatitis B virus is via

   A. contaminated water supply.

   B. body fluids, such as urine and semen.

   C. respiratory droplets.

   D. direct contact.

   E. infected insect vectors.

Correct answer = B. HBV is found at high levels in all body fluids, which results in transmission from mother to newborn, from sibling to sibling, through sexual intercourse, and by infection by virus-containing blood. Contaminated water or food is the typical source of HAV and HEV infection.

26.3 Hepatitis delta virus is unique in that

   A. infectivity requires an envelope protein provided by a helper virus.

   B. it has an RNA genome that is replicated by a replicase supplied by a coinfecting helper virus.

   C. its mRNA is transcribed by a transcriptase supplied by a helper virus.

   D. the virion contains a reverse transcriptase provided by a helper virus.

   E. it encodes a protein (HDAg) that replaces helper virus glycoproteins in the envelopes of helper virus particles.

Correct answer = A. The only function of the HBV helper is to supply the envelope. B: Genome replication requires a cell RNA polymerase, presumably modified by the HDV delta protein such that it can use the HDV RNA as a template. C: Transcription likewise depends on cell enzymes. D: The virion contains only the delta protein. E: HDAg is complexed with the RNA genome in the HDV virion and is not found in the HBV virion.

*"Everyone is out with the flu, the computers all have a virus, and the shredder just threw up."*

# Positive-strand RNA Viruses

# 27

## I. OVERVIEW

Viruses with a positive-strand RNA genome (that is, one that can serve as a messenger RNA in the infected cell) include the viral families Picornaviridae, Togaviridae, Flaviviridae, Caliciviridae, and Coronaviridae. The viruses in these families cause a broad spectrum of diseases, but share the following features: 1) they replicate in the cytoplasm; 2) genomic RNAs serve as messenger RNAs and are infectious; 3) genomic RNAs are non-segmented; 4) virions do not contain any enzymes; and 5) virus-specified proteins are synthesized as polyproteins that are processed by viral and cellular proteases, giving rise to individual viral proteins. Some positive-strand RNA viruses are enveloped; others are not. Figure 27.1 summarizes the positive-strand RNA viruses discussed in this chapter.

## II. FAMILY PICORNAVIRIDAE

Picornaviruses are small, naked (nonenveloped), icosahedral viruses (Figure 27.2), which contain a single-stranded, non-segmented RNA genome and four structural proteins. Picornaviridae are divided into five genera: enteroviruses, rhinoviruses, cardioviruses, aphthoviruses, and hepatoviruses. Cardioviruses cause encephalitis and myocarditis in mice, whereas aphthovirus is represented by the foot-and-mouth disease virus, which infects cattle. Enterovirus, rhinovirus, and hepatovirus cause a wide variety of clinical syndromes in humans.

> The most intensively studied picornavirus is poliovirus; however, what has been learned about the structure and replication of poliovirus also applies in large measure to the other viruses in this family.

### A. Genus Enterovirus

More than seventy enteroviruses have been identified. Currently, as new enteroviruses are identified, they are not assigned to one of these groups but are simply given numerical designations (for example, enterovirus 68, enterovirus 69, and so forth).

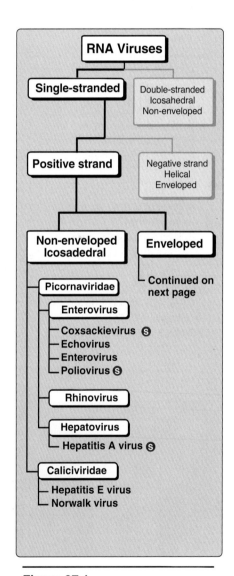

**Figure 27.1**
Classification of positive-strand RNA viruses (continued on next page). Ⓢ See p. 331 for summaries of these viruses.

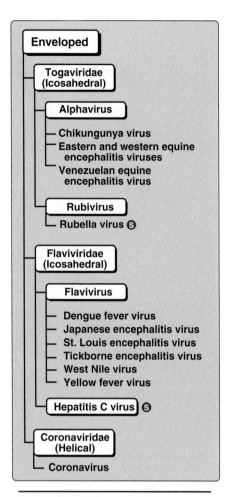

Enveloped

- Togaviridae (Icosahedral)
  - Alphavirus
    - Chikungunya virus
    - Eastern and western equine encephalitis viruses
    - Venezuelan equine encephalitis virus
  - Rubivirus
    - Rubella virus Ⓢ
- Flaviviridae (Icosahedral)
  - Flavivirus
    - Dengue fever virus
    - Japanese encephalitis virus
    - St. Louis encephalitis virus
    - Tickborne encephalitis virus
    - West Nile virus
    - Yellow fever virus
  - Hepatitis C virus Ⓢ
- Coronaviridae (Helical)
  - Coronavirus

**Figure 27.1** (continued)
Classification of positive-strand RNA viruses. Ⓢ See p. 331 for summaries of these viruses.

**Figure 27.2**
Poliovirus, a type of picornavirus, is one of the simplest and smallest viruses.

1. **Epidemiology:** Individuals are infected with enteroviruses by ingestion of contaminated food or water. Enteroviruses are stable at the low pH of the stomach, replicate in the gastrointestinal (GI) tract, and excreted in the stool. Thus, these viruses are said to be transmitted by the fecal-oral route. After replicating in the oropharynx and intestinal tract lymphoid tissue, enteroviruses can leave the intestine by entering the bloodstream, and thus spread to various target organs [for example, poliovirus spreads to the central nervous system (CNS)]. Although the great majority of infections are asymptomatic, infection, whether clinical or subclinical, usually results in protective immunity.

> Enteroviruses account for an estimated ten to fifteen million symptomatic infections per year in the United States.

2. **Viral replication:** Enteroviruses bind to specific receptors on host cell surfaces. For example, poliovirus binds to a receptor that is a member of the immunoglobulin supergene family of proteins. Cells lacking these specific receptors are not susceptible to infection.

   a. **Mechanism of genome replication:** This is the same process as described for Type I RNA viruses (see p. 239); namely, the incoming parental RNA serves as the template for a genome-size, negative-strand RNA, and this in turn serves as a template for multiple copies of progeny positive-strand RNA.

   b. **Translation:** Enterovirus RNA contains a single, long, open reading frame. Translation of this message results in the synthesis of a single, long polyprotein, which is processed by viral proteases into structural proteins and nonstructural proteins, including the viral RNA polymerase needed to synthesize additional copies of the viral genome.

3. **General clinical significance of enterovirus infections:** All enteroviruses can cause CNS disease. For example, they are currently the major recognizable cause of acute aseptic meningitis syndrome, which refers to any meningitis (infectious or noninfectious) for which the cause is not clear after initial examination plus routine stains and cultures of the cerebrospinal fluid (CSF).

> Viral meningitis is a common infection in the United States, with an estimated 75,000 cases each year.

Viral meningitis can usually be distinguished from bacterial meningitis because: 1) the viral disease is milder; 2) there is an elevation of lymphocytes in the CSF, rather than the elevated neutrophils seen in bacterial meningitis; and 3) the glucose concentration in the CSF is not decreased. Viral meningitis occurs mainly in the summer and fall, affecting both children and adults. The treatment is symptomatic, and the course of the illness is usually benign. Viruses can be isolated from the stool or from various target organs (CNS in fatal cases, or from conjunctival fluid in cases of conjunctivitis). Evidence of infection can also be obtained by demonstration of a rise in antibody titer against a specific enterovirus. No antiviral drugs are available for treatment of enterovirus infections.

4. **Clinical significance of poliovirus infection:** Poliomyelitis is an acute illness in which the poliovirus selectively destroys the lower motor neurons of the spinal cord and brainstem, resulting in flaccid, asymmetric weakness or paralysis. In the United States, no cases of paralytic poliomyelitis caused by wild-type poliovirus have occurred in more than twenty years. The few cases of polio that occur (less than ten per year) are all caused by the reversion to virulence of the virus in the live-attenuated Sabin polio vaccine (see below). In countries with low immunization rates, paralytic polio continues to occur, with significant numbers of cases in sub-Saharan Africa and southern Asia. However, the World Health Organization has set the goal of eradicating polio from the world within the next decade.

   a. **Transmission and pathogenesis:** Poliovirus infections may follow one of several courses: 1) asymptomatic infection, which occurs in 90 to 95 percent of cases and causes no disease and no sequelae; 2) abortive infection; 3) nonparalytic infection; or 4) paralytic poliomyelitis (Figure 27.3). The classic presentation of paralytic poliomyelitis is flaccid paralysis, most often affecting the lower limbs. This is a result of viral replication in, and destruction of, the lower motor neurons in the anterior horn of the spinal cord (Figure 27.4). Respiratory paralysis may also occur, following infection of the brain stem. Poliomyelitis should be considered in any unimmunized person with the combination of fever, headache, neck and back pain, asymmetric flaccid paralysis without sensory loss, and pleocytosis (an increase in the number of lymphocytes in the spinal fluid).

   b. **Prognosis:** Permanent weakness is observed in approximately two thirds of patients with paralytic poliomyelitis. Complete recovery is less likely when acute paralysis is severe; patients requiring mechanical ventilation because of respiratory paralysis rarely recover without some permanent disability.

   c. **Postpoliomyelitis syndrome:** Approximately twenty to thirty percent of patients who partially or fully recover from paralytic poliomyelitis experience a new onset of muscle weakness, pain, atrophy, and fatigue 25 to 35 years after the acute illness.

   d. **Treatment and prevention:** Specific antiviral agents for the treatment of poliomyelitis are not available. Management, therefore, is supportive and symptomatic. Vaccination is the only effective method of preventing poliomyelitis (see p. 40). Poliomyelitis can be prevented by either live-attenuated (Sabin) or killed (Salk) polio vaccines. These vaccines have

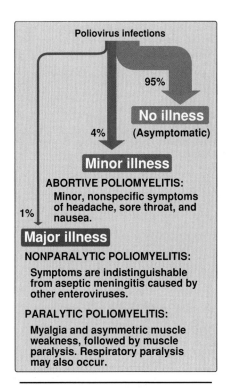

**Figure 27.3**
Clinical outcomes of infection with poliovirus.

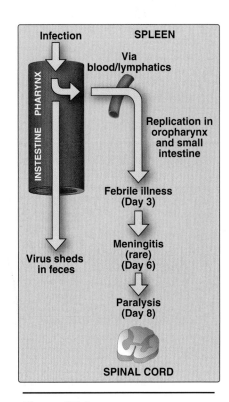

**Figure 27.4**
CNS invasion by poliovirus.

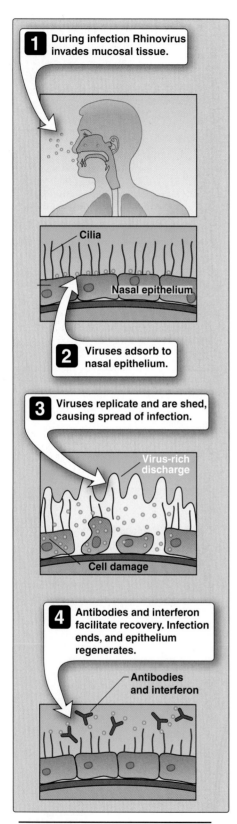

**Figure 27.5**
Pathogenesis of the common cold showing stages from infection to recovery.

led to the elimination of wild-type polio from Western Europe, Japan, and the Americas. [Note: Killed polio vaccine has no adverse effects, whereas live polio vaccine may undergo reversion to a virulent form while it multiplies in the human intestinal tract and cause vaccine-associated paralytic poliomyelitis in those receiving the vaccine.

> Since 1979, vaccine-associated poliomyelitis has accounted for all of the four to eight cases per year of paralytic poliomyelitis that have occurred in the United States.

5. **Clinical significance of coxsackievirus and echovirus infections:** These give rise to a large variety of clinical syndromes, including meningitis, upper respiratory infections, gastroenteritis, herpangina (severe sore throat with vesiculoulcerative lesions), pleurisy, pericarditis, myocarditis, and myositis.

6. **Clinical significance of enteroviruses 70 and 71 infections:** These have been associated with severe CNS disease. A particularly acute form of extremely contagious hemorrhagic conjunctivitis has also been associated with Enterovirus 70.

## B. Genus rhinovirus

Rhinoviruses cause the common-cold syndrome (Figure 27.5). They differ in two important respects from enteroviruses. First, whereas enteroviruses are acid-stable (they must survive the acid environment of the stomach), rhinoviruses are acid-labile. Second, rhinoviruses, which replicate in the nasal passages, have an optimal temperature for replication that is lower than that of enteroviruses. [Note: This permits rhinovirus to replicate efficiently at temperatures several degrees below body temperature.] Rhinovirus replication is similar to that of the poliovirus (see p. 284). There are more than 100 serotypes of rhinoviruses; therefore, development of a vaccine is impractical. Studies have shown that in addition to spread by respiratory droplets, rhinoviruses can also be spread by hand-to-hand contact. Thus, washing of hands at appropriate intervals can be a useful preventive measure.

## C. Genus hepatovirus

The sole member of this genus is hepatitis A virus (HAV). Although at one time HAV was also known as Enterovirus 72, sufficient differences have been found between HAV and the enteroviruses to warrant placing HAV in a genus by itself. HAV, of which there is only one serotype, causes viral hepatitis. As with the enteroviruses, transmission is by the fecal-oral route, and the virus is shed in the feces. For example, a common mode of transmission of the virus is through eating uncooked shellfish harvested from sewage-contaminated water. The main site of replication is the hepatocyte. Viral replication results in severe cytopathology, and liver function is significantly impaired (Figure 27.6). In contrast to most other picornaviruses, HAV grows poorly in tissue culture. The prognosis for patients with hepatitis A is generally favorable, and the development of persistent infection and chronic hepatitis is uncommon. Prevention depends on taking measures to avoid fecal contamination of food and water; therefore, HAV infection is most common in underdeveloped countries with poor sanitation (Figure 27.7). Immune globulin has been used for many years, mainly as postexposure prophylaxis. Vaccines prepared from whole virus inactivated with formaldehyde are now available.

# III. FAMILY TOGAVIRIDAE

The togaviruses are enveloped, icosahedral viruses that contain a positive-sense, single-stranded RNA genome and generally three structural proteins. The capsid (C) protein encloses the viral RNA, forming the nucleocapsid; the two other proteins (E1 and E2) are glycoproteins that form the hemagglutinin-containing viral spikes that project from the lipid bilayer. The family Togaviridae is divided into two genera—Alphavirus and Rubivirus.

## A. Genus alphavirus

The alphaviruses, of which there are approximately 26, are arthropod-borne viruses (arboviruses), which are transmitted to humans and domestic animals by mosquitoes. All alphaviruses share a common group antigen. [Note: Some arboviruses were initially isolated from horses, hence, the word "equine" in their names (see below).]

1. **Epidemiology and pathogenesis:** Alphaviruses have a broad host range, being able to replicate in organisms that are widely separated phylogenetically, such as mosquitoes and humans. Following inoculation of an Alphavirus by a mosquito, the patient is observed to have a viremia, following which the virus may be seeded in various target organs, for example, the CNS in the case of the encephalitis viruses.

2. **Viral replication:** Following attachment to the cell surface, the virus is internalized by receptor-mediated endocytosis. Like the picornaviruses, genome replication is as described for Type I RNA viruses (see p. 239).

3. **Clinical significance:** Several different clinical syndromes are associated with Alphavirus infections of humans. These include: 1) acute encephalitis (eastern and western equine encephalitis viruses); 2) acute arthropathy (Chikungunya virus); and 3) a febrile illness with a flulike syndrome (Venezuelan equine encephalitis virus). The majority of infections, however, are subclinical and can be diagnosed only by the demonstration of an immune response.

4. **Laboratory identification:** This is generally accomplished by the demonstration of a rise in antibody titer (that is, comparing acute and convalescent sera). In fatal cases of encephalitis, the virus may be isolated from the CNS.

5. **Prevention:** The most important measure for prevention of Alphavirus infection is control of the mosquito vector population. A Venezuelan equine encephalitis vaccine is available.

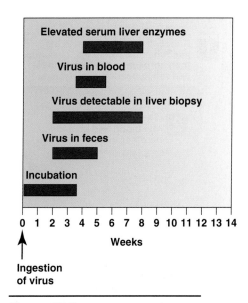

**Figure 27.6**
Time course of hepatitis A infection.

**Figure 27.7**
Distribution of hepatitis A virus infection worldwide.

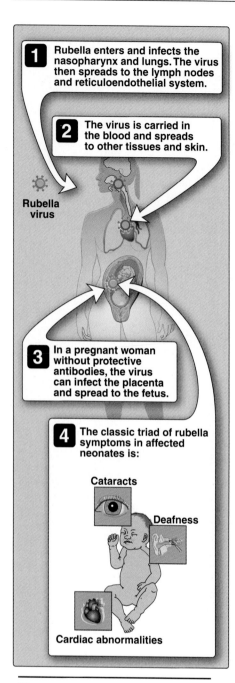

**1** Rubella enters and infects the nasopharynx and lungs. The virus then spreads to the lymph nodes and reticuloendothelial system.

**2** The virus is carried in the blood and spreads to other tissues and skin.

Rubella virus

**3** In a pregnant woman without protective antibodies, the virus can infect the placenta and spread to the fetus.

**4** The classic triad of rubella symptoms in affected neonates is:

Cataracts

Deafness

Cardiac abnormalities

**Figure 27.8**
Pathology of rubella virus infection.

## B. Genus rubivirus

The sole member of the Rubivirus genus is rubella virus. The structure and replication of rubella virus are basically as described for the alphaviruses (see p. 287). Respiratory secretions of an infected person are the primary vehicles for rubella virus transmission. Rubella causes a mild clinical syndrome that is characterized by a generalized maculopapular rash and occipital lymphadenopathy ["German measles", not to be confused with "measles" (rubeola), caused by the measles virus (see p. 313)]. In most cases, these symptoms may be hardly noticeable, and the infection remains subclinical. For this reason, the only reliable evidence for a prior infection with rubella virus is the demonstration of antirubella antibodies. The clinical significance of rubella lies not in the primary infection described above, but rather in the fact that when a woman is infected during pregnancy, there can be severe damage to the developing fetus, especially in the first trimester (congenital rubella). This damage can include congenital heart disease, cataracts, hepatitis, or abnormalities related to the CNS, such as mental retardation, motor dysfunction, and deafness (Figure 27.8). Fetal damage resulting from rubella infection is preventable by use of the live attenuated rubella vaccine (see p. 41) that is included with the routine childhood vaccinations. This vaccine, which has few complications, is effective in preventing congenital rubella because it reduces the reservoir of the virus in the childhood populations, and also ensures that women reaching childbearing age are immune to rubella infection. [Note: The vaccine should not be given to women who are already pregnant or to immunocompromised patients, including babies.]

 In the United States, rubella outbreaks often begin among infected persons from countries where rubella is not included in routine immunizations.

## IV. FAMILY FLAVIVIRIDAE

The members of this family are enveloped viruses that contain a single-stranded RNA genome and three structural proteins. The capsid (C) protein and the viral RNA form the icosahedral nucleocapsid; the other two proteins are envelope-associated. At the present time, the family Flaviviridae is divided into three genera: Flavivirus, Hepatitis C virus, and Pestivirus. [Note: The viruses in the genus Pestivirus (classical swine fever virus and bovine viral diarrhea virus) are of veterinary interest only.]

## A. Genus Flavivirus

The genus Flavivirus is composed of more than sixty viruses. These include many viruses of medical importance such as yellow fever, St. Louis encephalitis, Japanese encephalitis, dengue fever viruses, and West Nile virus, all of which are mosquito-transmitted. Tickborne encephalitis virus is, of course, transmitted by ticks. [Note: Like the viruses in the Alphavirus genus of the family Togaviridae (see p. 287), most of the viruses in this genus are thus arboviruses.] All of the viruses in the genus Flavivirus share a common group antigen.

1. **Epidemiology and pathogenesis:** As arboviruses, the medically important members of this genus are transmitted to humans by the bite of an infected mosquito or tick. These viruses are maintained in nature by replicating alternately in an arthropod vector and a vertebrate host. Figure 27.9 shows the global distributions of yellow fever and dengue fever.

2. **Replication:** Following attachment to the cell surface, the virus is taken up by receptor-mediated endocytosis (see Figure 23.9, p. 237). Replication of the viral RNA is as described for Type I RNA viruses (see p. 239). Only one species of viral mRNA—the genomic RNA—is found in infected cells. It is translated into a single, long polyprotein, which is processed by virus-coded and cellular proteases, giving rise to three structural and seven nonstructural proteins. Nucleocapsids are formed in the cytoplasm, and maturation of the viral particle occurs by envelopment of the nucleocapsid, not at the plasma membrane as with viruses in the family Togaviridae, but instead, at cytoplasmic golgi membranes. Virus particles then accumulate in vesicles, and are extruded when the vesicles move to the cell surface.

3. **Clinical significance:** Viruses in the genus Flavivirus are associated with several different clinical syndromes. These include: encephalitis (St. Louis encephalitis, Japanese encephalitis, and tickborne encephalitis viruses), hemorrhagic fever (yellow fever virus), and fever, myalgia, and rash (dengue viruses). [Note: Although there is little mortality associated with classic dengue fever, in certain parts of the world, such as Southeast Asia, a severe form of dengue infection occurs particularly in infants and young children. Called dengue hemorrhagic fever or dengue shock syndrome, it is associated with a significant mortality (ten percent or higher) if untreated.] Like dengue fever, West Nile fever is a mosquito-transmitted, acute, usually self-limited illness that presents chiefly with fever, malaise, lymphadenopathy, and rash. Infection may also result in aseptic meningitis or meningoencephalitis, especially in the elderly.

> The first outbreak of West Nile encephalitis in the United States occurred in the New York City area in the summer of 1999. It has occurred in other northeastern states in subsequent years.

4. **Laboratory identification:** A specific diagnosis is most often made by serologic means (that is, by demonstrating at least a fourfold rise in antibody titer, when comparing acute and convalescent sera). In some cases, virus isolation or demonstration of specific viral antigens is also feasible.

5. **Prevention:** A safe, highly effective, live attenuated vaccine for yellow fever has been available for many years. In China and Japan,

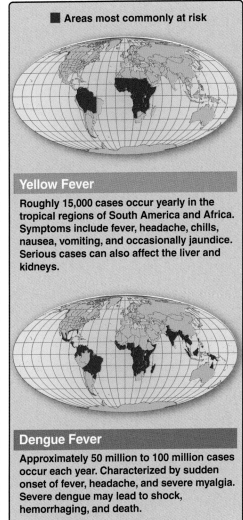

■ Areas most commonly at risk

**Yellow Fever**

Roughly 15,000 cases occur yearly in the tropical regions of South America and Africa. Symptoms include fever, headache, chills, nausea, vomiting, and occasionally jaundice. Serious cases can also affect the liver and kidneys.

**Dengue Fever**

Approximately 50 million to 100 million cases occur each year. Characterized by sudden onset of fever, headache, and severe myalgia. Severe dengue may lead to shock, hemorrhaging, and death.

**Figure 27.9**
Global distribution of yellow fever and dengue fever.

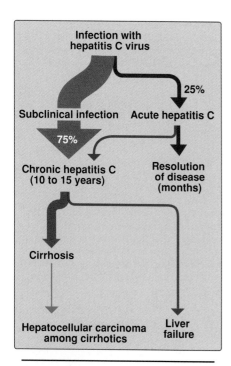

**Figure 27.10**
Natural history of infection with
hepatitis C virus.

**Figure 27.11**
Combination treatment with interferon
and ribavirin for chronic hepatitis C.
[Note: Patients receiving ribavirin
alone showed a biologic and histologic
response, but no decrease in
circulating virus.]

a formalin-inactivated Japanese encephalitis virus vaccine is used; in central Europe, a formalin-inactivated vaccine is widely used to prevent tickborne encephalitis. Another important method of prevention is vector control. In urban areas, elimination of breeding sites can dramatically reduce the population of *Aedes aegypti* mosquitoes, which serve as the vector for both yellow fever and dengue viruses.

### B. Hepatitis C viruses

Hepatitis C virus (HCV) was discovered in 1988 in the course of searching for the cause of non-A, non-B, transfusion-associated hepatitis. At that time, HCV accounted for ninety percent of the cases of non-A, non-B hepatitis. The hepatitis C viruses are heterogeneous and can be divided into six types on the basis of their nucleotide sequences.

1. **Transmission and pathogenesis:** Although HCV was initially identified as a major cause of posttransfusion hepatitis, intravenous drug users and patients on hemodialysis are also at high risk for infection with HCV. Tattoos are also a leading cause of HCV infection. In addition, there is evidence for sexual transmission of HCV, as well as for transmission from mother to infant. In the infected individual, viral replication occurs in the hepatocyte and probably also in mononuclear cells (lymphocytes and macrophages). Destruction of liver cells may result both from a direct effect of viral replication and from the host immune response.

2. **Clinical significance:** The majority of infections with HCV are subclinical, but about 25 percent of infected individuals present with acute hepatitis, including jaundice (Figure 27.10). More important, a significant proportion of infections progress to a chronic hepatitis and cirrhosis. Finally, some of these individuals go on to develop hepatocellular carcinoma many years after the primary infection.

3. **Laboratory identification:** A specific diagnosis can be made by demonstration of antibodies that react with a combination of recombinant viral proteins. Sensitive tests are also now available for detection of the viral nucleic acid by RT-PCR (PCR that amplifies a DNA copy—synthesized using reverse transcriptase—of the viral RNA, see p. 32).

4. **Treatment and prevention:** Tests to screen blood for HCV have been available for several years, so that HCV as a cause of transfusion-associated hepatitis is now unusual. Treatment of patients with chronic hepatitis by interferon-α is sometimes of benefit, but, in most cases, only for the period during which the patient is receiving the interferon. Treatment with interferon-α plus ribavirin provides a significantly improved response, and combination therapy is the treatment of choice (Figure 27.11). Chronic hepatitis resulting in severe liver damage may be an indication for a liver transplant.

## V. FAMILY CALICIVIRIDAE

Caliciviruses are small, nonenveloped, spherical particles. Each contains a single-stranded, nonsegmented RNA genome, and a single species of capsid protein. In contrast to the picornaviruses, the caliciviruses genome contains three open reading frames. Norwalk virus is the prototype human calicivirus. There are at least four strains of human caliciviruses.

### A. Caliciviruses

Norwalk virus replicates in the gastrointestinal tract and is shed in the stool. Infection by the Norwalk virus is by the fecal-oral route, following ingestion of contaminated food or water. Norwalk virus is a major cause of epidemic acute gastroenteritis, particularly at schools, camps, military bases, prisons, and similar settings. It affects primarily adults and school-age children, but not infants. The clinical presentation is characterized generally by nausea, vomiting, and diarrhea. Symptoms last 24 to 48 hours, and the disease is self-limited. Radioimmunoassays and ELISA tests are available for the detection of antiviral antibodies (see p. 28). No specific antiviral treatment is available. Careful attention to hand washing and measures to prevent contamination of food and water supplies should reduce the incidence of these infections.

### B. Hepatitis E virus (HEV)

HEV is a nonenveloped, single-stranded RNA virus. It is a major cause of enterically transmitted, water-borne hepatitis in developing countries. The peak incidence is in young adults, and the disease is especially severe in pregnant women, in whom death can result from HEV infection. Viral RNA can be detected in the feces of infected individuals by RT-PCR (see p. 30), and nearly all serologically confirmed epidemics of HEV can be attributed to fecally contaminated water. Apart from epidemic situations, the diagnosis of HEV cannot be made in an infected individual solely on clinical grounds. However, specific tests are available to detect antibodies to HEV. The signs and symptoms are similar to those seen with other forms of acute viral hepatitis, but like hepatitis A, progression to chronic hepatitis is not seen. Interestingly, in regions of the world where HEV is rarely, if ever, diagnosed, antibodies to HEV can still be found. No antiviral treatment nor vaccine is currently available.

## VI. FAMILY CORONAVIRIDAE

Coronaviruses are large, enveloped, pleomorphic particles, with a distinctive arrangement of spikes (peplomers) projecting from their surfaces. [Note: These projections have the appearance of a solar corona; hence, the name of the virus.] The coronavirus genome is the largest described for any RNA virus thus far. Human coronaviruses have been most commonly implicated in upper respiratory infections, such as the common cold syndrome.

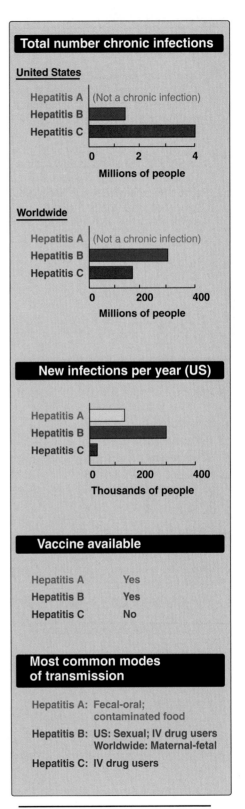

**Figure 27.12**
Summary of hepatitis A, B, and C.

## Study Questions

**Choose the ONE correct answer**

27.1  A company held an elaborate holiday dinner party for its 42 employees. Within three to four weeks, many of the banquet attendees complained of experiencing fatigue, fever, nausea, and dark urine, and were observed to be jaundiced. The group exhibited no bacterial infections in common. The employees who became ill had all eaten raw oysters at the party. The company doctor assayed a sample of the employees' blood for anti-hepatitis B antibodies, but all samples were negative for anti-HBsAg IgM. The causative agent consistent with this history is most likely:

A. hepatitis A virus.

B. hepatitis B virus.

C. hepatitis C virus.

D.  hepatitis D virus.

E. hepatitis E virus.

> Correct answer = A. Hepatitis A is transmitted by the fecal-oral route and is most frequently acquired by eating contaminated shellfish or by contact with a carrier. The symptoms that were exhibited by the party-goers are consistent with liver damage caused by, for example, hepatitis. Hepatitis B infection is excluded because of the negative test for antibodies. Hepatitis C infection is acquired most commonly by IV drug users, patients on dialysis, and individuals obtaining tattoos. Hepatitis D infection occurs only in combination with hepatitis B infection. Hepatitis E is a major cause of enterically transmitted, water-borne hepatitis in developing countries.

Questions 27.2 to 27.5:

Match the appropriate virus from the following list with the statement to which it most closely corresponds. Each virus can match one, more than one, or none of the statements.

A. Hepatitis A virus (HAV)

B. Coxsackie viruses

C. Hepatitis C virus (HCV)

D. Hepatitis E virus (HEV)

E. Yellow fever virus

F. Rubella virus

27.2 Intravenous drug users are at high risk for the virus

> Correct answer = C. Until the recent development of tests for the presence of HCV in blood, HCV was an important cause of transfusion-associated hepatitis. IV drug users are one of several groups still at high risk for infection with this virus.

27.3 Infection is caused by the bite of an infected mosquito

> Correct answer = E. Yellow fever virus is an arthropod-borne virus, which is transmitted by the bite of an infected *Aedes aegypti* mosquito. The virus does not spread from person to person.

27.4 Predisposes to hepatocellular carcinoma

> Correct answer = C. Unlike HAV, HCV infection has a strong tendency to lead to a chronic hepatitis and cirrhosis, often resulting after many years in hepatocellular carcinoma.

27.5 Causes congenital malformations

> Correct answer = F. Infection with rubella virus is generally of little consequence to the adult. The exception is the pregnant woman, in whom rubella virus infection can result in congenital malformations in the fetus. The risk is highest in the first trimester. These malformations can affect the CNS, the liver, the heart, and the eye.

*"We're pretty sure it's West Nile Virus."*

# Retroviruses and AIDS

# 28

## I. OVERVIEW

The family Retroviridae includes a large number of disease-producing animal viruses, several of which are of clinical importance to humans (Figure 28.1). Retroviridae are distinguished from all other RNA viruses by the presence of an unusual enzyme, reverse transcriptase, which converts a single-stranded RNA viral genome into double-stranded viral DNA. Because these viruses reverse the order of information transfer (RNA serving as a template for DNA synthesis, rather than the almost universal DNA serving as a template for RNA synthesis), they are are termed retroviruses. [Note: "Retro" is Latin for backwards.] Retroviridae are divided into seven genera on the basis of nucleotide sequence similarity and genome structure. The two genera of human interest are the genus Lentivirus, which includes human immunodeficiency viruses 1 and 2 (HIV-1 and -2), and the human T-cell lymphotrophic virus–bovine leukemia virus group (HTLV-BLV group), which contains human T-cell leukemia viruses 1 and 2 (HTLV-1 and -2). The lentiviruses cause neurologic and immunologic diseases, but do not have the oncogenic properties of the HTLV-BLV group. The oncogenic capacity of the animal retroviruses and the hope of identifying one or more of them as a cause of human cancer, were reasons for their initial investigation. The discovery that acquired immunodeficiency syndrome (AIDS) is also caused by a retrovirus (HIV) greatly increased the attention given to this family of viruses. In this chapter, a consideration of the features common to all retroviruses is presented, following which HIV and HTLV are discussed in detail.

## II. RETROVIRUS STRUCTURE

Despite their wide range of disease manifestations, all retroviruses are similar in structure, genome organization, and mode of replication. Retroviruses are enveloped particles (Figure 28.2). The viral envelope, formed from the host cell membrane, contains spiked knobs. These consist of a transmembrane protein, TM (fusion protein, also called gp41), which is linked to a surface protein, and SU (attachment protein, gp120) that binds to a cell receptor during infection. Host cell proteins, including the major histocompatibility complex class II proteins, are also found in the envelope. The virion has a cone-shaped, icosahedral core

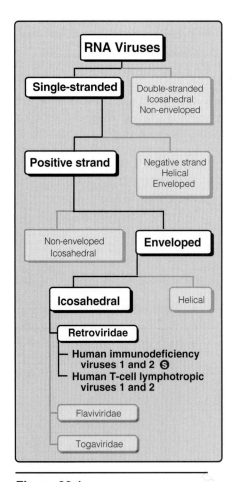

**Figure 28.1**
Classification of retroviruses that cause disease in humans. ⊙ See p. 331 for a summary of this virus.

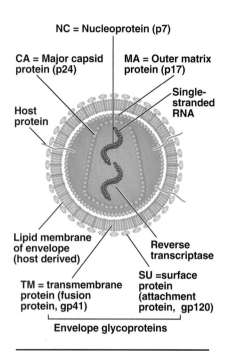

**Figure 28.2**
Structure of the human
immunodeficiency virus.

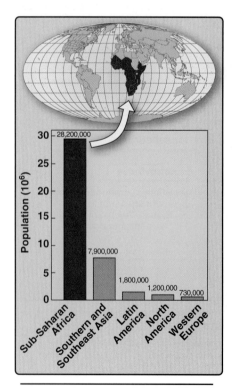

**Figure 28.3**
Estimated numbers of current HIV
infections or AIDS cases (2005).

containing the major capsid protein (CA also called p24). Between the capsid and the envelope is an outer matrix protein, MA (p17), which directs entry of the double-stranded DNA provirus into the nucleus, and is later essential for the process of virus assembly. There are two identical copies of the positive sense, single-stranded RNA genome in the capsid (that is, unlike other viruses, retroviruses are diploid). The RNA is tightly complexed with a basic protein, NC (p7), in a nucleocapsid structure that differs in morphology among the different retrovirus genera. [Note: The designation "gp41" refers to the structure of the molecule, which is a glycoprotein, whereas "p24" refers to a nonglycosylated protein.] Also found within the capsid are the enzymes reverse transcriptase and integrase (which are required for viral DNA synthesis and integration into the host cell chromosome) and protease (essential for virus assembly). A host cellular tRNA is hydrogen-bonded at the 5' end of each viral RNA molecule, where it functions as a primer for initiation of reverse transcription.

## III. HUMAN IMMUNODEFICIENCY VIRUS (HIV)

Acquired immune deficiency syndrome (AIDS) was first reported in the United States in 1981. The earliest cases of AIDS were seen in large urban centers, such as Los Angeles, San Francisco, and New York City. Clusters of young, male, homosexual patients exhibited a puzzling complex of symptoms, including severe pneumonia caused by *Pneumocystis jiroveci* (ordinarily a harmless eukaryotic organism), Kaposi sarcoma (ordinarily an extremely rare form of cancer), sudden weight loss, swollen lymph nodes, and general suppression of immune function. This constellation of signs and symptoms associated with illness came to be known as acquired immune deficiency syndrome (AIDS). Early attempts at understanding the disease focused on the possibility of immune suppression induced by chronic injectable drug use (IDU) or infection. Soon, however, cases were reported in nonhomosexual, non-IDU patients who had received blood or blood products by transfusion. By 1984, AIDS was recognized as an infectious disease caused by a virus, and eventually HIV was isolated from AIDS patients. In the decade after this initial recognition, AIDS killed more United States citizens than the Korean and Vietnam wars combined.

> At the beginning of the year 2000, more than 43,000,000 people worldwide were known to be infected with HIV. There were estimated to be about 5,000,000 new infections worldwide and 3,100,000 deaths due to AIDS in 2005.

Worldwide, new infections are almost equally distributed between men and women, with heterosexual activity accounting for the majority of cases. Although the United States and other developed countries have identified combinations of drugs that significantly slow the progression of AIDS, 95 percent of HIV-infected people live in developing countries where, for logistic and financial reasons, few have access to these drugs (Figures 28.3 and 28.4).

## A. Organization of the HIV genome

The HIV RNA genome contains three major genes: the *gag* gene that codes for CA, MA, and NC (core and matrix proteins), the *pol* gene that codes for reverse transcriptase, protease, integrase, and ribonuclease, and the *env* gene that codes for TM and SU (transmembrane and surface proteins). Genes for additional regulatory and accessory proteins of diverse function are located between the *pol* and *env* genes. At the 5' end of the viral RNA is a unique sequence, U5, which contains part of the site required for viral integration into the host cell chromosome and also the tRNA primer binding site for initiation of reverse transcription. At the 3' end of the viral RNA is the nucleotide sequence U3, which contains sequences that are important in the control of transcription of the DNA provirus (Figure 28.5). As with cellular mRNAs synthesized by RNA polymerase II, the 5' end of the viral RNA synthesized from proviral DNA has a methylated cap, and the 3' end has a poly-A tail.[1] At either end of the viral genome is a repeated sequence, R, which is involved in reverse transcription. Synthesis of the double-stranded DNA provirus results in duplication of the R and U sequences, producing two identical repeat units designated long terminal repeats (LTR). The genomic organization of the DNA provirus is illustrated in Figure 28.5. [Note: A brief overview of retrovirus replication is presented in Chapter 23 (see Figure 23.15, p. 241); additional details of some steps in the cycle are discussed below.]

## B. HIV Replication

The first phase of HIV replication, which includes viral entry, reverse transcription, and integration of the virus into the host genome, is accomplished by proteins provided by the virus. The second phase of replication, which includes the synthesis and processing of viral genomes, mRNAs, and structural proteins, uses the host cell machinery for transcription and protein synthesis. The end result of HIV replication in most cell types is cell death.

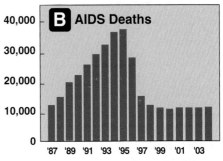

**Figure 28.4**
A. Incidence of AIDS in the United States. *Increase in 1993 resulted from several changes introduced in January 1993 in the case definition of AIDS.
B. Deaths due to AIDS in the United States. Data on deaths were unreliable until 1987.

**Figure 28.5**
HIV proviral genome. The *rev* and *tat* genes are divided into noncontiguous pieces, and the gene segments are spliced together in the RNA transcript.

[1]See p. 423 in *Lippincott's Illustrated Reviews: Biochemistry* (3rd ed.) for a discussion of the cap and poly-A tail of mRNA.

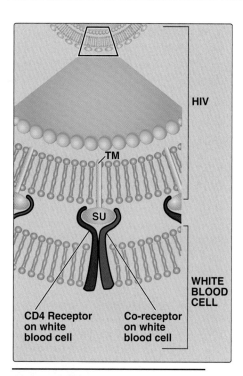

**Figure 28.6**
Binding of HIV to surface of lymphocyte.

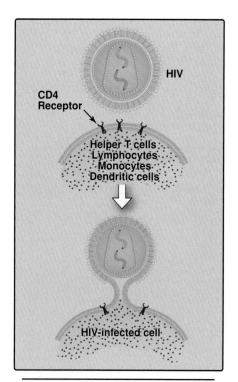

**Figure 28.7**
Attachment and entry of HIV virus.

1. **Attachment to a specific cell surface receptor:** Attachment is accomplished via the SU fragment of the *env* gene product on the surface of the HIV, which preferentially binds to a CD4 molecule (Figure 28.6). Thus, the virus infects helper T cells, lymphocytes, monocytes, and dendritic cells, which contain this protein in their cell membranes (Figure 28.7).

2. **Entry of virus into the cell:** An additional coreceptor—a chemokine receptor—is required for entry of the viral core into the cell (see Figure 28.6). [Note: A chemokine is a cytokine with chemotactic properties, produced by lymphocytes and macrophages.] Macrophages and T cells express different chemokine receptors that fulfill this function. Binding to a coreceptor activates the viral TM (fusion) glycoprotein, triggering fusion between the viral envelope and the cell membrane (Figure 28.8).

3. **Reverse transcription of viral RNA:** After entering the host cell, the HIV RNA is not translated. Instead, it is transcribed into DNA by reverse transcriptase—an RNA-directed DNA polymerase that enters host cells as part of the viral nucleocapsid (see Figure 28.8). A host cellular transfer RNA (tRNA) is hydrogen-bonded to a specific site on each viral RNA molecule, where it functions as a primer for initiation of reverse transcription. This process takes place in the cytoplasm, within the core structure. The viral reverse transcriptase first synthesizes a DNA-RNA hybrid molecule, then its RNase activity degrades the parental RNA molecule while synthesizing the second strand of DNA. This process results in duplication of the ends to form the long terminal repeats (LTR). The resulting linear molecule of double-stranded DNA is the provirus. LTRs at either end of the provirus contain promoter and enhancer sequences[2] that control expression of the viral DNA.

4. **Integration of the provirus into host cell DNA:** The provirus, still associated with virion core components, is transported to the nucleus with the aid of MA (matrix protein). There, viral integrase cleaves the chromosomal DNA and covalently inserts the provirus; the integrated provirus thus becomes a stable part of the cell genome (see Figure 28.8). The insertion is random with respect to the site of integration in the recipient DNA. Thus, HIV has two genomic forms; namely, single-stranded RNA present in the extracellular virus, and proviral double-stranded DNA within the cell.

5. **Transcription and translation of integrated viral DNA sequences:** The provirus is transcribed into a full-length mRNA by the cell RNA polymerase II. The genome-length mRNA has at least three functions: 1) Some copies will be the genomes of progeny virus, and are transported to the cytoplasm in preparation for viral assembly. 2) Some copies are translated to produce the virion

[2]See p. 442 in *Lippincott's Illustrated Reviews: Biochemistry* (3rd ed.) for a discussion of the role of promoters and enhancers in gene regulation.

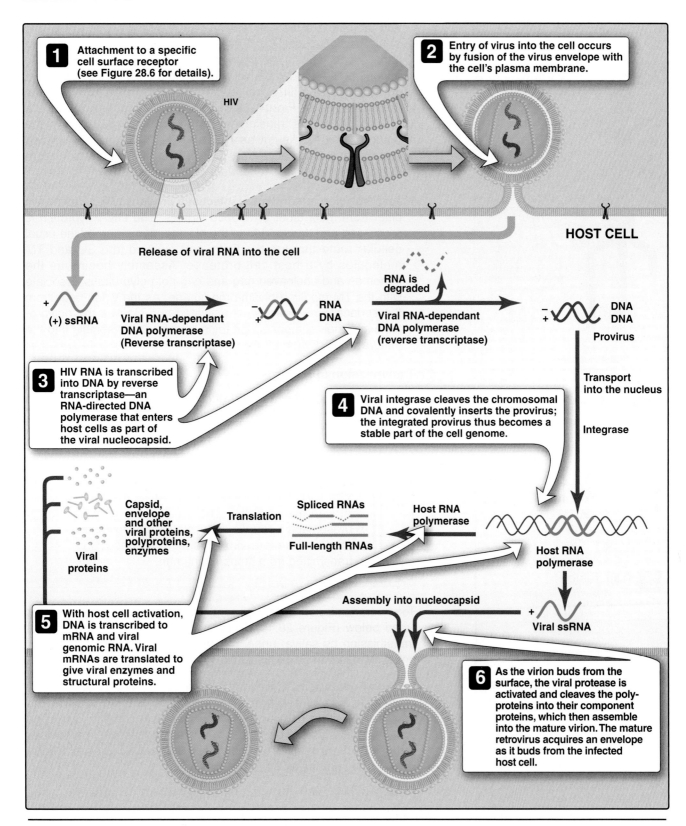

**Figure 28.8**
The HIV replication cycle.

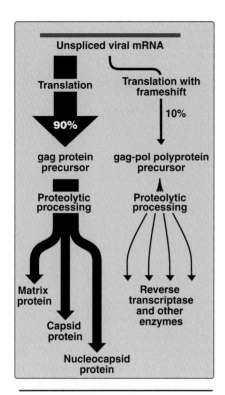

**Figure 28.9**
Processing of gag and gag-pol polyprotein precursor proteins by the viral protease.

**Figure 28.10**
Common modes of transmission of HIV.

gag proteins. Further, by reading past the stop codon at the end of the *gag* gene about one of twenty times, a gag-pol polyprotein is produced. This is the source of the viral reverse transcriptase and integrase that will be incorporated into the virion. 3) Still other copies of viral RNA are spliced, creating new translatable sequences (see Figure 28.8). In all retroviruses, one of the spliced mRNAs is translated into the envelope proteins. In the complex viruses, such as HIV and HTLV, additional spliced molecules produce accessory proteins that are important in regulating transcription and other aspects of replication.

6. **Assembly and maturation of infectious progeny:** These pathways differ from most other enveloped viruses. The env polyprotein is processed and transported to the plasma membrane by the usual cellular route through the Golgi and cleaved into SU and TM molecules by a host cell protease. Assembly begins as the genomes and uncleaved gag and gag-pol polyproteins associate with the TM-modified plasma membrane. As the virion buds from the surface, viral protease is activated and cleaves the polyproteins into their component proteins, which then assemble into the mature virion (Figure 28.9).

## C. Transmission of HIV

It is unclear how and where HIV originated. The virus was shown to be related to simian (monkey) immunodeficiency virus. It is speculated that the emergence of HIV began in the early 1950s, after the monkey virus mutated and began infecting humans.

> The first documented case of AIDS was in an African man in 1959. The initial infections were presumably sporadic and isolated until mutations produced a more virulent strain that was readily transmitted from human to human.

Today, transmission of HIV generally occurs by one of four routes listed below (Figure 28.10). There has been no firm evidence for transmission by saliva, urine, nonsexual contact in which blood is not exchanged, or by an insect bite.

1. **Sexual contact:** HIV, present in both semen and vaginal secretions, is transmitted primarily as cell-associated virus in the course of either homosexual or heterosexual contact. Disruption of mucosal surfaces by sexually transmitted diseases, particularly those such as syphilis and chancroid that result in genital ulcerations, may greatly facilitate HIV-1 infection.

2. **Transfusions:** HIV has been transmitted by transfusion with whole blood, plasma, clotting factors, or cellular fractions of blood.

3. **Contaminated needles:** Transmission can occur by inoculation with HIV-contaminated needles—either accidentally, or through use of shared needles or syringes by drug users.

**4. Perinatal transmission:** An HIV-infected woman has a fifteen to forty percent chance of transmitting the infection to her newborn, either transplacentally during passage of the baby through the birth canal, or via breast-feeding.

> ‖ Because of the high rates of HIV-1 infection in women of childbearing age in developing countries, perinatally acquired HIV-1 infection is responsible for approximately twenty percent of all AIDS cases in these areas.

Figure 28.11 compares the modes of transmission worldwide with those occurring in the United States.

### D. Pathogenesis and clinical significance of HIV infection

The pathology of HIV disease results from either tissue destruction by the virus itself or the host's response to virus-infected cells. In addition, HIV can induce an immunodeficient state that leads to opportunistic diseases that are rare in the absence of HIV infection. The progression from HIV infection to AIDS develops in fifty percent of HIV-infected individuals in an average of ten years, and, if untreated, it is uniformly fatal—generally within two years of diagnosis. However, there is a significant fraction (about ten percent) of HIV-infected individuals who have not developed AIDS after twenty years. Development from HIV infection to end-stage AIDS progresses through several phases (Figure 28.12).

**1. Initial infection:** After the acquisition of HIV, the initially infected cells are generally macrophages within the genital tract. From this initial localized infection, HIV disseminates via the blood, and virus may then localize in dendritic cells throughout the lymphoid tissue. From the surface of follicular dendritic cells, HIV can then infect CD4+ lymphocytes moving through the germinal centers of lymph nodes. This process creates a reservoir of chronically HIV-infected cells within the lymphatic tissue of the body.

**2. Acute phase viremia:** Several weeks after the initial infection with HIV, one third to two thirds of individuals experience an acute disease syndrome (also referred to as the primary infection) similar to infectious mononucleosis. During this period, there is a high level of virus replication occurring in CD4+ cells. Large amounts of virus and capsid protein (CA antigen) are present in the blood, and circulating antibody appears in one to ten weeks after the initial infection (seroconversion). A constant level of virus and virus-infected cells is maintained by a combination of replacement of the CD4+ cells killed by HIV infection with cells newly produced in lymphoid organs and the subsequent infection of these new cells with progeny virus. Lymph nodes also become infected during this time; they later serve as the sites of virus persistence during the asymptomatic period.

**Figure 28.11**
Modes of HIV transmission in United States compared with those worldwide. (A) In United States, the primary mode of HIV transmission is homosexual sex. Transmission in western Europe is similar to that in the United States. (B) In most of the world, transmission is primarily by heterosexual sex. [Note: Segment labeled "Other" includes perinatal transmission.]

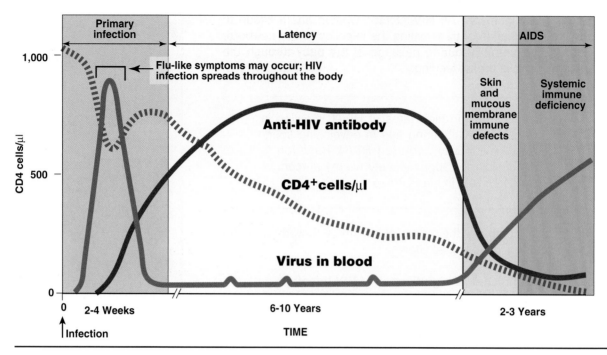

**Figure 28.12**
Typical time course of HIV infection.

3. **Latent period:** The acute phase viremia is eventually reduced significantly with the appearance of a HIV-specific cytotoxic T-lymphocyte response, followed by a humoral antibody response. A clinically asymptomatic or "latent" period lasting from months to many years follows the acute infection. During this latent period, the majority (ninety percent) of HIV proviruses are transcriptionally silent, so that only ten percent of the cells containing integrated HIV DNA also contain viral mRNA or viral proteins. There are transient peaks of viremia that are often correlated with stimulation of the immune system by infection with other pathogens or by immunization. Although there is continuous loss of those CD4+ cells in which HIV is replicating, active replacement through stem cell multiplication compensates for this loss, and the CD4+ count declines only slowly over a period of years. In addition, the host immune response is still sufficiently effective to maintain a relatively stable, low level of virus production. It has been estimated that $10^{11}$ virions and $10^9$ CD4 T cells are produced each day. Virus isolated during this period is also less cytopathic for CD4+ cells and replicates more slowly than does that isolated later during symptomatic AIDS. Despite the nearly normal levels of CD4+ cells, however, impairment of T-cell responses to specific antigens is evident. The infection remains relatively clinically asymptomatic as long as the immune system is functional.

> The actual level of virus replication in peripheral blood cells varies greatly among patients, and those with a higher steady-state viral load progress more rapidly to symptomatic AIDS and death.

**4. Clinical complications of HIV infection during the latent period:** During this period—whose length is variable, but lasts on average about ten years—there are multiple, nonspecific conditions, such as persistent, generalized lymphadenopathy (swollen lymph nodes), diarrhea, chronic fevers, night sweats, and weight loss. The more common opportunistic infections such as herpes zoster and candidiasis may occur repeatedly during this period, as well as when patients progress to AIDS. The CD4+ cell count remains normal or gradually declines, but is greater than 200/μl.

**5. Progression to AIDS:** The progression from asymptomatic infection to AIDS is not sudden, but in fact occurs as a continuum of clinical states. A number of virologic and immunologic changes occur that affect the rate of this progression. For example, coinfection with a number of the herpesviruses, such as human herpesvirus type 6 (see p. 255), can transactivate transcription from the silent HIV provirus, increasing HIV replication. Any stimulation of an immune response causing activation of resting T cells also activates HIV replication. Not only does this increase the number of infected CD4+ cells, but it also increases the opportunity to create generations of virus mutants. Eventually, a more highly cytocidal, more rapidly multiplying variant appears. In addition, these variants are often highly syncytium-inducing, promoting fusion between infected and previously uninfected cells. T-cell precursors in the lymphoid organs are also infected and killed, so the capacity to generate new CD4+ cells is gradually lost. The capacity to contain the infection is further compromised by the appearance of HIV mutants with altered antigenic specificity, which are not recognized by the existing humoral antibody or cytotoxic T lymphocytes. The eventual result of these accumulating, interacting factors is an increasingly rapid decline in CD4+ count, accompanied by loss of immune capacity.

> With the CD4+ count falling below 200/ml and the appearance of increasingly frequent and serious diseases and opportunistic infections ("AIDS-defining illnesses"), the patient is said to have AIDS.

**6. End-stage AIDS:** Nearly all systems of the body can be affected as a result of HIV infection, either by HIV itself or by opportunistic organisms. The weakening immune system leads to many complications including malignancies.

    **a. Spread of HIV to additional body sites:** Cell types other than CD4+ lymphocytes can be infected by HIV. Infection of these cells produces some of the additional manifestations of end-stage disease. Chief among these are infected cells of the monocyte-macrophage lineage, which are not killed as rapidly as CD4+ T cells and can transport the virus into other organs (Figure 28.13). For example, macrophages are the HIV-infected cells present in brains of patients with AIDS encephalopathy,

**Figure 28.13**
Pathogenesis of HIV.

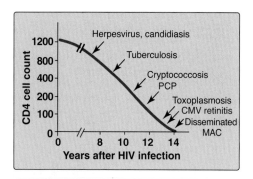

**Figure 28.14**
Pattern of opportunistic infections associated with declining CD4+ cell counts. CMV = Cytomegalovirus; MAC = *Mycobacterium avium* complex; PCP = *Pneumocystis jirovecci* pneumonia.

which typically evolves over a period of one year, with gradual deterioration resulting in severe dementia. This appears to be unrelated to CD4+ depletion, but rather to an expanded host range of variant HIV. The basis for damage to neuronal cells is, however, not known. Similarly, the wasting syndrome seen in late stages of AIDS is probably related to HIV-infected macrophages induced to produce various cytokines, especially tumor necrosis factor. Virus has also been found in Langerhans cells in the skin, dendritic cells in lymph nodes, and monocytes in bone marrow, but their significance in the disease process is not clear. The eye is another site affected by HIV infection itself, which produces focal areas of ischemia in the retina. HIV infection of blood cell progenitors in the bone marrow leads to the anemia seen in most AIDS patients.

b. **Opportunistic infections in AIDS:** Multiple recurrent bouts of infections with fungi, bacteria, and viruses occur as the CD4+ cell count declines (Figure 28.14). For example, the nervous system can be the site of opportunistic infections with *Toxoplasma*, *Cryptococcus*, JC virus, and *Mycobacteria*. The eye cannot only be infected with HIV, but also with opportunistic agents, the most prominent of which is cytomegalovirus (CMV)—a cause of retinal destruction. The lungs are also primarily affected by opportunistic infections, *P. jirovecci* pneumonia being one of the most common. Mycobacterial infections are also a common problem in the lung; for example, currently thirty percent of AIDS patients die from tuberculosis (see p. 186). Serious gastrointestinal tract illnesses are due to opportunistic pathogens, but these may be in concert with HIV infection. CMV colitis is a common problem, but HIV is often present as well. Protozoal parasitic diseases, as well as infections with gram-negative enteric bacteria are other sources of gastrointestinal disorders. The immune deficiency also provides the opportunity for latent herpesvirus infections to recur repeatedly or become chronic and spread extensively. Mucocutaneous candidiasis (for example, oral, esophageal, or vaginal) is an ongoing problem in AIDS patients as well. In fact, vaginal candidiasis is the most frequent reason HIV-infected females seek medical attention. (See Figure 28.16 for a summary of common AIDS-defining opportunistic infections.)

c. **Malignancies associated with AIDS:** A number of malignancies commonly arise in HIV-infected patients. The most characteristic neoplasm present in AIDS patients is Kaposi sarcoma (KS), which involves skin, mucous membranes, and deep viscera. Various lymphomas, including those of the CNS, are also common. These are probably the result of the immune compromise and not HIV itself. KS has been associated with human herpesvirus, type 8 (HHV-8, Figure 28.15). In AIDS patients, body cavity lymphomas are also usually associated with HHV-8 infection, whereas many other lymphomas are EBV-associated (see p. 268).

**Figure 28.15**
Herpesvirus 8 virions (arrows) associated with Kaposi sarcoma.

### E. Laboratory identification

1. **Demonstration of virus or virus components:** Amplification of viral RNA or DNA proviruses by the PCR technique (see p. 30) is the most sensitive method for early detection of virus in blood or tissue specimens. Recent adaptation of the technique to obtain quantitative estimates of viral load (measured, for example, as the amount of viral RNA per milliliter of blood plasma) now permit evaluation of the stage of the disease, effectiveness of a drug regimen, and prognosis. For purposes of initial screening of the blood supply, ELISA testing (see p. 28) for the CA (p24) antigen in serum can detect infection in individuals who are infectious but undetectable by screening for anti-HIV antibodies.

2. **Demonstration of immune response:** The usual screening procedure for HIV infection is a two-step process, used both for purposes of diagnosing individuals who may be infected and for protection of the blood supply. The first step in screening is an ELISA procedure (see p. 28) in which the serum sample is reacted with whole virus lysates or synthetic HIV peptides. The latter can detect antibody much earlier than the former and is now standard. At its most sensitive, there is still a 25-day window between the time that virus is first present in the blood and antibody can be detected. Although the ELISA test is highly specific, there are false-positives, so any positive result is confirmed using the Western blot technique.[3]

### F. Treatment

Because of the progressive nature of the disease, it is the HIV infection that is treated as the clinical problem, rather than focusing on the end stage—AIDS—alone. Virtually every step in the HIV replication cycle is a potential target for an antiviral drug, but only those directed against reverse transcriptase, viral protease, and viral fusion have thus far been used successfully (Figure 28.17). Used early in the infection, a combination of three different drugs administered together can reduce the plasma viral load to undetectable levels—at least temporarily.

1. **Strategy for multiple-drug therapy in treating HIV infections:** Unlike DNA polymerase, which makes few mistakes in the replication of DNA because of its proofreading activity, reverse transcriptase has no ability to proofread. Therefore, DNA synthesis by the viral reverse transcriptase produces many errors (about one per cycle of synthesis). This results in mutations in all of the HIV genes, and accumulation of a pool of mutant viruses in any individual patient. In the presence of an antiviral drug, there is strong selection for mutations that confer resistance to that drug, and the high mutation rate ensures that such mutations will occur. The answer to this therapeutic dilemma has been to use multiple drugs that act on different steps in the viral replication cycle because the probability of several different mutations occurring simultaneously in the appropriate genes in the same genome is low. In addition, certain drug combinations are synergistic, the effect on reducing viral load being considerably greater than merely the sum of the

**A Currently available drugs**

**Nucleoside/-tide reverse transcriptase inhibitors:**
- *Abacavir*
- *Didanosine*
- *Emtricitabine*
- *Lamivudine*
- *Stavudine*
- *Tenofovir*
- *Zalcitabine*
- *Zidovudine*

Nonnucleoside reverse transcriptase inhibitors:
- *Delavirdine*
- *Efavirenz*
- *Nevirapine*

**Protease inhibitors:**
- *Amprenavir*
- *Atazanavir*
- *Indinavir*
- *Lopinavir*
- *Nelfinavir*
- *Ritonavir*
- *Saquinavir*

Fusion inhibitor: • *Enfuvirtide*

**B Combination therapy**

Two nucleoside/-tide reverse transcriptase inhibitors
plus
One protease inhibitor

Two nucleoside/-tide reverse transcriptase inhibitors
plus
A non-nucleoside reverse transcriptase inhibitor

**Figure 28.16**
Highly active antiretroviral therapy (HAART).

[3]See p. 464 in *Lippincott's Illustrated Reviews: Biochemistry* (3rd ed.) for a discussion of the use of ELISA assay and Western blots in testing for HIV exposure.

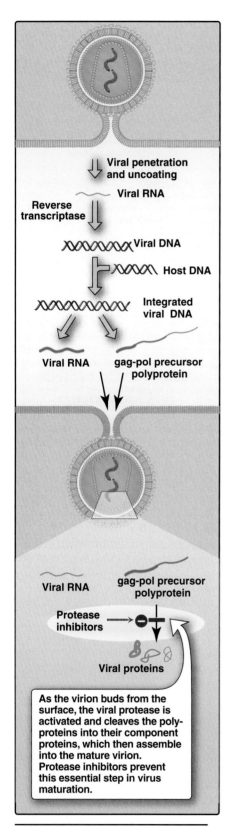

**Figure 28.17**
Role of HIV protease in viral
replication.

individual drug effects. The use of potent combination regimens can limit viral replication and dissemination to lymphoid tissue, creating a smaller reservoir of chronically infected cells, and limiting the potential for viral mutations (acquired during the replicative process) that could lead to acquisition of drug resistance. However, even this approach is not entirely effective because HIV also exhibits a relatively high rate of recombination, enabling mutations from two different genomes to be combined into one virus particle.

2. **Early therapy:** Approaches to therapy are evolving as more is learned about the nature of the disease. For example, it has been determined that the steady-state level of replicating virus in the plasma—the "viral load"—is a prognostic indicator of the rate of progression to AIDS. This has led to the principle that HIV infection should be treated as aggressively and as early as possible, minimizing the initial spread of the virus. Not only does this approach yield a lower steady-state level of virus, but it has the additional advantage of drugs being administered at a time when mutants are still rare, so that the drugs are more effective than they would be if given later in the infection.

3. **Highly active antiretroviral therapy:** Currently, combinations of various drugs described below that are given three at a time are being evaluated for efficacy, both in short-term reduction of viral load and/or increase in CD4+ cell count, and in long-term survival. Choice of a drug regimen is individualized based on criteria such as tolerability, drug-drug interactions, convenience/adherence, and possible baseline resistance. [Note: All such multiple-drug therapies are commonly referred to as "highly active antiretroviral therapy" or HAART (see Figure 28.17).] Unfortunately, whereas multidrug therapies can lower the viral load to undetectable levels, virus re-emerges if HAART is stopped, indicating that the HIV has not been eradicated. Therefore, with current drug therapy, HIV continues to exist in sanctuaries, such as the central nervous system (CNS), semen, or nonreplicating T-lymphocyte reservoirs. Thus, HIV infection is currently both chronic and incurable.

   a. **Nucleoside and nucleotide analog reverse transcriptase inhibitors:** Reverse transcriptase inhibitors prevent the copying of the HIV RNA genome into a proviral DNA genome. There are both nucleoside analogs and nonnucleoside inhibitors of the viral reverse transcriptase.[4] Nucleoside and nucleotide analogs inhibit primarily by serving as chain terminators after insertion into the growing DNA chain by the reverse transcriptase. Zidovudine (AZT), which is a pyrimidine analog, is an example of such a drug. Other examples include didanosine (ddI), zalcitabine (ddC), lamivudine (3TC), stavudine, emtricitabine, tenofovir, and abacavir.[5] Resistant mutants inevitably arise after long-term treatment with any one of these drugs; however, because cross-resistance is incomplete, AZT in combination with one of the other drugs has been successful in minimizing the effect of mutation. Significant adverse effects accompany use of these drugs; for example, macrocytic ane-

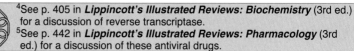
[4]See p. 405 in *Lippincott's Illustrated Reviews: Biochemistry* (3rd ed.) for a discussion of reverse transcriptase.
[5]See p. 442 in *Lippincott's Illustrated Reviews: Pharmacology* (3rd ed.) for a discussion of these antiviral drugs.

mia with AZT and peripheral neuropathy with ddI and ddC. The use of combined therapy in some cases permits less toxic doses to be administered.

b. **The nonnucleoside reverse transcriptase inhibitors** act by targeting the reverse transcriptase itself. They bind in a noncompetitive, reversible manner to a unique site on the enzyme, altering its ability to function. Their major advantage is their lack of effect on the host blood-forming elements and lack of cross-resistance with nucleoside analog reverse transcriptase inhibitors. A number of these drugs have been developed, including efavirenz, delaviridine, and nevirapine. Resistance to these compounds develops much more rapidly than that against the nucleoside analogs.

c. **Protease inhibitors:** The products of the *gag* and *pol* genes are translated initially into large polyprotein precursors that must be cleaved by the viral protease to yield the mature proteins. Protease inhibitors, which include ritonavir, nelfinavir, saquinavir, amprenavir, indinavir, and lopinavir interfere with the processing of the polyproteins in the budding virion and result in noninfectious particles (Figure 28.18). However, viral resistance develops if protease inhibitors are used alone. Further, lipodystrophy (redistribution of fat, so that the limbs become skinny and fat is deposited along the abdomen and the upper back) and hyperglycemia can occur with these drugs.

d. **Viral fusion inhibitor:** Enfuvirtide is a 36 amino acid peptide that binds to gp41 and inhibits the fusion of HIV with the membrane of the host cell.

4. **Effect of HAART on the incidence of opportunistic infections:** The incidence of opportunistic infections in AIDS patients is decreasing in response to widespread use of aggressive multidrug treatment. This is true for virtually all opportunistic infections (Figure 28.19).

5. **Perinatal treatment:** Zidovudine when administered to HIV-1–infected pregnant women during the second and third trimesters of pregnancy, followed by administration to the infants during the first six weeks of life, reduces risk of maternal-infant transmission of HIV-1 from approximately 23 percent to 8 percent. The availability of this effective intervention, which decreases perinatal transmission of HIV-1 has led to increased efforts to screen all pregnant women (with their consent) for the presence of HIV-1 infection. [Note: Postnatal transmission of HIV via breast milk can, however, occur.]

## G. Prevention

Due to lower availability of antiretroviral drugs in developing countries and lack of a vaccine, education concerning methods for preventing transmission of HIV is currently the primary means of preventing spread of the virus.

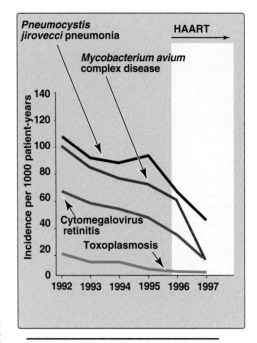

**Figure 31.18**
Incidence of selected opportunistic infections in patients with HIV infection. [Note: The shaded area labeled "HAART" indicates the period of wide availability of highly active anti-retroviral therapy (HAART). The decline in opportunistic infections after 1995 largely reflects the effect of HAART.]

**Figure 28.19**
Typical "cloverleaf" appearance of
nuclei of HTLV-1 infected adult
T-cell leukemic cells.

1. **Attempts to produce a vaccine:** An effective vaccine is not yet available despite intensive efforts to produce one. HIV has a high mutation rate, and antigenically distinct strains exist worldwide.

2. **Other measures:** Screening of the blood supply has nearly eliminated transmission by that route. Perinatal transmission can be reduced by nearly seventy percent with AZT therapy of the pregnant woman, followed by several weeks of AZT to the newborn. Strict adherence to standard precautions by healthcare workers can minimize risk in that setting.

> Is is recommended that physicians screen for HIV infection in all adolescents and adults at increased risk of HIV infection.

## IV. HUMAN T-CELL LYMPHOTROPHIC VIRUSES, TYPES 1 AND 2

HTLV-1 and -2 share about 65 percent nucleotide sequence homology, and therefore are genetically and biologically similar. However, their worldwide distribution is different. HTLV-1 has definitively been associated with a human malignant disease; adult T-cell leukemia (ATL); and a less common neurologic condition, HTLV-associated myelopathy (HAM). HTLV-2 infection causes a rare form of cancer, hairy cell leukemia.

### A. Transmission of HTLV

The distribution of HTLV infection varies greatly with geographic area and socioeconomic group. For example, the overall incidence of antibody in United States blood donors is about 1 in 2500, whereas about 25 percent of New York City intravenous drug users are infected with either HTLV-1 or -2. HTLV-2 infection is also high among the Native American population of the southwestern United States. HTLV transmission occurs primarily by cell-associated virus, via one of three routes. First, in highly endemic regions, mother to fetus or newborn is the most common mode of transmission. This is accomplished via infected lymphocytes either transplacentally or in breast milk. Second, infection can be transmitted sexually by infected lymphocytes contained in semen. Third, any blood products containing intact cells are also a potential source of infection. There is little evidence for transmission by cell-free fluids.

### B. Pathogenesis and clinical significance of adult T-cell leukemia

HTLV-1 infection both stimulates mitosis and immortalizes T lymphocytes, which acquire an "antigen-activated" phenotype. Following infection, the virus becomes integrated in the host cell as a provirus and transforms a polyclonal population of T cells. Although these cells all have an integrated provirus, there is no common integration site in different tumors. No HTLV mRNA is transcribed and no recognized oncogene is activated. However, in the course of continued multiplication over a period of many years, the infected T cells accumulate many chromosomal aberrations, leading to selection of monoclonal populations of cells that have an increasingly malignant phenotype (Figure 28.20). The majority of infected individuals are asymptomatic carriers who have an estimated one percent chance of developing adult T-cell leukemia (ATL) within their lifetime. ATL typically appears twenty to thirty years after initial infection, when an increasingly larger population of monoclonal malignant ATL cells develops and infiltration of various visceral organs by these cells occurs. There are accompanying serum chemistry abnormalities, and impairment of the immune system leads to opportunistic infections [for example, by human cytomegalovirus (see p. 263)], *P. jiroveci* (see p. 215), and/or various disseminated fungal and bacterial infections]. Median survival after appearance of acute ATL is about six months.

### C. Pathogenesis and clinical significance of HTLV-associated myelopathy

HTLV-associated myelopathy (HAM) is distinctly different from ATL in that it usually appears only a few years after infection. CNS involvement is indicated by: 1) the presence of anti-HTLV-1 antibody in the CSF; 2) lymphocytic infiltration and demyelination of the thoracic spinal cord; and 3) brain lesions. The lymphocyte count is normal, although there is a polyclonal nonmalignant fraction with integrated HTLV. HAM occurs with lower frequency than ATL among HTLV-infected populations. It is characterized by progressive spasticity and weakness of the extremities, urinary and fecal incontinence, hyperreflexia, and some peripheral sensory loss.

### D. Pathogenesis and clinical significance of hairy cell leukemia

This disease, caused by HTLV-2, is a rare, lymphocytic leukemia that is usually of B cell origin. It is characterized by malignant cells that look ciliated (Figure 28.21). These cells replace bone marrow and infiltrate the spleen, causing splenomegaly.

### E. Laboratory identification

Screening of blood donors for HTLV is done by ELISA or agglutination tests (see p. 28), but the existence of false-positives necessitates confirmatory testing by Western blotting. Test sensitivity is also a problem caused by the low and variable antibody titers in infected individuals.

### F. Treatment and prevention

The usual agents used in cancer chemotherapy have proven to be ineffective in treating ATL, and attempts to treat HAM have for the most part been equally unsuccessful. An estimated ten to twenty million people worldwide are infected with HTLV-1 or -2, and five percent of these will eventually develop either ATL or HAM. Screening of blood donors can effectively prevent transmission by transfusions, but the other modes of transmission could best be controlled by use of a vaccine. None is currently available for human use, but trials of experimental vaccines are in progress.

**Figure 28.20**
Appearance of hairy cell leukemia, a neoplasm of B lymphocytes caused by HTLV-2.

## Study Questions

**Choose the ONE correct answer**

28.1 Current approaches to therapy of AIDS involve the use of multiple drugs because

A. it is not known which one will be effective.

B. mutants resistant to any one drug appear rapidly, but the chance for appearance of mutants resistant to all of them is small.

C. all inhibit the same step in replication, thereby increasing their effectiveness.

D. this is the most effective means of curing cells of integrated HIV genomes.

E. each tends to neutralize the toxicity of the others.

Correct answer = B. The major problem with chemotherapy of AIDS is the high mutation rate of the virus, leading to rapid appearance of mutants resistant to any single drug. By choosing drugs that act at different steps in the replication cycle or with different mechanisms of action, mutations in each of the affected proteins would have to occur in the same virus genome. The chance for this to occur is considerably lower than for either one individually. D: There is no way known to cure cells of their integrated genomes. E: Whereas these drugs do not neutralize each other's toxicity, it is possible in some cases to use a lower dose of each of the drugs, decreasing the toxic adverse effects.

28.2 The "asymptomatic period" following the initial acute disease caused by HIV infection is characterized by

A. high levels of HIV replication in lymphoid tissue.

B. high levels of HIV replication in circulating T lymphocytes.

C. inability of the immune system to respond to antigenic stimuli.

D. absence of detectable HIV genomes or mRNA in circulating lymphocytes.

E. high titers of free virus in the blood.

Correct answer = A. During this period, a relatively large fraction of circulating lymphocytes can be shown to contain integrated HIV genomes, but a considerably smaller fraction have HIV mRNA, and virus replication occurs in relatively few cells. Infectious virus is largely confined to the lymphoid organs, although occasional bursts of viremia do occur, usually as the result of antigenic stimulation. The immune system retains its ability to respond to mitogenic stimuli generally, but there is some impairment of responses to specific antigens.

28.3 After infection of a cell by a retrovirus, synthesis of progeny genomes is carried out by

A. the DNA-dependent RNA polymerase activity of viral reverse transcriptase.

B. the retrovirus RNA-dependent RNA polymerase.

C. the host-cell DNA polymerase.

D. a host-cell RNA polymerase.

E. a complex of reverse transcriptase and a second virus protein that enables it to synthesize RNA rather than DNA.

Correct answer = D. Progeny virus RNA is synthesized by the same transcription process as that of cellular genes. A and E: Reverse transcriptase is involved only in the initial step, converting the infecting parental RNA genome into dsDNA. B: Unlike other RNA viruses, retroviruses do not encode an RNA-dependent RNA polymerase. C: The host cell DNA polymerase replicates the integrated provirus, but plays no role in synthesis of progeny.

*"Of course my cough is productive!"*

# Negative-strand RNA Viruses

# 29

## I. OVERVIEW

Medically important negative-strand RNA viruses are shown in Figure 29.1. They have several things in common: 1) they are all enveloped; 2) their virions contain an RNA-dependent RNA transcriptase that synthesizes viral mRNAs using the genomic negative-strand RNA as a template; 3) the genomic negative-strand viral RNAs are not infectious, in contrast to the genomic RNAs of positive-strand viruses (see p. 283); and 4) following entry and penetration, the first step in the replication of negative-strand RNA viruses is the synthesis of mRNAs, whereas with positive-strand RNA viruses, the first step in replication is translation of the incoming genomic RNA (see p. 239). Some negative-strand RNA viruses have segmented genomes, whereas others have nonsegmented genomes. Although most of these viruses replicate in the cytosol, the replication of influenza virus RNA (an orthomyxovirus) occurs in the nucleus.

## II. FAMILY RHABDOVIRIDAE

Rhabdoviruses are enveloped, bullet-shaped viruses (Figure 29.2). Each contains a helical nucleocapsid (see p. 235). The viruses in the family Rhabdoviridae known to infect mammals are divided into two genera: Lyssavirus (rabies virus, the rhabdovirus of greatest medical importance to humans), and Vesiculovirus [vesicular stomatitis virus (VSV), a virus of horses and cattle, and the best studied virus in this family]. Other rhabdoviruses infect invertebrates, plants, or other vertebrates.

### A. Epidemiology

A wide variety of wildlife, such as raccoons, skunks, squirrels, foxes, and bats, provide a reservoir for the rabies virus (Figure 29.3B). In third-world countries, domestic dogs and cats also constitute an important reservoir for rabies.

> Cases of human rabies are rare in the United States. However, in developing areas such as rural Africa and Asia, it is estimated that there are 55,000 deaths a year caused by rabies.

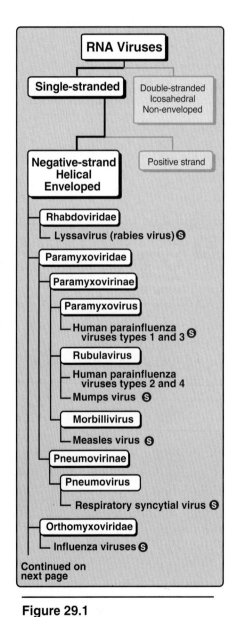

**Figure 29.1**
Classification of negative-strand RNA viruses (continued on next page). ⓢ See p. 331 for summaries of these viruses.

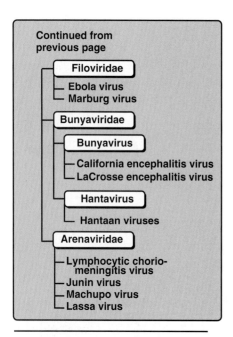

**Figure 29.1** (continued)
Classification of negative-strand
RNA viruses.

Humans are usually infected by the bite of an animal, but in some cases, infection is via an aerosol (for example, of droppings from infected bats).

 Sequence analysis of the viral RNA has shown that most human cases in the United States are from a bat strain of rabies virus.

### B. Viral replication

The genomic negative-strand RNA is nonsegmented. The virion contains five proteins, one of which, the G (for glyco-) protein, is an envelope protein that comprises viral spikes (see Figure 29.2). The rabies virion attaches via its glycoprotein spikes to cell-surface receptors. Entry into the cell is by receptor-mediated endocytosis, following which the viral envelope fuses with the endocytotic vesicle's membrane, releasing the viral nucleocapsid into the cytosol where replication occurs. Five different mRNAs are transcribed from the genomic RNA template by the virion's RNA-dependent RNA polymerase (transcriptase function), and each encodes one of five viral proteins. [Note: The polymerase that produces the mRNA also synthesizes positive-strand copies of the viral RNA template (replicase function), from which new negative-strand RNA genomic molecules can be transcribed.] This process is an example of the Type II virus genome replication described on p. 240. Viral structural proteins plus the negative-strand viral RNA form new helical nucleocapsids, which move to the cell surface. There, each nucleocapsid acquires its envelope by budding through a region of virus-modified plasma membrane (see Figure 23.16, p. 242).

### C. Pathology

Following inoculation, the virus may replicate locally, but then travels via the axoplasm of peripheral neurons to the brain, where it replicates primarily in the gray matter (Figure 29.3A). From the brain, the rabies virus can travel along autonomic nerves, leading to infection of the lungs, kidney, adrenal medulla, and salivary glands. [Note: Contamination of saliva potentially leads to further transmission of the disease; for example, through a bite from an infected animal.] The incubation period is extremely variable, depending on the host's resistance, amount of virus transferred, and distance of the site of initial infection from the central nervous system (CNS). Incubation generally lasts one to eight weeks, but may range up to several months or, in unusual cases, as long as several years following exposure. Clinical illness may begin with an abnormal sensation at the site of the bite, then progress to a fatal encephalitis, with neuronal degeneration of the brain and spinal cord. Symptoms include hallucinations, seizures, weakness, mental dysfunction, paralysis, coma, and finally death. Many, but not all, patients show the classic rabid sign of hydrophobia (in this case, "hydrophobia" refers to an infected individual's painful inability to swallow liquids, leading to avoidance). Once symptoms begin, death is inevitable.

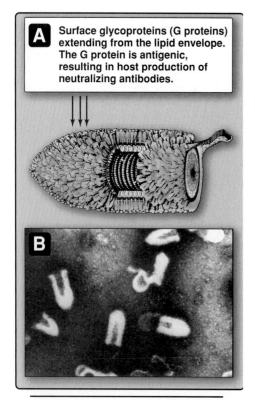

**Figure 29.2**
Rabies virus. A. Schematic drawing.
B. Electron micrograph.

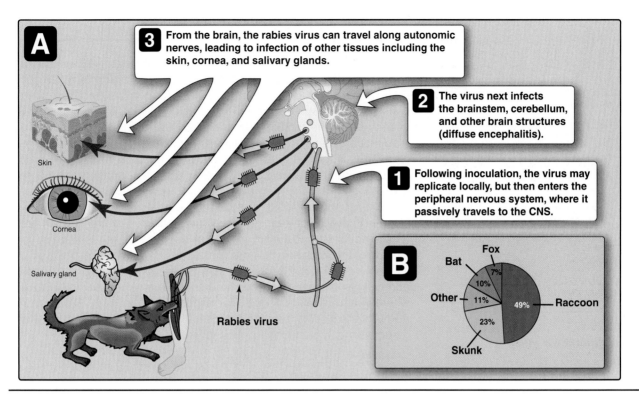

**Figure 29.3**
A. Schematic representation of pathogenesis of rabies infection. B. Wildlife rabies in the United States.

## D. Laboratory identification

Clinically, diagnosis rests on a history of exposure and signs and symptoms characteristic of rabies. However, a reliable history of exposure is often not obtainable, and the clinical presentation, especially in the initial stages, may not be characteristic. Therefore, a clinical diagnosis may be difficult. Postmortem, in approximately eighty percent of cases, characteristic eosinophilic cytoplasmic inclusions (Negri bodies) may be identified in certain regions of the brain, such as the hippocampus; these inclusion bodies are diagnostic of rabies (Figure 29.4). Prior to death, the diagnosis can be made by identification of viral antigens in biopsies of skin from the back of the neck or from corneal cells or by demonstration of the viral nucleic acid by RT-PCR (see p. 30).

## E. Treatment and prevention

Once an individual has clinical symptoms of rabies, there is no effective treatment. However, a killed rabies virus vaccine is available for prophylaxis. In the United States, this is generally the human diploid cell vaccine (HDCV). Preexposure prophylaxis is indicated for individuals at high risk because of the work they do (for example, for veterinarians). Postexposure prophylaxis refers to treatment instituted after an animal bite or exposure to an animal (or human) suspected of being rabid, and consists of thorough cleaning of the wound, passive immunization with antirabies immunoglobulin, and active immunization with the rabies vaccine (HDCV). Prevention of initial exposure is, however, clearly the most important mechanism for controlling human rabies.

**Figure 29.4**
An oval Negri body in a brain cell from a human rabies case.

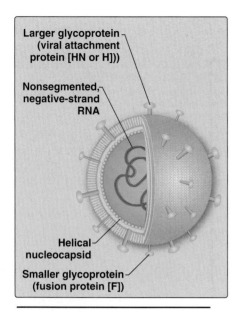

**Figure 29.5**
Model of paramyxovirus.

## III.  FAMILY PARAMYXOVIRIDAE

The members of the paramyxovirus family have recently been subdivided into two subfamilies (see Figure 29.1). First, the Paramyxovirinae, whose three genera include: 1) Paramyxovirus (parainfluenza viruses, which cause upper respiratory tract infections); 2) the Rubulavirus (mumps virus); and 3) the morbillivirus (measles virus). The second subfamily is the Pneumovirinae, which includes respiratory syncytial virus, a major respiratory tract pathogen in the pediatric population. Paramyxoviruses are spherical, enveloped particles that contain a nonsegmented, negative-strand RNA genome (Figure 29.5). Paramyxoviridae typically consist of a helical nucleocapsid, surrounded by an envelope that contains two types of integral membrane or envelope proteins. The first, the HN protein (H stands for hemagglutinin, and N for neuraminidase), is involved in the binding of the virus to a cell; measles virus lacks the neuraminidase activity. The second, the F protein (F stands for fusion), functions to fuse viral and cellular membranes, thus facilitating virus entry into the cytoplasm where viral replication occurs (see Figure 23.10, p. 237). Paramyxovirus mRNA transcription, genome replication, and viral assembly and release, resemble those of the rhabdoviruses (see p. 309).

### A.  Genus Paramyxovirus

The clinically important viruses in this genus are type 1 and type 3 human parainfluenza viruses (hPIV). They cause croup, pneumonia and bronchiolitis, mainly in infants and children. The term "parainfluenza" was first coined because infected individuals may present with influenza-like symptoms, and, like influenza virus, these viruses have both hemagglutinating and neuraminidase activities.

### B.  Genus Rubulavirus

This genus contains hPIV type 2 and type 4 and mumps virus.

1. **Type 2 and type 4 human parainfluenza viruses:** The clinical features of infection with parainfluenza virus type 2 are similar to those of types 1 and 3 viruses. Type 4 hPIV has been associated only with a mild upper respiratory tract illness, affecting both children and adults.

2. **Mumps virus:** Mumps used to be one of the commonly acquired childhood infections. Adults who escape the disease in childhood could also be infected. In the prevaccine period, mumps was the most common cause of viral encephalitis. Complete recovery, however, was almost always the rule. The virus is spread by respiratory droplets. Although about one third of infections are subclinical, the classic clinical presentation and diagnosis center on infection and swelling of the salivary glands, primarily the parotid glands (Figure 29.6). However, infection is widespread in the body and may involve not only the salivary glands but also the pancreas, CNS, and testes. Orchitis (inflammation of the testis) caused by mumps virus may cause sterility. A live, attenuated vaccine has been available for many years; this has resulted in a dramatic drop in the number of cases of mumps. [Note: Individuals who have had the disease develop lifelong immunity.]

**Figure 29.6**
Child with mumps showing swollen parotid gland.

## C. Genus Morbillivirus

Measles virus (MV) is the only virus in this genus that causes disease in humans. Other viruses in the genus morbillivirus are responsible for diseases in animals (for example, canine distemper virus). Measles virus differs in several ways from the other viruses in the family Paramyxoviridae.

1. **Viral replication:** The cellular receptor for measles virus is the CD46 molecule, a protein whose normal function is to bind certain components of complement. Although the viral attachment protein has hemagglutinating activity, it lacks neuraminidase activity. Hence, it is referred to as the H protein, rather than HN protein. A fusion (F) protein facilitates uptake of the virion. Measles virus replication in tissue culture and certain organs of the intact organism is characterized by the formation of giant multinucleate cells (syncytium formation), resulting from the action of the viral spike F protein.

2. **Pathology:** Measles virus is transmitted by sneeze- or cough-produced respiratory droplets. The virus is extremely infectious, and almost all infected individuals develop a clinical illness. Measles virus replicates initially in the respiratory epithelium and then in various lymphoid organs. Classically, measles (referred to previously as rubeola) begins with a prodromal period of fever, upper respiratory tract symptoms, and conjunctivitis. Two to three days later, specific diagnostic signs develop; first, Koplik spots (small white spots on bright red mucous membranes of the mouth and throat (Figure 29.7) and then a generalized macular rash, beginning at the head and traveling slowly to the lower extremities (Figure 29.8). Soon after the rash appears, the patient is no longer infectious. The major morbidity and mortality caused by measles are associated with various complications of infection, especially those affecting the lower respiratory tract and the CNS. The most important of these is postinfectious encephalomyelitis, which is estimated to affect 1 of 1,000 cases of measles, usually occurring within two weeks after the onset of the rash. This is an autoimmune disease associated with an immune response to myelin basic protein. Figure 29.9 shows the time course of measles virus infection.

> Children are particularly susceptible, especially those weakened by other diseases or malnutrition. Measles is, therefore, an important cause of childhood mortality in developing countries.

3. **Diagnosis:** In most cases, there is little difficulty in making a diagnosis of measles on clinical grounds, especially in an epidemic situation. The presence of Koplik spots provides a definitive diagnosis. If a laboratory diagnosis is necessary, it is usually made by demonstrating an increase in the titer of antiviral antibodies.

**Figure 29.7**
Koplik spots in the mouth caused by measles virus.

**Figure 29.8**
The measles rash consists of large, slightly raised lesions called maculopapules. These run into each other to form irregular blotches.

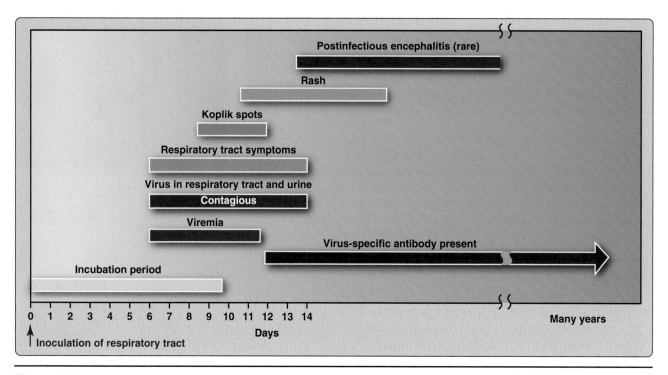

**Figure 29.9**
Time course of measles virus infection.

**4. Prevention:** Measles is usually a disease of childhood, and is followed by life-long immunity. A live, attenuated measles vaccine, which has been available for many years, has greatly reduced the incidence of the disease. Nevertheless, occasional outbreaks of measles continue to occur, especially in older children and young adults, possibly due to waning immunity. Thus, two doses of the vaccine, in the form of the measles-mumps-rubella (MMR) vaccine (see p. 39), are now recommended, the first at twelve to eighteen months, the second at four to twelve years.

### D. Genus pneumovirus

The one virus in this genus that is of medical importance is respiratory syncytial virus (RSV). RSV is the major viral respiratory tract pathogen in the pediatric population, and the most important cause of bronchiolitis in infants. RSV may also cause pneumonia in young children, an influenza-like syndrome in adults, and severe bronchitis with pneumonia in the elderly and organ transplant recipients. The viruses in the subfamily Pneumovirinae, genus Pneumovirus, are set apart from those in the other three genera in the Paromyxovirus family by a somewhat more complex genome and a larger number of virus-specific proteins. Nevertheless, the basic strategy of replication is as described for the other viruses in this family (see p. 312). RSV has one envelope protein that functions as an attachment protein and another that functions as a fusion protein; however, like measles virus, RSV lacks neuraminidase activity. RSV is transmitted by respiratory droplets or by contaminated hands carrying the virus to the nose or mouth. Repeated infections are common. A definitive diagnosis of RSV infection can be made only on the basis of laboratory findings, such as a rise in the titer of serum antibody or the demonstration of viral antigens in respiratory secretions. The only specific treatment is ribavirin, administered by aerosol, and this is only of moderate benefit. Hand-washing and avoidance of others with the infection are the major preventive measures.

## IV. FAMILY ORTHOMYXOVIRIDAE

Orthomyxoviruses are spherical, enveloped viruses containing a segmented, negative-strand RNA genome. Viruses in this family infect humans, horses, and pigs, as well as nondomestic water fowl, and are the cause of influenza. Orthomyxoviruses are divided into 3 types: influenza A, B, and C. Only influenza virus types A and B are of medical importance. Type A influenza viruses differ from type B viruses in that they have an animal reservoir and are divided into subtypes.

### A. Structure

Influenza virions are spherical, enveloped, pleomorphic particles (Figure 29.10). Two types of spikes project from the surface: one is composed of hemagglutinin (H protein) and the second of neuraminidase (N protein). [Note: This is in contrast to the paramyxoviruses, in which H and N activities reside in the same spike protein.] Both the H and N influenza proteins are integral membrane proteins. The M (matrix) proteins underlie the viral lipid membrane. The RNA genome, located in a helical nucleocapsid, is composed of eight distinct segments of RNA, six of which code for a single protein. Each nucleocapsid segment contains not only the viral RNA but also four proteins (NP, the major nucleocapsid protein, and three P proteins that are present in much smaller amounts than NP and are involved in synthesis and replication of viral RNA).

### B. Viral replication

There are two unusual features associated with synthesis and replication of influenza viral RNAs that distinguish the influenza viruses from the other RNA viruses discussed up to this point. First, the synthesis of influenza virus mRNAs and the replication of the viral genome, occur in the nucleus. This is in contrast to the replication of other RNA viruses, which occurs completely in the cytoplasm. [Note: The retroviruses are an exception to this generalization (see p. 295).] Second, compounds such as actinomycin D and α-amanitin, which inhibit the synthesis of eukaryotic RNA polymerase II[1] (Pol II) transcripts (messenger RNAs), inhibit the replication of influenza virus.

1. **Viral entry into the cell:** Influenza virus attaches to sialic acid residues on host cell glycoproteins or glycolipids. Entry then occurs via receptor-mediated endocytosis (see Figure 23.10, p. 237). Both the attachment and the fusion functions are associated with the H protein.

2. **Synthesis and translation of viral mRNAs:** The nucleocapsid segments are released into the cytosol, and, as with the other negative-strand RNA viruses, the viral genomic RNA serves as the

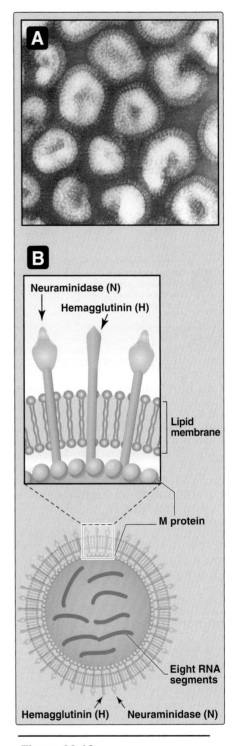

**Figure 29.10**
Influenza virus. A. Electron micrograph. B. Schematic drawing showing envelope proteins—called H and N spikes—that protrude from the surface.

[1]See p. 421 in *Lippincott's Illustrated Reviews: Biochemistry* (3rd ed.) for a discussion of RNA polymerase II.

**Figure 29.11**
"Cap snatching" by influenza virus prior to viral mRNA translation.

The figure contains the following labels:

1. Viral P proteins cleave 5'-terminal sequences—10 to 13 nucleotides long—from host cell mRNA.

5'    3'
CAP   Capped host cell mRNA

(–) Viral RNA

CAP

2. Oligonucleotide fragments are then used as primers for synthesis of viral mRNAs.

(–) Viral RNA

(+) Viral RNA

Translation to viral proteins in cytosol

3. Thus, each viral mRNA is composed of a short, 5'-sequence of RNA containing a methylated cap, which is host-derived, joined to a longer sequence of RNA, which is virus-encoded, and corresponds in length to the genome segment from which it was transcribed.

template for synthesis of viral mRNAs. Each of the eight genome segments directs the synthesis of one positive-strand mRNA. However, influenza virus is distinguished from the other negative-strand viruses in that, although the virions contain proteins that can transcribe mRNAs, these enzymes lack the ability to cap and methylate viral mRNAs. The synthesis of influenza virus mRNA, therefore, begins with "cap snatching," in which the viral P proteins cleave 5'-terminal sequences (ten to thirteen nucleotides long) from nascent host cellular Pol II transcripts that had been previously synthesized, capped, and methylated in the nucleus. The oligonucleotide fragments are then used as primers for the synthesis of the viral mRNAs (Figure 29.11). Thus, each viral mRNA is composed of a short, 5'-sequence of RNA containing a methylated cap that is host-derived, joined to a longer sequence of RNA that is virus-encoded and corresponds in length to the genome segment from which it was transcribed.

3. **Assembly and release of influenza virus particles:** Once the viral mRNAs are made and translated, the NP and the three P proteins move into the nucleus, whereupon replication of the eight genomic segments begins and progeny nucleocapsids are assembled. Meanwhile, certain regions of the plasma membrane become virus-modified by insertion of H and N proteins and alignment of the M protein on the inner side of the plasma membrane. The nucleocapsids move from the nucleus to the cytosol and, finally, to virus-modified regions of the plasma membrane, which they bud through, giving rise to extracellular viral particles (Figure 29.12). [Note: Viral release is facilitated by the N protein, which cleaves neuraminic acid on the cell surface.]

## C. Pathology and clinical significance

In humans, influenza is spread by respiratory droplets and is an infection solely of the respiratory tract (Figure 29.13). There is rarely viremia or spread to other organ systems. Destruction of respiratory epithelial cells is attributed to the host immune response, specifically cytotoxic T cells. Typically, influenza has an acute onset characterized by chills, followed by high fever, muscle aches (caused by circulating cytokines), and extreme drowsiness. The disease runs its course in four to five days, after which there is a gradual recovery. The most serious problems, such as development of pneumonia, occur in the very young, the elderly, and people with chronic cardiac or pulmonary disease or those who are immunodeficient.

> Reye syndrome is a rare and serious complication of viral infections in children, especially in those who have had chickenpox or influenza B. Aspirin, used to lower virus-induced fever, contributes to the appearance of this syndrome. Therefore, acetaminophen is usually recommended for fevers of unknown origin in children.

## D. The immunology of influenza viruses

When individuals are infected with influenza virus, antibodies are made against the various viral proteins. However, it is the antibodies made against the H protein that are neutralizing and the best index of protection. The antigenic properties of the influenza virus proteins are also important because they serve as the basis for the classification of influenza viruses.

**Figure 29.12**
Influenza virus budding from the surface of an infected cell (electron micrograph).

1. **Types and subtypes:** Influenza viruses are classified as types A, B, and C, depending on their inner proteins, mainly the M and NP proteins. Thus, all type A viruses share common internal antigens that are distinct from those shared by all type B viruses. Only the type A viruses are broken down into subtypes. The classification into subtypes depends on antigens associated with the outer viral proteins, H and N. Taking into consideration animal as well as human influenza viruses, 14 H and 9 N subtypes have been described. However, among human influenza viruses, only three H (H1, H2, and H3) and two N (N1 and N2) subtypes are found. Human influenza viruses are therefore designated, for example, as subtype H1N1, H2N2, and H3N2.

2. **Antigenic variability of influenza viruses:** In contrast to viruses such as polio or measles virus that have maintained antigenic stability since they were first isolated, influenza viruses have shown marked variation over the years in antigenic properties, specifically H and N proteins. Two distinct phenomena account for this observation: antigenic drift and antigenic shift.

   a. **Antigenic drift:** This refers to minor antigenic changes in H and N proteins that occur each year. Antigenic drift does not involve a change in the viral subtype. This phenomenon can be easily explained by random mutations in viral RNA and single or a small number of amino acid substitutions in H and N proteins.

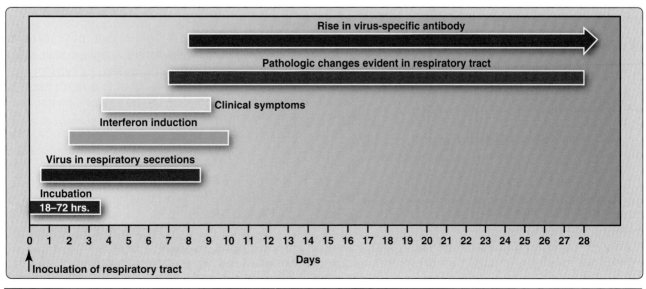

**Figure 29.13**
Time course of influenza A virus infection. The classic "flu syndrome" occurs early. Later, pneumonia may result from ascending bacterial infection.

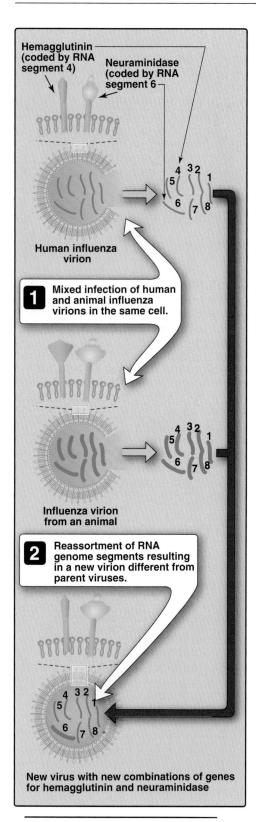

**Figure 29.14**
Mechanism of antigenic shift in influenza virus.

**b. Antigenic shift:** This phenomenon involves a much more dramatic change in the antigenic properties of the H and/or N proteins (Figure 29.14), and a change in subtype, for example, from H1N1 to H3N2. Antigenic shift occurs only infrequently, perhaps every ten or twenty years. For example, the appearance of a new, extremely virulent H1N1 virus, due presumably to antigenic shift, probably accounted for the pandemic of 1918–1919 that resulted in the death of an estimated twenty million people worldwide, including more than 500,000 in the United States (Figure 29.15). In 1957, antigenic shift again occurred, and H1N1 virus was replaced by subtype H2N2; in 1968, H2N2 was replaced by H3N2. Since 1977, multiple subtypes of influenza A have been circulating around the world.

> In most years, both type A and type B influenza viruses can be isolated from patients. Both type A and B viruses undergo antigenic drift, but only type A viruses show antigenic shift.

[Note: H5N1 (an avian flu virus strain) was first isolated in 1997 from a human. The virus affects individuals who live closely with domestic birds such as chickens. It has not been shown to be passed from human to human, but rather from bird to bird, including wild birds that migrate. The primary infections have been in Asia and the Middle East; as of March 2006, the virus has not been identified in the United States. Over fifty percent of reported cases have been fatal.]

**c. Consequences of antigenic variation:** When antigenic shift occurs and a new subtype of virus appears that has not been in circulation for many years, the immune systems of a large proportion of the population have never encountered that virus; these individuals are, therefore, immunologically unprotected. Thus, the conditions are set for an influenza epidemic or even pandemic (see Figure 29.15). Antigenic shift also means that the vaccine that was in use before the antigenic shift will not be effective in protecting against the new subtype of virus; therefore, it becomes necessary to develop a new vaccine as quickly as possible, incorporating the new virus subtype.

**d. The molecular basis of antigenic variation:** The dramatic changes associated with antigenic shift result from reassortment of viral RNA segments, a process observed with all RNA viruses having a segmented genome. Reassortment results when a cell is infected with two genetically distinct influenza viruses; the genomic RNAs of both parental viruses are replicated, and progeny viruses are assembled that contain genomic RNA segments from one of the parental viruses, and other genomic segments from the second parent (see Figure 29.14). In this way, new viruses can be generated that differ from both parents. Although all eight of the influenza virus RNA genome segments undergo reassortment, for antigenic shift to

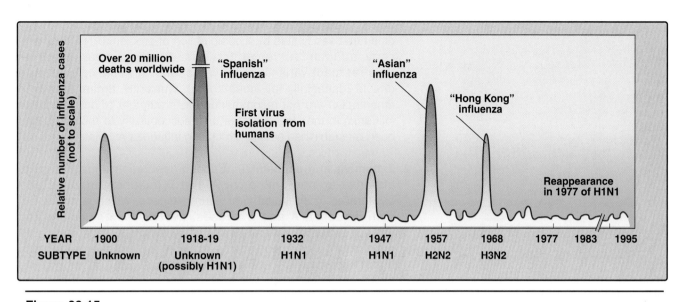

**Figure 29.15**
Time line showing the occurrence of some of the major outbreaks and antigenic shifts associated with type A influenza during the 1900s.

occur, it is the reassortment of the RNA segments that specify the mRNAs for H and N proteins (the proteins that define the antigenic subtypes) that is most critical. Where do the genes for the new viral subtypes come from? We know that influenza type A viruses are found in many different animals, including horses, pigs, and wild migrating water fowl. Furthermore, it has been demonstrated that reassortment can occur between influenza A viruses from different animal species and different avian species, including between mammalian and avian viruses. For example, in situations in which humans live in proximity to farm animals, there is opportunity for the generation of new, reassorted viral subtypes.

## E. Diagnosis

The collection of influenza-like symptoms described above can also be caused by other viruses (for example, respiratory syncytial virus, see p. 314). Therefore, a definitive diagnosis cannot be made on clinical grounds except in an epidemic situation. In most cases, it is not practical to make a specific laboratory diagnosis. However, if needed for surveillance purposes, for example, a widely performed and specific test is the quantitation of HI (hemagglutination inhibition) antibodies. This has the added advantage of identifying the subtype of the virus (see below). A more rapid diagnosis can be made by the demonstration of viral antigens in respiratory tract secretions.

## F. Treatment and prevention

1. **Amantadine and rimantadine:** First-generation antiviral agents effective against influenza A include two related drugs, amantadine and rimantadine. Both drugs stop viral uncoating by inhibition of the viral M2 membrane protein. These agents reduce both the duration and the severity of flu symptoms, but only if given early in infection. Given before the onset of symptoms, these drugs can

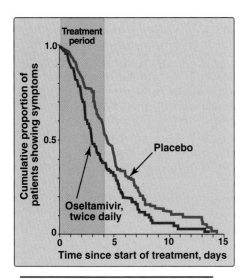

**Figure 29.16**
Time to alleviation of all symptoms
in influenza-infected patients.

**Figure 29.17**
Electron micrograph of Ebola virus.

also prevent disease. The usefulness of amantadine and rimantidine has been limited by a combination of problems: 1) lack of efficacy against influenza B virus, 2) rapid emergence of drug-resistant variants of the virus, and 3) neurologic adverse effects (especially for amantadine). Currently, amantadine and rimantadine are not recommended for treatment or prophylaxis of influenza in the United States until susceptibility to the drugs has been reestablished among circulating influenza A isolates.

2. **Zanamivir and oseltamivir:** Second-generation antiviral agents effective against influenza A and B include zanamivir and oseltamivir. They inhibit viral neuraminidase, which is present in both influenza A and B viruses. [Note: Neuraminidase—an enzyme essential for viral replication—cleaves terminal sialic acid residues from glycoconjugates to allow the release of the virus from infected cells.] The drugs are indicated for uncomplicated acute illness in adults and adolescents twelve years of age and older who have been symptomatic for no more than two days. Zanamivir must be taken by inhalation. In contrast, oseltamivir is well absorbed when administered orally, and has proven to be effective for symptomatic patients as well as for prophylaxis (for example, to prevent the spread of influenza in nursing homes). For maximum benefit, therapy should begin within two days of symptom onset. For example, oseltamivir taken within 24 hours of symptom onset shortened the duration of illness by about two days, with patients reporting feeling better within a day of starting treatment (Figure 29.16).

3. **Vaccine:** As useful as new therapies are, they are not a substitute for the vaccine. A vaccine consisting of formalin-inactivated influenza virus has been available for many years. It is recommended for the elderly and for people in high-risk groups, such as patients with chronic pulmonary or cardiac disease. It is of critical importance that the vaccine contain the specific subtypes of influenza virus that are in circulation at any given time.

> The circulating strains worldwide are monitored each season, and the following year's vaccine includes the principal strains recovered during the previous year—usually one type B influenza and two type A influenza strains.

## V. FAMILY FILOVIRIDAE

Filoviruses are pleomorphic viruses with unusual morphologies (Figure 29.17). They are generally seen as long, filamentous, enveloped particles that may be branched. Marburg virus was initially isolated in Germany and Yugoslavia from laboratory workers who became severely ill while preparing primary cell cultures from African green monkeys. Ebola virus was isolated from patients with hemorrhagic fever in Zaire and the Sudan. The two viruses are not related antigenically. Marburg and Ebola viruses cause severe hemorrhagic fever, characterized by widespread bleeding into the skin, mucous membranes, visceral organs, and the gastrointestinal tract. The mortality rate is high, often greater than fifty percent. Although the natural reservoir for these viruses is unknown, they can be transmitted to humans from infected monkeys and probably other animals or by exposure to blood or other body fluids from an infected patient. Outbreaks of hemorrhagic fever caused by these viruses continue to occur at irregular intervals. Laboratory identification is made by the demonstration of antiviral antibodies, for example, by ELISA assays (see p. 28). If virus can be recovered, the morphology of the particles is quite characteristic. There is no specific treatment for infections caused by these viruses. Strict barrier nursing techniques are essential when caring for infected individuals. Because of the hazards of working with filoviruses, they are studied in only a few reference laboratories around the world.

## VI. FAMILY BUNYAVIRIDAE

In the United States, the clinically most important viruses in this family are California encephalitis and LaCrosse viruses (genus, Bunyavirus), which cause meningitis and encephalitis, and the Hantaan viruses (genus, Hantavirus), which are associated with hemorrhagic fever with or without renal syndrome, and hantavirus pulmonary syndrome, a condition associated with high mortality. The viruses in this family are spherical, enveloped particles, with spikes projecting from the surface of the virions. Because the RNA genome is divided into three segments, reassortment of RNA segments between closely related viruses is possible. Arthropods serve as vectors for most viruses in the family Bunyaviridae that are transmitted to humans (Figure 29.18). However, because viruses in the genus Hantavirus do not have an arthropod vector, they are transmitted to humans by rodents via aerosols formed from their dried excretions. No effective antiviral agent is currently available.

## VII. FAMILY ARENAVIRIDAE

Arenaviruses are enveloped, spherical particles with a bipartite (two-segment) RNA genome that exists in virions as helical nucleocapsids. Both RNAs have an ambisense organization, which means that coding information is contained in both the genomic and antigenomic viral RNAs. Viral particles mature by budding from the plasma membrane. Viruses in this family are associated with chronic infections of rodents, and humans are infected by inhaling contaminated aerosols, eating food containing viral particles, or by exposure of open wounds to infected soil. Lymphocytic choriomeningitis (LCM) virus, a cause of viral meningitis, is a relatively benign infection with little mortality. In Latin America, Junin and Machupo viruses are associated with Argentine and Bolivian hemorrhagic fevers, respectively; these are diseases with mortality rates of 25 to thirty percent. In Africa, Lassa fever (caused by Lassa virus) is a severe infection that is associated with bleeding and an expected mortality rate of about fifteen percent. Ribavirin appears to be of benefit both in Lassa fever and hemorrhagic fevers. The most important measure in prevention, however, is rodent control.

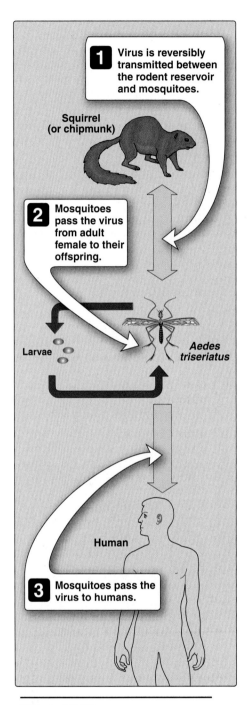

1 Virus is reversibly transmitted between the rodent reservoir and mosquitoes.

Squirrel (or chipmunk)

2 Mosquitoes pass the virus from adult female to their offspring.

Larvae

*Aedes triseriatus*

Human

3 Mosquitoes pass the virus to humans.

**Figure 29.18**
Transmission of California encephalitis virus.

# Study Questions

**Choose the ONE correct answer**

29.1 An ornithologist was on a three-month trip to study several species of birds living in a rain forest in South America. On the tenth day of her trip, she was bitten on the hand by an unusually aggressive bat. The scientist applied a topical antibiotic ointment and continued her research. Four weeks later, the scientist lost feeling in her hand. She shortly began experiencing high fever, periods of rigidity, difficulty in swallowing liquids, drooling, and disorientation. Death followed rapidly. A postmortem biopsy of her brain showed the presence of Negri bodies. These symptoms are consistent with the woman having died of

    A. California encephalitis virus.

    B. hantaan virus.

    C. ebola virus.

    D. rabies virus.

    E. lymphocytic choriomeningitis virus.

> Correct answer = D. Rabies virus is usually transmitted via the bite of an infected animal, and the woman's symptoms are consistent with those of rabies. California encephalitis virus, transmitted by arthropods, causes meningitis and encephalitis. Hantaan virus is transmitted through aerosols formed from dried rodent excretions. This virus causes hemorrhagic fever and severe pulmonary infections. Ebola virus can be transmitted by an animal, but infection causes severe hemorrhagic fever. Lymphocytic choriomeningitis virus is a cause of viral meningitis and a relatively benign infection with little mortality. Humans are infected by inhaling contaminated aerosols, or eating food containing viral particles, or by exposure of open wounds to infected soil.

29.2 From 1918 until 1956, the only subtype of influenza observed in humans was H1N1. In 1957, H1N1 was replaced by H2N2. This is an example of

    A. viral interference.

    B. phenotypic mixing.

    C. antigenic shift.

    D. antigenic drift.

    E. viral transformation.

> Correct answer = C. A marked antigenic change in the N protein, the H protein, or both is termed antigenic shift. In antigenic drift, there is also an antigenic change in one or both of these proteins, but the change is much less significant. With antigenic drift, although the H protein does change antigenically, H1 remains H1, for example.

*"Don't mind me, Richie—it's just the rabies talking."*

# Double-stranded RNA Viruses: the Reoviridae

# 30

## I. OVERVIEW

The single genus in the family that is of medical importance is the genus Rotavirus, which causes severe viral gastroenteritis primarily in infants and young children (Figure 30.1). Viruses in the family Reoviridae are spherical, non-enveloped particles that have an icosahedral structure. The viral genome consists of ten to twelve segments of double-stranded (ds) RNA. The virions contain all the enzymes needed to make positive-strand RNA transcripts, which are capped and methylated.[1] Reoviruses replicate completely in the cytoplasm. [Note: The name "reovirus" stands for respiratory and enteric orphan virus. Although an orphan virus is typically virus not known to be the cause of any disease, that is no longer the case for reoviruses. Echoviruses were also initially considered p. 283), but were soon discovered to cause a large number of clinical syndromes. Therefore, as far as viruses are concerned, being an orphan may be only a temporary state.]

## II. GENUS ROTAVIRUS

Rotaviruses, found in many mammalian species, often have a fairly broad host range. Rotaviruses have a characteristic morphology that distinguishes them from other reoviruses; namely, they have the appearance of wheels with spokes radiating from the center and a smooth outer rim (Figure 30.2). The particles also have a large number of channels connecting the outer surface of the virion to the inner core. It has been suggested that these channels are involved in the import of substrates needed for RNA transcription and the extrusion of newly synthesized RNA transcripts.

### A. Epidemiology

Rotaviruses are divided into seven serogroups (A through G) of which group A is the most important cause of outbreaks of disease in humans. Transmission of rotaviruses is via the fecal–oral route. There is a marked seasonal incidence associated with rotavirus infections, with the peak months in the United States being January through March. Because infectious particles are relatively stable, they can survive for extended periods on various surfaces.

 [1]See p. 423 in ***Lippincott's Illustrated Reviews: Biochemistry*** (3rd ed.) for a discussion of posttranscriptional modification.

**Figure 30.1**
Classification of double-stranded, nonenveloped RNA viruses.

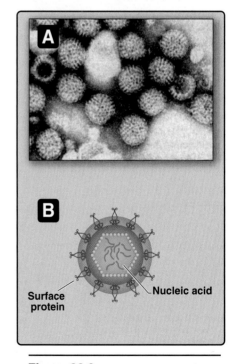

**Figure 30.2**
Structure of Rotavirus. A. Electron micrograph. B. Schematic drawing.

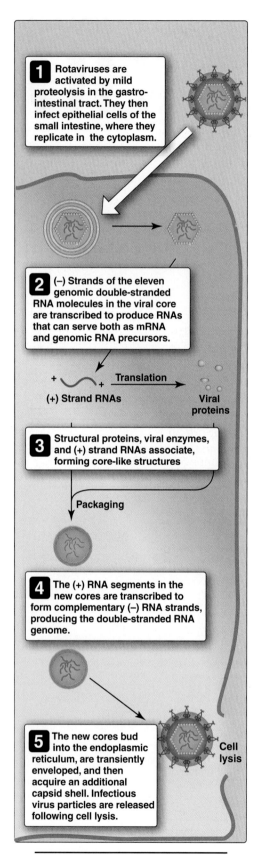

**Figure 30.3**
Replication of rotavirus.

Rotavirus infections account for about fifty percent of cases of severe diarrhea in infants and young children (up to two years of age).

## B. Viral replication

After attachment to and uptake by the host cell, rotaviruses become partially uncoated in a lysosome. The rotavirus genome has eleven segments of linear, double-stranded RNA, each of which codes for a single protein. Reassortment of the RNA segments can occur when a cell is infected with two different rotaviruses. The viral particles contain enzymes (such as RNA-dependent RNA polymerase) that are needed to synthesize positive-sense RNA transcripts with a 5' cap. These positive RNA strands function not only as mRNA, but also as templates for the synthesis of negative-strand RNA (see Figure 23.14, p. 241). After the negative-strand RNA is made, it stays associated with its positive-strand template, giving rise to a double-stranded RNA segment that is packaged in the virion. Rotaviruses are released following cell lysis rather than by budding through the membrane, thus accounting for the lack of a viral envelope. Figure 30.3 illustrates additional details of rotavirus replication.

## C. Clinical significance

Following ingestion, rotaviruses infect the epithelial cells of the small intestine, primarily the jejunum (Figure 30.4). [Note: Rotaviruses are able to reach the small intestine because they are resistant to the acid pH of the stomach.] The incubation period is usually 48 hours or less. Infection can be subclinical or may result in symptoms ranging from mild diarrhea and vomiting to severe, nonbloody, watery diarrhea with dehydration and loss of electrolytes. Although rotavirus infections are probably equally widespread around the world, the outcomes of infection vary significantly in different regions of the world. Despite the fact that more than ninety percent of children in the United States may have antibodies to rotaviruses by the age of three or four, mortality is low because patients who are severely ill are generally hospitalized, with fluid and electrolyte losses rapidly corrected.

In developing countries or areas where medical facilities or personnel may be lacking, the mortality is significant. For example, it is estimated that up to a million deaths per year worldwide result from rotavirus infection.

## D. Laboratory identification

Severe diarrhea, dehydration, and electrolyte loss can be due to a variety of causes. Accordingly, a definitive diagnosis cannot be made on clinical grounds alone. As with many other viral infections,

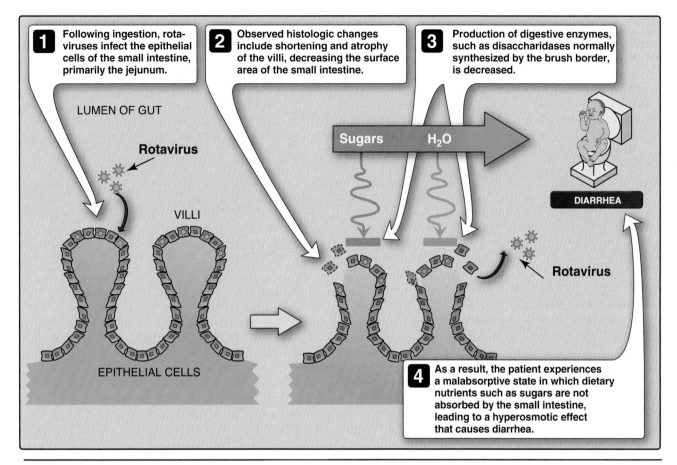

**1** Following ingestion, rotaviruses infect the epithelial cells of the small intestine, primarily the jejunum.

**2** Observed histologic changes include shortening and atrophy of the villi, decreasing the surface area of the small intestine.

**3** Production of digestive enzymes, such as disaccharidases normally synthesized by the brush border, is decreased.

LUMEN OF GUT

Rotavirus

VILLI

Sugars    H₂O

DIARRHEA

EPITHELIAL CELLS

Rotavirus

**4** As a result, the patient experiences a malabsorptive state in which dietary nutrients such as sugars are not absorbed by the small intestine, leading to a hyperosmotic effect that causes diarrhea.

**Figure 30.4**
Mechanism of rotavirus diarrhea.

identification can be made by using an ELISA test (see p. 30) or recognition of an increase in the titer of antiviral antibody in a patient's serum. Electron microscopy of stool specimens, although not a routine diagnostic measure, can aid in the identification of the virus because rotaviruses have a distinctive appearance (see Figure 30.2).

## E. Treatment and prevention

There is no specific antiviral drug appropriate for treatment of rotavirus infections. The most important clinical intervention is the rapid and efficient replacement of fluids and electrolytes, usually intravenously. Formulations are also being produced that can be used in developing countries so that fluids and electrolytes can be replaced orally. Two new oral vaccines using weakened live virus have been shown to be highly efficacious in protecting infants against severe rotavirus gastroenteritis and not associated with increased risk of intussusception (telescoping of one portion of the intestine into another). Prevention of rotavirus infections requires improved sanitation measures.

## Study Questions

**Choose the ONE correct answer**

30.1 The typical clinical syndrome associated with rotavirus infection is

    A. acute gastroenteritis of young adults.

    B. acute bronchiolitis of infants.

    C. acute hepatitis.

    D. nausea, vomiting, and diarrhea in infants and young children.

    E. acute paralytic syndrome.

> Correct answer = D. Rotaviruses infect and replicate in the gastrointestinal tract and typically affect infants and very young children. Although rotavirus infections are seen world-wide, there is significant mortality only in developing countries or in situations where good medical treatment (for example, fluid and electrolyte replacement), is not available.

30.2 Rotaviruses differ from polioviruses in that rotaviruses

    A. infect via the fecal-oral route.

    B. lack an envelope.

    C. can undergo genetic reassortment.

    D. do not contain any enzymes.

    E. have an icosahedral structure.

> Correct answer = C. Because rotaviruses contain a segmented genome, infection of a single cell with two different rotaviruses can result in genetic reassortment and the emergence of a new viral strain with some genomic segments from one parent and the remaining genomic segments from the other parent. Rotaviruses do contain the enzymes required to synthesize viral mRNAs. A, B, D, E: There are no differences between polioviruses and rotaviruses in these characteristics.

30.3 The diagnosis of a rotavirus infection

    A. can be made, in most cases, on the basis of the clinical presentation.

    B. can be made on the basis of an increase in antibody titer.

    C. is routinely made by electron microscopy of suitably treated stool samples.

    D. can only be made on epidemiologic grounds (for example, if there is an epidemic).

    E. must be made rapidly so that specific antiviral therapy is initiated as soon as possible.

> Correct answer = B. The diagnosis of rotavirus infection is readily made by serology (that is, by demonstrating a rise in antibody titer). There are also several tests available by which rotavirus antigens can be demonstrated in the stool. Although the diagnosis can be made by electron microscopy, it is not a routine procedure. The clinical presentation is not sufficiently distinctive to make the diagnosis, and there is no specific antiviral treatment for rotavirus infections.

*"I'll level with you. It's just a matter of time."*

# Unconventional Infectious Agents

# 31

## I. OVERVIEW

The designation "unconventional infectious agent" refers to a distinctive, transmissible, infectious agent that, although having some properties in common with viruses, does not fit the classic definition of a virus (Figure 31.1). One such highly unconventional infectious agent, the prion, has been strongly implicated as the causative agent of transmissible spongiform encephalopathies (TSEs). TSEs occurring in humans are designated as kuru, Creutzfeldt-Jakob disease (CJD), Gerstmann-Straussler syndrome (GSS), and fatal familial insomnia (FFI). Important TSEs of animals include scrapie in sheep, bovine spongiform encephalopathy (BSE) in cattle (popularly called "mad cow disease"), and chronic wasting disease (found in deer and elk). Histologically, these diseases are characterized by spongiform vacuolation of neuronal processes and gray matter, accumulation of a unique protein (as prion protein, or Pr; Figure 31.2), and, in certain cases, deposition in the brain of extracellular amyloid plaques composed of PrP. [Note: Such diseases are sometimes referred to as transmissible amyloidoses.]

## II. PRIONS

After an extensive series of purification procedures, scientists were astonished to find that the infectivity of the agent causing scrapie in sheep was associated with a single protein species, with no detectable associated nucleic acid. This infectious protein is designated the prion protein. It is relatively resistant to proteolytic degradation and, when infectious, tends to form insoluble aggregates of fibrils, similar to the amyloid found in other diseases of the brain.

### A. Presence of prion protein (PrP) in normal mammalian brain

A noninfectious form of PrP, having the same amino acid and gene sequences as the infectious agent, is present in normal mammalian brains on the surface of neurons and glial cells. It is referred to as $PrP^C$ (cellular prion protein). The function of noninfectious $PrP^C$ is unknown, however, it is highly conserved in nature, with the amino acid and gene sequences differing little in divergent mammalian species. The primary structure and posttranslational modifications of the normal and the infectious forms of the protein are closely related or identical. However, specific mutational changes of single amino acids at a few sites appear to be determinants of susceptibility to exogenous infection and the probability for spontaneous con-

**Figure 31.1**
Classification of unconventional infectious agents.

Fibrillar proteins accumulate in the brains of patients with transmissible spongiform encephalopathy.

**Figure 31.2**
Electron micrograph of fibrillar prion proteins.

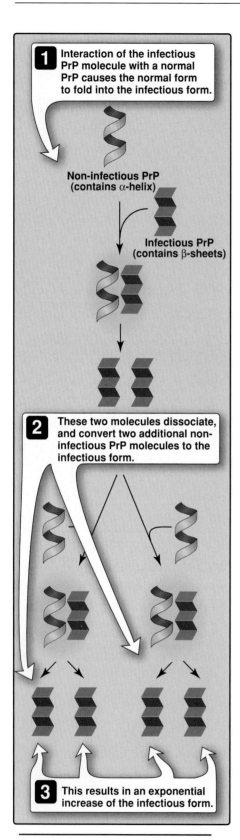

**1** Interaction of the infectious PrP molecule with a normal PrP causes the normal form to fold into the infectious form.

Non-infectious PrP (contains α-helix)

Infectious PrP (contains β-sheets)

**2** These two molecules dissociate, and convert two additional non-infectious PrP molecules to the infectious form.

**3** This results in an exponential increase of the infectious form.

**Figure 31.3**
One proposed mechanism for multiplication of the infectious prion agents.

version of the normal PrP$^C$ to the infectious form (PrP$^{Sc}$). The key to becoming infectious apparently lies in the three-dimensional conformation of the prion protein. It has been observed that a number of α-helices[1] present in noninfectious PrP$^C$ are replaced by β-sheets[2] in the infectious form. It is presumably this conformational difference that confers on infectious prions relative resistance to proteolytic degradation, and permits them to be distinguished from normal PrP$^C$ in infected tissue. A model for multiplication of the agent is shown in Figure 31.3.

## B. Epidemiology

The normal mode of transmission among animals (for example, among sheep in a flock infected with scrapie) has not been elucidated. It is clear, however, that several diseases of domestic animals have been transmitted via feed prepared from other diseased animals.

1. **Bovine spongiform encephalopathy:** BSE, commonly called mad cow disease, arose in British cattle presumably caused by their feed processed with animal parts prepared from diseased sheep and cattle. The obvious question raised by this occurrence is whether the BSE from infected cattle can be transmitted to humans. This was originally thought to carry negligible risk, but a study of infectious material from a cluster of histologically distinctive British CJD cases in unusually young patients (now referred to as "variant," or vCJD), indicated that animal-to-human transmission very likely did take place. Because the incubation time for symptoms to appear varies from four to forty years, the extent of a potential epidemic caused by BSE is unknown.

2. **Kuru:** An example of human-to-human transmission of a TSE is found in kuru, a disease in which the infectious agent is acquired by an individual's exposure to diseased brain tissue in the course of ritualistic cannibalism among members of a tribe in New Guinea. Infection occurs by consumption of contaminated brain tissue, or by inoculation through breaks in the skin following handling diseased tissue. With the cessation of cannibalism in the late 1950s, the disease is disappearing.

3. **Creutzfeldt-Jakob disease:** Of more general significance are the documented cases of iatrogenic (done unintentionally by a physician) transmission of Creutzfeldt-Jakob disease, for example, by use of prion-contaminated human pituitary-derived growth hormone prepared from individuals who died from CJD. Thus far, there has been no evidence of transplacental transmission, infection from blood products, or transmission by person-to-person contact. In about fifteen percent of CJD, the condition is inherited as a mutation in the PrP gene. However, the majority of CJD cases are sporadic and have an unknown etiology (that is, they occur with no known exposure or mutational change). The incidence of sporadic CJD is low—about one to two per million population—but in those families with a PrP mutation, an attack rate of 50 to 100 percent is seen in those carrying the mutation. In contrast to CJD, all cases classified as GSS or FFI have involved inheritance of specific PrP mutations. Despite the inherited nature of the disease, however, brain tissues from these patients are infectious.

[1,2]See pp. 16-17 in *Lippincott's Illustrated Reviews: Biochemistry* (3rd ed.) for a discussion of the α-helix and β-sheet.

## C. Pathology

Extracerebral exposure to prions results in significant multiplication of prions in lymphoreticular and other peripheral tissues early after infection, but it is invasion of the central nervous system (CNS) that results in the typical clinical effects. The basis for the pathogenic consequences of abnormal PrP$^{Sc}$ deposition has not been clarified. Diseased brain tissue is characterized by accumulation of abnormal PrP$^{Sc}$ in the form of amyloid fibrils in cytoplasmic vesicles of neurons (see Figure 31.2) and in the form of extracellular amyloid plaques. There is, in addition, extensive vacuolation within neurons, neuronal loss, and astroglial proliferation. The extensive destruction results in the characteristic spongiform appearance of gray matter in histologic sections.

> Whereas TSE amyloid plaques are morphologically similar to those of Alzheimer disease, the PrP gene is located on a different chromosome than the gene for the Alzheimer amyloid-b-protein precursor, and there is no nucleotide or amino acid homology between the two.

## D. Clinical significance

Transmissible spongiform encephalopathies are a group of progressive, ultimately fatal, neurodegenerative diseases affecting humans and a number of animal species. The disease process is fundamentally the same in all TSEs, but their clinical manifestations and histopathologies differ. TSEs also share some similarities with conventional infectious diseases, but their differences are striking (Figure 31.4).

1. **Molecular basis of inherited TSEs:** In each inherited TSE, specific, single amino acid substitutions or insertions of nucleotide repeat sequences are found in the PrP gene. These are thought to increase greatly ($10^6$-fold) the probability of transition to the infectious conformation. In the spontaneously occurring, sporadic disease (that is, with no known exposure to infectious material and no inheritance of a mutated PrP gene), it is proposed that the altered folding occurs randomly with low probability; however, once formed, the abnormal PrP$^{Sc}$ acquires both the ability to "multiply," as well as the properties of an infectious agent. It has been recognized, however, that certain amino acid substitutions at one specific site increase susceptibility to infection.

2. **Major symptoms:** All TSEs involve deposition of the PrP$^{Sc}$ protein. In the inherited forms, each PrP$^{Sc}$ mutation is associated with a characteristic clinical phenotype. For example, the most prominent features of CJD are rapidly progressive dementia and behavioral disturbances, ending in death within one year. In GSS, ataxia is the more prominent feature, with death resulting in two to six years. FFI, also fatal within one year, has the additional symptom of uncontrollable insomnia. Although there is some difference in

**Similarities**

- Bacteria
- Fungi
- Protozoa
- Viruses
- Prions

- They all can be transmitted to a healthy individual by inoculation with diseased tissue.
- They all can multiply in the infected host.
- There are characteristic and reproducible pathologic changes and clinical dysfunction in the diseased host.
- Strains differing in virulence and species specificity can be recovered from different hosts.

**Differences**

- Prions

- Compared with conventional infectious agents, prions are extremely resistant to inactivation by UV light and X-rays and to chemical agents that inactivate viruses or bacteria.
- No humoral immune or inflammatory response is observed during the course of the TSE disease.
- No virus-like particles can be seen by electron microscopy or isolated from diseased tissues.
- Certain TSEs, unlike conventional infectious diseases, can be inherited.

**Figure 31.4**
Similarities and differences between conventional and unconventional agents. TSE = Transmissible spongiform encephalopathies.

age of onset, all human TSEs (with the exception of BSE-associated vCJD) occur relatively late in life, typically between the ages of forty and sixty years.

### E. Laboratory identification

A presumptive diagnosis can be made on clinical grounds, but there is some overlap with other dementing illnesses. Routine laboratory tests of serum and cerebral spinal fluid (CSF) are generally normal. The presence of infectious PrP$^{Sc}$ in peripheral lymphatic tissue provides specimens for analysis without the need for brain biopsy. Currently, however, the definitive diagnosis of these diseases is by postmortem histopathologic examination of brain sections.

### F. Treatment and prevention

TSEs are invariably fatal, and no treatment is currently available that can alter this outcome. The unusually high resistance of the infectivity to most disinfecting agents makes prevention of transmission by the usual infection control procedures ineffective. Current recommendations for decontamination of a CJD brain specimen are autoclaving at 132°C, plus immersion in either undiluted sodium hypochlorite or 1N sodium hydroxide. With respect to preventing possible transfer of BSE to humans, all animals showing signs of illness are destroyed, and preparation of animal feed from internal organs of potentially infected animals has ceased.

## Study Questions

**Choose the ONE correct answer**

31.1 A patient with symptoms of Creutzfeldt-Jacob disease caused by eating contaminated beef would most likely exhibit which of the following

   A. circulating antibodies specific for bovine CNS antigens.

   B. DNA copies of the bovine infectious agent integrated into chromosomes of the patient's diseased CNS tissue.

   C. cytotoxic T lymphocytes directed against CNS-specific antigens found in both cattle and humans.

   D. amyloid deposits that have bovine rather than the human amino acid sequences.

   E. lack of any bovine-specific protein or nucleic acid or an immune response.

> Correct answer = E. A and C: An important characteristic of the prion diseases is that there is no unique immune response to either the prion or to CNS antigens. B: A second distinguishing feature of these agents is the absence of a detectable nucleic acid genome. D: The amyloid deposits found in these diseases are composed of the diseased host's proteins, and not of proteins from the source of the infection.

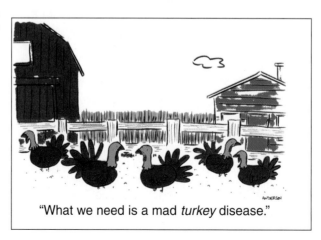

"What we need is a mad *turkey* disease."

# Quick Review of Clinically Important Microorganisms

# 32

## I. OVERVIEW

Although all of the microorganisms presented in this volume have clinical significance, some play a more critical role than do others in the pathology of disease in the United States. This chapter presents a summary of these particularly important microorganisms, using icons to aid the reader in retaining the morphology and classification of the microorganisms. The classifications of bacteria and viruses continues to be presented in pie charts, in which each segment represents a general class of microorganisms ( Figure 32.1A and B). One section of the bacterial pie chart is labeled "Other," and represents any of several microorganisms specifically covered in different chapters. At the top of each box in which a new organism is introduced in this summary chapter, a "pie wedge" is pulled out with an arrow pointing to it. This indicates the general group of bacteria or viruses to which the organism belongs, according to the definitions in  Figure 32.1A or B. The name in large type above the arrow in the **bacteria** section is the name of the **genus** to which the organism(s) listed below the arrow belong (exceptions will be noted in the text). In the **virus** section, the names in large type above the arrow refer to the **family** of which the individual viruses listed below the arrow are members. [Note: Only the bacteria and viruses that are summarized in this chapter are listed below the arrows. Additional organisms belonging to the same genus or family are described in the body of the text.] The order of the microorganisms in this chapter is presented alphabetically in  Figure 32.2.

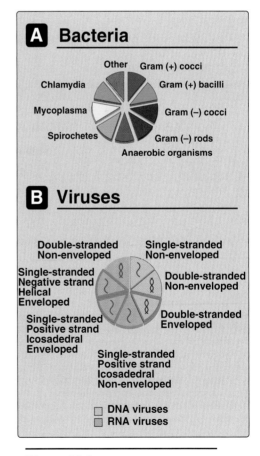

**Figure 32.1**
Representations of medically important bacteria and viruses.

## BACTERIA

## VIRUSES

**FIGURE 32.2**

Alphabetical listing of microorganisms summarized in this chapter. Page numbers refer to location in this chapter.

## BACTERIA

### Bacillus species

***Bacillus anthracis***

## Common characteristics

- **Gram-positive**
- **Blunt-ended bacilli that occur singly, in pairs, or frequently in long chains**
- **Form endospores—oval and centrally located**
- **Nonmotile; has capsule that is antiphagocytic**
- **Facultative or strictly aerobic organisms**
- **Culture on blood agar**

### Pathogenesis/Clinical Significance

*B. anthracis* infects primarily domestic herbivores such as sheep, goats, and horses. Infection usually occurs through contact with infected animal products or spore-contaminated dust that is inoculated through incidental skin abrasions or is inhaled. *B. anthracis* spores are highly resistant to physical and chemical agents, and may remain viable for many years in contaminated pastures or animal materials. *B. anthracis* produces two plasmid-coded exotoxins: edema factor, which causes elevation of intracellular cAMP leading to severe edema, and lethal factor, which causes additional adverse effects. The *B. anthracis* capsule is essential for full virulence.

- **Cutaneous anthrax**

    Upon introduction of organisms or spores that germinate, a papule develops. It rapidly evolves into a painless, black, severely swollen "malignant

[*B. anthracis* is is continued on the next page.]

### Treatment and Prevention

- **Treatment:** *B. anthracis* is sensitive to penicillin, doxycycline and ciprofloxacin. However, these antibiotics are effective in cutaneous anthrax only when administered early in the course of the infection.

- **Prevention:** Because of the resistance of endospores to chemical disinfectants, autoclaving is the only reliable means of decontamination. A cell-free vaccine is available for workers in high-risk occupations.

### Laboratory Identification

- Cultured on blood agar, *B. anthracis* forms large, grayish, nonhemolytic colonies with irregular borders.

- A direct immunofluorescence assay aids in the identification of the organism.

## *Bacillus anthracis* (continued)

| Pathogenesis/Clinical Significance | Treatment and Prevention | Laboratory Identification |
|---|---|---|

pustule", which eventually crusts over. The organisms may invade regional lymph nodes, and then the general circulation, leading to a fatal septicemia. The overall mortality rate in untreated cutaneous anthrax is about twenty percent.

● **Pulmonary anthrax ("wool-sorter's disease")**

Caused by inhalation of spores, this disease is characterized by progressive hemorrhagic pneumonia and lymphadenitis (inflammation of the lymph nodes), and has a mortality rate approaching 100 percent if untreated.

● **Gastrointestinal form of anthrax**

This unusual form of anthrax is caused by ingestion of spores, for example, by eating raw or inadequately cooked meat containing *B. anthracis* spores. This is the portal of entry commonly seen in animals.

# Bordetella species
## *Bordetella pertussis*

# Common characteristics

● **Gram-negative**
● **Small coccobacilli that grow singly or in pairs**
● **Encapsulated**
● **Aerobic**
● **Culture on Regan-Lowe agar**

| Pathogenesis/Clinical Significance | Treatment and Prevention | Laboratory Identification |
|---|---|---|

*B. pertussis* is transmitted primarily by droplets spread by coughing. The organism survives only briefly in the environment. *B. pertussis* binds to ciliated epithelium in the upper respiratory tract. There the bacteria produce a variety of toxins and other virulence factors that interfere with ciliary activity, eventually causing the death of these cells.

● **Pertussis ("whooping cough")**

The incubation period for this disease ranges from one to three weeks. The disease can be divided into two phases: 1) the **catarrhal phase**, which begins with relatively nonspecific symptoms, and then progresses to include a dry, nonproductive cough; and 2) the **paroxysmal phase**, in which the cough worsens, causing paroxysms of coughing followed by a "whoop" as the patient inspires rapidly. Large amounts of mucus are typically produced. During the three-to-four week convalescent period, secondary complications, such as encephalopathy, seizures, and/or pneumonia, may occur.

● **Treatment:** Erythromycin is the drug of choice for *B. pertussis* infections, both as chemotherapy and as chemoprophylaxis for household contacts. Trimethoprim-sulfamethoxazole is an alternative choice for erythromycin treatment failures.

● **Prevention:** Two forms of vaccine are currently available (one of killed whole cells, and one that is acellular, containing purified *B. pertussis* proteins). Both are formulated in combination with diphtheria and tetanus toxoids.

● *B. pertussis* from nasopharyngeal samples can be cultured on selective agar such as Regan-Lowe medium, where the organism produces pinpoint, hemolytic colonies.

● More rapid diagnosis may be accomplished using a direct fluorescent antibody test to detect *B. pertussis* in smears of nasopharyngeal specimens.

# Borrelia species
### *Borrelia burgdorferi*

## Common characteristics

● Gram-negative, but some stain poorly and need to be visualized by other means

● Long, slender, flexible, spiral- or corkscrew-shaped rods

● Organisms are highly motile

● Difficult and time-consuming to culture

| Pathogenesis/Clinical Significance | Treatment and Prevention | Laboratory Identification |
|---|---|---|

*B. burgdorferi* is transmitted to humans by the bite of a small tick (genus *Ixodes*), which must feed for at least 24 hours to deliver an infectious dose. Deer, mice, other rodents, and birds serve as reservoirs for the spirochete. The organism is not spread from human to human.

● **Lyme disease**

The first stage of the disease begins 3 to 22 days after a tick bite, with a characteristic red, circular rash with a clear center (erythema chronicum migrans) appearing at the site of the bite. Flu-like symptoms can accompany the rash. The organism spreads via the lymph or blood to musculoskeletal sites, the skin, central nervous system, heart, and other organs. Weeks to months after the initial symptoms, the second stage of the disease begins with symptoms such as arthritis, arthralgia, cardiac complications, and neurologic complications such as meningitis. The third stage begins months to years later, with chronic arthritis and progressive central nervous system disease.

● **Treatment:** Cephalosporins, amoxicillin, or doxycycline are useful in treating the early stages of Lyme disease. If arthritic symptoms have already appeared, longer courses of antibiotics are used.

● **Prevention:** A ninety percent effective vaccine is currently available. The best prevention is wearing clothing that limits skin exposure to ticks, and using insect repellent.

● Samples of blood can be treated with Giemsa or Wright stain to visualize the large, loosely coiled *B. burgdorferi* when present.

● The polymerase chain reaction used to assist in detection of *B. burgdorferi* in body fluids provides the most definitive test.

● *B. burgdorferi* infection can be diagnosed serologically, but the number of false positives can outnumber the true positives.

# Brucella species
### *Brucella abortus*
### *Brucella canis*
### *Brucella melitensis*
### *Brucella suis*

## Common characteristics

● Gram-negative

● Small coccobacilli, arranged singly or in pairs

● Unencapsulated

● Aerobic, intracellular parasites

● Culture on blood agar

| Pathogenesis/Clinical Significance | Treatment and Prevention | Laboratory Identification |
|---|---|---|

Brucellosis is a chronic, lifelong infection in animals. Organisms localize in reproductive organs (male and female), and are shed in large numbers, for example, in milk and urine. Transmission to humans usually occurs either through direct contact with infected animal tissues or ingestion of unpasteurized milk or milk products. Human-to-human transmission is rare.

Brucellae typically enter the body through cuts in the skin or through the GI tract. They are transported via the lymphatic system to the regional lymph nodes, where they survive and multiply within host phagocytes. They are then carried by the blood to organs that are involved in the reticuloendothelial system, including the liver, spleen, kidneys, bone marrow, and other lymph nodes. Lipopolysaccharide is the major virulence factor.

● **Brucellosis (undulant fever)**

Symptoms of brucellosis are nonspecific and flu-like (malaise, fever, sweats, anorexia and GI symptoms, headache, and back pains), and may also include depression. Untreated patients may develop an undulating pattern of fever. Brucellosis may involve any of a variety of organ systems, including the GI tract, and the skeletal, neurologic, cardiovascular, and pulmonary systems.

● **Treatment:** Combination therapy involving doxycycline and either streptomycin or gentamicin is recommended for brucellosis. Prolonged treatment (for example, six weeks) is generally necessary to prevent relapse and to reduce the incidence of complications.

● A detailed history is often crucial because of the nonspecific symptoms.

● The organism can be cultured from blood and other body fluids, or from tissue specimens, but isolation of the organism is difficult and time consuming.

● Serologic tests for agglutinating antibodies are diagnostically useful. Titers greater than 1:160 and rising are considered indicative of brucella infection.

# Campylobacter species

*Campylobacter jejuni*

# Common characteristics

- Gram-negative
- Curved, spiral, or S-shaped rods
- Single, polar flagellum results in characteristic darting motion
- Microaerophilic
- Do not ferment carbohydrates
- Culture on selective medium (blood agar containing antibiotics to inhibit growth of other fecal flora)

| Pathogenesis/Clinical Significance | Treatment and Prevention | Laboratory Identification |
|---|---|---|
| *C. jejuni* is widely distributed in nature, existing as part of the normal flora of many vertebrate species, including both mammals and fowl, wild and domestic. Transmission is via the fecal/oral route through direct contact, or exposure to contaminated meat (especially poultry) or to contaminated water.<br><br>*C. jejuni* infects the intestine, where it can cause ulcerative, inflammatory lesions in the jejunum, ileum, or colon. Although cytotoxins and enterotoxins have been identified, the role of these molecules in disease has not been established.<br><br>● **Acute enteritis**<br>*C. jejuni* is the leading cause of food-borne disease in the United States. Symptoms may be both systemic (fever, headache, myalgia) and intestinal (abdominal cramping and diarrhea, which may or may not be bloody). *C. jejuni* is a cause of both traveler's diarrhea and pseudoappendicitis. Rare complications include septic abortion, reactive arthritis, and Guillain-Barre syndrome. | ● **Treatment:** Diarrhea should be treated symptomatically (fluid and electrolyte replacement). If disease is severe, ciprofloxacin is the drug of choice.<br><br>● **Prevention:** No vaccine or preventive drug is available. Good hygiene, avoiding contaminated water, pasteurizing milk and milk products, and thoroughly cooking potentially contaminated food (for example, poultry) is important in prevention of infection. | ● Presumptive diagnosis can be made on the basis of finding curved organisms with rapid, darting motility in a wet mount of feces. |

# Chlamydia species

*Chlamydia pneumoniae*
*Chlamydia psittaci*
*Chlamydia trachomatis*

# Common characteristics

- Not routinely stained with Gram stain
- Small, round to ovoid organisms
- Envelope consists of two lipid bilayers
- Obligate intracellular parasites, the organisms replicate in endocytic vacuoles, creating characteristic cytoplasmic inclusion bodies

*Chlamydia pneumoniae*

| Pathogenesis/Clinical Significance | Treatment and Prevention | Laboratory Identification |
|---|---|---|
| *C. pneumoniae* is generally transmitted by respiratory droplets. *Chlamydia* are energy parasites, and require exogenous ATP and NAD$^+$ for growth. They acquire these compounds by replicating inside host cells.<br><br>● **Community-acquired respiratory infection**<br>*C. pneumoniae* is a significant cause of respiratory infections worldwide, causing pharyngitis, laryngitis, bronchitis, and interstitial pneumonia. Epidemic outbreaks have been reported. | ● **Treatment:** Doxycycline and erythromycin are the drugs of choice.<br>● **Prevention:** No vaccine or preventive drug is available. | ● Neither serologic tests nor recovery by culturing is routinely available. |

[*CHLAMYDIA* SPECIES ARE CONTINUED ON THE NEXT PAGE]

## *Chlamydia psittaci*

| Pathogenesis/Clinical Significance | Treatment and Prevention | Laboratory Identification |
|---|---|---|
| ● **Psittacosis (ornithosis)**<br><br>This is a zoonotic disease transmitted to humans by inhalation of dust contaminated with respiratory secretions or feces of infected birds (such as parrots). *C. psittaci* infection of humans targets the respiratory tract, causing a dry cough, flu-like symptoms, and pulmonary infiltrates. Enlargement of the liver and spleen frequently occurs. | ● **Treatment:** Tetracycline and doxycycline are the drugs of choice. Erythromycin therapy is the alternative treatment, but may be less efficacious in severe cases. | ● Demonstration of a rise in antibody titer, using either complement fixation or indirect immunofluorescence tests, can aid in diagnosis. |

## *Chlamydia trachomatis*

| Pathogenesis/Clinical Significance | Treatment and Prevention | Laboratory Identification |
|---|---|---|
| ● **Nongonococcal urethritis (NGU)**<br><br>*C. trachomatis* is the major causal agent of NGU, which is the most common sexually transmitted bacterial disease in the United States. It is transmitted by personal contact, and affects both sexes. Repeated or chronic exposure to *C. trachomatis* can lead to sterility and ectopic pregnancy. Women may develop **pelvic inflammatory disease (PID)**.<br><br>● **Trachoma**<br><br>*C. trachomatis* causes eye infections (**chronic keratoconjunctivitis**) with symptoms that range from simple irritation of the eye to blindness. This disease is widely prevalent in developing countries. It is transmitted by personal contact with infected humans or contaminated surfaces, and by flies.<br><br>● **Inclusion conjunctivitis of the newborn (ICN)**<br><br>Infants born to mothers infected with *C. trachomatis* can become infected during passage through the birth canal. This can lead to an acute, purulent conjunctivitis that is usually self-healing.<br><br>● **Lymphogranuloma venereum (LGV)**<br><br>*C. trachomatis* causes LGV, an invasive, sexually transmitted disease that is uncommon in the United States, but is endemic in Asia, Africa, and South America. LGV is characterized by transient papules on the external genitalia, followed in one to two months by painful swelling of inguinal and perirectal lymph nodes. Regional lymphatic drainage can become blocked. | ● **Treatment:** Azithromycin, erythromycin, and tetracyclines such as doxycycline are useful in treating chlamydial infections. [Note: Erythromycin is used for young children and pregnant women.]<br><br>● **Prevention:** No vaccine is available. Erythromycin or silver nitrate in ointment or eyedrops is applied prophylactically to newborns' eyes, especially those at risk. Proper precautions should be taken during sexual contact to prevent transmission of NGU. | ● Microscopic examination of infected cells stained with direct fluorescent antibodies reveals characteristic cellular cytoplasmic inclusions.<br><br>● Nucleic acid hybridization using a DNA probe for chlamydial ribosomal RNA genes can detect *C. trachomatis* with a high degree of sensitivity.<br><br>● An enzymatic immunoassay that detects chlamydial lipopolysaccharides is also available. |

# Clostridia species

### Clostridium botulinum
### Clostridium difficile
### Clostridium perfringens
### Clostridium tetani

# Common characteristics

● **Gram-positive**

● **Large, blunt-ended rods that produce endospores**

● **Most species are motile**

● **Obligate anaerobe**

● **Culture anaerobically on blood agar**

## *Clostridium botulinum*

| Pathogenesis/Clinical Significance | Treatment and Prevention | Laboratory Identification |
|---|---|---|
| *C. botulinum* is found in soil and aquatic sediments. Its spores contaminate vegetables, meat, and fish. *C. botulinum* exotoxin inhibits the release of acetylcholine at the neuromuscular junctions, preventing contraction and causing flaccid paralysis.<br><br>● **Botulism (food poisoning) and floppy baby syndrome**<br><br>Caused by ingestion of exotoxin, leading to flaccid paralysis, vomiting, and diarrhea. Death can occur due to respiratory paralysis. *C. botulinum* colonizes the large intestine, producing exotoxin that is slowly absorbed. Lethargy, poor muscle tone, and constipation result. | ● **Treatment:** Antitoxin (horse antiserum) that neutralizes unbound botulinum toxin should be administered as soon as possible in suspected botulinal intoxication.<br><br>● **Prevention:** Proper food preservation techniques prevent the production of the clostridial exotoxin. | ● *C. botulinum* toxin can be detected in food, intestinal contents, or serum by mouse inoculation with or without neutralizing antiserum.<br><br>● The organism can be cultured and identified by standard anaerobic methods. |

[CLOSTRIDIA SPECIES ARE CONTINUED ON THE NEXT PAGE.]

## Clostridium difficile

| Pathogenesis/Clinical Significance | Treatment and Prevention | Laboratory Identification |
|---|---|---|
| *C. difficile* is found as a normal but minor component of the flora of the large intestine. Its spores can contaminate indoor as well as outdoor environments. *C. difficile* can overgrow in the colon of an individual on antibiotics that deplete the normal flora.<br><br>*C. difficile* enterotoxin A causes excessive fluid secretion and an inflammatory response in the colon. Toxin B is a cytotoxin that disrupts protein synthesis, causing lysis of host cells.<br><br>● **Pseudomembranous colitis**<br>Caused by toxins A and B, this condition is characterized by watery, explosive diarrhea and pseudomembrane formation in the colon. | ●**Treatment:** Discontinue the predisposing drug, and replace fluids and electrolytes. *C. difficile* is resistant to many antibiotics. Oral administration of vancomycin or metronidazole may be added in severe cases.<br><br>● **Prevention:** No vaccine or preventive drug is available. | ● The enterotoxin can be detected in stool samples using the ELISA test for exotoxins A and B.<br><br>● The presence of a pseudomembrane in the colon can be detected by endoscopy. |

## Clostridium perfringens

| Pathogenesis/Clinical Significance | Treatment and Prevention | Laboratory Identification |
|---|---|---|
| *C. perfringens* is part of the normal flora of the vagina and gastrointestinal tract. Its spores are found in soil. *C. perfringens* alpha toxin is a phospholipase C (lecithinase) that causes lysis of endothelial and blood cells. The bacterium produces at least eleven additional exotoxins that have hemolytic or other cytotoxic and necrotic effects.<br><br>● **Myonecrosis (gas gangrene)**<br>Spores germinate in open wounds such as those caused by GI tract surgery, burns, puncture wounds, and war wounds, and produce cytotoxic factors. Fermentation of tissue carbohydrates causes formation of gas bubbles. As the disease progresses, increased capillary permeability leads to exotoxins being carried by the circulation from the damaged tissues to other organs, resulting in systemic effects such as shock, renal failure, and intravascular hemolysis. Untreated myonecrosis is uniformly fatal.<br><br>● **Acute food poisoning**<br>This condition is caused by the generation of spores in improperly cooked food, resulting in the production of enterotoxin that disrupts ion transport in the lower portion of the small intestine. This causes loss of fluid and intracellular proteins.<br><br>● **Anaerobic cellulitis**<br>This is clostridial infection of connective tissue in which bacterial growth spreads rapidly along fascial planes. | ● **Treatment of gas gangrene:** Immediate treatment and wound debridement or amputation, and exposure of the wound to hyperbaric oxygen are important mechanisms for treating the infection. High doses of penicillin G or doxycycline should be administered.<br><br>● **Treatment of food poisoning:** Clostridial food poisoning is usually self-limiting and requires only supportive care.<br><br>● **Prevention:** No vaccine or preventive drug is available. Prevention of food poisoning is a matter of appropriate food handling practices. | ● When specimens from diseased tissue are Gram stained, large, gram-positive rods are observed.<br><br>● When cultured anaerobically on blood agar, *C. perfringens* produces a unique double-zone of β-hemolysis.<br><br>● Other diagnostic biochemical tests are available that measure such characteristics as sugar fermentation and organic acid production. |

## Clostridium tetani

| Pathogenesis/Clinical Significance | Treatment and Prevention | Laboratory Identification |
|---|---|---|
| *C. tetani* spores are common in soil. *C. tetani* exotoxin, tetanospasmin, binds irreversibly, penetrating neurons and blocking neurotransmitter release at inhibitory synapses. This causes severe, prolonged muscle spasms.<br><br>● **Tetanus ("lockjaw")**<br>Caused by *C. tetani* spores infecting a puncture wound, a severe burn or postsurgical incision. In the early stages, the jaw muscles are affected, so that the mouth cannot open (**trismus** or "lockjaw"). Gradually, other voluntary muscles become involved. Death is usually the result of paralysis of the chest muscles, leading to respiratory failure. | ● **Treatment:** Preferred treatment is with human hyperimmune (tetanus immune) globulin. Alternative treatment is with horse antitoxin. Sedatives and muscle relaxants are administered, and proper ventilation should be maintained. *C. tetani* is sensitive to penicillin.<br><br>● **Prevention:** Inactivated tetanus toxoid (formalin-inactivated toxin) is given as part of the DPT vaccine (D=diphtheria toxoid; P=pertussis antigen). | ● Diagnosis is based on clinical findings, because laboratory identification is difficult (*C. tetani* is difficult to culture, and frequently, few organisms can be isolated from infected tissue). |

# Corynebacterium species
## *Corynebacterium diphtheriae*

## Common characteristics

- Gram-positive; stain unevenly
- Small, slender, pleomorphic rods that form characteristic clumps that look like Chinese characters or a picket fence
- Nonmotile and unencapsulated
- Most species are facultative anaerobes
- Culture aerobically on selective medium such as Tinsdale agar

### Pathogenesis/Clinical Significance

*C. diphtheriae* is found on the skin, and in the nose, throat, and nasopharynx of carriers and patients with diphtheria. The organism is spread primarily by respiratory droplets.

Diphtheria is caused by the local and systemic effects of a single exotoxin that inhibits eukaryotic protein synthesis. This toxin inactivates eukaryotic polypeptide chain elongation factor EF-2 by ADP-ribosylation, thus terminating protein synthesis. [Note: The structural gene for the toxin is coded for by a bacteriophage; only those strains of *C. diphtheriae* that are lysogenic for this phage can produce toxin and are therefore virulent.]

- **Diphtheria**

  This life-threatening disease begins as a local infection, usually of the throat. The infection produces a distinctive thick, grayish, adherent exudate (called a pseudomembrane) that is composed of cell debris from the mucosa, and inflammatory products. The exudate coats the throat and may extend into the nasal passages or respiratory tract where it sometimes obstructs the airways, leading to suffocation. Generalized symptoms are due to dissemination of the toxin. Although all human cells are sensitive to diphtheria toxin, major clinical effects involve the heart (myocarditis may lead to congestive heart failure and permanent heart damage) and peripheral nerves (neuritis of cranial nerves and paralysis of muscle groups such as those that control movement of the palate or the eye).

### Treatment and Prevention

- **Treatment:** A single dose of horse serum antitoxin inactivates any circulating toxin, although it does not affect toxin that is already bound to a cell-surface receptor. [Note: Serum sickness caused by a reaction to the horse protein may cause complications.] Eradication of the organism is accomplished with any of several antibiotics, such as erythromycin or penicillin.

- **Prevention:** Immunization with toxoid, usually administered in the DPT triple vaccine (together with tetanus toxoid and pertussis antigens) should be started in infancy. Booster injections of diphtheria toxoid (with tetanus toxoid) should be given at approximately ten-year intervals throughout life.

### Laboratory Identification

- The initial diagnosis and decision to treat for diphtheria must be made based on clinical observation, because no reliable, rapid laboratory test is available.

- *C. diphtheriae* can be cultured on selective media such as Tinsdale agar, which contains potassium tellurite, an inhibitor of other respiratory flora. The organism can then be tested for toxin production using an immunologic precipitin reaction.

# Enterococcus species
## *Enterococcus faecalis*
## *Enterococcus faecium*

## Common characteristics

- Gram-positive
- Round-to-ovoid in shape, occurring in pairs or chains
- α- or nonhemolytic colonies
- Catalase-negative
- Grow in 6.5 percent NaCl; culture on bile-esculin agar

### Pathogenesis/Clinical Significance

*Enterococcus faecalis* and *Enterococcus faecium* are part of the normal fecal flora.

- **Nosocomial infections:** Enterococci are frequent causes of such infections—especially in intensive care units. Under conditions where host resistance is lowered, or where the integrity of the gastrointestinal or genitourinary tract has been disrupted, enterococci can spread to normally sterile sites, causing urinary tract infections, bacteremia/sepsis, subacute bacterial endocarditis, biliary tract infection, or intraabdominal abscesses.

### Treatment and Prevention

- **Treatment:** A combination of a penicillin and an aminoglycoside, or the glycopeptide vancomycin is used to treat enterococcal infections. Newer antibiotics, such as the combination of quinupristin and dalfopristin, are used to threat vancomycin-resistant infections.

- **Prevention:** No vaccine is available against enterococci. Careful attention to hand washing and other cleanliness measures among hospital personnel can significantly decrease the incidence of nosocomial infections.

### Laboratory Identification

- Enterococci are distinguished from the non-Group D streptococci by their ability to survive in 6.5 percent sodium chloride. They can also hydrolyze the polysaccharide esculin in the presence of bile.

# Escherichia species
## *Escherichia coli*

# Common characteristics

● **Gram-negative**

● **Short rods**

● **Facultative anaerobe**

● **Ferments glucose and a wide range of carbohydrates**

● **Catalase-positive, oxidase-negative**

● **Culture on MacConkey agar**

| Pathogenesis/Clinical Significance | Treatment and Prevention | Laboratory Identification |
|---|---|---|

*E. coli* is part of the normal flora in the colon of humans and other animals, but can be pathogenic both within and outside the gastrointestinal tract. *E. coli* species possess three types of antigens, O, K, and H. Pili facilitate the attachment of the bacterium to human epithelial surfaces. Diseases caused by *E. coli* can be gastrointestinal and/or extraintestinal.

● **Urinary tract infections (UTI)**

*E. coli* is the most common cause of UTIs, especially in women. Symptoms include dysuria, urinary frequency, hematuria, and pyuria.

● **Diarrhea**

Several categories of diarrhea are caused by different strains of *E. coli*. Among the most prevalent are the following:

**Enterotoxigenic *E. coli* (ETEC):** This organism is a common cause of "**traveler's diarrhea**" in developing countries. It infects only humans, with transmission occurring through food and water contaminated with human waste, or by person-to-person contact. ETEC colonizes the small intestine, and in a process mediated by an enterotoxin that stimulates increased cAMP production, causes prolonged hypersecretion of chloride ions and water while inhibiting the reabsorption of sodium. The gut becomes full of fluid, resulting in significant watery diarrhea over a period of several days.

**Enteropathogenic *E. coli* (EPEC):** This organism is an important cause of diarrhea in infants, especially in developing countries. The newborn becomes infected during birth or *in utero*. EPEC attaches to mucosal cells in the small intestine, causing destruction of microvilli and development of characteristic lesions. Watery diarrhea results, which may become chronic.

**Enterohemorrhagic *E. coli* (EHEC):** EHEC binds to cells in the large intestine, and produces an exotoxin (**verotoxin**) that destroys microvilli, causing a severe form of copious, bloody diarrhea (**hemorrhagic colitis**) and acute renal failure (**hemolytic uremic syndrome**). Serotype O157:H7 is the most common strain of *E. coli* that produces verotoxin. The primary reservoir of EHEC is cattle. Therefore the possibility of infection can be greatly decreased by thoroughly cooking ground beef and pasteurizing milk.

● **Meningitis in infants**

*E. coli* and group B streptococci are the leading causes of neonatal meningitis. Newborns lack IgM, and therefore are particularly susceptible to *E. coli* sepsis, which can result in the organism's being carried to the brain.

● **Treatment for UTIs:**
Trimethoprim-sulfamethoxazole or a fluoroquinolone, such as ciprofloxacin, are the drugs of choice. [Note: Isolated microorganisms must be tested for antibiotic sensitivity because multiple drug resistance, carried by transmissible plasmids, is common.]

● **Treatment for meningitis:** The combination of a cephalosporin, such as cefotaxime, plus gentamicin is usually recommended.

● **Treatment for diarrhea:**
Antibiotics cited above shorten the duration of the disease. Patients with diarrhea must be rehydrated and their electrolytes replaced.

● **Prevention:** No vaccine or preventive drug is available. Diarrhea can be prevented by taking precautions in food and water consumption. Spread of infection between people can be controlled by hand washing and disinfection.

● *E. coli* can be cultured on differential medium such as MacConkey agar.

● Carbohydrate fermentation patterns are observed, for example, most strains of *E. coli* ferment lactose, produce gas during glucose fermentation, and show a positive test for mannitol fermentation.

# Francisella species
## *Francisella tularensis*

# Common characteristics

- **Gram-negative**
- **Small, pleomorphic coccobacillus with a lipid-rich capsule**
- **Facultative intracellular parasite**
- **Strict aerobe**
- **Primarily pathogen of animals**
- **Rarely cultured**

## Pathogenesis/Clinical Significance

The host range of *F. tularensis* is broad, and includes wild and domestic mammals, birds, and house pets. A number of biting or blood-sucking arthropods serve as vectors. Transmission is thus by contact with infected animal tissues, contaminated water, or an arthropod bite. Tularemia is an occupational risk for veterinarians, hunters and trappers, domestic livestock workers, and meat handlers.

*F. tularensis* is an intracellular parasite that can survive and multiply within host macrophages as well as in other cells. After cutaneous inoculation, *F. tularensis* multiplies locally, producing a papule that ulcerates after several days. Organisms spread from the local lesion to the regional lymph nodes, where they cause enlarged, tender nodes that may suppurate. From the lymph nodes, the organisms spread via the lymphatic system to various organs and tissues, including lungs, liver, spleen, kidneys, and the CNS.

- **Tularemia**

  Tularemia varies in severity from mild to fulminant and fatal. Onset of symptoms is usually abrupt. The most common symptoms are flu-like (chills, fever, headache, malaise, anorexia, and fatigue), although respiratory and gastrointestinal symptoms may also occur. Ulcers may result from contact with animal products or from insect bites (ulceroglandular tularemia). Lymphadenopathy is characteristic.

## Treatment and Prevention

- **Treatment:** The drug of choice for treatment of tularemia is streptomycin or, as an alternate, gentamicin.
- **Prevention:** Avoiding insect vectors and taking precautions when handling wild animals or animal products are the best means of prevention of *F. tularensis* infection.

## Laboratory Identification

- Clinical presentation and history consistent with possible exposure is of primary importance in the diagnosis of tularemia. Confirmation of the clinical diagnosis is most commonly made serologically.
- The organism is rarely cultured.

# Haemophilus species
## *Haemophilus influenzae*

# Common characteristics

- **Gram-negative**
- **Pleomorphic in shape, ranging from small coccobacilli to long, slender filaments**
- **Obligate parasite, requiring hemin and NAD+ for growth**
- **Culture on chocolate agar containing hemin and NAD+**

## Pathogenesis/Clinical Significance

*H. influenzae* is a normal resident of the human upper respiratory tract, and may also colonize the conjunctiva and genital tract. Transmission is by respiratory droplets.

*H. influenzae* may be unencapsulated, or may produce a capsule (capsular type b is associated with the most serious, invasive disease). After attaching to and colonizing the respiratory mucosa, the infection can become systemic, with bacteria spreading via the blood to the central nervous system.

- **Bacterial meningitis**

  *H. influenzae* is a leading cause of bacterial meningitis, especially in infants and very young children.

  [*H. INFLUENZAE* IS CONTINUED ON THE NEXT PAGE.]

## Treatment and Prevention

- **Treatment:** Antibiotic sensitivity testing should be done to determine appropriate antibiotic. Generally, a third-generation cephalosporin such as cefotaxime or ceftriaxone is effective in the treatment of meningitis. The combination of ampicillin plus sulbactam is also used.
- **Prevention:** A conjugated vaccine against *H. influenzae* capsular polysaccharide type b (Hib) is administered to infants. Rifampin is given prophylactically.

## Laboratory Identification

- *H. influenzae* can be cultured on chocolate agar containing hemin (factor X) and NAD+ (factor V).
- Capsular swelling (quellung reaction) can be observed, and the capsule can be identified by immunofluorescent staining.
- Capsular antigen can also be detected in CSF or other body fluids using immunologic techniques.

*Haemophilus influenzae* (continued)

| Pathogenesis/Clinical Significance | Treatment and Prevention | Laboratory Identification |
| --- | --- | --- |

● **Upper respiratory tract infections**

*H. influenzae* is a major cause of otitis media, sinusitis, and epiglottitis, primarily in children.

● **Pneumonia**

This organism causes pneumonia, particularly of the elderly or immuno-compromised individuals.

# Helicobacter species
### *Helicobacter pylori*

# Common characteristics

● **Gram-negative**

● **Curved or spiral rods**

● **Multiple polar flagella give the organism rapid, corkscrew motility**

● **Urease-positive**

● **Culture on selective medium containing antibiotics to inhibit growth of other fecal flora**

| Pathogenesis/Clinical Significance | Treatment and Prevention | Laboratory Identification |
| --- | --- | --- |

*H. pylori* is unusual in its ability to colonize the stomach, where low pH normally protects against bacterial infection. Transmission is thought to be from person to person (the organism has not been isolated from food or water). Untreated, infections tend to be chronic and life-long.

*H. pylori* colonizes gastric mucosal cells in the stomach, surviving in the mucous layer that coats the epithelium. The organism is noninvasive, but recruits and activates inflammatory cells, thus causing a chronic inflammation of the mucosa. *H. pylori* secretes urease, producing ammonium ions that neutralize stomach acid in the vicinity of the organism, thus favoring bacterial multiplication. Ammonia can damage the gastric mucosa, and may also potentiate the effects of a cytotoxin produced by *H. pylori*.

● **Acute gastritis**

Initial infection with *H. pylori* results in decreased mucous production, and leads to acute gastritis. Both **duodenal ulcers** and **gastric ulcers** are closely correlated with infection by *H. pylori*. The organism appears to be a risk factor for development of **gastric carcinoma** and **gastric B-cell lymphoma**.

● **Treatment:** Elimination of *H. pylori* requires combination therapy with two or more antimicrobials due to rapid appearance of resistant strains. A typical regimen includes tetracycline plus metronidazole plus bismuth salts.

● **Prevention:** No vaccine or preventive drug is available.

● Characteristic corkscrew movement can be seen in smears of biopsied gastric mucosa.

● Urease-positivity can be measured by a breath test (radioactively labeled urea is cleaved by bacterial enzyme, releasing radioactive $CO_2$ in expired breath).

● Serologic tests are available, including ELISA for serum antibodies to *H. pylori*.

# Legionella species
## *Legionella pneumophila*

# Common characteristics

- Gram-negative (faintly staining)
- Slender rod in nature; coccobacillary in clinical material
- Facultative, intracellular parasite
- Organisms are unencapsulated with monotrichous flagella
- Culture on specialized medium

## Pathogenesis/Clinical Significance

*L. pneumophila's* normal habitats are water and soil, and the organism can colonize cooling towers, humidifiers, air conditioners, and water distribution systems. The organism is chlorine tolerant, and thus survives water treatment procedures.

Infections generally result from inhalation of aerosolized organisms. The resulting pathology is therefore initially confined primarily to the respiratory tract. Macrophages phagocytose the *L. pneumophila*, but the phagosome fails to fuse with a lysosome. Instead, the organisms multiply within this protected environment until the cell ruptures, releasing increased numbers of infectious bacteria.

### ● Legionnaires' disease

This is an acute lobar pneumonia with multisystem symptoms. Predisposing factors include immunocompromise, pulmonary compromise (due, for example, to heavy smoking or chronic lung disease), and debilitation brought on by excessive alcohol consumption, age, or surgery. Pneumonia (associated with a cough that is only slightly productive) is the predominant symptom. Watery, nonbloody diarrhea occurs in 25 to 50 percent of cases. Nausea, vomiting, and neurologic symptoms may also occur.

### ● Pontiac fever

This is an influenza-like illness that characteristically infects otherwise healthy individuals. Recovery is usually complete within one week.

## Treatment and Prevention

- **Treatment:** Macrolides, such as erythromycin or azithromycin, are the drugs of choice for legionnaire's disease. Fluoroquinolones are also effective. No specific therapy is required for Pontiac fever.

- **Prevention:** No vaccine or preventive drug is available. Measures such as flushing the water supply with extremely hot water decrease the chance of contamination.

## Laboratory Identification

- Culture *L. pneumophila* from respiratory secretions using buffered charcoal yeast extract enriched with L-cysteine, iron, and α-ketoglutarate.

- Serologic tests include a direct fluorescent antibody test and a radioimmunoassay for *L. pneumophila* antigen in the urine.

- Hybridization with *L. pneumophila* ribosomal RNA using a DNA probe is also available.

---

# Leptospira species
## *Leptospira interrogans*

# Common characteristics

- Gram-negative, but stains poorly, and needs to be visualized by other means
- Long, very slender, flexible, spiral- or corkscrew-shaped rods
- Highly motile
- Culture on specialized medium

## Pathogenesis/Clinical Significance

A number of wild and domestic animals serve as reservoirs for *L. interrogans*. Transmission to humans occurs following ingestion of food or water contaminated, for example, by animal urine containing the spirochete. These organisms can survive for several weeks in stagnant water, but are sensitive to drying.

### ● Leptospirosis

Different strains of *L. interrogans* are found worldwide, and cause leptospirosis, known under various local names such as **infectious jaundice**, **marsh fever**, **Weil's disease**, and **swineherd's disease**. Fever occurs about one to two weeks after infection, and *L. interrogans* is present in the blood. The organisms next infect various organs, particularly the liver and kidneys, resulting in jaundice, hemorrhage, and tissue necrosis. Large numbers of leptospira are shed into the urine by the diseased kidneys. The second phase of the disease involves a rise in IgM antibody titer accompanied by aseptic meningitis. Hepatitis frequently occurs.

## Treatment and Prevention

- **Treatment:** Penicillin G or a tetracycline such as doxycycline are used during early stages of the infection.

- **Prevention:** No vaccine is available. Doxycycline is effective prophylactically. Prevention of exposure to contaminated water, and rodent control, can both help decrease the chance of infection.

## Laboratory Identification

- *L. interrogans* does not stain well. However, the organisms can sometimes be observed in a fresh blood smear by dark-field microscopy.

- *L. interrogans* can be detected by serologic agglutination tests.

# Listeria species
### *Listeria monocytogenes*

# Common characteristics

- **Gram-positive, staining darkly**
- **Slender, short rods, sometimes occurring as diplobacilli or in short chains**
- **Intracellular parasites**
- **Catalase-positive**
- **Distinctive tumbling motility in liquid medium**
- **Grow facultatively on a variety of enriched media**

## Pathogenesis/Clinical Significance

*Listeria* species are widespread among animals in nature. Infections with the pathogenic *L. monocytogenes* may occur as sporadic cases or in small epidemics which are usually food-borne (dairy products, ground meats, and poultry).

*L. monocytogenes* is a facultative, intracellular parasite. It attaches to and enters a variety of mammalian cells by phagocytosis. Once inside the cell, it escapes from the phagocytic vacuole by producing a membrane-damaging toxin, **listeriolysin**. *Listeria* grows in the cytosol, and stimulates changes in cell function that facilitate its direct passage from cell to cell.

- **Listeriosis**

  Septicemia and meningitis are the most commonly reported forms of listeria infection. The organism can be transmitted from an infected mother to her newborn (*Listeria* is a relatively common cause of newborn meningitis), or to the fetus, initiating abortion. Immunocompromised individuals, especially those with defects in cellular immunity, are susceptible to serious, generalized infections.

## Treatment and Prevention

- **Treatment:** A variety of antibiotics have been successfully used to treat *L. monocytogenes* infections, including ampicillin or trimethoprim plus sulfamethoxazole.
- **Prevention:** No vaccine is available against *L. monocytogenes*. Prevention of *Listeria* infections can be accomplished by proper food preparation and handling.

## Laboratory Identification

- *L. monocytogenes* can be isolated from blood, cerebrospinal fluid, and other clinical specimens.
- On blood agar, the organism produces a small colony surrounded by a narrow zone of β hemolysis.
- *Listeria* species can be distinguished by morphology, positive motility, and the production of catalase.

# Mycobacterium species
### *Mycobacterium leprae*
### *Mycobacterium tuberculosis*

# Common characteristics

- **Not colored by Gram stain due to lipid-rich cell walls**
- **Long, slender, nonmotile rods**
- **Aerobic**
- **Resistant to drying**
- **Culture *M. tuberculosis* on specialized medium such as Lowenstein-Jensen agar; *M. leprae* does not grow in culture**

### *Mycobacterium leprae*

## Pathogenesis/Clinical Significance

*M. leprae* has low infectivity. It is transmitted from human to human through prolonged contact, for example between exudates of a leprosy patient's skin lesions, and the abraded skin of another individual. No *M. leprae* toxins or virulence factors are known.

- **Hansen disease (leprosy)**

  Leprosy is a chronic granulomatous condition of peripheral nerves and skin. There are two clinical forms: **tuberculoid leprosy**, in which destructive lesions due to the host's cell-mediated immune response occur as large macular plaques in cooler body tissues such as skin (especially nose and outer ears), testicles, and in superficial nerve endings; and **lepromatous leprosy**, in which the cell-mediated immune response is severely depressed, and the disease becomes slow but progressive, with large numbers of organisms in the lesions and blood.

[*MYCOBACTERIUM* SPECIES ARE CONTINUED ON THE NEXT PAGE.*]

## Treatment and Prevention

- **Treatment for tuberculoid form:** Dapsone plus rifampin.
- **Treatment for lepromatous form:** Clofazamine. Both forms require long-term antibiotic treatment.
- **Prevention:** No preventive drug is available. Vaccination with BCG shows some protective effects in leprosy.

## Laboratory Identification

- **Tuberculous leprosy:** Organisms in clinical samples are very rare; diagnosis relies on clinical findings and the histology of biopsy material.
- **Lepromatous leprosy:** Acid-fast stains of skin scrapings from nasal mucosa or other infected areas can show the presence of *M. leprae*.

## *Mycobacterium tuberculosis*

| Pathogenesis/Clinical Significance | Treatment and Prevention | Laboratory Identification |
|---|---|---|

*M. tuberculosis* survives and grows in host macrophages, where it can remain viable but quiescent for decades. Immunosuppression can lead to reactivation. *M. tuberculosis* produces no demonstrable endo- or exotoxins.

Tuberculosis is the principal chronic bacterial disease in humans, and is the leading cause of death from infection worldwide. Transmission is by aerosol droplets produced by coughing, and depends on crowded conditions and poor ventilation.

● **Tuberculosis:**

Tubercles (productive granulomatous lesions) form in the lung following infection by *M. tuberculosis*. Their formation is mediated by the host immune response. The lesion may arrest and become fibrotic and calcified, or it can break down, resulting in spread of the infection via the lymph and bloodstream. *M. tuberculosis* can seed different tissues, causing, for example, chronic pneumonitis, tuberculous osteomyelitis, or tuberculous meningitis. If active tubercles develop throughout the body, this serious condition is known as miliary (disseminated) tuberculosis.

● **Treatment:** A long course of combined antibiotic treatment (six months or more) with isoniazid, ethambutol, streptomycin, and/or pyrazinamide (these drugs are usually used in mixtures) is required for a cure.

● **Prevention:** Bacille Calmette-Guerin vaccine (BCG) is available, and is used for tuberculin-negative individuals under sustained heavy risk of infection. Isoniazid is used prophylactically, for example, for individuals who are tuberculin-positive but asymptomatic, and who need immunosuppressive therapy for other illnesses.

● Acid-fast bacteria can be observed in clinical specimens treated with Ziehl-Neelsen stain.

● Nucleic acid probes can be used to detect *M. tuberculosis* DNA that has been amplified by PCR.

● The organism can be cultured on specialized media such as Lowenstein-Jensen agar.

# Mycoplasma species
### *Mycoplasma pneumoniae*

## Common characteristics

● **Not seen with Gram stain because it lacks peptidoglycan cell walls**

● **Plastic, pleomorphic shape (neither rods nor cocci)**

● **Three-layer (trilaminar) cell membrane contains sterols**

● **Colonies may have "fried egg" appearance**

● **Rarely cultured for diagnostic purposes**

| Pathogenesis/Clinical Significance | Treatment and Prevention | Laboratory Identification |
|---|---|---|

*M. pneumoniae* is found as part of the normal flora of the human mouth and and genitourinary tract. It is transmitted by respiratory droplets.

*M. pneumoniae* has a membrane-associated cytoadhesin (P1) that binds to ciliated bronchial epithelial cells, and inhibits ciliary action. This results in an inflammatory response in bronchial tissues. *M. pneumoniae* produces no exo- or endotoxins.

● **Primary atypical pneumonia:**

This disease of the lower respiratory tract is the best-known form of *M. pneumoniae* infection. It is also referred to as "walking pneumonia" because the signs and symptoms may be minimal, and the patient usually remains ambulatory throughout the illness. *M. pneumoniae* infection also causes bronchitis, pharyngitis, and nonpurulent otitis media. The highest incidence of disease occurs in older children and young adults (six to twenty years old).

● **Treatment:** Doxycycline and erythromycin are the drugs of choice.

● Serologic tests such as complement fixation antibodies to *M. pneumoniae* are the most widely used procedures for establishing an identification of primary atypical pneumonia.

● *M. pneumoniae* is difficult and expensive to culture.

● Commercially available DNA probes can be used to detect *M. pneumoniae* RNA in sputum specimens.

# Neisseria species

*Neisseria gonorrhoeae*
*Neisseria meningitidis*

# Common characteristics

- Gram-negative
- Kidney bean–shaped diplococci
- Piliated
- Oxidase-positive
- Aerobic
- Culture on Thayer-Martin agar

## *Neisseria gonorrhoeae*

| Pathogenesis/Clinical Significance | Treatment and Prevention | Laboratory Identification |
|---|---|---|
| The normal habitat of *N. gonorrhoeae* is the human genital tract. It is usually transmitted during sexual contact, but can also be transmitted during the passage of a baby through an infected birth canal.<br><br>*N. gonorrhoeae* is highly sensitive to dehydration, and is unencapsulated. Bacterial proteins (pili and outer membrane proteins) enhance the attachment of the bacterium to host epithelial and mucosal cell surfaces, such as those of the urethra, rectum, cervix, pharynx, or conjunctiva, followed by colonization. Pilin confers resistance to phagocytosis, and an IgA protease protects against opsonization; pili and the IgA protease are the organisms' most important virulence factors.<br><br>● **Gonorrhea**<br>Gonorrhea is a very commonly reported infectious disease in the United States. In males, symptoms include urethritis, purulent discharge, and pain during urination. In females, infection is usually localized to the endocervix, often causing a purulent vaginal discharge. If the woman's disease progresses to the uterus, **gonococcal salpingitis** (which may lead to tubal scarring and infertility), **pelvic inflammatory disease** (PID), and fibrosis can occur. Alternatively, the infection may be asymptomatic.<br><br>● **Ophthalmia neonatorum**<br>This is a purulent conjunctivitis acquired by a newborn during passage through the birth canal of a mother infected with gonococcus. If untreated, acute conjunctivitis can lead to blindness.<br><br>● **Septic arthritis**<br>Blood-borne (disseminated) *N. gonorrhoeae* are the most common cause of infectious arthritis in sexually active adults. | ● **Treatment for uncomplicated gonorrhea:** Ceftriaxone is currently the antibiotic of choice. A tetracycline, such as doxycycline, is added when *Chlamydia* is a suspected co-pathogen. Spectinomycin is used for resistant organisms, and in patients allergic to cephalosporins.<br><br>● **Treatment for ophthalmia neonatorum:** Tetracycline or erythromycin is instilled into newborns' eyes to eradicate both *N. gonorrhoeae* and *Chlamydia trachomatis* (if present).<br><br>● **Prevention:** No vaccine or preventive drug is available. Newborns whose eyes are at risk for infection with *N. gonorrhoeae* are treated prophylactically with tetracycline or erythromycin. Taking precautions during sex (that is, using condoms) can prevent transmission of the disease. | ● Gram-negative diplococci are visible within neutrophils in urethral exudates.<br><br>● Oxidase-positive cultures grow on Thayer-Martin agar under increased oxygen tension.<br><br>● *N. gonorrhoeae* ferments glucose but not maltose. |

## *Neisseria meningitidis*

| Pathogenesis/Clinical Significance | Treatment and Prevention | Laboratory Identification |
|---|---|---|
| *N. meningitidis* is one of the most frequent causes of meningitis. Transmission is via respiratory droplets, and pili allow the attachment of *N. meningitidis* to the nasopharyngeal mucosa.<br><br>The meningococcal polysaccharide capsule is antiphagocytic, and is therefore the most important virulence factor aiding in maintenance of the infection. *N. meningitidis* also makes IgA protease (see *N. gonorrhoeae*). | ● **Treatment:** Penicillin G, cefotaxime, and ceftriaxone are the drugs of choice. | ● Under the light microscope, *N. meningitidis* obtained from CSF appear as gram-negative diplococci, often in association with polymorphonuclear leukocytes. |

[*N. MENINGITIDIS* IS CONTINUED ON THE NEXT PAGE.]

### *Neisseria meningitidis* (continued)

| Pathogenesis/Clinical Significance | Treatment and Prevention | Laboratory Identification |
|---|---|---|

● **Meningitis**

The epithelial lining of the nasopharynx normally serves as a barrier to bacteria. If meningococci penetrate that barrier and enter the blood stream they rapidly multiply, causing **meningococcemia**. This septicemia can result in intravascular coagulation, circulatory collapse, and potentially fatal shock (for which the bacterial endotoxin is largely responsible). If *N. meningitidis* crosses the blood-brain barrier it can infect the meninges, causing an acute inflammatory response that results in a purulent **meningitis**. The initial fever and malaise can rapidly evolve into severe headache, rigid neck, vomiting, and sensitivity to bright light. Coma can occur within a few hours.

● **Waterhouse-Friderichsen syndrome**

This syndrome is an acute, fulminating meningococcal septicemia seen mainly in young children. It is associated with adrenal hemorrhage.

● **Prevention:** A capsular vaccine for serogroups A and C is effective, and is used routinely by the military or during an outbreak of meningococcal serogroup A or C in the civilian population. Unfortunately, the polysaccharide of serogroup B does not elicit an effective immune response.

● **Prophylaxis:** Rifampin can be used to treat family members or other close associates of an infected individual.

● *N. meningitidis* can be cultured on chocolate agar.

● The organism is oxidase-positive, and ferments glucose and maltose in an atmosphere of five percent $CO_2$.

---

# Pseudomonas species
### *Pseudomonas aeruginosa*

# Common characteristics

● **Gram-negative**

● **Encapsulated, motile rods (polar flagella)**

● **Obligate aerobe**

● **Oxidase-positive**

● **Produces diffusible green and blue pigments**

● **Oxidizes but does not ferment carbohydrates such as lactose**

● **Culture on MacConkey agar**

| Pathogenesis/Clinical Significance | Treatment and Prevention | Laboratory Identification |
|---|---|---|

*P. aeruginosa* is widely distributed in nature (soil, water, plants, animals). It may colonize healthy humans without causing disease, but is also a significant opportunistic pathogen, and a major cause of nosocomial infections. *P. aeruginosa* is regularly a cause of nosocomial pneumonia, nosocomial infections of the urinary tract, surgical sites, severe burns, and of infections of patients with cystic fibrosis, or those who are undergoing either chemotherapy for neoplastic diseases or antibiotic therapy for other infections. *P. aeruginosa* can grow in distilled water, laboratory hot water baths, hot tubs, wet IV tubing, and other water-containing vessels. This explains why the organism is responsible for so many nosocomial infections.

*P. aeruginosa* disease begins with attachment and colonization of host tissue. Virtually any tissue/organ may be affected. Pili mediate adherence, and extracellular proteases, cytotoxin, hemolysins, and pyocyanin promote tissue damage and local invasion and dissemination of the organism. Systemic disease is promoted by an antiphagocytic capsule, and endo- and exotoxins.

● **Localized infections:**

Localized *P. aeruginosa* infections may occur in the eye, ear, skin, urinary tract, respiratory tract, gastrointestinal tract, and central nervous system. In most cases, localized infections have the potential to lead to disseminated infection.

● **Systemic infection**

The gastrointestinal tract is a particularly common site for penetration. The resulting systemic infections may include bacteremia, secondary pneumonia, bone and joint infections, endocarditis, and infections of the skin/soft tissue or central nervous system.

● **Treatment:** Resistance to a variety of antibiotics is common in this species, therefore antimicrobial therapy often requires a combination of bactericidal antibiotics such as an aminoglycoside and an antipseudomonal β-lactam.

● **Prevention:** No vaccine or preventive drug is available. Prevention of burn wound infection requires the use of topical silver sulfadizine.

● *P. aeruginosa* does not ferment lactose, and is oxidase positive.

● *P. aeruginosa* produces colorless colonies on MacConkey agar. Cultured organisms produce blue (pyocyanin) and fluorescent green (pyoverdin) pigments.

# Rickettsia species
## *Rickettsia rickettsii*

# Common characteristics

- **Gram-negative, but stain poorly**
- **Small, rod-like or coccobacillary in shape**
- **Grow only inside living host cells**
- **Transmitted by infected tick**
- **Not routinely cultured because of obligate intracellularity**

| Pathogenesis/Clinical Significance | Treatment and Prevention | Laboratory Identification |
|---|---|---|

*R. rickettsii* is transmitted to humans by the bite of an infected wood or dog tick. It parasitizes endothelial cells lining the capillaries throughout the circulatory system, ultimately killing the host cell. This results in the formation of focal thrombi in various organs including the skin. A variety of small hemorrhages and hemodynamic disturbances create the symptoms of illness.

### ● Rocky Mountain spotted fever

This disease is characterized by high fever, malaise, and a prominent rash that begins on the palms and soles, and then spreads to cover the body. The rash can progress from macular to petechial or frankly hemorrhagic. Untreated, infection can lead to myocardial or renal failure. The disease occurs most frequently in children and teenagers, but mortality rates are highest (five to thirty percent) among individuals older than forty years of age.

- **Treatment:** Doxycycline and chloramphenicol are the drugs of choice for *R. rickettsii* infections, provided the drugs are administered early in the illness. Because the principal diagnostic methods await the demonstration of seroconversion, a decision to treat must be made on clinical grounds, together with a history or suspicion of contact with a tick.

- **Prevention:** No antirickettsial vaccine is licensed in the United States, and no preventive drug is available. Prevention depends on vector control, wearing proper clothing that minimizes bare skin, and immediate removal of attached ticks.

- Serologic procedures rely on the demonstration of a rickettsia-specific antibody response during the course of infection.

- Indirect fluorescent antibody tests using rickettsia-specific antibodies are available, primarily in reference laboratories.

---

# Salmonella species
## *Salmonella typhi*
## *Salmonella typhimurium*

# Common characteristics

- **Gram-negative rods**
- **Facultative anaerobes**
- **Ferment glucose and a wide range of carbohydrates, but most strains of salmonella do not ferment lactose**
- **Catalase-positive, oxidase-negative**
- **Culture on MacConkey agar**

### *Salmonella typhi*

| Pathogenesis/Clinical Significance | Treatment and Prevention | Laboratory Identification |
|---|---|---|

*S. typhi* is transmitted between humans, without animal or fowl reservoirs. Infection is via the oral/fecal route, generally through food or water contaminated by human feces. Young children and the elderly are particularly susceptible to *Salmonella* infections, as are individuals in crowded institutions or living conditions.

*S. typhi* causes disease by attaching to and invading macrophages of the intestinal lymphoid tissue (Peyer's patches). The bacteria replicate rapidly within these cells, and eventually spread to the reticuloendothelial system (including both liver and spleen, which become enlarged), and potentially to the gall bladder.

### ● Enteric (typhoid) fever

This is a severe, life-threatening systemic illness, characterized by fever and, frequently, by abdominal symptoms. About thirty percent of patients have a faint, maculopapular rash on the trunk (termed "rose spots"). After one to three weeks of incubation, *S. typhi* can enter the blood, the resulting bacteremia causing fever, headache, malaise, and bloody diarrhea. Bacterial endotoxin can cause encephalopathy, myocarditis, or intravascular coagulation. Perforations of the intestine can lead to hemorrhage. Some infected individuals may become chronic carriers for periods as long as years due to persistent residual infection of the gallbladder. Public food handlers or health care deliverers who are carriers can present a serious public health problem (remember "Typhoid Mary"!).

- **Treatment:** Ceftriaxone and fluoroquinolones such as ciprofloxacin are the first-line drugs of choice.

- **Prevention:** A vaccine is available, but less than seventy percent of those given the vaccine are protected. Prevention requires maintaining proper hygiene and cooking food thoroughly.

- *S. typhi* can be isolated from blood, feces, bone marrow, urine, or tissue from rose spots.

- *S. typhi* can be cultured on MacConkey agar, where it produces colorless, non–lactose-fermenting colonies.

- Serologic tests for antibodies against O antigen in patient's serum also aid in the diagnosis.

[*SALMONELLA* SPECIES ARE CONTINUED ON THE NEXT PAGE.]

## *Salmonella typhimurium*

| Pathogenesis/Clinical Significance | Treatment and Prevention | Laboratory Identification |
|---|---|---|
| *S. typhimurium* (and other *Salmonella* species that cause enterocolitis) reside in the gastrointestinal tracts of humans, other animals, and fowl. They are transmitted through contaminated food products, or via the oral/fecal route.<br><br>● **Enterocolitis (gastroenteritis, food poisoning)**<br>Contaminated poultry products including eggs are the primary vehicle for infection of humans by *S. typhimurium*, although raw milk and pets such as turtles also transmit the disease. *Salmonella* adhere to and invade enterocytes of both the small and large intestine, causing a profound inflammatory response. Within 10 to 48 hours after ingestion, nausea, vomiting, abdominal cramps, and diarrhea ensue. Diarrhea usually ends spontaneously within a week. | ● **Treatment:** Fluid and electrolyte replacement are important if diarrhea is severe. Antibiotics are not normally used except in immuno-compromised individuals to prevent systemic spread of the infection.<br><br>● **Prevention:** No vaccine or preventive drug is available. Prevention is accomplished by proper sewage disposal, correct handling of food, and good personal hygiene. | ● Organisms isolated from stool samples produce colorless colonies on MacConkey agar. |

# Shigella species
### *Shigella sonnei*

# Common characteristics

● **Gram-negative rods**

● **Facultative anaerobes**

● **Ferment glucose and a wide range of carbohydrates, but most strains of salmonella do not ferment lactose**

● **Catalase-positive, oxidase-negative**

● **Culture on Hektoen agar**

| Pathogenesis/Clinical Significance | Treatment and Prevention | Laboratory Identification |
|---|---|---|
| *S. sonnei* is typically spread from person to person, with contaminated stools serving as a major source of organisms. Flies and contaminated food or water can also transmit the disease. The organism has a low infectious dose (less than 200 viable organisms are sufficient to cause disease). Therefore secondary cases within a household are common, particularly under conditions of crowding and/or poor sanitation.<br><br>*S. sonnei* invades and destroys the mucosa of the large intestine, but rarely penetrates to the deeper intestinal layers. The organism produces an exotoxin (**Shiga toxin**) with enterotoxic and cytotoxic properties.<br><br>● **Bacillary dysentery (shigellosis)**<br>This disease is characterized by diarrhea with blood, mucus, and painful abdominal cramping. The disease is generally most severe in the young and elderly, and among malnourished individuals, in whom shigellosis may lead to severe dehydration and even death. | ● **Treatment:** Antibiotics such as ciprofloxacin or azithromycin can reduce the duration of illness and the period of shedding organisms, but usage is controversial because of widespread antibiotic resistance.<br><br>● **Prevention:** Protection of the water and food supplies and personal hygiene are crucial for preventing *Shigella* infections. Vaccine development is currently experimental. | ● During acute illness, organisms can be cultured from stools using Hektoen agar or other media specific for intestinal pathogens. |

# Staphylococcus species

*Staphylococcus aureus*
*Staphylococcus epidermidis*
*Staphylococcus saprophyticus*

# Common characteristics

● **Gram-positive, staining darkly**
● **Round cocci tending to occur in bunches like grapes**
● **True facultative anaerobic organisms**
● **Cultured on enriched media containing broth and/or blood**

## *Staphylococcus aureus*

### Pathogenesis/Clinical Significance

*S. aureus* is part of the normal flora of certain mucous membranes (for example, the anterior nares, vagina), and of the skin. It is also, however, the most virulent of the staphylococci.

Infection occurs during penetration of the skin (for example, due to a wound, or during surgery), typically resulting in an abscess. Subsequent disease can be caused by the actual infection, by toxins in the absence of infection (toxinosis), or by a combination of infection and intoxication. Important *S. aureus* virulence factors include: 1) cell wall virulence factors that can promote binding to mucosal cells and exert antiopsonic (and therefore antiphagocytic) effects; 2) cytolytic exotoxins (including hemolysins); 3) superantigen exotoxins, including enterotoxins (which cause food poisoning), toxic shock syndrome toxin, and exfoliative toxin (which causes scalded skin syndrome in children, and also bullous impetigo). The most common diseases caused by *S. aureus* are the following.

● **Localized skin infections**

These include 1) small, superficial abscesses involving sweat or sebaceous glands, or hair follicles (for example, the common **sty**); 2) subcutaneous abscesses (**furuncles** or **boils**) that form around foreign bodies such as splinters; and 3) larger, deeper infections (**carbuncles**) that can lead to bacteremia.

● **Diffuse skin infection–impetigo (pyoderma)**

This is a superficial, spreading, crusty skin lesion generally seen in children.

● **Deep, localized infections**

*S. aureus* is the most common cause of acute and chronic infection of the bone marrow (**osteomyelitis**), and also the most common cause of arthritis resulting from acute infection of the joint space ("**septic joint**").

● **Other infections**

*S. aureus* can cause **acute endocarditls**, **septicemia**, and severe, **necrotizing pneumonia**. [Note: *S. aureus* is one of the most common causes of hospital-acquired (nosocomial) infections. Progression to septicemia is often a terminal event.]

● **Toxinoses**

**Toxic shock syndrome** is caused by strains of *S. aureus* that produce a specific, absorbable toxin. The syndrome results in high fever, rash, vomiting, diarrhea, hypotension, and multiorgan involvement (especially GI, renal, and/or hepatic damage). Staphylococcal **gastroenteritis** is caused by ingestion of food contaminated with toxin produced by *S. aureus*. **Scalded skin syndrome** (mild cases are sometimes called **bullous impetigo**) involves the appearance of superficial bullae resulting from the action of an exfoliative toxin that attacks the intercellular adhesive of the stratum granulosum, causing marked epithelial desquamation.

[STAPHYLOCOCCUS SPECIES ARE CONTINUED ON THE NEXT PAGE]

### Treatment and Prevention

● **Treatment:** Serious *S. aureus* infections require aggressive treatment, including incision and drainage of localized lesions as well as systemic antibiotics. Acquired antibiotic resistance determinants are frequently present, complicating the choice of drug. For example, nearly all *S. aureus* isolates are resistant to penicillin G, and methicillin-resistant *S. aureus* (MRSA) are becoming prevalent in hospital isolates. Nafcillin and oxacillin have replaced penicillin G because they are β-lactamase resistant. Vancomycin is also used to treat MRSA, but strains resistant to this drug are emerging.

● **Prevention:** No vaccine or preventive drug is available. Infection control procedures such as barrier precautions, washing of hands, and disinfection of fomites are important in the control of nosocomial *S. aureus* epidemics.

### Laboratory Identification

● *S. aureus* stains strongly positive with Gram stain, and cells appear in grape-like clusters.
● *S. aureus* is catalase- and coagulase-positive.
● *S. aureus* forms deep yellow, hemolytic colonies on enriched media.

## *Staphylococcus epidermidis*

| Pathogenesis/Clinical Significance | Treatment and Prevention | Laboratory Identification |
|---|---|---|
| *S. epidermidis* is part of the normal flora of the skin and anterior nares.<br><br>● **Important cause of infections from prosthetic implants**<br>Surgical implants, such as heart valves and catheters, are easily infected by *S. epidermidis*. Cell envelope factors that facilitate attachment to plastic surfaces act as virulence factors. | ● **Treatment:** Acquired drug resistance by *S. epidermidis* is even more frequent than with *S. aureus*. Vancomycin sensitivity remains the rule, but vancomycin-resistant isolates have been reported.<br><br>● **Prevention:** No vaccine or preventive drug is available. | ● *S. epidermidis* stains strongly positive with Gram stain. The cocci appear in grape-like clusters.<br><br>● The organism produces white, nonhemolytic colonies on enriched agar. It is coagulase-negative, and novobiocin-sensitive. |

## *Staphylococcus saprophyticus*

| Pathogenesis/Clinical Significance | Treatment and Prevention | Laboratory Identification |
|---|---|---|
| *S. saprophyticus* is part of the normal vaginal flora.<br><br>● **Cystitis in women**<br>*S. saprophyticus* is a frequent cause of cystitis in women. [Note: A urinary coagulase-negative staphylococcus is often presumed to be *S. saprophyticus*; novobiocin resistance can be used for confirmation.] | ● **Treatment:** *S. saprophyticus* tends to be sensitive to most antibiotics, even penicillin G.<br><br>● **Prevention:** No vaccine or preventive drug is available. | ● *S. saprophyticus* stains strongly positive with Gram stain. The cocci appear in grape-like clusters.<br><br>● The organism produces white, nonhemolytic colonies on enriched agar. It is coagulase-negative and novobiocin-resistant. |

# Streptococcus species
### *Streptococcus agalactiae*
### *Streptococcus pneumoniae*
### *Streptococcus pyogenes*

# Common characteristics

● **Gram-positive**

● **Ovoid to spherical in shape, occurring as pairs or chains**

● **Nonmotile, catalase-negative**

● **Most are facultative anaerobes, but grow fermentatively even in the presence of oxygen**

● **Culture on blood agar**

## *Streptococcus agalactiae*

| Pathogenesis/Clinical Significance | Treatment and Prevention | Laboratory Identification |
|---|---|---|
| *S. agalactiae* is a group B streptococcus. It is found normally in the vaginocervical tract of female carriers, and the urethral mucous membranes of male carriers, as well as in the GI tract (especially the rectum). Transmission occurs from an infected mother to her infant at birth, and venereally among adults.<br><br>*S. agalactiae's* polysaccharide capsule is antiphagocytic, which allows the bacterium to infect tissue and induce an inflammatory response.<br><br>● **Meningitis and septicemia in neonates**<br>Infection occurs as the infant traverses the birth canal. *S. agalactiae* is a leading cause of these syndromes in neonates, with a high mortality rate.<br><br>● **Infections of adults**<br>*S. agalactiae* is an occasional cause of endometritis in postpartum women, and of septicemia or pneumonia in individuals with impaired immune systems. | ● **Treatment:** All isolates remain sensitive to penicillin G and ampicillin, which are still the antibiotics of choice. In life-threatening infections, an aminoglycoside can be added to the regimen.<br><br>● **Prevention:** No vaccine or preventive drug is available. | ● Samples of blood, cervical swabs, sputum, or spinal fluid can be cultured on blood agar. Group B streptococci are β-hemolytic, with larger colonies and less hemolysis than group A streptococci.<br><br>● *S. agalactiae* can hydrolyze sodium hippurate, and is catalase-negative. |

[*STREPTOCOCCUS* SPECIES ARE CONTINUED ON THE NEXT PAGE.]

## Streptococcus pneumoniae

| Pathogenesis/Clinical Significance | Treatment and Prevention | Laboratory Identification |
|---|---|---|

*S. pneumoniae* (formerly called *Diplococcus pneumoniae*, and referred to as "pneumococcus") is the most common cause of pneumonia and otitis media, and an important cause of meningitis and bacteremia/sepsis. *S. pneumoniae* is carried in the nasopharynx of many healthy individuals. Infection can be either endogenous (in a carrier who develops impaired resistance to the organism) or exogenous (by droplets from the nose of a carrier).

Virulence factors include the polysaccharide capsule, which is antiphagocytic, and the cell-associated enzymes, pneumolysin and autolysin.

### ● Acute bacterial pneumonia

Pneumonia, caused most frequently by *S. pneumoniae*, is a leading cause of death in the aged and those whose resistance is impaired. It is frequently preceded by an upper or middle respiratory viral infection, which predisposes to *S. pneumoniae* infection of pulmonary parenchyma. Mechanisms include increased volume and viscosity of secretions that are more difficult to clear, and secondary inhibition of the action of bronchial cilia by viral infection.

### ● Otitis media

Characterized by earache, this is the most common bacterial infection of children, and *S. pneumoniae* is its most common cause.

### ● Meningitis

*S. pneumoniae* is a common cause of meningitis. This disease has a high mortality rate, even when treated appropriately.

● **Treatment:** Penicillin G has been the drug of choice, but resistant strains are regularly seen. Most resistant strains remain sensitive to vancomycin; these antibiotics are therefore the agents of choice for invasive infections by penicillin-resistant strains of *S. pneumoniae*.

● **Prevention:** An anti-pneumococcal capsular polysaccharide vaccine that immunizes against 23 serotypes of *S. pneumoniae* is indicated for the protection of high-risk individuals over two years of age.

● Under the light microscope, gram-positive *S. pneumoniae* appear as encapsulated, lancet-shaped organisms, occurring in pairs (hence the former name, "diplococcus").

● Samples obtained from a nasopharyngeal swab, blood, pus, sputum, or spinal fluid can be cultured on blood agar. The colonies are α-hemolytic.

● Capsular swelling (quellung reaction) is observed when the pneumococci are treated with type-specific antiserum.

## Streptococcus pyogenes

| Pathogenesis/Clinical Significance | Treatment and Prevention | Laboratory Identification |
|---|---|---|

*S. pyogenes* is a Group A streptococcus that has as its habitat infected patients, and also healthy human carriers, in whom the organism resides on skin and mucous membranes (especially the nasopharynx). Most common sources of contagion are via aerosol from a carrier or someone who has streptococcal pharyngitis, or from direct contact with a skin carrier or a patient with impetigo.

*S. pyogenes* causes some of the most rapidly progressive infections known, causing **cellulitis** (diffuse spreading inflammation) anywhere in the body. It also causes postinfectious sequelae, including rheumatic fever and acute glomerulonephritis. Like *Staphylococcus aureus*, *S. pyogenes* secretes a wide range of exotoxins.

### ● Acute pharyngitis or pharyngotonsillitis

*S. pyogenes* is the most common bacterial cause of sore throats, especially in patients two to twenty years old; pharyngitis (for example, **strep throat**) is the most common type of *S. pyogenes* infection. [Note: Release of pyrogenic exotoxin to which the patient does not have antibodies leads to an extensive rash, and the syndrome designated **scarlet fever**.]

### ● Acute rheumatic fever

This autoimmune disease can occur two to three weeks after initiation of pharyngitis. This disease is caused by cross-reactions between antigens of the heart and joint tissues, and streptococcal antigen.

### ● Impetigo

This is a contagious, pus-forming infection of the skin, in which a thick, yellowish crust forms—usually on the face. It usually affects children, and can cause severe and extensive lesions on the face and limbs.

● **Treatment:** Drainage and debridement are very important in treating necrotizing fasciitis/myositis. Antibiotics are used for all Group A streptococcal infections. *S. pyogenes* has not acquired resistance to penicillin G, which remains the antibiotic of choice for acute streptococcal disease. For the penicillin-allergic patient, a macrolide such as clarithromycin or azithromycin is the preferred drug.

● **Prevention:** There is no vaccine against *S. pyogenes*. Rheumatic fever is prevented by rapid eradication of the organism by antibiotic treatment early in the infection.

● Specimens obtained from throat swabs, pus and lesion samples, sputum, blood, or spinal fluid can be cultured on sheep blood agar. *S. pyogenes* forms characteristic small, opalescent colonies surrounded by a large zone of β-hemolysis.

● Serologic tests are used to detect a patient's antibody titer to streptolysin-O (ASO test).

● *S. pyogenes* is highly sensitive to bacitracin, and diagnostic disks with a very low concentration of the antibiotic inhibit growth in culture.

[*STREPTOCOCCUS PYOGENES* IS CONTINUED ON THE NEXT PAGE.]

## Streptococcus pyogenes (continued)

| **Pathogenesis/Clinical Significance** | **Treatment and Prevention** | **Laboratory Identification** |
| --- | --- | --- |

### ● Erysipelas

Affecting all age groups, patients with erysipelas suffer from a fiery red, advancing erythema, especially on the face or lower limbs.

### ● Puerperal sepsis

This infection is initiated during, or following soon after, the delivery of a newborn. A disease of the uterine endometrium, patients suffer from a purulent vaginal discharge, and are often very ill systemically, with high fever.

### ● Invasive group A streptococcal (GAS) disease

Patients have a deep local invasion with or without necrosis. (The involvement of **necrotizing fasciitis/myositis** led to the term "**flesh-eating bacteria**.") GAS disease often spreads rapidly, even in otherwise healthy individuals, leading to bacteremia and sepsis.

# Treponema species
## *Treponema pallidum*

# Common characteristics

● Gram-negative, but some stain poorly and need to be visualized by other means

● Long, slender, flexible, spiral- or corkscrew-shaped rods

● Organisms are highly motile

● Does not grow in culture

| **Pathogenesis/Clinical Significance** | **Treatment and Prevention** | **Laboratory Identification** |
| --- | --- | --- |

*T. pallidum* is a human parasite, transmitted primarily by sexual contact, where the infectious lesion is generally on the skin or mucous membranes of the genitalia.

*T. pallidum* secretes the enzyme hyaluronidase, which disrupts the ground substance, thus facilitating the spread of infection. They have endoflagella (axial filaments) that lie beneath the outer sheath of the organism, providing motility.

### ● Syphilis

*T. pallidum* multiplies at the site of initial infection, and spreads via the lymph to the blood. Within two to ten weeks, a hard ulcer (**chancre**) forms. Up to ten weeks later, secondary lesions appear. These consist of a red **maculopapular rash**, seen primarily on the palms and soles, and pale, moist papules, seen primarily in the anogenital region (there they are called **condylomas**), the armpits, and the mouth. Both primary and secondary lesions are rich in *T. pallidum* organisms, and are extremely infectious, but both heal spontaneously. Secondary lesions may be accompanied by systemic involvement, such as **syphilitic hepatitis**, **meningitis**, **nephritis**, or **chorioretinitis**. In approximately forty percent of infected individuals, the disease progresses to a tertiary stage, characterized by degenerative changes in the nervous system, cardiovascular lesions, and/or development of granulomatous lesions (**gummas**) in the liver, skin, and bones.

### ● Congenital syphilis

A pregnant woman with syphilis can transmit *T. pallidum* through the placenta to her fetus after the first ten to fifteen weeks of pregnancy. Infection can cause death and spontaneous abortion of the fetus, or cause it to be stillborn. Those infants that live develop the symptoms of congenital syphilis, including a variety of central nervous system and structural abnormalities.

● **Treatment:** Penicillin G is still the drug of choice. Erythromycin or tetracycline can be used for penicillin-allergic patients.

● **Prevention:** No vaccine or preventive drug is available, and protection from syphilis depends on safe sexual practice. Treatment of a woman with appropriate antibiotics during pregnancy prevents congenital syphilis.

● *T. pallidum* cannot be seen in a gram-stained smear; a dark-field examination of a clinical sample can show motile spirochetes.

● *T. pallidum* has not been cultured *in vitro*.

● Serologic tests include the nontreponemal antigen tests (BDRL, RPR, and Wasserman tests), and treponemal antibody tests (FTA-ABS, TPI, and TPHA tests).

# Vibrio species
## *Vibrio cholerae*

# Common characteristics

- Gram-negative
- Short, curved, rod-shaped
- Rapidly motile due to single polar flagellum
- Facultative anaerobes
- Growth of many vibrio strains requires or is stimulated by NaCl
- Culture on blood or MacConkey agar

## Pathogenesis/Clinical Significance

*V. cholerae* is transmitted by contaminated water and food. There are no known animal reservoirs, nor animal or arthropod vectors. Outbreaks of *V. cholerae* infection have been associated with raw or undercooked seafood harvested from contaminated waters.

Following ingestion, *V. cholerae* infects the small intestine. Adhesion factors are important for colonization and virulence. The organism is noninvasive, and causes disease through the action of an enterotoxin (**cholera toxin**) that causes the activation of adenylate cyclase by ADP-ribosylation. This initiates an outpouring of fluid into the intestine.

### • Cholera

Full-blown cholera is characterized by massive loss of fluid and electrolytes from the body. After an incubation period ranging from hours to a few days, profuse watery diarrhea (**rice-water stools**) begins. Untreated, the death from shock may occur in hours to days, with the death rate exceeding fifty percent.

## Treatment and Prevention

- **Treatment:** Replacement of fluids and electrolytes is crucial in preventing shock, and does not require bacteriologic diagnosis. Antibiotics such as doxycycline can shorten the duration of diarrhea and excretion of the organism.

- **Prevention:** Public health measures that reduce fecal contamination of water supplies and food, and adequate cooking of foods, can minimize transmission.

## Laboratory Identification

- *V. cholerae* from a stool sample grows on standard, nonselective media such as blood and MacConkey agars. Thiosulfate-citrate-bile salts-sucrose (TCBS) medium can enhance isolation.

- *V. cholerae* is oxidase-positive.

---

# Yersinia species
## *Yersinia pestis*

# Common characteristics

- Gram-negative
- Small rod that stains bipolarly
- Nonmotile, encapsulated
- Culture on MacConkey or CIN (selective) agar

## Pathogenesis/Clinical Significance

*Y. pestis* is endemic in a variety of mammals, both urban and sylvatic, and is distributed worldwide. Infection is transmitted by fleas, which serve to maintain the infection within the animal reservoir. Humans are generally accidental and dead-end hosts. The organism can also be transmitted by ingestion of contaminated animal tissues, or via the respiratory route.

Organisms are carried by the lymphatic system from the site of inoculation to regional lymph nodes, where they are ingested by phagocytes. *Y. pestis* multiplies in these cells. Hematogenous spread of bacteria to other organs or tissues may occur, resulting in hemorrhagic lesions at these sites.

### • Bubonic (septicemic) plague

The incubation period (from flea bite to development of symptoms) is generally two to eight days. Onset of nonspecific symptoms, such as high fever, chills, headache, myalgia, and weakness that proceeds to prostration, is characteristically sudden. Within a short time, the characteristic, painful **buboes** develop—typically in the groin, but they may also occur in axillae or on the neck. Blood pressure drops, potentially leading to septic shock and death.

### • Pneumonic plague

If plague bacilli reach the lungs, they cause a purulent pneumonia that is highly contagious, and, if untreated, is rapidly fatal.

## Treatment and Prevention

- **Treatment:** Streptomycin is the drug of choice; gentamicin and tetracycline are acceptable alternatives. Because of the potential for overwhelming septicemia, rapid institution of antibiotic therapy is crucial. Supportive therapy is essential for patients with signs of shock.

- **Prevention:** A formalin-killed vaccine is available for those at high risk of acquiring plague. For individuals in enzootic areas, efforts to minimize exposure to rodents and fleas is important.

## Laboratory Identification

- Laboratory identification can be made by a gram-stained smear, and culture of an aspirate from a bubo (or sputum in the case of pneumonic plague).

- The organism grows on both MacConkey and blood agars, although colonies grow somewhat more slowly than do those of other Enterobacteriaceae.

# VIRUSES

## Adenoviridae
### Adenoviruses

## Common characteristics

- ● **Double-stranded, linear DNA**
- ● **Nonenveloped, icosahedral**
- ● **Replicates in nucleus, killing host cell**

| Pathogenesis/Clinical Significance | Treatment and Prevention | Laboratory Identification |
|---|---|---|

The site of the clinical syndrome caused by adenovirus infection is generally related to the mode of virus transmission. Adenoviruses are primarily agents of respiratory disease, and are transmitted via the respiratory route. Those associated specifically with gastrointestinal disease are transmitted by the fecal-oral route, whereas ocular infections are transmitted by virus-contaminated hands, ophthalmologic instruments, or swimming pools.

- ● **Respiratory tract diseases**

    The most common manifestation of adenovirus infection of infants and young children is **acute febrile pharyngitis**, characterized by a cough, sore throat, nasal congestion, and fever. Acute respiratory disease occurs primarily in epidemics among new military recruits, and is facilitated by fatigue and crowded conditions. These syndromes may progress to true viral pneumonia, which in infants has a mortality rate of about ten percent.

- ● **Ocular diseases**

    If both the respiratory tract and the eyes are involved, the syndrome is referred to as **pharyngoconjunctival fever**. A similar follicular conjunctivitis may occur as a separate, self-limiting disease. A more serious infection is **epidemic keratoconjunctivitis** in which the corneal epithelium is also involved, and which may be followed by corneal opacity lasting several years. The epidemic nature of this disease arises in part from transmission by improperly sterilized ophthalmologic instruments.

- ● **Gastrointestinal diseases**

    Most of the human adenoviruses multiply in the GI tract, and can be found in stools. However, these are generally asymptomatic infections. Two serotypes have been associated specifically with **infantile gastroenteritis**, and have been estimated to account for five to fifteen percent of all viral diarrheal disease in children.

- ● **Treatment:** No antiviral agents are currently available for treating adenovirus infections.

- ● **Prevention:** A live, attenuated adenovirus vaccine is used to prevent epidemic respiratory disease in the military population. Although not known to be associated with human malignancies, the oncogenicity of the adenoviruses in experimental animals has inhibited the use of adenovirus vaccines on a wider scale.

- ● Isolation of virus for identification is not done on a routine basis, but may be desirable in cases of epidemic disease, or a nosocomial outbreak, especially in the nursery.

- ● Identification of the adenovirus serotype can be done by neutralization or hemagglutination inhibition using type-specific antisera.

- ● Enteric adenoviruses are detected by direct test of stool specimens by ELISA.

## Picornaviridae
### Coxsackievirus
### Hepatitis A virus (p. 3566)
### Poliovirus (p. 364)

## Common characteristics

- ● **Positive-strand, single-stranded, nonsegmented RNA genome**
- ● **Non-enveloped, icosahedral**
- ● **Genomic RNAs serve as messenger RNAs and are infectious**
- ● **Virions do not contain any enzymes**

[COXSACKIEVIRUS IS CONTINUED ON THE NEXT PAGE]

## Coxsackievirus

| Pathogenesis/Clinical Significance | Treatment and Prevention | Laboratory Identification |
|---|---|---|
| Coxsackieviruses are members of the genus Enterovirus. Individuals are infected with coxsackieviruses by ingestion of contaminated food or water, or inhalation of aerosols containing the virus. These viruses are stable in the low pH of the stomach, replicate in the GI tract, and are excreted in the stool (fecal-oral route). Coxsackieviruses also replicate in the oropharynx. They are carried by the blood to peripheral tissues, including the heart and central nervous system.<br><br>● **Coxsackievirus infections**<br>These give rise to a large variety of clinical syndromes including upper respiratory infections, meningitis, gastroenteritis, herpangina (intense swelling of the throat), pleurisy, pericarditis, myocarditis, and myositis. | ● **Treatment:** No antiviral agents or vaccines are currently available for treating coxsackievirus infections. | ● Viruses can be isolated and cultured from the stool or from various target organs.<br><br>● Evidence of infection can also be obtained by demonstration of a rise in antibody titer. |

# Herpesviridae

**Epstein-Barr virus**
**Herpes simplex virus, Type 1 (p. 358)**
**Herpes simplex virus, Type 2 (p. 358)**
**Human cytomegalovirus (p. 359)**
**Human herpesvirus, Type 8 (p. 360)**
**Varicella-zoster virus (p. 366)**

# Common characteristics

● **Linear, double-stranded DNA genome**

● **Replicate in the nucleus**

● **Envelope contains antigenic, species-specific glycoproteins**

● **In the tegument between the envelope and capsid are a number of virus-coded enzymes and transcription factors essential for initiation of the infectious cycle**

● **All herpesviruses can enter a latent state following primary infection, to be reactivated at a later time**

## Epstein-Barr virus

| Pathogenesis/Clinical Significance | Treatment and Prevention | Laboratory Identification |
|---|---|---|
| Most transmission of Epstein-Barr virus (EBV) occurs by intimate contact with saliva that contains virus.<br><br>EBV replicates in mucosal epithelium. The virus then spreads to the lymph nodes, where it infects B cells. EBV next travels via the blood to other organs, particularly targeting liver and spleen. The B cell infection is an abortive one, leading to B cell proliferation, accompanied by nonspecific increases in total IgM, IgG, and IgA.<br><br>● **Infectious mononucleosis (IM)**<br>The "atypical lymphocytosis" characteristic of infectious mononucleosis is caused by the active cytotoxic T cell response to the EBV antigens expressed by infected B cells. The typical IM syndrome appears after an incubation period of four to seven weeks, and includes pharyngitis, lymphadenopathy, and fever. Headache and malaise often precede and accompany the disease, which may last several weeks. Throughout life, healthy EBV carriers continue to have episodes of asymptomatic virus shedding.<br><br>● **Association with Burkitt lymphoma and other human neoplastic diseases**<br>EBV infection has been found to be associated with Burkitt lymphoma, nasopharyngeal carcinoma, and Hodgkin disease. The exact role played by the EBV in these diseases is not clear. | ● **Treatment:** Although acyclovir inhibits EBV replication, none of the antiherpes drugs have been effective in modifying the course or severity of IM due to EBV, or in preventing development of EBV-related B cell malignancies.<br><br>● **Prevention:** No vaccine or preventive drug is available. | ● The classic diagnostic test for EBV-associated mononucleosis is detection of heterophile antibodies that agglutinate sheep and horse red blood cells.<br><br>● Serologic tests, such as immunofluorescence reactions or ELISA to detect antibodies specific for viral proteins, are used to evaluate the stage of disease.<br><br>● Detection of EBV DNA or RNA by hybridization, or of viral antigens using immunohistochemical techniques, can be done with cell homogenates. |

## Picornaviridae

### Coxsackievirus (p. 354)
### Hepatitis A virus
### Poliovirus (p. 364)

## Common characteristics

● **Positive-strand, single-stranded, nonsegmented RNA genome**

● **Non-enveloped, icosahedral**

● **Genomic RNAs serve as messenger RNAs and are infectious**

● **Virions do not contain any enzymes**

## Hepatitis A virus

| Pathogenesis/Clinical Significance | Treatment and Prevention | Laboratory Identification |
|---|---|---|
| Hepatitis A virus (HAV) is a member of the genus hepatovirus. It is the most common cause of viral hepatitis in the United States. Transmission is by the fecal-oral route, and the virus is shed in the feces. For example, a common mode of transmission of the virus is through eating uncooked shellfish harvested from sewage-contaminated water. Transmission via blood (similar to HBV transmission) is rare.<br><br>● **Hepatitis A ("infectious hepatitis")**<br><br>HAV infections are most commonly seen among children, especially those living in crowded accommodations such as summer camps. The main site of replication is the hepatocyte, where infection results in severe cytopathology, and liver function is severely impaired. The prognosis for patients with HAV is generally favorable, and development of persistent infection and chronic hepatitis is uncommon. | ● **Treatment:** Immune globulin is used as postexposure prophylaxis. No antiviral agents are currently available for treating HAV infections.<br><br>● **Prevention:** Vaccines prepared from whole virus inactivated with formaldehyde are now available. Immune globulin has been used for many years, mainly as postexposure prophylaxis. Prevention of HAV infection requires taking measures to avoid fecal contamination of food and water. | ● HAV grows poorly in tissue culture.<br><br>● Evidence of infection can be gained by the demonstration of a rise in antibody titer. |

## Hepadnaviridae

### Hepatitis B virus

## Common characteristics

● **Circular DNA, partly single-stranded, partly double-stranded, non–covalently closed genome, with four overlapping genes**

● **Enveloped, icosahedral nucleocapsid**

● **Multifunctional reverse transcriptase/DNA polymerase in virion**

● **Viral antigens: the capsid protein (hepatitis B capsid antigen, HBcAg), the envelope protein (hepatitis B surface antigen, HBsAg), and a variant of HBcAg (HBeAg) that is secreted by infected cells**

| Pathogenesis/Clinical Significance | Treatment and Prevention | Laboratory Identification |
|---|---|---|
| Infectious hepatitis B virus (HBV) is present in all body fluids of an infected individual. Therefore, blood, semen, saliva, mother's milk, etc. serve as sources of infection. In the United States, HBV is most frequently contracted by sexual intercourse or by IV drug use. In areas of high endemicity in third-world countries, the majority of the population becomes infected at or shortly after birth from a chronically infected mother or from infected siblings.<br><br>The primary cause of hepatic cell destruction is the cell-mediated immune response by HLA–I-restricted cytotoxic (CD8) T lymphocytes, which react specifically with fragments of the nucleocapsid proteins—HBcAg and HBeAg—expressed on the infected hepatocyte membrane.<br><br>● **Acute hepatitis**<br><br>In about two thirds of individuals infected with HBV, the primary infection is asymptomatic, even though such patients may later develop symptomatic chronic liver disease. In acute HBV infections, there is an incubation period of between 45 and 120 days, followed by a preicteric (prejaundice) period lasting several days to a week. This is characterized by mild fever, malaise, anorexia, myalgia, and nausea. The acute, icteric | ● **Treatment:** For acute hepatitis, treatment has traditionally been largely supportive. Lamivudine (3TC), a drug used in HIV therapy, is also licensed for treatment of HBV infections. It is a reverse transcriptase inhibitor, which has significantly depressed liver damage and serum levels of HBV antigen. Unfortunately, when treatment is discontinued, HBV reappears. | ● Hepatitis is established using liver function tests.<br><br>● Viral antigens and antiviral antibodies are detected using serologic techniques such as ELISA and RIA.<br><br>● Presence of IgM anti-HBc accompanied by HBsAg is a specific indicator of HBV infection. |

[HEPATITIS B IS CONTINUED ON THE NEXT PAGE]

## Hepatitis B virus (continued)

| Pathogenesis/Clinical Significance | Treatment and Prevention | Laboratory Identification |

phase then follows, and lasts for one to two months. It is during this phase that dark urine, due to bilirubinuria and jaundice, are evident. There usually is also an enlarged and tender liver. During the acute phase, large quantities of viral antigens, nucleic acids, and antiviral antibodies appear in the blood. In eighty to ninety percent of adults, a convalescent period of several more months is followed by complete recovery. Following resolution of the acute disease (or asymptomatic infection), about two to ten percent of adults, and over eighty percent of infants, remain chronically infected.

● **Fulminant hepatitis**

In one to two percent of acute symptomatic cases, much more extensive necrosis of the liver occurs during the initial acute illness. This is accompanied by high fever, abdominal pain, and eventual renal dysfunction, coma, seizures, and, in about eight percent of cases, death.

● **Primary hepatocellular carcinomas (HCC; hepatomas)**

HCC is one of the major causes of death due to malignancy worldwide. Approximately eighty percent of HCCs occur in chronically HBV-infected individuals. However, the mechanisms relating HBV infection and HCC are not understood. Clinically, a patient with HCC exhibits weight loss, right upper-quadrant pain, fever, and intestinal bleeding.

● **Prevention:** A vaccine is available that is constructed against the HBsAg. It is recommended as one of the routine infant immunizations, and also for adults in health care professions, or with life-styles that present a high risk of infection. Hepatitis B immunoglobulin is prepared from the blood of donors having a high titer of anti-HBs antibody. It provides passive immunization for individuals accidentally exposed to HBV, and for infants born to women who are HBV-positive.

# Flaviviridae

Hepatitis C viruses

# Common characteristics

● **Positive-strand, single-stranded, nonsegmented RNA genome**

● **Enveloped, icosahedral nucleocapsid**

● **Genomic RNAs serve as messenger RNAs and are infectious**

● **Virions do not contain any enzymes**

| Pathogenesis/Clinical Significance | Treatment and Prevention | Laboratory Identification |

Hepatitis C viruses (HCV) have in the past been the primary cause of non-A, non-B, transfusion-associated hepatitis. Tests to screen blood for HCV have been available for several years, so that HCV as a cause of transfusion-associated hepatitis is now unusual. This group of viruses is heterogeneous, and can be divided into several types. Transmission is via blood—through transfusion, intravenous drug use, and renal dialysis treatment. In addition, there is evidence of sexual transmission, as well as transmission from mother to child.

● **Hepatitis C**

HCV replication occurs in the hepatocyte, and probably also in mononuclear cells (lymphocytes and macrophages). Destruction of liver cells may result both from a direct effect of viral replication, and from the host immune response. The majority of infections with HCV are subclinical, but about 25 percent of infected individuals present with acute hepatitis including jaundice. More important, a significant proportion of infections progress to a chronic hepatitis and cirrhosis. Some of these individuals go on to develop hepatocellular carcinoma many years after the primary infection. Concomitant chronic infection with HBV results in more severe disease.

● **Treatment:** Treatment of patients with chronic hepatitis with α-interferon is sometimes of benefit, but in most cases, only for the period during which the patient is receiving the interferon. Chronic hepatitis caused by HCV that results in severe liver damage may be an indication for a liver transplant.

● **Prevention:** No vaccine or preventive drug is available at this time.

● A specific diagnosis can be made by demonstration of antibodies that react with a combination of recombinant viral proteins.

● Sensitive tests are also now available for detection of viral RNA, for example, by polymerase chain reaction (PCR) amplification of reverse-transcribed HCV cDNA.

# Herpesviridae

**Epstein-Barr virus (p.4 355)**
**Herpes simplex virus, Type 1**
**Herpes simplex virus, Type 2**
**Human cytomegalovirus**
**Human herpesvirus, Type 8**
**Varicella-zoster virus (p. 366)**

# Common characteristics

● **Enveloped DNA viruses**

● **Linear, double-stranded DNA genome**

● **Herpesviruses replicate in the nucleus**

● **Envelope contains antigenic, species-specific glycoproteins**

● **In the tegument between the envelope and capsid are a number of virus-coded enzymes and transcription factors essential for initiation of the infectious cycle**

● **All herpesviruses can enter a latent state following primary infection, to be reactivated at a later time**

## Herpes simplex virus, type 1

| Pathogenesis/Clinical Significance | Treatment and Prevention | Laboratory Identification |
|---|---|---|
| Herpes simplex virus type 1 (HSV-1) has a relatively rapid, cytocidal growth cycle. HSV-1 establishes latency in trigeminal ganglia after oropharyngeal infection. Transmission of HSV-1 is by direct contact with virus-containing secretions (usually saliva), or with lesions on mucosal surfaces. <br><br> ● **Primary HSV-1 infections** <br><br> The virus multiplies in the nuclei of epithelial cells on the mucosal surface onto which it has been inoculated—most frequently, that of the oropharyngeal region. Vesicles or shallow ulcers containing infectious HSV-1 are produced, primarily in the oropharynx. These cause sore throat, fever, gingivitis, and anorexia. The most common symptomatic HSV-1 infections of the upper body are **gingivostomatitis** in young children, and **tonsillitis** and **pharyngitis** in adults. Infection of the eye by HSV-1 can cause severe **keratoconjunctivitis**. [Note: HSV-1 infections of the eye are the second most common cause of corneal blindness in the United States (after trauma).] If HSV-1 infection spreads to the CNS, frequently fatal **encephalitis** can occur. In immunocompetent individuals, HSV-1 infection remains localized due to cytotoxic T cells that recognize HSV-specific antigens on the surface of infected cells, and kills them before progeny virus has been produced. <br><br> ● **Latent HSV-1 infections** <br><br> A life-long latent infection is usually established in the trigeminal ganglia as a result of entry of infectious virions into sensory neurons that end at the site of infection. Recurrent HSV-1 infections may be asymptomatic, but result in viral shedding in secretions. If symptoms occur, they usually include **herpes labialis** (formation of "**cold sores**" or "**fever blisters**") around the lips. | ● **Treatment:** Herpesviruses encode considerably more enzymatic activities and regulatory functions than do viruses with smaller genomic size. A number of these activities duplicate the functions of cell enzymes, but because they are virus-specific, they provide excellent targets for anti-viral agents that are relatively non-toxic for the cell. Acycloguanosine (acyclovir) is selectively effective against HSV because it becomes an active inhibitor only after initially being phosphorylated by the HSV-coded thymidine kinase. The drug cannot cure a latent infection, but can minimize or prevent recurrences. Other inhibitors active against HSV DNA synthesis include famciclovir, foscarnet, and topically applied penciclovir. <br><br> ● **Prevention:** No vaccine or preventive drug is available. | ● Cell tissue culture inoculated with a sample of vesicle scraping, fluid, or genital swab shows gross cytopathic changes in several days; individual infected cells can be detected within 24 hours by use of immunofluorescence or immunoperoxidase staining with antibodies against viral early proteins. <br><br> ● Viral DNA (amplified by PCR) can be detected in clinical samples, including CSF in patients with HSV encephalitis. |

## Herpes simplex virus, type 2

| Pathogenesis/Clinical Significance | Treatment and Prevention | Laboratory Identification |
|---|---|---|
| Herpes simplex virus, type 2 (HSV-2) has a relatively rapid, cytocidal growth cycle. HSV-2 establishes latency in sacral or lumbar ganglia. Transmission of HSV-2 generally occurs by sexual contact, or by infection of a newborn during birth. <br><br> ● **Primary HSV-2 infections** <br><br> Primary genital tract lesions are similar to those of the oropharynx caused by HSV-1, but the majority of these infections are asymptomatic. When symptomatic, local symptoms such as pain and itching, and systemic symptoms of fever, malaise, and myalgias may be more severe than those that accompany primary oral cavity infections. <br><br> [HERPES SIMPLEX VIRUS, TYPE 2 IS CONTINUED ON THE NEXT PAGE.] | ● **Treatment:** Acycloguanosine (acyclovir) is selectively effective against HSV because it becomes an active inhibitor only after initially being phosphorylated by the HSV-coded thymidine kinase. The drug cannot cure a latent infection, but can minimize or prevent recurrences. Other inhibitors active against HSV DNA synthesis include famciclovir, foscarnet, cidofovir, and topically applied penciclovir. | ● Cell tissue culture inoculated with a sample of vesicle scraping, fluid, or genital swab shows gross cytopathic changes in several days; individual infected cells can be detected within 24 hours by use of immunofluorescence or immunoperoxidase staining with antibodies against viral early proteins. |

## Herpes simplex virus, type 2 (continued)

| Pathogenesis/Clinical Significance | Treatment and Prevention | Laboratory Identification |
|---|---|---|

### ● Primary HSV-2 infections (cont.)

Vesiculoulcerative lesions on the female's vulva, cervix, and vagina or the male's penis can be very painful. Neonatal herpes is contracted by the baby during birth. If untreated, a disseminated infection results, often involving the CNS, leading to a high mortality rate. [Note: Infection in utero appears to occur only rarely.]

### ● Latent HSV-2 infections

HSV-2 remains latent in the sacral ganglia. Reactivation of HSV-2 genital infection occurs frequently, and may be asymptomatic. However, the infected individual sheds virus during the reactivation period regardless of symptoms, and can transmit the virus to a sexual partner during that period.

● **Prevention:** No vaccine or preventive drug is available. Prevention of HSV transmission is enhanced by avoidance of contact with potential virus-shedding lesions and by safe sexual practices. Neonatal HSV can be prevented by delivery via cesarean section.

● Viral DNA (amplified by PCR) can be detected in clinical samples, including CSF in patients with HSV encephalitis.

## Human cytomegalovirus

| Pathogenesis/Clinical Significance | Treatment and Prevention | Laboratory Identification |
|---|---|---|

Human cytomegalovirus (HCMV) is transmitted by infected individuals through their tears, urine, saliva, semen or vaginal secretions, and breast milk. HCMV can also cross the placenta.

HCMV replicates initially in epithelial cells of the respiratory and GI tracts, followed by viremia and infection of all organs of the body. In symptomatic cases, kidney tubule epithelium, liver, and CNS, in addition to the respiratory and GI tracts, are most commonly affected. HCMV has a relatively slow replication cycle, with the formation of characteristic multinucleated giant cells, thus the name "cytomegalo-". Latency is established in nonneural tissues, primarily lymphoreticular cells, and glandular tissues.

### ● HCMV infectious mononucleosis

Whereas most HCMV infections occur in childhood, primary infection as an adult may result in a mononucleosis syndrome that is clinically identical to that caused by Epstein-Barr virus. It is estimated that about eight percent of infectious mononucleosis (IM) cases are due to HCMV. The major distinguishing feature of HCMV IM is the absence of the heterophile antibodies that characterize IM caused by EBV.

### ● Cytomegalic inclusion disease

HCMV is the most common intrauterine virus infection. Of infants born to women experiencing their first HCMV infection during pregnancy, 35 to 50 percent will become infected, of which 10 percent will be symptomatic. The severity of the latter, referred to as cytomegalic inclusion disease, ranges from fetal death to various degrees of damage to liver, spleen, blood-forming organs, and components of the nervous system (a common cause of hearing loss and mental retardation).

### ● HCMV infection of immunosuppressed transplant recipients

Such individuals are multiply at risk from 1) HCMV present in the tissue being transplanted, 2) virus carried in leukocytes in the associated blood transfusions, and 3) reactivation of endogenous latent virus. The resulting infection can cause destruction of GI tract tissues, hepatitis, and pneumonia, the latter being a major cause of death in bone marrow transplant recipients.

### ● HCMV infection of AIDS patients

Invasive opportunistic HCMV infections are common in AIDS patients. These become increasingly important as CD4+ lymphocyte counts and immune competence decline. Any organ systems can be affected, but pneumonia, and blindness due to HCMV retinitis, are especially common. Encephalitis and dementia, esophagitis, enterocolitis, and gastritis are other significant problems.

● **Treatment:** Treatment of HCMV infections is indicated primarily in immunocompromised patients. Acyclovir is ineffective because HCMV lacks a thymidine kinase. Ganciclovir is used for invasive infections of transplant recipients and AIDS patients. Cidofovir is used for ganciclovir-resistant mutants. Foscarnet can be used in combination with ganciclovir, or as an alternate treatment when resistant mutants appear.

● **Prevention:** No vaccine or preventive drug is available.

● Serologic diagnosis using ELISA techniques can distinguish primary from recurrent infection, by demonstrating either IgG seroconversion, or the presence of HCMV-specific IgM.

● Determination of the presence and amount of viral DNA or proteins in white blood cells is used to evaluate invasive disease.

● Presence of extracellular virus in urine or saliva may simply be due to an asymptomatic recurrence.

## Human herpesvirus, type 8

| Pathogenesis/Clinical Significance | Treatment and Prevention | Laboratory Identification |
|---|---|---|
| Genome analysis of a virus recovered from cells of Kaposi sarcoma revealed it to be a member of the human herpes family, human herpesvirus type 8 (HHV-8), also called Kaposi sarcoma-associated herpes virus (KSHV). In contrast to the other human herpesviruses, HHV-8 infection appears to be relatively infrequent in the normal, healthy population. <br><br> ● **Kaposi sarcoma** <br><br> The virus has been detected in over ninety percent of patients with Kaposi sarcoma, and in several other types of vascular tumors and lymphomas found in AIDS patients. Antibodies to HHV-8 antigens are found primarily in the populations that are at risk for HIV infection, suggesting that at least one route for transmission is exchange of body fluids. | ● **Treatment:** Various drugs are currently being evaluated for use against HHV-8/Kaposi sarcoma. <br><br> ● **Prevention:** No vaccine or preventive drug is available. | ● DNA hybridization following PCR amplification of viral DNA isolated from clinical samples can be used to provide a definitive diagnosis. <br><br> ● Antibody status of the infected individual can be determined serologically. |

# Retroviridae
Human Immunodeficiency Virus

# Common characteristics

● **Single-stranded, positive-sense, linear RNA—two copies per virion (diploid)**

● **Viral envelope contains glycoprotein that undergoes antigenic variation**

● **Virion contains reverse transcriptase**

| Pathogenesis/Clinical Significance | Treatment and Prevention | Laboratory Identification |
|---|---|---|
| Human immunodeficiency virus (HIV) is a nononcogenic retrovirus. Transmission occurs mainly by one of three routes: 1) sexually (it is present in both semen and vaginal secretions); 2) with blood or blood products (whole blood, plasma, clotting factors, and cellular fractions of blood by transfusion, or by inoculation with HIV-contaminated needles); and 3) perinatally (either transplacentally, during passage through the birth canal, or in breast feeding). <br><br> The specific HIV cell surface receptor is the CD4 molecule, located primarily on helper T cells. HIV enters the cell by fusion of the virus envelope with the plasma membrane. Reverse transcription takes place in the cytoplasm, with the viral RNA-dependent reverse transcriptase first synthesizing a DNA-RNA hybrid molecule, then degrading the parental RNA while replacing it with a second strand of DNA. The resulting linear molecule of double-stranded DNA is the provirus. It is transported to the nucleus and is randomly inserted into the host chromosome by viral enzymes. The integrated DNA is translated into viral mRNAs that code for viral proteins, and also will be packaged into progeny virus. Assembled virions bud through the plasma membrane. Production of virus is a continuous process, eventually killing the host cell. <br><br> ● **Human immunodeficiency virus infection** <br><br> Several weeks after the initial infection, one third to two thirds of individuals experience symptoms similar to those of infectious mononucleosis, during which there is a very high level of virus replication in CD4+ cells. Lymph nodes become infected, which are the sites of virus persistence during the asymptomatic period. The acute phase viremia resolves into a clinically asymptomatic or "latent" period lasting from months to many years. This period is characterized by persistent generalized lymphadenopathy, diarrhea, and weight loss. | ● **Treatment:** Inhibitors of viral reverse transcriptase include both nucleoside and non-nucleoside reverse transcriptase inhibitors. They prevent the establishment of HIV infection. Inhibitors of the viral protease delay the production of progeny virus. Administering combinations of these drugs delays the appearance of resistant mutants, therefore three or four drugs are given at the same time. This is referred to as "highly active anti-retroviral therapy" or HAART. <br><br> ● **Prevention:** No vaccine is available. Perinatal transmission can be reduced with zidovudine (AZT) therapy of the pregnant woman, followed by several weeks of AZT to the newborn. Prevention can be achieved by screening blood and tissues prior to transfusion or transplant, using condoms during sexual intercourse, and strict adherence to the universal precautions by health care workers | ● Amplification of viral RNA or DNA proviruses by the PCR technique is the most sensitive method for detection of virus in blood or tissue specimens. <br><br> ● For purposes of screening the blood supply, ELISA testing for the p24 (CA) antigen in serum can detect infection about a week earlier than tests for antibody. <br><br> ● For screening individuals, the ELISA procedure is also used to detect antibodies in serum; any positive results must be confirmed using the Western blot technique. |

[HUMAN IMMUNODEFICIENCY VIRUS IS CONTINUED ON THE NEXT PAGE]

### Human immunodeficiency virus (continued)

| Pathogenesis/Clinical Significance | Treatment and Prevention | Laboratory Identification |
|---|---|---|

● **Acquired immunodeficiency syndrome (AIDS):**

The progression from asymptomatic infection to AIDS occurs as a continuum of progressive clinical states. The number of infected CD4+ cells decreases, and T cell precursors in the lymphoid organs are infected and killed, so the capacity to generate new CD4+ cells is gradually lost. Cells of the monocyte/macrophage lineage are also infected, and transport the virus into other organs, including the brain. When the CD4+ count falls below 200/µl, and increasingly frequent and serious opportunistic infections appear, the syndrome is defined as AIDS.

# Orthomyxoviridae
## Influenza virus

# Common characteristics

● **Negative-strand RNA genome**

● **Spherical, enveloped, pleomorphic virus**

● **RNA is segmented into eight pieces, each of which codes for a single protein**

● **Virion has two types of membrane protein spikes: H protein (hemagglutinin) and N protein (neuraminidase)**

● **Virion contains RNA polymerase**

| Pathogenesis/Clinical Significance | Treatment and Prevention | Laboratory Identification |
|---|---|---|

Influenza is spread by respiratory droplets, and is an infection solely of the respiratory tract. There is rarely a viremia, or spread to other organ systems.

Influenza viruses are classified as types A, B, and C, depending on the antigenicity of their inner proteins (only A and B are of medical importance). Type A viruses are further broken down into subtypes based on antigens associated with the outer viral proteins, H and N. Influenza viruses have shown marked variation over the years in their antigenic properties, specifically of the H and N proteins. This variation is due primarily to antigenic shift.

● **Influenza (the "flu")**

Following inhalation of influenza virus particles, respiratory epithelial cells are destroyed by the host immune response, specifically, cytotoxic T cells. Typically, influenza has an acute onset characterized by chills, followed by a high fever, muscle aches, and extreme drowsiness. The disease runs its course in four to five days, after which there is a gradual recovery. The most serious problems, such as pneumonia, occur in the very young, the elderly, and people with chronic cardiac or pulmonary disease, or who are immunodeficient.

● **Reye syndrome**

This is a rare and serious complication of viral infections in children, especially in those who have had chicken pox or influenza. Aspirin used to lower the virus-induced fever may contribute to the appearance of this syndrome. Therefore, acetaminophen is usually recommended for fevers of unknown origin in children.

● **Treatment:** Amantidine and rimantadine prevent the influenza virus from uncoating. They reduce both the duration and severity of flu symptoms in type A influenza infections, but only if given early in infection. Influenza viruses readily develop resistance to these compounds. Zanamivir and oseltamivir are newer drugs that inhibit viral neuraminidase—an enzyme required for release of virus from infected cells.

● **Prevention:** A vaccine consisting of formalin-inactivated influenza virus is available. It is of critical importance that the vaccine contain the specific subtypes of influenza virus present in the population that year. Given before the onset of symptoms, amantidine and rimantidine can also prevent disease, and are useful for treating high-risk groups.

● Quantitation of HI (hemagglutination inhibition) antibodies can be done for surveillance purposes.

● Demonstration of viral antigens in respiratory tract secretions is a more rapid method for diagnosis of influenza infection.

# Paramyxoviridae

**Measles virus**
**Mumps virus**
**Parainfluenza virus (p. 363)**
**Respiratory syncytial virus (p. 365)**

# Common characteristics

● Nonsegmented, negative-strand RNA

● Spherical, enveloped viruses

● Some contain RNA polymerase in their virions

● Envelope contains F (fusion) protein that allows virus to enter cells via a fusion process, rather than by receptor-mediated endocytosis

## Measles virus

| Pathogenesis/Clinical Significance | Treatment and Prevention | Laboratory Identification |
|---|---|---|
| Measles virus is transmitted by sneeze- or cough-produced respiratory droplets. The virus is extremely infectious, and almost all infected individuals develop a clinical illness.<br><br>● **Measles**<br><br>Measles virus replicates initially in the respiratory epithelium, and then in various lymphoid organs. Classic measles begins with a prodromal period of fever, upper respiratory tract symptoms, and conjunctivitis. Two to three days later, Koplik spots develop in the mouth and throat, and a generalized macular rash appears, beginning at the head and traveling slowly to the lower extremities. Soon after the rash appears, the patient is no longer infectious. A rare complication occurring within two weeks after the onset of the rash is **postinfectious encephalomyelitis** —an autoimmune disease. Children are particularly susceptible, especially those weakened by other diseases or hunger. | ● **Treatment:** No antiviral drugs are available for measles.<br><br>● **Prevention:** A live, attenuated measles vaccine is available; it is usually administered in the form of the measles-mumps-rubella (MMR) vaccine. | ● Demonstration of an increase in the titer of antiviral antibodies can be used in the diagnosis of measles. |

## Mumps virus

| Pathogenesis/Clinical Significance | Treatment and Prevention | Laboratory Identification |
|---|---|---|
| Mumps virus is spread by respiratory droplets.<br><br>● **Mumps**<br><br>Although about one third of infections are subclinical, the classic clinical presentation and diagnosis center on infection and swelling of the salivary glands, primarily the parotid glands. However, mumps virus can enter the bloodstream, causing widespread infection. This may involve not only salivary glands, but also the pancreas, CNS, and testes. Male sterility occasionally occurs, due to bilateral infection of the testes (orchitis). | ● **Treatment:** No antiviral drugs are available for mumps.<br><br>● **Prevention:** A live, attenuated vaccine is available; it is usually administered in the form of the measles-mumps-rubella (MMR) vaccine. | ● Virus may be recoverable from saliva, blood, CSF, or urine, and can be cultured.<br><br>● Serologic tests detect antiviral antibody in the blood. |

# Papovaviridae

Papillomavirus

## Common characteristics

- **Double-stranded, circular DNA**
- **Nonenveloped, icosahedral**
- **Over seventy types of human papilloma viruses currently recognized**

| Pathogenesis/Clinical Significance | Treatment and Prevention | Laboratory Identification |
|---|---|---|
| Transmission of human papillomavirus (HPV) infection requires direct contact with infected individuals or contaminated surfaces. All human papillomaviruses induce **hyperplastic epithelial lesions**; they infect either cutaneous (keratinizing) or mucosal (squamous) epithelium. The HPVs within each of these tissue-specific groups have varying potentials to cause malignancies. There are: 1) a small number of virus types that produce lesions having a high risk of progression to malignancy, such as in the case of **cervical carcinoma**; 2) other virus types produce mucosal lesions that progress to malignancy with lower frequency, causing, for example, **anogenital warts** (**condyloma acuminatum**, a common sexually transmitted disease) and **laryngeal papillomas** (the most common benign epithelial tumors of the larynx); 3) in those individuals with a genetic predisposition for the inability to control the spread of warts, some virus types cause multiple cutaneous warts that do not regress, but spread to many body sites (**epidermodysplasia verruciformis**)—these lesions give rise with high frequency to **squamous cell carcinomas** several years after initial appearance of the original warts; and 4) still other virus types that are associated only with benign lesions, for example, **common, flat**, and **plantar warts**. | • **Treatment:** Cutaneous warts generally require surgical removal or destruction of the wart tissue with liquid nitrogen, laser vaporization, or cytotoxic chemicals. Interferon, given orally, is effective in causing regression of laryngeal papillomas. When injected directly into genital warts, interferon is effective in about half of the patients. Cidofovir is also effective as a topical application.<br><br>• **Prevention:** The primary means of prevention is avoidance of contact with wart tissue. In the case of genital tract warts, procedures for prevention of sexually transmitted diseases should be employed, but are not always effective. | • Diagnosis of cutaneous warts generally involves no more than visual inspection.<br><br>• Typing of human papillomavirus is done either by immunoassays for viral antigens, or by DNA hybridization.<br><br>• Human papillomavirus cannot be cultured in the laboratory. |

# Paramyxoviridae

**Measles virus (p. 362)**
**Mumps virus (p. 362)**
**Parainfluenza virus**
**Respiratory syncytial virus (p. 365)**

## Common characteristics

- **Nonsegmented, negative-strand RNA**
- **Spherical, enveloped viruses**
- **Some contain RNA polymerase in their virions**
- **Envelope contains F (fusion) protein that allows virus to enter cells via a fusion process, rather than by receptor-mediated endocytosis**

## Parainfluenza virus

| Pathogenesis/Clinical Significance | Treatment and Prevention | Laboratory Identification |
|---|---|---|
| There are four clinically important human parainfluenza viruses (hPIV), designated hPIV types 1 to 4. They are called "parainfluenza" because individuals may present with influenza-like symptoms, and like influenza, the viruses have both hemagglutinating and neuraminidase activity. (Unlike influenza, these activities are not subject to antigenic shift.)<br><br>Infection by these viruses is spread by respiratory droplets, and is confined to the respiratory tract.<br><br>• **Respiratory tract infections**<br>Parainfluenza viruses cause **croup, pneumonia**, and **bronchiolitis**, mainly in infants and children. They are also a cause of the "**common cold**" in individuals of all ages. | • **Treatment:** No antiviral drugs are recommended for these infections. Symptoms can be treated as necessary.<br><br>• **Prevention:** No vaccine or preventive drug is available. | • Serologic tests for antibody to the virus can aid in the diagnosis of parainfluenza virus infection. |

# Picornaviridae

Coxsackievirus (p. 354)
Hepatitis A virus (p. 356)
Poliovirus

## Common characteristics

● **Positive-strand, single-stranded, nonsegmented RNA genome**

● **Non-enveloped, icosahedral**

● **Genomic RNAs serve as messenger RNAs and are infectious**

● **Virions do not contain any enzymes**

## Poliovirus

| Pathogenesis/Clinical Significance | Treatment and Prevention | Laboratory Identification |
|---|---|---|
| Poliovirus is a member of the genus Enterovirus. Individuals are infected with poliovirus by ingestion of contaminated food or water. Enteroviruses are stable in the low pH of the stomach, replicate in the GI tract, and are excreted in the stool (fecal-oral route). After replicating in the oropharynx and intestinal tract lymphoid tissue, poliovirus can enter the bloodstream and spread to the central nervous system.<br><br>● **Poliomyelitis**<br><br>The great majority of poliovirus infections are asymptomatic. The classic presentation in those poliovirus-infected individuals who become ill is that of **flaccid paralysis**, most often affecting the lower limbs. This is due to viral replication in, and destruction of, the lower motor neurons in the anterior horn of the spinal cord. **Respiratory paralysis** may also occur, following infection of the brain stem. | ● **Treatment:** No antiviral agents are currently available for treating poliovirus infections.<br><br>● **Prevention:** A killed poliovirus vaccine (Salk) that is injected, and a live, attenuated poliovirus vaccine (Sabin) that is given orally are available, and have led to the elimination of wild-type polio from Western Europe, Japan, and the Americas. The few cases that occur in the United States are either brought from other countries, or are caused by vaccine strains of virus that have reverted to a virulent form. | ● Poliovirus can be isolated and cultured from the stool or cerebral spinal fluid.<br><br>● Evidence of infection can also be obtained by demonstration of a rise in antibody titer. |

# Rhabdoviridae

Rabies virus

## Common characteristics

● **Negative-strand, single-stranded, non-segmented RNA genome**

● **Enveloped, helical nucleocapsid**

● **Virus is bullet-shaped**

● **Virion contains RNA-dependent RNA polymerase**

| Pathogenesis/Clinical Significance | Treatment and Prevention | Laboratory Identification |
|---|---|---|
| Rabies virus is a member of the genus Lyssavirus. A wide variety of wildlife, such as raccoons, skunks, squirrels, foxes, and bats, provide a reservoir for the virus. In developing countries, domestic dogs and cats also constitute an important reservoir for rabies. Humans are usually infected by the bite of an animal, but in some cases, infection is via an aerosol, for example, of droppings from infected bats.<br><br>● **Rabies**<br><br>Following inoculation, the virus may replicate locally, but then travels via the axoplasm of peripheral neurons to the brain, where it replicates primarily in the gray matter. From the brain, the rabies virus can travel along autonomic nerves, leading to infection of the lungs, kidney, adrenal medulla, and salivary glands. The incubation period is extremely variable, but generally lasts one to eight weeks. Symptoms of the infection include hallucinations, seizures, weakness, mental dysfunction, paralysis, coma, and finally death from a fatal encephalitis with neuronal degeneration of the brain and spinal cord. Once symptoms begin, death is inevitable. Many, but not all, patients show the classic rabid sign of hydrophobia—a painful inability to swallow liquids, leading to avoidance. | ● **Treatment:** Once an individual has clinical symptoms of rabies there is no effective treatment.<br><br>● **Prevention:** Preexposure prophylaxis, which is indicated for individuals at high risk (for example, veterinarians) consists of administration of a killed virus vaccine. In the United States, this is generally the human diploid cell vaccine (HDCV). Postexposure prophylaxis is instituted after an animal bite or exposure to an animal suspected of being rabid. It consists of both passive immunization with antirabies immunoglobulin and active immunization with HDCV. | ● Diagnosis rests on a history of exposure and signs and symptoms characteristic of rabies. However, a reliable history of exposure is often not obtainable, and the initial clinical presentation may vary. Therefore, a clinical diagnosis may be difficult.<br><br>● Postmortem, characteristic cytoplasmic inclusions (Negri bodies) may be seen in regions of the brain such as the hippocampus. |

# Paramyxoviridae

### Measles virus (p. 362)
### Mumps virus (p. 362)
### Parainfluenza virus (p. 363)
### Respiratory syncytial virus

## Common characteristics

● **Nonsegmented, negative-strand RNA**

● **Spherical, enveloped viruses**

● **Some contain RNA polymerase in their virions**

● **Envelope contains F (for fusion) protein that allows virus to enter cells via a fusion process, rather than by receptor-mediated endocytosis**

## Respiratory syncytial virus

| Pathogenesis/Clinical Significance | Treatment and Prevention | Laboratory Identification |
|---|---|---|
| Respiratory syncytial virus (RSV) is transmitted by respiratory droplets, or by contaminated hands carrying the virus to the nose or mouth. Repeated infections are common.<br><br>● **Respiratory tract infections**<br>RSV is the major viral respiratory tract pathogen in the pediatric population, and the most important cause of **bronchiolitis** in infants. It may also cause **pneumonia** in young children, an **influenza-like syndrome** in adults, and **severe bronchitis with pneumonia** in the elderly. RSV does not spread systemically. | ● **Treatment:** The only specific treatment for RSV infection is ribavirin, administered by aerosol, which is only of moderate benefit.<br><br>● **Prevention:** No vaccine or preventive drug is available. Spread of infection between people can be controlled by hand-washing and avoiding others with the infection. | ● Demonstration of an increase in the titer of antiviral antibodies or demonstration of viral antigens in respiratory secretions can provide a definitive diagnosis of RSV infection. |

# Togaviridae

### Rubella virus

## Common characteristics

● **Positive-strand, single-stranded, nonsegmented RNA genome**

● **Enveloped, icosahedral nucleocapsid**

● **Genomic RNAs serve as messenger RNAs and are infectious**

● **Virions do not contain any enzymes**

| Pathogenesis/Clinical Significance | Treatment and Prevention | Laboratory Identification |
|---|---|---|
| Rubella virus is a member of the genus rubivirus. The virus is transmitted via respiratory secretions from an infected individual.<br><br>● **German measles**<br>This is a mild clinical syndrome (not to be confused with rubeola, caused by the measles virus). The infection is characterized by a generalized maculopapular rash, and occipital lymphadenopathy. In most cases, these symptoms may be hardly noticeable, and the infection remains subclinical.<br><br>● **Congenital rubella**<br>The major clinical significance of rubella is that when a pregnant woman is infected with the virus, there can be significant damage to the developing fetus, especially in the first trimester. This damage can include congenital heart disease, cataracts, hepatitis, or abnormalities related to the CNS, such as mental retardation, motor dysfunction, and deafness. | ● **Treatment:** No antiviral drugs are presently in use.<br><br>● **Prevention:** Fetal damage due to rubella infection is preventable by use of the live, attenuated rubella vaccine that is included with the routine childhood vaccinations. This vaccine is effective, has few complications, and ensures that when women reach childbearing age, they are immune to rubella infection. The vaccine should not be given to women who are already pregnant or to immunocompromised patients, including young babies. | ● A diagnosis of rubella infection can be made by measuring a rise in antibody titer.<br><br>● Pregnant women with anti-rubella IgM antibody are presumed to have been recently exposed to the virus. |

# Herpesviridae

Epstein-Barr virus (p. 355)
Herpes simplex virus, Type 1 (p. 358)
Herpes simplex virus, Type 2 (p. 358)
Human cytomegalovirus (p. 359)
Human herpesvirus, Type 8 (p. 360)
Varicella-zoster virus

# Common characteristics

- Enveloped DNA viruses

- Linear, double-stranded DNA genome

- Herpesviruses replicate in the nucleus

- Envelope contains antigenic, species-specific glycoproteins

- In the tegument between the envelope and capsid are a number of virus-coded enzymes and transcription factors essential for initiation of the infectious cycle

- All herpesviruses can enter a latent state following primary infection, to be reactivated at a later time

## Varicella-zoster virus

| Pathogenesis/Clinical Significance | Treatment and Prevention | Laboratory Identification |
|---|---|---|

### Pathogenesis/Clinical Significance

Varicella-zoster virus (VZV) has a relatively rapid, cytocidal growth cycle, and establishes latency in sensory nerve ganglia.

Transmission of VZV is usually via respiratory droplets, which results in initial infection of the respiratory mucosa, followed by spread to the regional lymph nodes. From there, progeny virus enters the bloodstream, undergoes a second round of multiplication in cells of the liver and spleen, and is disseminated throughout the body by infected mononuclear leukocytes.

- **Varicella ("chickenpox")**

  Following infection of a normal, healthy child, the first symptoms include fever, malaise, headache, and abdominal pain. Next is appearance of the virus-containing vesicles ("pox") characteristic of the disease. These begin on the scalp, face, or trunk about 10 to 23 days after exposure, causing severe itching, and then proceed to the extremities and mucous membranes, such as the oropharynx, conjunctiva, and vagina. The infected individual is contagious from one to two days before appearance of the vesicles. Varicella is more serious in adults and immunocompromised patients, potentially causing pneumonia, fulminant hepatic failure, and varicella encephalitis. Fetal infection during pregnancy is uncommon, but can result in multiple developmental anomalies.

- **Zoster ("shingles")**

  Due to the disseminated nature of the primary infection, latency is established in multiple sensory ganglia, the trigeminal and dorsal root ganglia being most common. On reactivation, there is substantial multiplication and horizontal spread of virus among the cells in the ganglion. Viral destruction of sensory ganglia leads to the pain associated with acute zoster. Debilitating postherpetic neuralgia and abnormal sensory phenomena may last as long as several months. The likelihood of reactivation increases with age and with depressed cellular immune competence.

### Treatment and Prevention

- **Treatment for varicella:** Varicella in normal children does not require treatment. Treatment of primary varicella in immunocompromised patients, adults, and neonates is warranted by the severity of the disease. Acyclovir has been the drug of choice. Newer drugs—famciclovir and valacyclovir—have greater activity against VZV.

- **Treatment for zoster:** Oral acyclovir reduces the time course and acute pain of zoster, but has little or no effect on the subsequent postherpetic neuralgia. Famciclovir, given early in the acute phase of zoster, decreases acute pain and the time to resolution of lesions, and also shortens the duration of postherpetic pain.

- **Prevention:** A live, attenuated vaccine is recommended as one of the routine childhood vaccines. It is also indicated for nonimmune adults who are at risk of contagion. Varicella-zoster immune globulin can protect neonates and immunocompromised individuals who have been exposed to chickenpox or zoster lesion fluid.

### Laboratory Identification

- Cell tissue culture inoculated with a sample of vesicle fluid shows gross cytopathic changes in several days; individual infected cells can be detected within 24 hours by use of immunofluorescence or immunoperoxidase staining with antibodies against viral early proteins.

- More rapid diagnosis can be made by reacting epithelial cells scraped from the base of vesicles with the stains described above, or doing in situ hybridization with VZV-specific DNA probes.

# Disease Summaries

# 33

## I. OVERVIEW

The chapter describes diseases caused by organisms that have common features, including their modes of transmission or clinical syndrome associated with the disease. This summary is guided, in part, by the frequency of disease as reported to the Centers for Disease Control and Prevention (CDC) which monitors the incidence of more than fifty notifiable disease, most of them organism-specific (Figure 33.1). [Note: A notifiable disease is one for which regular, frequent, and timely information regarding individual cases is considered necessary for prevention and control of the disease.] For example, data reported to the CDC show sexually transmitted diseases—diseases that have sexual contact as a common mode of transmission—are among the most common infectious diseases in the United States. However, some diseases included in this chapter are not reported by the CDC. These diseases are monitored by institutions, such as hospitals, where the reporting is as much clinical syndrome as it is by organism. For example, a hospital keeps track of its nosocomial urinary tract infections or ventilator-associated pneumonias.

## II. SEXUALLY TRANSMITTED DISEASES

*Chlamydia* remains the most commonly reported infectious disease in the United States and its incidence is slowly increasing. Women, especially young women, are hit hardest by *Chlamydia*. Gonorrhea is the second most commonly reported infectious disease in the United States. Although the disease rate is falling to historic lows, the occurrence of drug resistance is on the rise. Other sexually transmitted agents are described in Figures 33.2.

**Figure 33.1**
Reported cases of some notifiable diseses in the United States, 2004. [1]Invasive disease.

# Sexually Transmitted Diseases

## A Prevalence of common bacterial diseases

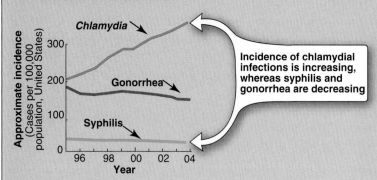

Incidence of chlamydial infections is increasing, whereas syphilis and gonorrhea are decreasing

## B Classification of bacterial pathogens

## Chlamydia trachomatis

- *C. trachomatis* is the major causal agent of sexually transmitted bacterial disease in the United States. It affects both sexes. Transmission is by close personal contact (for example, during birth, or sexual contact). Men develop **nongonococcal urethritis** and possible other infections (for example, of the prostate or rectum). Women develop infection of the cervix, which may progress to **pelvic inflammatory disease**. Repeated or chronic exposures to *C. trachomatis* can lead to sterility and ectopic pregnancy. A clinically distinct infection causing adenopathy, with destructive lesions on genitalia and adjacent tissue, is called **lymphogranuloma venereum**.

- *C. trachomatis* is an obligate intracellular parasite. It uses adhesins to attach to susceptible host cell membrane receptors on mucous membranes. It replicates in phagocytic vesicles, eventually killing the host cell.

Urethritis

Chlamydial cervicitis

Chlamydial conjunctivitis

Trachoma

## Neisseria gonorrhoeae

- *N. gonorrhoeae* causes **gonorrhea**. It is transmitted by sexual contact. In males, symptoms include infection of the urethra (**gonococcal urethritis**), purulent discharge, and pain during urination. In females, infection is usually localized to the endocervix, often causing a purulent vaginal discharge. If the woman's disease progresses to the uterus, **gonococcal salpingitis** (which may lead to tubal scarring and infertility), **pelvic inflammatory disease**, and fibrosis can occur. Alternatively, the infection may be asymptomatic in women.

- *N. gonorrhoeae* is highly sensitive to cool temperatures and dehydration. Bacterial proteins (pili and outer membrane proteins) enhance the attachment of the bacterium to host epithelial and mucosal cell surfaces, such as those of the urethra, rectum, cervix, pharynx, or conjunctiva, causing colonization and infections.

Gonococcal urethritis

Gonococcal ophthalmia neonatorum

**BACTERIA**

**Figure 33.2** (continued on the next page)
Characteristics of sexually transmitted diseases (STD): bacterial pathogens.

# Sexually Transmitted Diseases

## Treponema pallidum

- *T. pallidum* infection causes **syphilis**. It is transmitted primarily by sexual contact, in which the infectious lesion is generally on the skin or mucous membrane of the genitalia. Within two to ten weeks after infection, a painless, hard ulcer (**chancre**) forms. Up to ten weeks later, a secondary rash occurs that may be accompanied by systemic involvement, such as syphilitic hepatitis, meningitis, nephritis, or chorioretinitis. In about 40 percent of infected individuals, a tertiary stage occurs after a latent (asymptomatic) period. Tertiary syphilis is characterized by degenerative changes in the nervous system, cardiovascular lesions, and granulomatous lesions (gummas) in the liver, skin, and bones.

- *T. pallidum* can be transmitted across the placenta of an infected woman to her fetus, causing death and spontaneous abortion of the fetus, or causing it to be stillborn. Those infants that live have the symptoms of congenital syphilis, which include a variety of central nervous system (CNS) and structural abnormalities.

Primary syphilis chancres of the penis       Secondary syphilis

A gumma of tertiary syphilis

## Ureaplasma urealyticum

- *U. urealyticum* causes **nongonococcal urethritis**, particularly in men. The organism has a high colonization rate among sexually active men and women.

- In women, *U. urealyticum* causes **postpartum fever** and **chorioamnionitis**. The organism has been isolated from cases of endometritis and from vaginal secretions of women who undergo premature labor or deliver low-birth-weight babies. These infants are often colonized, and *U. urealyticum* has been isolated from the infant's lower respiratory tract and the CNS, both with and without evidence of inflammatory response.

Non-gonococcal urethritis

## Haemophilus ducreyi

- *H. ducreyi* causes **chancroid (soft chancre)**, a sexually-transmitted, ulcerative disease. Chancroid is a major health problem in developing countries, and its incidence is increasing in the United States. *H. ducreyi* infection causes painful, ragged ulcers on the genitalia, and lymphadenopathy may occur. Untreated, this progresses to formation of a bubo (a swollen, painful lymph node), which then suppurates.

- Open genital sores facilitate the transmission of HIV, and *H. ducreyi* infection is frequently associated with AIDS.

Chancroid

**BACTERIA**

**Figure 33.2** (continued on the next page)
Characteristics of sexually transmitted diseases: bacterial pathogens.

# Sexually Transmitted Diseases

## Candida albicans

● *C. albicans* is a yeast that is part of the normal body flora, which can be found in the skin, mouth, vagina, and intestines. It can also be introduced to the body, for example, during sexual contact. Overgrowth of candida (**candidiasis**) occurs when competing bacterial flora are eliminated, for example, by antibacterial antibiotics. Unlike *Trichomonas vaginalis*, which requires that the vagina have a pH of about 6.0 for growth, *C. albicans* grows at the normal vaginal pH of 4.0.

● **Vulvovaginal candidiasis** is a common clinical syndrome, often seen both in the physician's office and at STD clinics. This syndrome causes itching and burning pain of the vulva and vagina, accompanied by a white discharge that is usually thick, and curd-like.

Vulvovaginal candidiasis

**FUNGUS**

## Trichomonas vaginalis

● *T. vaginalis* causes **trichomoniasis**, the most common protozoal urogenital tract infection of humans. The disease is largely sexually transmitted. In females, it causes inflammation of the mucosal tissue of the vagina, vulva, and cervix, accompanied by a copious, yellowish discharge. Less commonly, it infects the male urethra, prostate, and seminal vesicles, producing a white discharge.

● The optimum pH for growth of *T. vaginalis* is about 6.0; therefore, the organism does not thrive in the normal, acidic vagina, which has a pH of about 4.0. Abnormal alkalinity of the vagina favors acquisition of the disease.

*Trichomonas vaginalis*

**PROTOZOAN**

### A  Prevalence of common viral diseases

Human papillomavirus

Herpes simplex virus

HIV

```
0            500,000          1,000,000
   New cases  per year in the United States
```

### B  Classification of viral pathogens

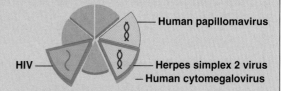

HIV

Human papillomavirus

Herpes simplex 2 virus
Human cytomegalovirus

## Herpes simplex virus type 2

● HSV-2 transmission generally occurs by sexual contact or by infection during birth. The nonperinatal infection causes **genital tract lesions**, most of which are asymptomatic. When symptomatic, local pain and itching and systemic symptoms of fever, malaise, and myalgias may occur. Vesiculoulcerative lesions on the vulva, cervix, and vagina, or the penis, can be painful. **Neonatal herpes** is contracted by a baby during birth. If untreated, a disseminated infection results, often involving the CNS, leading to a high mortality rate.

● HSV-2 has a relatively rapid, cytocidal growth cycle that establishes latency in nerve ganglia. Reactivation of HSV-2 genital infection occurs frequently and is often asymptomatic. The infected person sheds virus during the reactivation period regardless of symptoms and can transmit the virus to a sexual partner during that period.

Herpes simplex lesions

**VIRUSES**

**Figure 33.2** (continued on the next page)
Characteristics of sexually transmitted diseases: fungi, protozoa, and viruses.

# Sexually Transmitted Diseases

VIRUSES

## Human papillomavirus

- Infection by certain HPV causes **anogenital warts** (**condylomata acuminata**) and **periungual verruca vulgaris**. Transmission is through sexual contact or from mother to baby during birth.

- Lesions appear around the external genitalia, on the cervix, and/or inside the urethra or vagina, four to six weeks after infection. Some HPV infections are benign, but several types have been implicated as causes of cervical cancer.

Condyloma acuminatum    Periungual verruca vulgaris (on a finger)

A single renal tube contains large intranuclear virus inclusion bodies that have a typical "owl-eye" appearance.

## Human cytomegalovirus

- HCMV is the most common intrauterine viral infection. It is also the most common viral infection of neonates. HCMV is transmitted by infected individuals through tears, urine, saliva, semen or vaginal secretions, and breast milk. Of infants born to women experiencing their first HCMV infection during pregnancy, 35 percent to 50 percent will become infected, of which 10 percent will be symptomatic (**cytomegalic inclusion disease**). Manifestations of the latter can include various degrees of damage to liver, spleen, blood-forming organs, and components of the nervous system (a common cause of hearing loss and mental retardation) or fetal death. Invasive opportunistic HCMV infections are common in AIDS patients. Such infections are also a danger to transplant recipients and other immunocompromised individuals.

- HCMV replicates initially in epithelial cells, usually of the respiratory and GI tracts. This is followed by viremia and infection of all organs of the body. Latency is established in non-neural tissues, primarily lymphoreticular cells and glandular tissues.

Cytomegalovirus infection. Section of kidney taken at autopsy from a three-month-old boy.

**Opportunistic Infections of AIDS**

Cryptococcus present in the cerebrospinal fluid.    Oral thrush, or candidiasis

## Human immunodeficiency virus

- HIV infects CD4+ T-cells, T cell precursors, and cells of the monocyte/macrophage lineage, resulting in a state of immunodeficiency. Transmission of HIV occurs by three routes: 1) sexually (virus is present in both semen and vaginal secretions); 2) via blood or blood products; and 3) perinatally. Several weeks after the initial infection, some individuals experience symptoms similar to infectious mononucleosis. The acute-phase viremia resolves into a clinically asymptomatic latent period lasting from months to many years. The progression from asymptomatic infection to **acquired immunodeficiency syndrome** occurs as a continuum of progressive clinical states. Infected cells of the monocyte/macrophage system transport the virus into other organs including the brain. Death usually occurs from opportunistic infections, such as those shown to the right.

- HIV is a nononcogenic retrovirus. It binds to a surface CD4 molecule, located primarily on helper T cells. HIV enters the cell by fusion of the virus envelope with the plasma membrane, followed by reverse transcription. This results in formation of a molecule of double-stranded DNA that is integrated into a host cell chromosome. Progeny virus are produced continuously, and the process eventually kills the host cell.

Cytomegalovirus retinitis    Pneumocystis pneumonia

Kaposi sarcoma    Hairy leukoplakia

**Figure 33.2** (continued)
Characteristics of sexually transmitted diseases: viruses.

# FOOD POISONING (bacterial)

## A Common causes of food poisoning

*Campylobacter* species

*Salmonella* species

*Shigella* species

*Clostridium perfringens*

0    5    10    15%

Incidence (per 100,00 populaton) of diagnosed foodborne infections in the United States (2000)

## B Classification of pathogens

| *Staphylococcus aureus* | GRAM (+) COCCI (Ch. 9) |

*Escherichia coli*
*Campylobacter jejuni*
*Salmonella* species
*Shigella* species    GRAM (–) RODS (Ch. 12)

*Clostridium botulinum*
*Clostridium perfringens*    GRAM (+) RODS (Ch. 14)

## C Common complaints[1]

**DYSURIA LUMBAR PAIN**

**NAUSEA AND VOMITING**

**GI DISTURBANCES**

**FEVER**

### Campylobacter jejuni

● *C. jejuni* is the leading cause of foodborne disease in the United States. It also causes traveler's diarrhea and pseudoappendicitis. *C. jejuni* is transmitted to humans primarily via the fecal-oral route—through direct contact, exposure to contaminated meat (especially poultry), or contaminated water supplies.

● *C. jejuni* infects the intestine, and it can cause ulcerative, inflammatory lesions in the jejunum, ileum, or colon. In otherwise healthy individuals, it typically causes an acute enteritis following a one- to seven-day incubation. The disease lasts days to several weeks, and generally is self-limiting. Symptoms may be both systemic (fever, headache, myalgia) and intestinal (abdominal cramping and diarrhea, which may or may not be bloody). Bacteremia may occur, most often in infants and the elderly.

### Salmonella species

● Nontyphoidal *Salmonella* serotypes, particularly *S. typhimurium* and *S. enteritidis*, cause a localized gastroenteritis in which the symptoms result from causative bacteria proliferating in the intestine of affected individuals. Transmission is usually via food, especially chickens, eggs, and egg products.

● These organisms all produce exotoxins. Wide-spread antibiotic resistance among these organisms requires sensitivity testing to determine the appropriate antibiotic treatment, if any is given.

### Shigella species

● *Shigella* species cause shigellosis (bacillary dysentery)—a human intestinal disease that occurs most commonly among young children. Shigellae are typically spread from person to person, with food or water contaminated with fecal material serving as a major source of organisms.

● Shigellae invade and destroy the mucosa of the large intestine. The resulting bacillary dysentery is characterized by diarrhea with blood, mucus, and painful abdominal cramping. The disease is generally most severe in the very young and elderly, and among malnourished individuals, in whom shigellosis may lead to severe dehydration, and sometimes death.

### Clostridium species

● *Clostridium perfringens* is a major cause of food poisoning in the United States. The occurrence of clinical symptoms requires a large inoculum of $10^8$ organisms or greater. Therefore, a typical episode of clostridial food poisoning involves cooking that fails to inactivate spores, followed by holding the food for several hours under conditions that allow bacterial germination and several cycles of growth.

● *Clostridium perfringens* secretes various exotoxins, enterotoxins, and hydrolytic enzymes that facilitate the disease process. Symptoms involved in clostridial food poisoning typically include nausea, abdominal cramps, and diarrhea, occurring eight to eighteen hours after eating contaminated food. Fever is absent and vomiting rare. The attack is usually self-limited, with recovery within one to two days.

● *Clostridium botulinum* causes botulism. A neurotoxin produced by the bacteria results in flaccid paralysis. Contact with the organism itself is not required; hence, the disease is a pure intoxication.

**Figure 33.3** (continued on the next page)

Disease summary of some major organisms causing bacterial food poisoning.
[1]Other complaints may include headache and myalgias.

# FOOD POISONING (bacterial)

## Staphylococcus aureus

● *S. aureus* gastroenteritis is caused by ingestion of food containing the bacterial enterotoxin. Often contaminated by a food-handler, these foods tend to be protein-rich (for example, egg salad, cream pastry) and improperly refrigerated.

● The toxin stimulates the vomiting center in the brain by binding to neural receptors in the upper gastrointestinal tract. Symptoms such as nausea, vomiting, and diarrhea are acute following a short incubation period (less than six hours). The attack is usually self-limiting.

## D Therapy[2]

| | |
|---|---|
| *Campylobacter jejuni* | Ciprofloxacin or azithromycin in severe cases |
| *Clostridium* species | None |
| *Escherichia coli 0157:H7* *Escherichia coli,* enterotoxigenic | Antibiotics are contraindicated. Ciprofloxacin in severe cases |
| *Shigella* species | Ciprofloxacin in severe cases |
| *Staphylococcus aureus* | None |
| *Salmonella* species | Antibiotics not indicated unless extraintestininal spread; ciprofloxacin indicated for invasive disease |

## Escherichia coli

● *E. coli* is part of the normal flora of the colon, but can be pathogenic both inside and outside of the GI tract. Transmission of intestinal disease is commonly by the fecal-oral route, with contaminated food (such as beef and unpasteurized milk) and water serving as the vehicles.

● Several types of intestinal infections with *E. coli* have been identified. These differ in their pathogenic mechanisms. Among the most important are: 1) enterotoxigenic *E. coli* (ETEC)—a common cause of traveler's diarrhea in developing countries. ETEC colonizes the small intestine and produces enterotoxins. These cause prolonged hypersecretion of chloride ions and water by the intestinal mucosal cells while inhibiting the reabsorption of sodium, resulting in significant watery diarrhea over a period of several days. 2) Enterohemorrhagic *E. coli* (EHEC) binds to cells in the large intestine, where it produces an exotoxin (verotoxin) that destroys microvilli, causing a severe form of copious, bloody diarrhea (hemorrhagic colitis) in the absence of mucosal invasion or inflammation. Serotype O157:H7 is the most common strain of *E. coli* that produces verotoxin.

**Figure 33.3** (continued)
Disease summary of major organisms causing bacterial food poisoning. [2]Adequate fluid and electrolyte replacement and maintenance are key to managing diarrheal illnesses.

## III. FOOD POISONING (bacterial)

Food poisoning results from eating food contaminated with organisms or toxins (Figure 33.3). Food poisoning tends to occur at picnics, school cafeterias, and large social functions. These are situations in which food may be left unrefrigerated or food preparation techniques are not clean. Food poisoning often occurs from undercooked meats or dairy products that have remained at room temperature for extended periods.

In patients with food poisoning, fluid consumption is important to avoid dehydration.

Children with diarrhea may be given an over-the-counter electrolyte product. Solid foods should not be eaten until the diarrhea has passed, and dairy should be avoided, which can worsen diarrhea.

Intravenous fluid may be indicated in patients with severe diarrhea who are unable to drink fluids (for example, caused by nausea or vomiting)

Most patients spontaneously recover from the most common types of food poisoning within a couple of days.

Antibiotic therapy is usually not indicated, except in cases of severe illness.

Infants and elderly people have the greatest risk for food poisoning. It is estimated that foodborne gastroenteritis causes 76 million illnesses, 318,574 hospitalization, and 4,316 deaths in the United States.

# URINARY TRACT INFECTIONS

## A Common causes of UTI[1]

Escherichia coli

Staphylococcus saprophyticus

Klebsiella

Proteus

Pseudomonas aeruginosa

0  10  20  30  40  50  60  70  80  90
**Approximate prevalence (%)**

## B Classification of pathogens

Staphylococcus saprophyticus          GRAM (+) COCCI (Ch. 8)

Escherichia coli
Klebsiella
Proteus
Pseudomonas aeruginosa          GRAM (–) RODS (Ch. 13)

## Escherichia coli

● *E. coli* is the most common cause of urinary tract infections (UTI), including cystitis and pyelonephritis. Women are particularly at risk for infection. Transmission is frequently from the patient's flora.

● Uncomplicated cystitis (the most commonly encountered UTI) is caused by uropathogenic strains of *E. coli*, characterized by P fimbriae (an adherence factor). Complicated UTI (pyelonephritis) often occurs in settings of obstructed urinary flow, and may be caused by nonuropathogenic strains of *E. coli*. UTI require treatment with antibiotics.

## Staphylococcus saprophyticus

● *S. saprophyticus* is a frequent cause of cystitis in women, probably related to its occurrence as part of normal vaginal flora. It is also an important agent of hospital-acquired infections associated with the use of catheters.

● *S. saprophyticus* is a coagulase-negative staphylococcal species. It tends to be sensitive to most antibiotics, even penicillin G. It can be distinguished from most other coagulase-negative staphylococci by its natural resistance to novobiocin.

## C Common complaints

**DYSURIA LUMBAR PAIN**

**FEVER**

**CHILLS**

## Other enterobacteria

● Other genera of Enterobacteriaceae, such as *Klebsiella*, *Enterobacter*, *Proteus*, and *Serratia*, which can be found as normal inhabitants of the large intestine, include organisms that are primarily opportunistic and often nosocomial pathogens. They all frequently colonize hospitalized patients, especially in association with antibiotic treatment, indwelling catheters, or invasive procedures, causing extra-intestinal infections such as those of the urinary tract.

● These organisms produce exotoxins. Wide-spread antibiotic resistance among these organisms necessitates sensitivity testing to determine the appropriate antibiotic treatment.

## Pseudomonas aeruginosa

● *P. aeruginosa* is a significant opportunistic pathogen, and a major cause of hospital-acquired (nosocomial) infections such as UTI, particularly in patients who have been subjected to catheterization, instrumentation, surgery, or renal transplantation or to prior antibiotic therapy.

● *P. aeruginosa* disease begins with attachment and colonization of host tissue. Pili on the bacteria mediate adherence, and glycocalyx capsule reduces the effectiveness of normal clearance mechanisms. Host tissue damage facilitates adherence and colonization. Because pseudomonas infections typically occur in patients with impaired defenses, aggressive antimicrobial therapy is generally required.

**Figure 33.4** (continued on the next page)
Disease summary of urinary tract infections. [1]Uncomplicated cystitis.

**Figure 33.4** (continued)
Disease summary of urinary tract infections.

## IV. URINARY TRACT INFECTIONS

Urinary tract infections (UTIs) most commonly affect either the lower urinary tract (acute cystitis or infection of urethra, bladder) or, less frequently, the upper urinary tract (acute pyleonephritis or infection of kidney). UTIs are termed "uncomplicated" when there is no underlying condition that increases the risk of infection, such as obstruction or urologic dysfunction.

> Most patients with UTI have uncomplicated cystitis, which is one of the most common infections in the United States, especially in sexually active women.

*Escherichia coli* is the most common cause of uncomplicated cystitis and pyelonephritis (70 to 95 percent of infections, Figure 33.4). Fecal contamination can lead to entry of an organism such as *E. coli* (one of the most common organisms found in stool) into the urethra. These bacteria then move up into the bladder (and sometimes ascend into the kidney), producing infection. UTIs occur much more frequently in women as a result of the proximity of the urethral opening to the anus and the shorter length of the urethra before it opens into the bladder in women.

*Staphylococcus saprophyticus* as a causative agent is a distant second to *E. coli*, causing 5 to 20 percent of infections. *S. saprophyticus*, although less common than *E. coli*, often presents as a more aggressive disease with approximately one half of the patients showing involvement in the upper urinary tract. These patients are also more likely to have recurrent infection.

Patients with uncomplicated UTI usually present with dysuria, urinary frequency, urinary urgency and/or suprapubic pains. Pyuria (the production of urine that contains white blood cells) is commonly found in UTIs. Fever or flank tenderness could indicate pyelonephritis. If the features suggestive of vaginitis or urethritis described above are present, a pelvic examination and appropriate cultures should be performed.

> The causative bacteria for UTIs are rather predicable, making routine urine cultures unnecessary.

The risk of UTI, both cystitis and pyelonephritis, can be increased by several factors, especially sexual intercourse, particularly with a new sexual partner. The use of spermicides, particularly in combination with a diaphragm, also increases the risk of a woman developing a UTI.

# BACTERIAL MENINGITIS

## A Overview of common causes of bacterial meningitis in adults[1]

Streptococcus pneumoniae

Neisseria meningitidis

Haemophilus influenzae

Streptococcus agalactiae

Listeria monocytogenes

0   10   20   30   40   50   60

**Approximate prevalence (%)**

## B Classification of pathogens

| Streptococcus agalactiae Streptococcus pneumoniae | GRAM (+) COCCI (Ch. 9) |
| Listeria monocytogenes | GRAM (+) BACILLI (Ch. 10) |
| Neisseria meningitidis | GRAM (–) COCCI (Ch. 11) |
| Haemophilus influenzae | GRAM (–) RODS (Ch. 13) |

## C Common complaints[2]

**HEADACHE ALTERED MENTAL STATUS**

**FEVER**

**STIFF NECK**

**PHOTOPHOBIA**

## Streptococcus pneumoniae

- *S. pneumoniae* is an important cause of meningitis and pneumonia. It is carried in the nasopharynx of many healthy individuals. Infection can be either endogenous (in a carrier who develops impaired resistance to the organism) or exogenous (by droplets from the airway of a carrier).

- *S. pneumoniae* infections can result in a bacteremia leading to infection of several sites in the human body, including the CNS. This meningitis has a high mortality rate, even when treated appropriately. *S. pneumonia* is the most common cause of bacterial meningitis in adults.

## Neisseria meningitidis

- *N. meningitidis* is a common cause of meningitis. Transmission is via respiratory droplets. Pili allow the attachment of *N. meningitidis* to the nasopharyngeal mucosa.

- If meningococci penetrate the epithelial lining of the nasopharynx and enter the bloodstream they rapidly multiply, causing meningococcemia. If *N. meningitidis* crosses the blood-brain barrier, it can infect the meninges, causing an acute inflammatory response that results in a purulent meningitis. The initial fever and malaise can rapidly evolve into severe headache, rigid neck, vomiting, and sensitivity to bright light. Coma can occur within a few hours. *N. meningitidis* is the most common cause of bacterial meningitis between the ages of 2 and 18 years.

## Haemophilus influenzae

- *H. influenzae* is a normal resident of the human upper respiratory tract. Transmission is by respiratory droplets.

- After attaching to and colonizing the respiratory mucosa, the infection can become systemic, with bacteria spreading via the blood to the CNS. *H. influenzae* has been a leading cause of bacterial meningitis, especially in infants and young children. A conjugated vaccine against *H. influenzae* capsular polysaccharide type b is now administered to infants, and has lowered dramatically the number of meningitis cases attributable to this organism.

## Streptococcus agalactiae

- *S. agalactiae* causes meningitis and septicemia in neonates. It is found normally in the vaginocervical tract of female carriers and the urethral mucous membranes of male carriers, as well as in the GI tract (especially the rectum). Transmission occurs during birth and venereally among adults.

- Infection of an infant occurs as it traverses the birth canal. *S. agalactiae* infection is a leading cause of neonatal meningitis, and it has a high mortality rate.

## Listeria monocytogenes

- *L. monocytogenes* infections are common in the elderly, pregnant women, their fetuses or newborns, and immunocompromised individuals for whom listeria is a common cause of meningitis. Listeria infections, which may occur as sporadic cases or in small epidemics, are usually foodborne, with the organism entering the body via the GI tract.

**Figure 33.5** (continued on the next page)
Characteristics of organisms causing bacterial meningitis.

[1]*Escherichia coli* is a major cause of meningitis in the newborn. Viral meningitis is more common than the bacterial form and generally—but not always— less serious. Viral meningitis is often caused enteroviruses and sometimes herpes simplex virus.
[2]Other complaints include chills and cardiac arrhythmias.

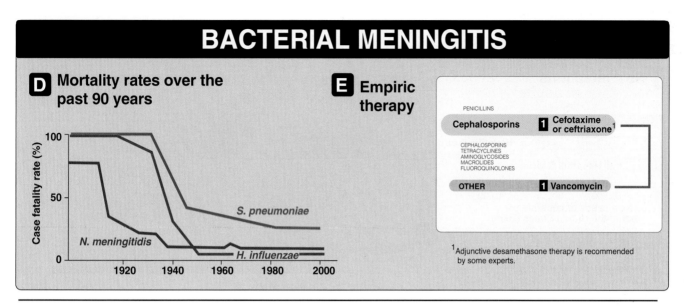

**Figure 33.5** (continued)
Characteristics of organisms causing bacterial meningitis.

## V. MENINGITIS

Bacterial meningitis is a medical emergency that requires immediate diagnosis and treatment. Untreated disease shows a mortality approaching 100 percent and, even with optimal therapy, there is a high failure rate.

Virtually all patients with community-acquired bacterial meningitis show at least one of the classic triad of symptoms—fever, neck stiffness, and altered mental status (Figure 33.5). These symptoms can develop over several hours, or they may take 1 to 2 days. Other symptoms may include nausea, vomiting, discomfort looking into bright lights, confusion, and sleepiness.

> *Streptococcus pneumoniae* and *Neisseria meningitidis* are responsible for 80% of all cases of bacterial meningitis.

Initial blood tests are positive in 50 to 75 percent of adults with bacterial meningitis. A specimen of cerebrospinal fluid (CSF) should be obtained for cell count and differential, glucose and protein concentration, Gram stain, and culture. Characteristic findings in bacterial meningitis include decreased glucose con- centration, elevated protein and white blood cell count in the CSF. Some patients may require computed tomography (CT) scan as a precaution before lumbar puncture.

Therapy for bacterial meningitis requires bactericidal antimicrobial agents that can cross the blood-brain barrier into the CSF. Most patients should be treated with intravenous antibiotics. Oral antibiotics should be used with caution because the dose and tissue levels tend to be considerably lower than with parenteral agents. Antibiotic therapy should be initiated immediately after lumbar puncture. If imaging is performed before lumbar puncture, therapy should be initiated before the patient is sent for neuroimaging.

> Delay in the initiation of anti- microbial therapy increases the risk of death or brain damage.

Initial therapy may be empiric. However, the availability of Gram stain of organisms in the CSF should guide the selection of intravenous antibiotics. Antibiotic therapy should also be reviewed once the CSF culture and in vitro susceptibility studies are available.

# HEPATITIS

## A New infections[1]

Hepatitis A virus
Hepatitis B virus
Hepatitis C virus

0     30,000     60,000     90,000
New cases of hepatitis per
year in the United States (2004)

**Flaviviridae** (Ch. 27)
● Hepatitis C

**Hepadnaviridae** (Ch. 26)
● Hepatitis B

**Picornaviridae** (Ch. 27)
● Hepatitis A

**Caliciviridae** (Ch. 27)
● Hepatitis E

## B Chronic infections

Hepatitis A virus not a chronic infections

Hepatitis B virus
Hepatitis C virus

0        1        2        3
Chronic infection in the
United States (2004)
(millions)

## C Common complaints

**NAUSEA AND VOMITING**

**FLANK PAIN**

108
104
100
98  Normal
94

**FEVER**

**ALT BILIRUBIN**

**ELEVATED LIVER ENZYMES; JAUNDICE**

## HEPATITIS B

● Hepatitis B virus (HBV) is a hepadnavirus and the only human hepatitis virus that has a DNA genome. A unique feature of HBV is that the viral DNA replicates via an RNA intermediate. HBV is enveloped.

● Infectious HBV is present in all body fluids of an infected individual, including blood, semen, saliva, mother's milk. In the United States, HBV is most frequently contracted by adults through sexual intercourse or by intravenous (IV) drug use. In developing countries, it is transmitted primarily from mother to infant.

● The primary cause of hepatic cell destruction by HBV is the specific reaction of HLA-I-restricted cytotoxic T lymphocytes with viral HBc and HBe antigens expressed on the infected cell's membrane. HBV infections can be acute (accompanied by mild fever, malaise, and myalgia, followed by jaundice and bilirubinuria, with an enlarged and tender liver) or chronic. Chronic carriers may be asymptomatic, but have a higher risk of developing severe chronic hepatitis, leading to progressive liver damage that may include cirrhosis and/or hepatocellular carcinoma.

● A highly effective vaccine produced in genetically engineered yeast cells is now available. It is included among routine childhood immunizations.

## Hepatitis A

● Hepatitis A virus (HAV) is a picornavirus, with a linear, single-stranded, positive-sense RNA genome. The capsid is nonenveloped.

● Transmission is by the fecal-oral route. The main site of replication is the hepatocyte, where infection results in severe cytopathology and liver function is severely impaired. The prognosis for patients with HAV is generally favorable and development of persistent infection and chronic hepatitis is uncommon.

● Prevention of infection requires taking sanitary measures. Immune globulin has been used for many years, mainly as postexposure prophylaxis. A formalin-inactivated whole virus vaccine is available.

## Hepatitis C

● Hepatitis C virus (HCV) is a member of the Flaviviridae. It has a linear, single-stranded, positive-sense RNA genome. HCV is enveloped.

● HCV was a major cause of post-transfusion hepatitis ("non-A, non-B"). IV drug users and patients on hemodialysis are also at high risk for infection with HCV. The virus can be transmitted sexually and from mother to infant.

● HCV replication occurs in hepatocytes and mononuclear cells. Both viral replication and the host immune response contribute to destruction of liver cells. Most infections are subclinical, but about 25 percent of infected individuals present with acute hepatitis, including jaundice. A significant proportion of infections progresses to a chronic hepatitis and cirrhosis, and some of these individuals develop hepatocellular carcinoma. Coinfection with HBV is often present in those manifesting these more serious consequences. Combination treatment with ribavirin plus interferon provides a higher rate of success in eradicating viral infection in adults than does interferon alone.

**Figure 33.6** (continued on the next page)
Characteristics of hepatitis. [Note: ALT = alanine aminotransferase.]
[1]No cases of hepatitis E have been reported in the United States.

# HEPATITIS

## HEPATITIS D

- Hepatitis D virus (HDV, or delta agent) is found in nature only as a result of coinfection with HBV, and it requires HBV to serve as a helper virus for infectious HDV production. HDV has a circular, single-stranded negative-sense RNA genome and an envelope in which protein is provided by HBV.
- HDV can be transmitted by the same routes as HBV. Pathologically, liver damage is essentially the same as in other viral hepatitides, but the presence of HDV usually results in more extensive and severe damage. No specific treatment for HDV infection is available.

## HEPATITIS E

- Hepatitis E virus (HEV) is a calicivirus, with a linear, single-stranded, positive-sense RNA genome. HEV is non-enveloped.
- HEV is a major cause of enterically transmitted, waterborne hepatitis in developing countries.[1] The peak incidence is in young adults, and the disease is especially severe in pregnant women, in whom death can result from HEV infection.
- No antiviral treatment or vaccine is currently available.

| | Drug | Vaccine |
|---|---|---|
| Hepatitis A | None | As an inactivated virus vaccine which offers 99 percent effective immunization against hepatitis A virus infection. Neutralizing antibodies persist for more than 3 years. |
| Hepatitis B | Lamivudine<br>α-Interferon<br>Adefovir<br>Entecavir | Recombinant hepatitis B vaccine is a noninfectious subunit viral vaccine. The vaccine is derived from hepatitis B surface antigen (HBsAg) produced through recombinant DNA techniques from yeast cells. Following a 3-dose series, immunity lasts approximately 5 to 7 years. |
| Hepatitis C | α-Interferon<br>Ribavirin | None |

**Figure 33.6** (continued )
Characteristics of hepatitis.

## VI. HEPATITIS

Hepatitis is inflammation of the liver. The disease can be caused by infections from parasites, bacteria, or viruses (such as hepatitis A, B, or C, Figure 33.6). Liver damage can also result from alcohol, drugs, or poisonous mushrooms. Hepatitis A, B, and C are clinically the most important forms of viral liver disease.

 Hepatitis A does not lead to chronic infection. Infection provides life-long immunity

Persons at risk of hepatitis B infection include 1) individuals with multiple sex partners; 2) men who have sex with men; 3) sex contacts of infected persons; 4) injection drug users; and 4) household contacts of chronically infected persons.

 Death from chronic hepatitis B occurs in 15 to 25 percent of chronically infected persons.

Most hepatitis C infections result from illegal injection drug use. Transfusion-associated cases occurred prior to blood donor screening; now occurs in less than one per 2 million transfused units of blood. Fifty percent of those with hepatitis C go on to have chronic liver disease and, possibly, liver failure (cirrhosis) or liver cancer.

 Hepatitis C is the number one reason for receiving a liver transplant in the United States.

# COMMUNITY-ACQUIRED PNEUMONIA[1]

## A  Common pathogens[2]

*Streptococcus pneumoniae*

*Haemophilus influenzae*

*Staphylococcus aureus*

Viruses

0   10   20   30   40   50   60
**Approximate prevalence (%)**

## B  Classification of pathogens

GRAM (+) COCCI

*Staphylococcus aureus*
*Streptococcus pneumoniae*

Parainfluenza viruses
Influenza virus types A and B
Respiratory syncytial virus

OTHER GRAM (–) BACILLI

*Haemophilus influenzae*

**SINGLE-STRANDED, NEGATIVE STRAND, HELICAL, ENVELOPED, RNA VIRUSES**

## C  Common complaints[2]

CHEST PAIN DYSPNEA

108
104
100   Normal
98
94

FEVER

CHILLS

COUGH

## *Streptococcus pneumoniae*

● Most common cause of pneumonia; leading cause of death in the aged and those with impaired resistance.

● Carried in nasopharynx of many healthy individuals; infection may, therefore, be endogenous or exogenous (by droplets from the nose of a carrier).

● A prior virus infection (for example, with influenza virus) that causes increased volume and viscosity of bronchial secretions and inhibition of the action of the bronchial cilia predisposes the patient to secondary infection by *S. pneumoniae.*

## *Haemophilus influenzae*

● Transmission is by respiratory droplets.

● *H. influenzae* causes pneumonia, especially in the elderly and immunocompromised individuals.

● After attaching to and colonizing the respiratory mucosa, the infection can become systemic, with bacteria spreading via the blood to the CNS.

## *Staphylococcus aureus*

● *S. aureus* infections are most common in IV drug users, the elderly, in people with a recent influenza virus infection, and in individuals with cystic fibrosis.

● *S. aureus* is transmitted by respiratory droplets. If it infects the lungs it causes severe, necrotizing pneumonia. Cell wall virulence factors promote binding to mucosal cells.

## Influenza virus Types A and B

● Influenza, spread by respiratory droplets, is an infection solely of the respiratory tract.

● Following inhalation of influenza virus particles, infected respiratory epithelial cells are destroyed by cytotoxic T cells.

● Pneumonia following a bout of influenza occurs in the young, the elderly, and people with chronic cardiac or pulmonary disease, or those who are immunodeficient. Pneumonia can be caused by influenza virus, or by secondary infection with bacteria, such as *S. pneumoniae.*

## Parainfluenza viruses

● Human parainfluenza viruses Types 1–4 cause influenza-like symptoms.

● Infection by these viruses is spread by respiratory droplets and is confined to the respiratory tract.

● Human parainfluenza viruses cause pneumonia, as well as croup and bronchiolitis, mainly in infants and children.

## Respiratory syncytial virus

● Transmission is by respiratory droplets or by contaminated hands carrying the virus to the nose or mouth.

● RSV is the major viral respiratory tract pathogen in the pediatric population. It may cause pneumonia in young children and severe bronchitis with pneumonia in the elderly.

**Figure 33.7** (continued on the next page)
Characteristics of community-acquired pneumonia.
[1] Disease may be "typical" or "atypical." "Typical" pneumonia is characterized by shaking chills, purulent sputum, and x-ray abnormalities that are proportional to the physical symptoms. "Atypical" pneumonia is characterized by insidious onset, scant sputum and x-ray abnormalities greater than predicted by physical symptoms.
[2] Other pathogens include Legionella, *Mycoplasma pneumoniae, Chlamydia pneumoniae,* and gram-negative bacilli. Other complaints include anorexia, headache, nausea, diarrhea, and vomiting.

# COMMUNITY-ACQUIRED PNEUMONIA

**D** **Outpatient, oral empirc therapy**
(seven to ten days)

PENICILLINS
CEPHALOSPORINS
**Tetracyclines** **1** Doxycycline
AMINOGLYCOSIDES
**MACROLIDES** **1** Clarithromycin
or azithromycin
**Fluoroquinolones** **1** Ciprofloxacin
OTHER

**Figure 33.7** (continued)
Characteristics of community-acquired pneumonia.

## VII. COMMUNITY-ACQUIRED PNEUMONIA

The term "community-acquired pneumonia" refers to a pneumonia in a previously healthy person who acquired the infection outside a hospital (or a long-term care facility).

Typical pneumonia usually is caused by bacteria (left hand column of Figure 37.7) and tends to be the most serious and, in adults, the most common cause of pneumonia. Atypical pneumonia usually is caused by the influenza virus, *Mycoplasma*, *Chlamydia*, *Legionella*, adenovirus, or other unidentified microorganisms. The patient's age is the main distinguishing factor between typical and atypical pneumonia; young adults are more prone to atypical causes, and very young and older persons are more predisposed to typical causes.

> *Streptococcus pneumoniae* is the most common cause of community-acquired bacterial pneumonia.

Respiratory viruses are the most common causes of pneumonia in young children, peaking between the ages of 2 and 3. By school age, *Mycoplasma pneumoniae* becomes more common.

Tests for a microbial diagnosis are usually not done in outpatients because most patients with community-acquired pneumonia are treated empirically, based on the most common pathogens associated with the condition.

Choosing between outpatient and inpatient treatment is a crucial decision because of the possible risk of death. Many infected individuals can be treated as outpatients with oral antibiotics. In the presence of an underlying chronic disease or severe symptoms, the patient will likely require hospitalization for intravenous antibiotics and oxygen therapy. Infants and the elderly are more commonly admitted for treatment of pneumonia. With treatment, most patients will improve within two weeks.

> Elderly or debilitated patients who fail to respond to treatment may die from respiratory failure.

Pneumococcal vaccine prevents *Streptococcus pneumoniae*. Flu vaccine prevents pneumonia and other infections caused by influenza viruses. It must be given yearly to protect against new viral strains. Hib vaccine prevents pneumonia in children from *Haemophilus influenzae* type b.

# "ATYPICAL" PNEUMONIA[1]

## A Common pathogens[2]

*Mycoplasma pneumoniae*

*Chlamydia pneumoniae*

*Legionella pneumophila*

Viruses

0   10   20   30   40   50   60
**Approximate prevalence (%)**

## B Classification of pathogens

**DOUBLE-STRANDED NON-ENVELOPED DNA VIRUSES**

*Chlamydia pneumoniae*

*Mycoplasma pneumoniae*

GRAM (–) RODS

*Legionella pneumophila*

Influenza viruses

Respiratory syncytial virus

Adeno-viruses

**SINGLE-STRANDED NEGATIVE STRAND HELICAL ENVELOPED, RNA VIRUSES**

## *Mycoplasma pneumoniae*

● Most common cause of primary atypical pneumonia (also called "walking pneumonia" because the patient usually remains ambulatory throughout the illness). The highest incidence of disease occurs in older children and young adults (6 to 20 years old). *M. pneumoniae* infection of the lower respiratory tract is transmitted by respiratory droplets.

● P1 protein (a cytoadhesin) allows *M. pneumoniae* to adhere tightly to the cell surface of host ciliated bronchial epithelial cells, inhibiting ciliary action. Patches of affected mucosa desquamate causing an inflammatory response in bronchial tissues.

## *Chlamydia pneumoniae*

● *C. pneumoniae* is a major cause world-wide of atypical pneumonia, as well as community-acquired respiratory infections such as pharyngitis, laryngitis, and bronchitis. Transmission from human to human occurs primarily by the aerosol route.

● *C. pneumoniae* is an obligate intracellular parasite. It uses adhesins to attach to susceptible host cell membrane receptors, usually in columnar or transitional epithelia. They replicate in phagocytic vesicles, eventually killing the host cell.

## *Legionella pneumophila*

● *L. pneumophila* causes Legionnaires disease—an atypical pneumonia with multisystem symptoms. Infections generally result from inhalation of contaminated aerosol from commercial water handling systems, such as air conditioners. Human-to-human transmission does not occur.

● *L. pneumophila* replicates in cells of the monocyte-macrophage system in the alveoli, causing a necrotizing, multifocal pneumonia. )

## C Common complaints[2]

HEADACHE

108
104
100  Normal
98
94

FEVER

COUGH

MYALGIA

## Influenza viruses

● Influenza epidemics regularly occur worldwide. Influenza infections are the most significant causes of viral pneumonia in adults. Influenza, spread by respiratory droplets, is an infection solely of the respiratory tract. There is rarely a viremia or spread to other organ systems.

● Following inhalation of influenza virus particles, infected ciliary respiratory epithelial cells desquamate and lose their ability to mechanically clear the respiratory tract. This results in various respiratory complaints, which may include bacterial pneumonia.

## Respiratory syncytial virus (RSV)

● RSV is the major viral respiratory tract pathogen in the pediatric population and the most important cause of bronchiolitis and pneumonia in infants under one year of age. It also causes atypical pneumonia in young children, an influenza-like syndrome in adults, and severe bronchitis with pneumonia in the elderly. RSV is transmitted by respiratory droplets or by contaminated hands carrying the virus to the nose or mouth. Repeated infections are common.

● Infection by RSV causes necrosis of epithelial cells in the alveoli, bronchioles, and bronchi. Mucus, dead cells, and fibrin clog the airways.

## Adenovirus

● Adenoviruses cause outbreaks of lower respiratory tract infections, especially in crowded environments such as military bases. Adenoviruses are generally spread by respiratory droplets. Infected infants most commonly suffer from febrile pharyngitis, Acute respiratory disease occurs primarily in epidemics among new military recruits. These respiratory syndromes can progress to true pneumonia.

● Adenoviruses replicate well in epithelial cells, the replicative infection resulting in cell death. Systemic infections are rare.

**Figure 33.8** (continued on the next page).
Characteristics of atypical pneumonia.

[1]"Atypical" pneumonia is characterized by insidious onset, scant sputum and x-ray abnormalities greater than predicted by physical symptoms.
[2]Other pathogens include *Chlamydia psittaci*, *Pneumocystis jiroveci*, varicella-zoster virus, and parainfluenza viruses.

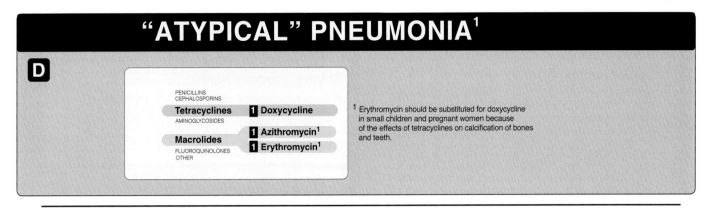

**Figure 33.8** (continued)
Characteristics of atypical pneumonia (continued).

## VIII. ATYPICAL PNEUMONIA

Pneumonia is often divided into "typical" pneumonia caused by pyogenic bacteria such as *Streptococcus. pneumoniae* or *Haemophilus influenzae*, and "atypical" pneumonia caused by organisms such as *Mycoplasma pneumoniae*, *Chlamydia pneumoniae* and *Legionella pneumophilia* (Figure 33.8).

Atypical pneumonia caused by *Mycoplasma pneumoniae* and *Chlamydia pneumoniae* usually cause milder forms of pneumonia. It is characterized by a more drawn out course of symptoms unlike other forms of pneumonia that can come on more quickly with more severe early symptoms. In contrast, pneumonia caused by *Legionella pneumophilia* occurs particularly among the elderly and those with chronic diseases and weakened immune systems. It is associated with a higher mortality rate.

> Atypical pneumonias: 1) exhibit a nonlobar, patchy, ill-defined infiltrate on chest radiography; and 2) failure to show a causative organism on Gram stain or culture of sputum as routinely performed.

Despite the identification of multiple causative organism, *Mycoplasma pneumoniae* is responsible for more cases of this syndrome than any other single organism.

Mycoplasma pneumonia often affects younger people and may be associated as anemia, rashes, and neurologic syndromes.

Chlamydial pneumonia is usually mild with a low mortality rate. In contrast, atypical pneumonia caused by *Legionella* accounts for 2-6 percent of pneumonias and has a higher mortality rate.

Elderly individuals, smokers, and people with chronic illnesses and weakened immune systems are at higher risk for atypical pneumonia. Contact with contaminated aerosol systems (like infected air conditioning systems) has also been associated with pneumonia caused by *Legionella*.

Patients with atypical pneumonia can generally be treated with empirical antibiotic therapy as outpatients. Severe cases of atypical pneumonia, especially common with pneumonia caused by *Legionella*, may require intravenous antibiotics and oxygen supplementation.

> Empiric treatment of community-acquired pneumonia should always include treatment for atypical organisms.

There are no proven methods for preventing atypical pneumonia, and no vaccinations are available.

# Diseases of the Eye

## Herpes Simplex Virus

● Herpes simplex virus types 1 and 2 are the most common causes of **infectious keratitis** (infection of the cornea leading to **corneal ulcers**) in developed countries. Symptoms include a red eye with moderately severe pain, tearing, decreased visual acuity, and photophobia. The infection usually involves only one eye. HSV keratitis may be **primary** (symptoms ranging from subclinical to conjunctivitis with vesicular eruption of the eyelid and potential corneal ulcers) or **recurrent** (more common than primary keratitis, especially in the immunocompromised, in whom symptoms generally include mild irritation and photophobia). [Note: The conjunctiva is a thin, translucent, mucous membrane that lines the eyelid and covers the white portion of the eyeball. Viral conjunctivitis is more common than bacterial conjunctivitis in developed countries.] Treatment involves application of topical antiherpes agents, such as trifluridine.

● Other herpesviruses also cause eye infections. For example, cytomegalovirus infection is particularly dangerous in AIDS patients, in whom it causes a variety of diseases. One of these syndromes can cause blindness if untreated (for example, with ganciclovir or foscarnet). Varicella-zoster virus (VZV) is also dangerous for AIDS patients, causing **acute retinal necrosis** that is treated with acyclovir. In non-AIDS patients, VZV reactivation can cause **herpes zoster**.

## Adenovirus

● Adenovirus infection is a common cause of **acute conjunctivitis**, especially in children. This infection may occur while the child is experiencing acute febrile pharyngitis, in which case the syndrome is referred to as **pharyngoconjunctival fever**. Adenoviruses may be transmitted via the hands, contaminated eyedrops, or insufficiently chlorinated swimming pools. Adenoviral conjunctivitis usually resolves after seven to ten days without therapy.

● A more serious infection is **epidemic keratoconjunctivitis**, which involves formation of a painful ulcer of the corneal epithelium. The ulcer may result in corneal opacity lasting several years. The epidemic nature of this disease arises in part from transmission by improperly sterilized ophthalmologic instruments. No antiviral agents are currently available for adenovirus infections.

## *Staphylococcus aureus*

● *S. aureus*, a member of the normal flora of the body, is a major cause of infections of the eyelid and cornea. For example, *S. aureus* can infect the glands of the eyelid, resulting in the production of a **sty**—a painful red swelling on the margin of the eyelid. Treatment consists of warm compresses applied regularly and topical antibiotic ointment (for example, bacitracin ointment).

## *Staphylococcus aureus* (continued)

● *S. aureus* is an important cause of **chronic bacterial conjunctivitis**, leading to **keratitis**. The organism invades the cornea following trauma that causes a break in the corneal epithelium. The resulting ulcers are painful and must be treated with antibiotic drops. (See p. 138)

## *Neisseria gonorrhoeae*

● *N. gonorrhoeae* is the most common cause of **hyperacute bacterial conjunctivitis**—the most severe form of conjunctivitis. Untreated, it can lead to keratitis and corneal perforation. Ceftriaxone can be used to treat gonococcal conjunctivitis.

● **Ophthalmia neonatorum** (ON) refers to any conjunctival inflammation of the newborn. It is acquired by the infant during its passage through the birth canal of a mother infected with gonococcus. [Note: Gonococci are the most serious infectious cause of ON, although *Chlamydia* are the most common cause.] If untreated, acute conjunctivitis may lead to blindness. Treatment is with doxycycline or erythromycin—antibiotics that also eradicate *Chlamydia trachomatis*, if present.

## *Chlamydia trachomatis*

● *C. trachomatis*, serotypes A, B, Ba, and C cause chronic keratoconjunctivitis (**trachoma**) that often results in blindness. Trachoma is a leading cause of blindness in endemic areas of northern India, the Middle East, and North Africa. Trachoma is transmitted by personal contact, for example, by eye-to-eye via droplets, by contaminated surfaces touched by hands and conveyed to the eye, or by flies. Because of persistent or repeated infection over several years, the inflammatory response with attendant scarring leads to permanent opacities of the cornea and distortion of eyelids.

● Over 50 percent of infants born to women infected with *C. trachomatis* serotypes D–K will contract **ophthalmia neonatorum** (see *N. gonorrhoeae*, above) on passage through the birth canal. The most common presentation is **inclusion conjunctivitis of the newborn**. This acute, purulent conjunctivitis (named for the inclusion bodies seen in infected conjunctival epithelial cells) usually heals without permanent damage to the infant's eye. Treatment is with oral erythromycin. Individuals of any age may develop a **transient purulent inclusion conjunctivitis** due to *C. trachomatis* serotypes D–K. Such individuals are often found to be genitally infected as well. Treatment includes any of a number of broad-spectrum antibacterial agents, such as azithromycin, erythromycin, or tetracycline (in patients older than 8 years.

## Figure 33.9
Examples of bacteria and viruses that cause diseases of the eye.
Other viruses causing eye diseases include influenza virus and rubella virus. Other bacteria causing eye diseases include *Staphylococcus pneumoniae*, *Streptococcus pyogenes*, *Haemophilus* species, *Pseudomonas aeruginosa*, *Treponema pallidum*, and *Mycobacterium tuberculosis*.

## IX. DISEASES OF THE EYE

Trachoma is the most prevalent eye infection in the world (Figure 33.9). However, physicians in developed countries are more likely to encounter patients with: 1) conjunctivitis (or pink eye), marked by pus or watery discharge and crust on the eyelashes; 2) styes, an abscess in the follicle of an eyelash; and 3) blepharitis, inflammation of the eyelids. Conjunctivitis, a condition which is often treated with antibiotics even though a minority of cases are caused by bacterial infection. Although it has characteristic signs, herpes simplex keratitis can be misdiagnosed as conjunctivitis.

## X. OPPORTUNISTIC INFECTIONS OF HIV

Individuals with advanced human immunodeficiency virus (HIV) infection are vulnerable to infections and malignancies called "opportunistic infections" because they take advantage of the opportunity offered by a weakened immune system (Figure 33.10). The clinical symptoms of HIV infection are mainly caused by the emergence of opportunistic infections and cancers that the immune system would normally prevent.

Infections that are rarely seen in those with with normal immune systems are deadly to those with HIV.

Different opportunistic infections typically occur at different stages of HIV infection. Patient with early HIV disease can develop tuberculosis, malaria, bacterial pneumonia, herpes zoster, staphylococcal skin infections and septicemia. These are diseases that can affect individuals with normal immune systems, but occur at a much higher rate with HIV secondary infections.

When the immune system is very weak due to advanced HIV disease, opportunistic infections such as *Pneumocystis jiroveci*, toxoplasmosis, and cryptococcosis develop. Many of the opportunistic infections that occur at this late stage can be fatal.

The development of highly active antiretroviral therapies (HAART, p. 303) has greatly decreased the morbidity and mortality from HIV.

HAART is effective in preventing opportunistic infections and should be considered for all HIV-infected persons.

However, certain patients are unable to take HAART, and others have not responded to HAART regimens. Such patients will benefit from prophylaxis against opportunistic infections. In addition, prophylaxis against specific opportunistic infections continues to provide survival benefits even among persons who are receiving HAART.

With HAART, antimicrobial prophylaxis for opportunistic infections need not be lifelong.

Antiretroviral therapy can restore immune function. The period of susceptibility to opportunistic processes continues to be accurately indicated by CD4+ T lymphocyte counts for patients receiving HAART. Stopping prophylactic regimens can simplify treatment, reduce toxicity and drug interactions, lower cost of care, and potentially facilitate adherence to antiretroviral regimens.

# OPPORTUNISTIC INFECTIONS OF HIV

## A Bacteria

### Mycobacterium avium complex

● *Mycobacterium avium-intracellulare complex* (MAC) is a complex of acid-fast bacilli, serotypes of which infect birds and various mammals. MAC is ubiquitous, thus individuals can easily acquire a MAC infection.

● In the United States, **disseminated (miliary) disease** caused by MAC is the most common systemic bacterial infection in AIDS patients and is responsible for significant morbidity. Serious pulmonary diseases include **chronic bronchitis** and **pneumonia**. **Cervical lymphadenitis**, **chronic osteomyelitis**, and **renal or skin infections** can occur. Clinical presentation usually includes fevers, night sweats, chills, and weight loss. In AIDS patients undergoing HAART treatment, cases of MAC-caused disease have sharply declined.

● Diseases caused by the MAC complex are particularly refractory to chemotherapy. Because of the large number of resistant variants, treatment of disease and prevention of reinfections requires two to four drugs given simultaneously. Current regimens include azithromycin or clarithromycin with or without rifabutin. Relapses are common.

Skin infection (A)

Pneumococcal pneumonia (B)

Tuberculosis (C)

### Mycobacterium tuberculosis

● Once a disease mainly of the elderly, clinical tuberculosis has become more prevalent among younger individuals (25 to 44 years old) and among children. In the United States, the increase is attributed to the high prevalence of mycobacterial disease in AIDS patients (for whom it is a major health threat) and the increase in immigrants, particularly from southeast Asia.

● Transmission occurs when patients with active pulmonary tuberculosis shed large numbers of organisms by coughing. The organisms are resistant to desiccation and can remain viable in the surroundings for a long time. Individuals with a depressed immune system—especially those who are HIV positive—are particularly susceptible to infection.

● In the primary disease, *M. tuberculosis* survives and grows within host cells such as macrophages, which can carry the organisms to additional sites. Productive (granulomatous) lesions known as tubercles can develop at those sites. In AIDS patients, as their immunity wanes, the primary infection is generally progressive, and one or more of the tubercles may expand, leading to destruction of tissue and clinical illness, for example, **chronic pneumonitis**, **tuberculous osteomyelitis**, or **tuberculous meningitis**. If active tubercles develop throughout the body, the condition is known as **miliary (disseminated) tuberculosis**. Reactivation of preexisting tubercles is caused by an impairment in immune status, such as that seen in AIDS.

● Because of the large number of drug-resistant strains of *M. tuberculosis*, treatment includes two or more drugs to prevent outgrowth of resistant strains. Principal drugs used include isoniazid, ethambutol, and/or pyrazinamide. The BCG antituberculosis vaccine should not be given to AIDS or other immuno-suppressed individuals because it contains live organisms, and has occasionally appeared to become virulent.

### Streptococcus pneumoniae

● *S. pneumoniae* (pneumococci) are gram-positive, nonmotile, encapsulated cocci that tend to occur in pairs (diplococci). They can be found in the nasopharynx of many healthy individuals. *S. pneumoniae* can be spread endogenously (if the carrier develops impaired resistance to the organism) or exogenously (by droplets from the nose of a carrier).

● *S. pneumoniae* is the most common bacterial respiratory pathogen in HIV-positive patients. The *S. pneumoniae* cell-associated virulence factors autolysin and pneumolysin contribute to its pathogenicity. The organism causes acute bacterial pneumonia and is a leading cause of death. *S. pneumoniae* also causes bacteremia/sepsis and meningitis.

● Most *S. pneumoniae* strains resistant to penicillin G remain sensitive to third generation cephalosporins and vancomycin.

**Figure 33.10** (continued on next page)
Organisms causing opportunistic infections in patients infected with human immunodeficiency virus (HIV).
[Note: Other opportunistic bacterial species include *Haemophilus influenzae* (pneumonia), *Campylobacter* species (diarrhea), *Shigella* species (diarrhea and bacteremia).] HAART = highly active antiviral therapy.

# OPPORTUNISTIC INFECTIONS OF HIV

## A Bacteria (continued)

### Salmonella species

● Salmonella are flagellated, motile, gram-negative bacilli, routinely found in the GI tract of humans and other animals. Salmonella are transmitted most frequently by the fecal-oral route—often with food as an intermediary—but can also be transmitted to humans by pets such as turtles. *S. typhimurium* is of particular concern because it is increasingly drug-resistant.

● *Salmonella* invade epithelial cells of the small intestine. In immunocompromised hosts, the infection can become systemic with disseminated foci. In HIV-infected individuals, a high-grade bacteremia can occur, in which *Salmonella* seeds distant organs, and in older patients, promotes atherosclerotic plaque. Fever can persist for one to two weeks. *Salmonella* infections also cause severe gastroenteritis, characterized by nausea, vomiting, and diarrhea.

● The treatment for *Salmonella* infections in an immunocompromised host is typically ciprofloxacin. Alternative treatments (depending on drug-resistance) include ampicillin or trimethoprim-sulfamethoxazole. In patients with AIDS, relapse is a major problem. Therefore, months of therapy are required.

←— *Salmonella* species (D)

Pulmonary histoplasmosis (E) →

## B Fungi

### Candida species

● *Candida albicans* and other *Candida* species are part of the normal body flora. They are found in the skin, mouth, vagina, and intestines. **Candidiasis** is the most common fungal infection of HIV-positive individuals. The presence of esophageal candidiasis is a hallmark of the progression from HIV infection to AIDS.

● Candidiasis is generally limited to oral, esophageal, or vaginal mucosa. **Oral candidiasis (thrush)** presents as raised, white plaques on the oral mucosa, tongue, or gums. The plaques can become confluent and ulcerated and can spread to the esophagus (an indicator of full-blown AIDS). **Vaginal candidiasis** presents as itching and burning pain of the vulva and vagina, accompanied by a thick or thin white discharge. Vaginal candidiasis frequently reoccurs. **Systemic candidiasis** is rare.

● Candidiasis is treated with fluconazole or itraconazole. However, azole-resistant strains of candida require alternative treatment, for example, with amphotericin B.

←— Oral candidiasis (F)

### Histoplasma capsulatum

● *H. capsulatum* is a soil fungus that is found worldwide, but is most prevalent in central North America. The organism produces spores that, when airborne, enter the lungs and germinate into yeast-like cells. These yeast cells are engulfed by macrophages in which they multiply.

● In healthy individuals, pulmonary infections with *H. capsulatum* may be acute but self-limiting. In HIV-infected persons, nearly all cases are disseminated at the time of diagnosis. Dissemination results from invasion of cells of the reticuloendothelial system, which distinguishes this organism as the only fungus to exhibit intracellular parasitism. **Disseminated histoplasmosis** causes fever, weight loss, hypertension, and pulmonary distress. If untreated, it can lead to respiratory and liver failure.

● *H. capsulatum* infection is treated with itraconazole, with amphotericin B as an alternative. Life-long maintenance therapy may be required to prevent reoccurrence of the disease.

### Cryptococcus neoformans

● *C. neoformans* is a yeast that is found world-wide. It is especially abundant in soil containing bird droppings. Its spores are inhaled.

● In healthy persons, cryptococcosis is generally a mild, subclinical lung infection. In AIDS patients, **cryptococcosis** is the second most common fungal infection and potentially the most serious. In these individuals, the infection often disseminates to the brain and meninges, causing **meningitis**—frequently with fatal consequences. Presenting symptoms include fever, headache, and malaise. Patients are often forgetful and lethargic.

● Cryptococcal meningitis is treated with fluconazole, with amphotericin B as an alternative. This therapy should be continued lifelong to prevent reoccurrence of the infection.

└— Cutaneous cryptococcosis (G)

**Figure 33.10** (continued on next page)
Organisms causing opportunistic infections in patients infected with human immunodeficiency virus (HIV). [Note: Other opportunistic fungal infections include aspergillosis and coccidioidomycosis.]

# OPPORTUNISTIC INFECTIONS OF HIV

## C Other

### *Pneumocystis jiroveci*

- *P. jiroveci* is a unicellular eukaryote whose taxonomic status and life cycle are still uncertain. It is the most common opportunistic pathogen in AIDS patients.

- *P. jiroveci* causes frequently fatal **pneumonia (PJP)**. Before the use of immunosuppressive drugs and the AIDS epidemic, PJP was a rare disease. It is almost 100 percent fatal if untreated.

- Prophylaxis with trimethoprim-sulfamethoxazole is recommended for HIV-infected patients with fewer than 200 CD4+ cells/µl. However, individuals infected with HIV who are undergoing treatment with HAART have shown a significant decrease in incidence of PJP.

### *Cryptosporidium* species

- *Cryptosporidium* is an intracellular parasite that inhabits the epithelial cells of the villi of the lower small intestine. The source of infection is often the feces of domestic animals and farm run-off has been implicated as a source of cryptosporidium contamination of drinking water.

- Infection of healthy individuals may be asymptomatic or may cause mild cases of diarrhea, which are generally self-limiting. However, in AIDS patients, the infection may be severe and intractable. **Cryptosporidiosis** causes diarrhea that varies from mild to a fulminant, persistent cholera-like illness. Patients experience nausea, vomiting, abdominal pain, and weight loss.

- In AIDS patients, no treatment for cryptosporidiosis has proven completely effective, although paramomycin has provided some improvement.

Pneumocystis pneumonia

*Toxopolasma gondii*

Cryptosporidium species

Kaposi sarcoma

## D Parasites

### *Toxoplasma gondii*

- *T. gondii* is a sporozoan, distributed worldwide, which infects all vertebrate species, although the definitive host is the cat. Transmission is by accidental ingestion of oocysts present in cat feces, eating raw or undercooked meat, congenitally from an infected mother, or from a blood transfusion. Rapidly growing *T. gondii* trophozoites establish early, acute infections. Slowly growing trophozoites encyst in muscle and brain tissue and in the eye.

- *T. gondii* infections of healthy humans are asymptomatic and common, but they are the most common cause of **focal encephalitis** in AIDS patients. **Toxoplasmosis** in this population is usually due to reemergence of encysted organisms, rather than from new, exogenous infection. Clinical presentation of encephalitis can include weakness, confusion, seizures, or coma. Disseminated toxoplasmosis can involve the heart, skeletal muscle, lung, colon, and other organs.

- *T. gondii* infection is treated with a combination of sulfadiazine and pyrimethamine. Lifelong secondary prophylaxis involves sulfadiazine plus pyrimethamine.

## E Viruses

### Human herpesvirus type 8

- Human herpesvirus type 8 (HHV-8) (also known as Kaposi sarcoma-associated herpesvirus) is a member of the Herpesviridae family. It is enveloped, with a double-stranded DNA genome. Interestingly, its genome encodes a number of human cell-derived genes related to growth regulation, including cytokines, cytokine receptors, growth factors, and a factor that inhibits apoptosis.

- In the United States, antibodies to HHV-8 antigens are found primarily in the same populations at risk for HIV infection, leading to the conclusion that the primary mode of transmission is sexual. The frequency of perinatal transmission of HHV-8 appears low.

- HHV-8 has been detected in over ninety percent of patients with Kaposi sarcoma (KS), but in less than one percent of non-KS tissues. KS was the most common neoplasm in AIDS patients, but has essentially disappeared from those HIV-infected individuals with access to HAART treatment. There is no established independent drug treatment for HHV-8 infected individuals.

**Figure 33.10** (continued on the next page)
Organisms causing opportunistic infections in patients infected with human immuodeficiency virus (HIV).

# OPPORTUNISTIC INFECTIONS OF HIV

## E Viruses (continued)

### Herpes simplex virus

● Herpes simplex virus (HSV) types 1 and 2 are members of the Herpesviridae family. They are enveloped, with a double-stranded DNA genome. Initial infection with HSV is by direct contact with virus-containing secretions, or with lesions on mucosal surfaces. HSV can also be transmitted during a baby's journey down the birth canal. HSV coinfection of patients with HIV infection occurs frequently, probably because of their similar modes of transmission. For example, 95 percent of homosexual men with AIDS are seropositive for HSV.

● Initial replication of the virus is in epithelial cells of the mucosal surface onto which they have been inoculated. In individuals with depressed immune systems, the virus reproduces and can be transported to various sites in the body. It also establishes lifelong latent infections in the regional ganglia.

● Reactivation of latent virus leading to invasive HSV infections in AIDS patients becomes increasingly important as CD4+ lymphocyte counts decline. Herpetic ulcers occur on the face, hand, or genitals, and oral ulcers occur. Recurrence of genital herpes can be more frequent and severe in HIV-infected persons.

● If primary or recurrent herpes episodes are particularly frequent and/or severe, acyclovir or, alternatively, famciclovir can be administered.

Herpes simplex infection

Cytomegalovirus retinitis

JC virus particles from an infected oligodendrocyte nucleus

### JC virus

● JC virus (JCV) is a member of the Papovaviridae family, Polyomavirinae subfamily. It is a nonenveloped virus containing supercoiled, double-stranded, circular DNA.

● As HIV-infected individuals become increasingly immunocompromised, approximately five percent of them will develop **progressive multifocal leukoencephalopathy (PML)**—so called because the lesions are restricted to the white matter of the brain. In PML, reactivated JCV carries out a cytocidal infection of the brain's oligodendrocytes. This leads to demyelination caused by loss of capacity of myelinated cells to maintain their sheaths. Early development of impaired speech and mental capacity is rather rapidly followed by paralysis and sensory abnormalities, with death commonly occurring within three to six months of the initial symptoms.

● JCV is transmitted by droplets from the upper respiratory tract of infected persons and possibly through contact with their urine. The virus spreads from the upper respiratory tract to the kidneys, where it may persist in an inactive state in the tubular epithelium of healthy individuals.

● A regimen of HAART plus cidofovir is currently showing some promise in patients experiencing PML. Because infection with JCV is nearly universal and asymptomatic, and PML represents reactivation of latent virus in the immunocompromised host, there are no viable preventive measures at present.

### Human cytomegalovirus

● Human cytomegalovirus (HCMV) is a member of the Herpesviridae family. It is enveloped, with a double-stranded DNA genome. Initial infection with HCMV commonly occurs during childhood. Transmission is via body fluids such as tears, urine, saliva, milk, semen, and vaginal secretions or organ transplants, and by blood transfusions. HCMV can also be transmitted transplacentally. HCMV coinfection of patients with HIV infection occurs frequently, probably because of their similar modes of transmission.

● Initial replication of the virus in epithelial cells of the respiratory and GI tracts is followed by viremia and infection of all organs of the body, including the kidney tubule epithelium, liver, CNS, and respiratory and GI tracts. The virus establishes latency, predominantly in the monocytes and macrophages, among other cells.

● Reactivation of latent virus leading to invasive HCMV infections in AIDS patients becomes increasingly frequent as CD4+ lymphocyte counts decline. Any organ system can be affected, but blindness due to HCMV chorioretinitis is especially common, developing in more than twenty percent of AIDS patients whose CD4+ count is less than 50/μl. Encephalitis and dementia, esophagitis, enterocolitis, and gastritis are other significant problems caused by HCMV. In addition, coinfection with HCMV may accelerate the progression of AIDS. At autopsy, ninety percent of AIDS patients are shown to be infected with HCMV. However, the incidence of HCMV chorioretinitis has been significantly decreased in HIV-infected individuals being treated with HAART.

● The drug regimen for both primary prophylaxis (when recommended) and prevention of recurrence of HCMV infections in AIDS patients includes ganciclovir, cidofovir, and/or foscarnet. Oral valganciclovir is currently undergoing successful clinical trials for the treatment of HCMV chorioretinitis.

**Figure 33.10** (continued)
Organisms causing opportunistic infections in patients infected with human immunodeficiency virus (HIV).
[Note: Other opportunistic viral infections include shingles and oral hairy leukoplakia.]

# SINUSITIS (BACTERIAL)

**A** **Common pathogens²**

*Streptococcus pneumoniae*
*Haemophilus influenzae*
*Staphylococcus aureus*
Anaerobes
*Moraxella catarrhalis*

0        15        30
**Approximate prevalence (%)**

**B** **Classification of pathogens**

GRAM (+) COCCI

*Staphylococcus aureus*
*Streptococcus pneumoniae*

GRAM (–) COCCI

ANAEROBES

*Moraxella catarrhalis*

*Haemophilus influenzae*

OTHER GRAM (–) BACILLI

**C** **Common complaints¹**

NASAL CONGESTION

NASAL DISCHARGE

COUGH

FACIAL PAIN OR PRESSURE

**D** **Empirc therapy²**
(seven to ten days)

Penicillin  **1**  Amoxicillin/ clavulanate
Cephalosporins  **1**  Cefpodoxim or cefdinir

TETRACYCLINES
AMINOGLYCOSIDES
MACROLIDES

Fluoroquinolones  **1**  Levofloxacin or moxifloxacin

OTHER

**Figure 33.11**
Characteristics of bacterial sinusitis.
¹Other symptoms include maxillary tooth discomfort, hyposmia (diminished sense of smell), headache, fever (nonacute), halitosis, fatigue, ear pain, and ear fullness.
²Experts vary widely in their recommendations for antibiotics.

## XI. BACTERIAL SINUSITIS

Acute sinusitis is an infection of one or more of the paranasal (alongside the nose) sinuses. A viral infection accompanying the common cold is the most frequent cause of acute sinusitis. Viral infection is also the most common predisposing condition associated with acute bacterial sinusitis. However, only approximately two percent of viral sinusitis is complicated by acute bacterial sinusitis. There appear to be no signs and symptoms of acute respiratory illness that are both sensitive and specific in making the distinction between bacterial and viral infection. Bacterial sinusi-

tis is usually a self-limited disease, with 75 percent of cases resolving without treatment in one month. However, untreated acute bacterial sinusitis are at risk of developing intracranial and orbital complications as well as chronic sinus disease.

Viral sinusitis is associated with the presence of rhinovirus, parainfluenza, and influenza viruses in sinus aspirates. Other viruses which cause acute respiratory disease can also presumably produce viral sinusitis.

# OTITIS MEDIA (ACUTE)

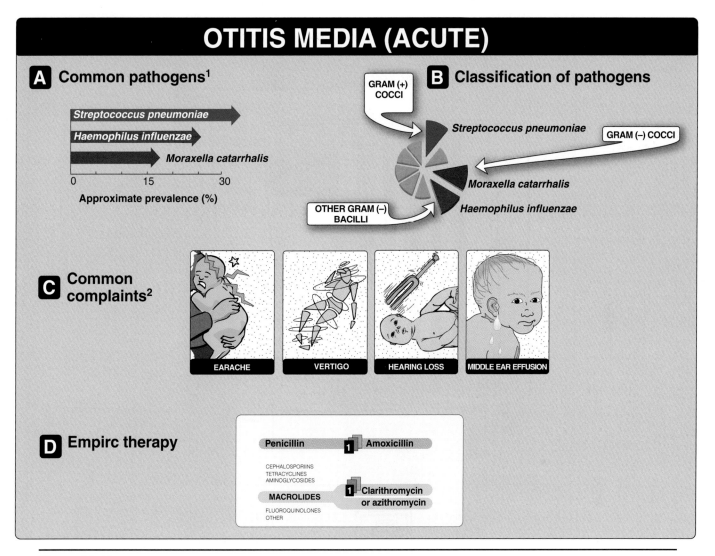

## A Common pathogens[1]

Streptococcus pneumoniae
Haemophilus influenzae
Moraxella catarrhalis

0        15        30
Approximate prevalence (%)

## B Classification of pathogens

GRAM (+) COCCI
Streptococcus pneumoniae
GRAM (–) COCCI
Moraxella catarrhalis
OTHER GRAM (–) BACILLI
Haemophilus influenzae

## C Common complaints[2]

EARACHE | VERTIGO | HEARING LOSS | MIDDLE EAR EFFUSION

## D Empirc therapy

Penicillin — 1 Amoxicillin

CEPHALOSPORIINS
TETRACYCLINES
AMINOGLYCOSIDES

MACROLIDES — 1 Clarithromycin or azithromycin

FLUOROQUINOLONES
OTHER

**Figure 33.12**
Some characteristics of acute bacterial otitis media.
[1]Other pathogens include *staphylococcus aureus*, Group A streptococcus, and *pseudomonas aeruginosa*.
[2]Nonspecific symptoms and signs include fever, irritability, headache, apathy, anorexia, vomiting and diarrhea.

## XII  OTITIS MEDIA

Otitis media is one the most frequent diagnosis in sick children visiting physicians' offices and accounts for almost one third of all antibiotic prescriptions for children in the United States.

Acute otitis media is characterized by the presence of fluid in the middle ear accompanied by acute signs of illness, and usually occurs in young children. Fluid may persist for weeks to months after the onset of signs of acute otitis media despite appropriate therapy. Whenever fluid fills the middle ear space, there is some loss of hearing, which may lead to problems of development of speech, language. and cognitive abilities in the child.

Otitis media often follows a upper respiratory tract viral infection or allergy that results in congestion of the respiratory mucosa of the nose, nasopharynx, and eustachian tube. Congestion of the mucosa in the eustachian tube causes an obstruction which can lead to accumulation of secretions produced by the mucosa of the middle ear. These secretions have no way to exit and accumulate in the middle ear space. Viruses and bacteria that colonize the upper respiratory tract can reach the middle ear and may result in suppuration (formation of pus) with clinical signs of acute otitis media.

"I've called in a specialist for your boil."

# Illustrated Case Studies

# 34

## I. OVERVIEW

These extended case studies complement the basic information presented in Chapters 1 to 31. They reinforce basic principles of clinical microbiology, such as the role of a Gram stain, and the patient's history in instituting effective antimicrobial therapy—concepts useful in answering examination questions, and in the clinics. Most of the cases provide clinical information obtained from a single patient; a few cases describe a composite of typical features derived from several patients.

## Case 1: Man with necrosis of the great toe

This 63-year-old man with a long history of diabetes mellitus was seen in consultation because of an abrupt deterioration in his clinical status. He was admitted to the hospital for treatment of an ulcer, which had been present on his left great toe for several months. Figure 34.1 shows a typical example of perforating ulcer in a diabetic man.

Because of the inability of medical therapy (multiple courses of oral antibiotics) to resolve the ulcer, he underwent amputation of his left leg below the knee. On the first postoperative day he developed a temperature of 101°F,

and on the second postoperative day he became disoriented and his temperature reached 105.2°F. His amputation stump was mottled with many areas of purplish discoloration, and the most distal areas were quite obviously necrotic (dead). Crepitus (the sensation of displacing gas when an area is pressed with the fingers) was palpable up to his patella. An X-ray of the left lower extremity showed gas in the soft tissues, extending beyond the knee to the area of the distal femur. A Gram stain of a swab from the necrotic tissue is shown in Figure 34.2.

**Figure 34.1**
Perforating ulcer of the great toe.

**Figure 34.2**
Gram stain of material swabbed from deep within a crepitant area. There are numerous polymorphonuclear leukocytes and many large gram-positive bacilli, as well as a few gram-negative bacilli and cocci.

34.1 Based on the morphology of the gram-positive organisms, their most likely identification is:

   A. *Streptococcus pyogenes*.

   B. *Escherichia coli*.

   C. *Actinomyces israelii*.

   D. *Clostridium perfringens*.

   E. *Staphylococcus aureus*.

> Correct answer = **D** (*Clostridium perfringens*), which is a rather large, gram-positive bacillus. **A** (*Streptococcus pyogenes*) cannot be correct because it is a gram-positive coccus, not a bacillus. **B** (*Escherichia coli*) is incorrect because it is a gram-negative rod, not gram-positive. **C** (*Actinomyces israelii*) is, in fact a gram-positive bacillus, but it is thin to the point of being described as filamentous, and characteristically branched, and therefore, is essentially impossible to mistake for a *Clostridium*. **E** (*Staphylococcus aureus*) is gram-positive, but a coccus, not a bacillus.

The patient was treated with massive intravenous doses of aqueous penicillin G, together with intravenous gentamicin. He underwent an above-knee amputation of his leg and, after a very stormy period of hectic fever and hypotension, he began to improve. Cultures from deep within his necrotic amputation stump grew *Clostridium perfringens* and *Pseudomonas aeruginosa*. Throughout his course his hemoglobin, which was tested repeatedly while he was very ill, remained stable.

**Discussion:** This patient had *Clostridium perfringens* gas gangrene, one of the dreaded complications that may follow lower extremity amputation in diabetics. Diabetics sometimes require amputation of part or all of a lower extremity because the blood supply to these limbs is reduced by accelerated atherosclerosis, which occludes blood vessels. The resulting dead or dying tissue has very low oxygen tension, which greatly favors the growth of anaerobes. *Clostridium perfringens* colonizes the area around the anus, and may extend onto the lower extremities. If the amputation is low enough it may leave behind tissue whose blood supply is compromised to the point that oxygen tension in the remaining stump favors the growth of anaerobes. The elaboration, by *Clostridium perfringens*, of large amounts of gas that are not absorbed by the tissues allows the clostridial organisms to spread along fascial planes, which are separated by the pressure of the gas as the clostridium grows. Thus the gas acts as a "virulence factor", which makes this organism quite ferocious.

The reason that the physicians were worried about the stability of the patient's hemoglobin is that another virulence factor of *Clostridium perfringens* is an exotoxin (the α-toxin) with lecithinase activity. Since red blood cell membranes are rich in lecithin, this toxin, which is secreted by the bacteria directly into the bloodstream, destroys red blood cell membranes, causing cells to lyse. Patients who die of overwhelming *Clostridium perfringens*

infection may have sufficient red blood cells destroyed so rapidly that the resulting anemia is itself fatal.

For those who might have wondered what the *Pseudomonas aeruginosa* was doing in the wound, it probably got there by being selected out by the antibiotics that the patient received prior to his surgery, during the attempts at treating his ulcer medically. Antibiotics exert great pressure on the microbial flora of the skin and bowel. Less resistant organisms on his skin and in his bowel were replaced by those, such as *Pseudomonas aeruginosa*, which could withstand many antibiotics. Anaerobic infections tend to be mixed with facultative anaerobic and aerobic bacteria, as this one was.

## Case 2: Adult conjunctivitis

This 15-year-old boy was admitted because of pain and redness of his left eye, which had lasted for four days. He had always been well. Four days prior to medical evaluation he awoke with pain in his left eye, accompanied by a thick yellow discharge of the conjunctiva. He saw an ophthalmologist, who obtained a culture of the yellow discharge, and prescribed tobramycin ophthalmic antibiotic drops, which the patient began to use the same day.

The patient's eye remained severely inflamed after four days of treatment with eye drops (Figure 34.3). The conjunctiva was very swollen and injected (the blood vessels were very dilated). At a follow-up visit on the fourth day of treatment, the patient reported minimal improvement in his symptoms. The culture taken at the first visit had grown a gram-negative diplococcus that fermented only glucose.

A swab of the yellow discharge from this patient's eye would have the appearance of Figure 34.4 on Gram stain, with numerous polymorphonuclear leukocytes, several con-

**Figure 34.3**
Inflamed eye of patient.

**Figure 34.4**
Gram-stain of discharge from eye.

taining kidney bean–shaped, gram-negative diplococci whose longer dimension is side-by-side with that of its mate in the pair.

34.2  Based on the morphology and fermentation characteristics of the organism that grew in the culture, the most likely etiology of this eye infection is:

    A. *Escherichia coli.*

    B. *Neisseria gonorrhoeae* (gonococcus).

    C. *Neisseria meningitidis* (meningococcus).

    D. *Streptococcus pneumoniae* (pneumococcus).

    E. *Staphylococcus aureus.*

> The correct answer is **B** (*Neisseria gonorrhoeae*). It is a gram-negative diplococcus whose only sugar fermentation is glucose, and it is known to cause serious ocular infections when it is placed directly in the eye (see below). **A** (*Escherichia coli*) is incorrect because *Escherichia coli*, while gram-negative, is a bacillus and not a coccus. **C** (*Neisseria meningitidis*) is not acceptable because, although it is a gram-negative diplococcus, it ferments both maltose *and* glucose, eliminating it from consideration based on the information available. **D** (*Streptococcus pneumoniae*) is wrong because it is a gram-*positive* diplococcus and not a gram-*negative* diplococcus. **E** (*Staphylococcus aureus*) is incorrect because it is a gram-*positive* coccus and is characteristically arranged in clusters, not in pairs.

The patient was treated with ceftriaxone, and his eye cleared dramatically. At the time of his second visit to the ophthalmologist he was asked whether he had had any genital symptoms. He related that he had had a purulent (full of pus) discharge from his penis for several days before the onset of his ocular symptoms. He wasn't sure whether his current female sexual partner had been having any vaginal discharge.

34.3  The most likely source from which this organism entered the patient's eye is:

    A. his unwashed hands after touching a toilet seat.

    B. his unwashed hands after touching his penis.

    C. kissing his girlfriend's cheek.

    D. a public swimming pool.

    E. a dry cotton towel that he used to dry his face.

> The correct answer is **B** (his penis). *Neisseria gonorrhoeae* most commonly causes urethritis (inflamed urethra) in males, and it is most probable that this patient inadvertently rubbed his eyes with his hands after contaminating them with material from his penis. **A** is unlikely because gonococci do not survive very well on inanimate objects (**fomites**) and, although many an unfaithful husband or boyfriend would like his partner to believe that toilet seats are good sources of acquiring gonorrhea, it just doesn't happen that way. **C** (his girlfriend's cheek) is very unlikely because facial skin is seldom involved with gonorrhea and he would have had to rub his eye directly on an infectious lesion to get *Neisseria gonorrhoeae* into it. **D** (a swimming pool) is very unlikely because of the dilution effect of the water in a pool and the probable inhibition of the growth of gonococci, which are very fastidious, by chlorine or other antibacterial substances in a public swimming pool. **E** is incorrect because *Neisseria gonorrhoeae* is very susceptible to drying and because cotton contains fatty acids that actually inhibit this organism. In fact, it is recommended that swabs which are used to obtain material for gonococcal cultures **not** be made of cotton. In addition, the environmental fragility of the gonococcus is such that it is important that specimens for gonococcal culture be transferred promptly from the patient either to the definitive culture plate or to a reliable transfer medium until they can be inoculated onto culture plates. This is especially true for a specimen taken from an eye, because other fastidious organisms, such as haemophilus species, may cause conjunctivitis that is clinically indistinguishable from that caused by *Neisseria gonorrhoeae*.

**Discussion:** This patient had adult gonococcal conjunctivitis. In this syndrome the gonococcus is carried from a genital discharge to the patient's own eye by his or her hands. In newborns who acquire gonococcal eye infections by passing through the uterine cervix and vagina of mothers with active gonorrhea, the syndrome is called "ophthalmia neonatorum." Topical therapy with antibiotic drops is inadequate to treat gonococcal conjunctivitis, an infection that requires therapy with a systemically administered (for example, intravenous or intramuscular) antibiotic. If proper treatment is not given, the organism may invade more deeply into the eye, causing it to rupture. If this patient's urethritis had been treated earlier, his ocular infection might have been prevented. Figure 34.5 summarizes the chronology of the case.

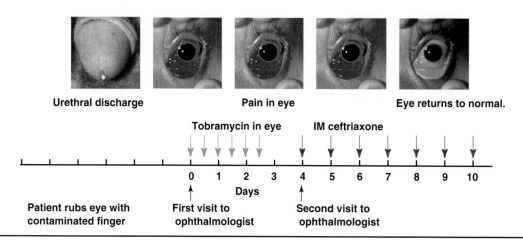

Urethral discharge          Pain in eye          Eye returns to normal.

Tobramycin in eye          IM ceftriaxone

0    1    2    3    4    5    6    7    8    9    10

Days

Patient rubs eye with          First visit to          Second visit to
contaminated finger          ophthalmologist          ophthalmologist

**Figure 34.5**
Summary of case.

## Case 3: Gas within a bulla

This 60-year-old woman was seen in consultation because of a skin lesion and fever that had been present for 24 hours. She had been in failing health for many years because of chronic active hepatitis. Recently, because of progression of liver disease, oral prednisone at a dose of 60 mg daily had been begun. The day prior to admission to the hospital she developed fever and chills, and she was admitted for intravenous antibiotics. When she arrived at the hospital, she complained of pain in her right knee and thigh.

Physical examination revealed a stuporous woman (unresponsive to verbal stimuli, barely responsive to painful stimuli). The temperature was 100°F. Remarkable findings, in addition to her mental status, included edema of the right thigh and leg, and areas of erythema (redness due to tiny dilated blood vessels in the skin) of both thighs and legs. On the medial aspect of the right lower extremity, proximal

and distal to the knee, there was an area of purpura (hemorrhage into the skin, Figure 34.6). Within this area there were bullae (large blisters), one of which was filled with red fluid. At the top of the fluid in this bulla there floated many tiny bubbles. (Figure 34.7) There was marked asterixis of the hands (a flapping tremor indicative of metabolic encephalopathy that, in a stuporous patient, can be elicited by holding the wrists in slight extension).

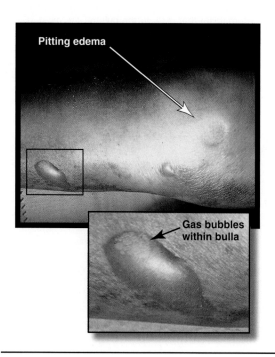

Pitting edema

Gas bubbles
within bulla

**Figure 34.7**
Close-up of the area in Figure 34.6, showing the bulla with bubbles. To the right is a depression caused by thumb pressure, illustrating pitting edema.

Bulla

**Figure 34.6**
Erythema of the thighs and legs and a patch of purpura, proximal and distal to the right knee. Within the more distal purpuric area is a bulla.

**Figure 34.8**
Gram stain of the bulla fluid shows gram-negative organisms, probably rods. The shorter forms probably represent rods seen at an angle, from their ends.

Because of the presence of a cellulitis with purpura, and a bulla with cherry-red fluid and gas, a presumptive diagnosis of *Clostridium perfringens* sepsis was made, with the plan being to treat the patient with very high doses of penicillin G. However, Gram stain of the fluid aspirated from the bulla revealed the appearance seen in Figure 34.8.

34.4  The organism seen in this Gram stain is most likely to be:

A. *Clostridium perfringens*

B. *Streptococcus pyogenes*

C. *Escherichia coli*

D. *Neisseria meningitidis*

E. *Lactobacillus casei*

> The correct answer is **C** (*Escherichia coli*), which is the only gram-negative rod on the list. **A** (*Clostridium perfringens*) is associated with gas-forming infections and bullae filled with red fluid, but it is a gram-positive rod. Skin infections due to **B** (*Streptococcus pyogenes*) may also form bullae, some even with reddish fluid. But *Streptococcus pyogenes* is a gram-positive coccus, not a gram-negative rod. **D** (*Neisseria meningitidis*) is a gram-negative organism associated with purpuric skin lesions, but it is a coccus (usually seen in pairs) and not a rod. **E** (*Lactobacillus casei*) is a gram-positive rod that is seldom involved in invasive disease.

To the surprise of the consultant, this patient did not have a clostridial infection. *Escherichia coli* alone grew from blood cultures and from the bulla fluid. It turned out to be susceptible to all the antibiotics against which it was tested, including ampicillin and gentamicin, but this information was not available for 48 hours. She was empirically treated with ampicillin, clindamycin, and gentamicin, beginning as soon

as the results of the Gram stain were available. However, the morning after the initial consultation visit, in spite of treatment with two drugs effective against her *E. coli*, she died in hepatic failure.

**Discussion:** This patient illustrates many important clinico-microbiologic points. First, many organisms may cause similar-appearing clinical lesions, so that as much hard microbiological data as possible must be collected prior to treatment. This allows assessment of the efficacy of therapy on grounds that may go beyond clinical responses (such as reduction of fever). The Gram stain was the initial tip that, despite the clinical appearance of the lesion, this was not a gram-positive anaerobic process but a gram-negative process, allowing optimal antibiotic selection within minutes of assessment of the patient. Second, this patient reminds us that not all gas-forming infections are due to the notorious clostridial genus. Gas is produced by the metabolism of a wide variety of microorganisms of quite varied morphologies. With *E. coli*, gas does not accumulate as it does with clostridial species because the gas produced by *E. coli* is mainly carbon dioxide, which is absorbed by the tissues almost as fast as it is produced by the microorganism. Culture is necessary for speciation and to allow antibiotic susceptibility testing. Finally, the patient died even though she was treated quite promptly with the right drugs. It was reassuring to have cultures that proved the *in vitro* efficacy of her antibiotic regimen. It is probable that her underlying liver disease was so advanced that this episode of sepsis caused her to go into irreversible hepatic coma. In addition, the steroid therapy may have interfered with her ability to fight off any infection. Although her physicians were dismayed at her death, they could feel confident that she did not die because of inadequate antibiotic therapy or incorrect antibiotic choices. The appropriateness of the initial antibiotic regimen resulted from the clinical-microbiologic correlation of the lesion and the Gram stain.

## Case 4: Man with a rash

This 25-year-old man was admitted to the hospital for shortness of breath, which had been present for one day. He had been well until three days before admission, in mid-June, when he developed sneezing, and a runny and stuffy nose. The next day he noted a non-productive cough. Red blotches were observed on his face the following day, at which time the patient began to complain of retro-orbital headache and feverishness. One day later there was more rash on his face, and it had spread to his arms and trunk. Progressive malaise and shortness of breath prompted hospital admission.

There had been no known tick exposure. At age three months the patient's mother was told that an illness with rash, which the patient had, was measles. He had never received a dose of measles vaccine.

34.5 The illness in the differential diagnosis that prompted the question about tick exposure is:

    A. Dengue fever.

    B. Measles (rubeola).

    C. German measles (rubella).

    D. Meningococcemia.

    E. Rocky Mountain spotted fever.

> The correct answer is **E** (Rocky Mountain spotted fever), which is the only tick-borne disease on this list. This patient's rash made the physician of record think of Rocky Mountain spotted fever, especially because it occurred in June, when ticks are quite active in many areas of the United States. (See below for further elaboration on this point.) **A** (Dengue fever) is, in fact, a disease carried by an arthropod vector, but the vector of dengue fever is a mosquito and not a tick. **B** (measles), **C** (German measles), and **D** (meningococcemia) are not vector-borne, but are transmitted by inhalation of contagious material that may be breathed out by an infected individual into ambient air, a simpler and rather more direct mode of transmission.

On physical examination the temperature was 100°F, the pulse 84 beats per minute, and the respirations mildly labored at a rate of 22 per minute. (Normal respiratory rate is somewhere between 14 and 18. It takes real work to breathe at 22 per minute, and this is often quite obvious when you look at a patient, for which reason the respirations are described as "labored.") The skin was warm and dry. The face was completely erythematous (red, but

**Figure 34.9**
Extensive erythematous maculopapular rash covering the trunk and extremities. Not shown are the patient's face, on which the lesions were so confluent that his entire face was erythematous, and back, which had many large confluent areas of erythema.

blanching upon pressure) and there was an erythematous maculopapular (flat spots and raised bumps) rash on the trunk and extremities (Figure 34.9), with large confluent areas on the back. Similar lesions were present on the palms. There were shotty (the size of shot (ammunition for a shot gun)) anterior cervical and supraclavicular lymph nodes. The conjunctivae were hyperemic (too red, from dilated blood vessels) along the outer margins of the lids. The throat was extremely hyperemic. The buccal mucosa contained several raised white spots, each the size of a grain of salt, opposite the lower molars. The chest was resonant and clear. The remainder of the physical examination was unremarkable.

The white blood cell count was 3100/µl (lower than the lower limit of normal, which in many laboratories is 4000/µl), with a differential of 70% polymorphonuclear leukocytes, 22% band forms, 7% lymphocytes, 1% monocytes. (These results are very suggestive of a viral infection.) The partial pressure of oxygen in arterial blood, with the patient breathing air enriched to make its oxygen content 24%, was 110 mm Hg (abnormally low, for such a high percentage of oxygen in inspired air at sea level). The chest film revealed interstitial infiltrates (not involving the actual alveolar spaces, but mainly the interalveolar septa) in both lower lobes.

Because of clinical suspicions raised by the history and physical examination, antibodies against rubeola virus were measured, with the following results:

| Complement fixation | Hemagglutination inhibition |
|---|---|
| Hospital day three | |
| <1: 8 | 1:20 |
| Ten days later | |
| 1:64 | 1:80 |

Using acute and convalescent phase sera for a retrospective immunologic diagnosis, the presence of at least a fourfold rise in these antibodies is considered conclusive proof that the illness, which is clinically compatible with measles, was, in fact, measles, and not one of its late spring/early summer mimics, such as Rocky Mountain spotted fever, an enterovirus infection, or early meningococcemia.

34.6 The clinical clues that would make the consultant consider measles prominently in the differential diagnosis included all of the following EXCEPT:

    A. the pattern of spread of the rash.

    B. the presence of the white spots on the buccal mucosa.

    C. the appearance of the illness in June.

    D. the interstitial pneumonia.

    E. the relatively low total white blood cell count.

The correct answer is **C** (appearance of the illness in June). Unlike many vector-borne illnesses, measles in the United States is a disease of cooler weather, quite typically the winter. While it is not impossible to see measles in June (after all, this patient got it in June), it is not among the data that would heighten suspicion that an illness is measles. The other answers are incorrect because they are data that do heighten the suspicion of measles: **A** (the pattern of spread of the rash) is very typical of the way in which measles evolves on the skin, that is, from the face to the trunk and extremities, in contrast to Rocky Mountain spotted fever, which classically begins at the periphery (wrists and ankles) and spreads centripetally; **B** (the white spots on the buccal mucosa) were Koplik spots, an enanthem (mucosal rash) that is felt to be pathognomonic (distinctly characteristic) of measles; **D** (interstitial pneumonia), while nonspecific, is quite compatible with an illness such as measles, which characteristically causes an interstitial "giant cell" pneumonia, interfering with the transport of oxygen across the alveolar septa into the pulmonary capillaries; **E** (the relatively low white blood cell count) is also what is expected in many viral illnesses, including measles.

**Discussion:** This patient had serologically proven measles at age 25. He somehow had escaped laws requiring measles immunization for entry into school, perhaps because he was thought to have had actual measles in infancy. Whether he actually had measles at age three months will never be known with certainty, but it is unlikely. Because of the very high degree of immunity to measles in adults of his mother's age, the presence of specific maternal antimeasles antibody, crossing the placenta into his circulation, should have protected him from measles for many months after his birth. On the other hand, if he did actually have measles at age three months, it is unlikely that he would have acquired durable immunity to this virus, owing to the immaturity of the immune system in so young an infant.

Koplik spots

**Figure 34.10**
Koplik spots.

However, this patient had Koplik spots (Figure 34.10). In the setting of a compatible febrile illness with rash, Koplik spots are very good evidence of measles. Serologic evidence was obtained because, at the time of his illness, in his state of residence, the measles situation was unstable, and the State Health Department was very interested in unassailable proof that a suspicious illness was, in fact, measles. Whereas viral cultures could have been obtained, serologic evidence was used to prove the etiology of this patient's illness, for reasons of convenience and cost. This is a common practice for documenting the viral etiology of diseases in the clinical setting.

This lucky patient gradually improved, and was discharged from the hospital. Many individuals with measles, especially adults and very young children, suffer severe illness with measles, often with serious immediate complications (such as bacterial pneumonia) and long-term sequelae that involve the central nervous system.

## Case 5: Woman with cough

This 39-year-old woman was admitted with fever and cough, which had been present for several days. She had daily cough productive of green sputum (indicating the presence of inflammatory cells, most probably polymorphonuclear leukocytes), and was treated with inhaled bronchodilators for what was believed to be asthma. The patient had a long history of productive cough (cough yielding sputum) and in 1976, invasive studies documented bronchiectasis (a condition in which inflammation has caused permanent dilation of the walls of bronchi). She was treated with antibiotics, and had no further physician contact until 1982, when she developed pneumonia. This resolved with antibiotics.

In 1991 (two years prior to the current admission) she again developed pneumonia. Noninvasive studies, including computerized tomographic (CT) scan of the chest, confirmed bronchiectasis of the left lower lobe and lingula. The patient's physicians believed that there was also bronchiectasis elsewhere in the lungs. With antibiotics this pneumonia resolved, and for several months prior to this admission she took cefaclor, an oral second-generation cephalosporin, one out of every four weeks. This was changed to azithromycin (a macrolide with antimicrobial spectrum broader than that of erythromycin). Shortly before admission, because of increasing fever and productive cough, the antimicrobial regimen was again changed, this time to trimethoprim-sulfamethoxazole. Her symptoms became worse, and she agreed to be admitted to the hospital. There was no exposure to dusts, fumes, danders, or toxins. A parrot was the only house pet.

34.7 Pets are sometimes important sources of infection to their owners. The organism that is most closely associated with parrots is:

    A. *Pasteurella multocida.*

    B. *Mycobacterium marinum.*

    C. *Francisella tularensis.*

    D. *Chlamydia psittaci.*

    E. *Coxiella burnetii.*

> The correct answer is **D** (*Chlamydia psittaci*). This organism, which does not grow in ordinary culture media, is closely associated with many types of birds, not only the "psittacine" birds (parrots, parakeets) from which it gets its specific name. The birds need not appear ill to be capable of transmitting *C. psittaci* to humans. The other choices are all associated with animals or their environments, but not birds. **A** (*Pasteurella multocida*) is found in the mouths of animals, especially cats and dogs, and is a gram-negative rod. **B** (*Mycobacterium marinum*) is an acid-fast bacillus that infects traumatic wounds that are sustained in salt or brackish water. **C** (*Francisella tularensis*) is classically associated with handling freshly killed rabbits, although it has also been acquired from other mammals. **E** (*Coxiella burnetii*) is categorized with the *Rickettsiae* and causes Q fever, an infection that may occur after exposure to livestock (for example, parturient sheep).

**Figure 34.11**
Gram stain of sputum shows many filamentous, branched, gram-positive rods. The fine caliber and the prominent presence of branching are important distinguishing morphologic characteristics.

The patient's temperature was 103°F. She was alert and in no distress. Examination of the chest revealed it to be normally resonant throughout, with diffuse coarse wheezes (musical sounds indicating constriction of bronchi and consistent with, but not diagnostic of, asthma). There was mild clubbing of the fingers and toes (bulbous swellings of the distal digits seen in patients with a variety of chronic illnesses, especially those involving the lungs).

The chest film revealed right lower lobe pneumonia. Gram stain of expectorated sputum revealed many filamentous, branched gram-positive rods. (Figure 34.11) These failed to grow in cultures but had grown, aerobically, from sputum cultured in 1991.

34.8 From this Gram stain, the possible genera into which the organism fits include:

    A. *Candida.*

    B. *Nocardia.*

    C. *Clostridium.*

    D. *Actinomyces.*

    E. *Pseudomonas.*

> Both **B** (*Nocardia*) and **D** (*Actinomyces*) are correct answers, as both are gram-positive filamentous rods with prominent branching. Their fine, threadlike (filamentous) diameter distinguishes them immediately from the much larger fungal genera, such as **A** (*Candida*). Multiple overlapping pseudohyphae of *Candida* species may appear to be branches, but their much larger size makes their identity as fungi, and not bacteria, quite evident. **C** (*Clostridium*) is, indeed, a gram-positive rod, but it is not branched, and its width is much greater than that of *Nocardia* or *Actinomyces*. **E** (*Pseudomonas*) can't be correct for many reasons, the most important of which is that it is a gram-negative rod.

The patient was treated with high doses of trimethoprim-sulfamethoxazole, intravenously at first. It was then given orally, because of the decrease in her temperature and marked improvement in her cough. Subsequent Gram stains of her sputum showed near-disappearance of the filamentous gram-positive rods (that had been identified as *Nocardia asteroides* in 1991).

**Discussion:** The *Nocardia* had probably never been eradicated from her lungs in 1991, and had most likely smoldered there until it finally reached a quantity adequate to cause symptoms and radiographic changes of pneumonia. The absence of treatment effective against *Nocardia*, after resolution of the 1991 pneumonia, made this very likely to occur. Bronchiectasis made this patient's mucociliary clearance mechanisms ineffective, allowing persistence of bacteria in areas that are normally sterile. *Nocardia* may be quite tenacious under these circumstances, making it necessary to maintain this patient, probably for years, on a regimen that will at least suppress the organism to levels that do not make her ill.

It should be noted that expectorated sputum is not usually cultured for anaerobes, since there would be contamination of the sputum with mouth flora, heavy in anaerobes, on its way from lungs to collection container. Documentation of an anaerobe, such as *Actinomyces*, as the cause of a lung lesion requires that the specimen be obtained without passing through the mouth. One way to do this is to pass a needle through the chest wall, under CT scan guidance, directly into the lesion. This was never done to this patient, whose filamentous branched gram-positive rod did not grow in sputum obtained during this episode of pneumonia. It was, after all, not cultured anaerobically, so that *Actinomyces*, if present, would not have grown. But her physicians felt confident that *Nocardia* was the culprit, for two reasons: 1) *Nocardia* was what had been in her sputum previously, and 2) there was a clear response to trimethoprim-sulfamethoxazole, which would not be expected to have a significant effect on *Actinomyces*. Unfortunately, not every organism that causes disease, including *Nocardia*, will be successfully grown in cultures every time. That (and the rapid availability of the presumptive answer) is why Gram stain is such an important tool in the clinical application of microbiology.

## Case 6: Woman with swollen wrist

This 25-year-old woman was admitted because of swelling and pain of her left wrist of ten days' duration. She had always been well. Twelve days before admission she was bitten on the left hand by her pet cat. Two days later she developed pain, redness, and swelling of her hand, and her physician treated her with oral cloxacillin (a penicillin derivative, active against *Staphylococcus aureus* and *Streptococcus pyogenes*, with the ability to withstand staphylococcal β-lactamase). After transient improvement

in her symptoms and signs of inflammation, she became worse, so that by the time of admission she was unable to close her fingers or move her wrist. In addition, she noted evening fevers as high as 100.2°F.

On physical examination her temperature was 99.7°F. The left wrist and thenar eminence were erythematous (red, but with blanching of the redness on pressure, indicating dilation of cutaneous blood vessels—the "rubor" of the classic signs of inflammation). There was markedly reduced range of motion, both extension and flexion, of the fingers. Extension and flexion of the wrist were limited to just a few degrees. The patient's wrist and hand are shown in Figure 34.12.

The white blood cell count was 13,000/µL, with a marked increase in the percentage of immature granulocytes (the "left shift" of an acute inflammatory process). Gram stain of the wrist fluid, which was cloudy when aspirated, revealed sheets of polymorphonuclear leukocytes and many gram-negative rods (Figure 34.13).

**Figure 34.13**
Gram stain of wrist fluid. There are innumerable ("sheets") polymorphonuclear leukocytes and many gram-negative rods.

34.9 From among the following, the gram-negative rod that is most commonly associated with cat bites is:

    A. *Pasteurella multocida*.

    B. *Bartonella henselae*.

    C. *Streptobacillus moniliformis*.

    D. *Streptococcus pyogenes*.

    E. *Lactobacillus casei*.

The correct answer is **A** (*Pasteurella multocida*), a gram-negative rod that frequents the mouths of some animals, particularly cats, but also dogs. The extreme sharpness of feline teeth causes enormous pressure at the site of the puncture during a bite, allowing inoculation of the organism deep into tissues. **B** (*Bartonella henselae*) is incorrect, although it is a gram-negative rod associated with exposure to cats. In immunocompetent hosts, the principal condition caused by this organism, which is carried mainly on the paws of cats, is cat scratch disease, whose

**Figure 34.12**
The thenar eminence is swollen, and the patient is only able to flex and extend her wrist and fingers minimally, due to pain. This photo was taken just prior to removal of wrist joint fluid from a point within the circle on the volar aspect of the wrist.

name implies transmission by cat scratches not cat bites. **C** (*Streptobacillus moniliformis*) is also a gram-negative rod, pleomorphic, which is most commonly acquired by the bite or scratch of rats or mice. While it may be carried—and transmitted—by carnivores that prey on these rodents, it is less characteristically associated with cat-induced injuries than with rat or mouse exposure. The simplest reason that **D** (*Streptococcus pyogenes*) is wrong is that it is a gram-positive coccus, not a gram-negative rod. Likewise, **E** (*Lactobacillus casei*) cannot be a correct answer because it is a gram-positive rod, and not gram-negative.

Culture of the wrist joint fluid yielded *Pasteurella multocida* and *Pseudomonas aeruginosa*. The patient underwent open debridement of her wrist, which showed extensive damage of the joint space and tendons in the vicinity of the joint space. With intravenous penicillin G (aimed at the *Pasteurella multocida*) and gentamicin (aimed at the *Pseudomonas aeruginosa*), together with intensive physical therapy, she had complete recovery of flexion and extension of her wrist and fingers.

**Discussion:** *Pasteurella multocida* is a notorious cause of infection induced by animal bites, especially those of cats. It has a propensity to invade osteoarticular tissues, which are often very near to the point at which the animal bites. Serious illness has occurred in newborns who have been licked by the family cat, presumably due to inoculation of *Pasteurella multocida* onto the infant, and invasion of the bloodstream because of the immaturity of the neonatal immune system. It is important to make the clinical association of animals and *Pasteurella multocida*, since this organism is resistant to a number of antibiotics, yet sensitive to penicillin G, which ordinarily would not be used to treat infection due to most gram-negative rods.

## Case 7: Man with endophthalmitis

This 66-year-old man with non–insulin-dependent diabetes mellitus had been feeling well until one week earlier. At that time he noted the sudden onset of shaking chills lasting about 20 minutes, associated with low back pain that radiated into the medial aspect of both thighs. These episodes occurred several times over the next few days. About two days after the onset of these chills he developed pain, swelling, and erythema (redness that blanches with pressure, due to dilation of superficial blood vessels as part of the inflammatory response (rubor)) of his left hand. The next day he noted a "black spot" obscuring his vision on his right eye, progressing over the next day to complete loss of vision in his right eye. His ophthalmologist found a hypopyon (collection of pus in the anterior chamber) and treated him with a subconjunctival injection of gentamicin (an aminoglycoside antibiotic) 80 mg, methylprednisolone (a glucocorticoid anti-inflammatory agent) 40 mg, topical gentamicin, and atropine (an anticholinergic to keep the pupil dilated) eye drops. The patient's diabetes had been well controlled with chlorpropamide (a sulfonylurea oral

hypoglycemic agent) and diet. There was no history of trauma to the eye.

The pain in his back and his left hand became worse the next day, and the following day, because the hypopyon was much worse, the ophthalmologist admitted the patient to the hospital. The anterior chamber was opaque (Figure 34.14) and the intraocular pressure was increased.

**Figure 34.14**
The patient's right eye at the time of admission to the hospital. The cornea is cloudy and there is a collection of white blood cells (hypopyon) behind it in the anterior chamber.

Physical examination revealed the temperature to be 97.8°F, the pulse regular at 90 beats per minute, and the blood pressure 160/90 mm Hg. The cornea of the right eye was opaque, with a dense hypopyon along its lower half. The retina could not be visualized behind this hypopyon. The left hand revealed erythema, swelling, warmth, tenderness, and very decreased range of motion of the third, fourth, and fifth metacarpo-phalangeal (MCP) joints (Figure 34.15). There was a small, healing laceration of the left shin.

**Figure 34.15**
The patient's left hand at the time of admission to the hospital. The lateral three MCP joints are swollen, with erythema especially visible over the fourth MCP joint.

**Figure 34.16**
Gram stain of the anterior chamber fluid taken at the time of admission to the hospital. There are polymorphonuclear leukocytes and many gram-positive cocci, some distorted to an elongated shape.

The white blood cell (WBC) count was 16,500/µl (normal 5,000 to 10,000), with 78% polymorphonuclear leukocytes, 20% band forms, and 2 lymphocytes (a "left shift" toward immature granulocytes, consistent with an acute inflammatory process). Gram stain of fluid aspirated from the anterior chamber of the right eye (Figure 34.16) revealed many polymorphonuclear leukocytes and large numbers of gram-positive cocci, some irregular in shape (a reflection of partial efficacy of the injected gentamicin, which was injuring these organisms without killing them). Blood cultures taken at the time of hospitalization yielded gram-positive cocci in long chains (Figure 34.17) that were identified as *Streptococcus agalactiae*. The same organism grew from cultures of the anterior chamber fluid.

**Figure 34.17**
Gram stain of organisms grown from blood cultures. These are gram-positive cocci in chains, consistent with *Streptococcus* species.

Day 5

Day 12

**Figure 34.18**
Top: The patient's right eye after 5 days of intravenous penicillin G, showing persistence of the hypopyon and intense chemosis (edema of the conjunctiva, which has swelled to the point that it is hanging over the lower eyelid). Bottom: The patient's right eye after 10 days of intravenous penicillin G, with resolution of the chemosis but persistence of corneal opacification.

34.10 *Streptococcus agalactiae* is also known by its Lancefield group which is:

   A. Group A
   B. Group B
   C. Group C
   D. Group D
   E. Group G

> The correct answer is **B** (Group B). Since *Streptococcus agalactiae* is in Group B, all of the other choices are incorrect.

This patient went on to have a stormy course, with intense pain in his eye, where the inflammation increased for several days before it started to improve (Figure 34.18).

He was found on further study to have infective endocarditis (an infection of a heart valve, with growths of bacteria, called "vegetations," which may break off into the arterial circulation). He thus had "showers" of bacteria-laden material in his arterial tree, explaining his low back pain, the acute arthritis of his left hand, and the very active infection of his eye. The "portal of entry" of this bacterial infection was most probably the laceration of his shin. Diabetics are more likely to harbor *Streptococcus agalactiae* on their skin, especially on the lower extremities. Because his diabetes impaired his ability to contain a localized infection, he was more prone to having the bacteria that contaminated the laceration invade his bloodstream, from which some of them colonized a heart valve and, from there, further seeded tissues with end-artery circulation (eye, hand, vertebral column). He was treated with a total of six weeks of intravenous aqueous penicillin G, 4 million units every 4 hours, and he eventually got better, but the vision in his right eye was permanently lost.

## Case 8: Man with fever and paraplegia

This 32-year-old man complained of fever and myalgias (muscle pain) for one week. He had always been in good health. In late July he visited a grassy area of rural New Jersey. Two days later he developed diarrhea, fever, malaise (a general feeling of not being well), and a rash. He saw a physician three days after the onset of these symptoms and, because of elevated serum transaminase levels, was told he had hepatitis. The diarrhea had stopped, and he now complained of headache, primarily frontal and retro-orbital (over and behind the eyes).

There was no travel outside New Jersey, and there was no history of injecting drug use, multiple sexual partners, or homosexual contact.

On examination he was well-developed, well-nourished, and comfortable. His temperature was 103.5°F, his pulse 120 beats per minute (a rapid heart rate consistent with his fever). The conjunctivae were injected (bloodshot), and the

**Figure 34.19**
Top: The patient's ankle, showing numerous, tiny, cutaneous hemorrhages (petechiae). Bottom: The patient's right hand showing edema to the extent that he cannot flex his fingers further than shown in this photo.

pharynx slightly more red than normal. A diffuse, confluent, erythematous macular rash covered the back and chest (red, but blanching when pressed (erythematous) and not raised above the level of surrounding skin (macular)). The liver was slightly enlarged, with a total span measuring 13 cm. Its edge was tender (painful to the touch of the examiner). The muscles of the patient's arms and legs were also tender. Numerous petechiae were present on the extremities, as shown in Figure 34.19. His hands were edematous, preventing him from closing them into a fist (see Figure 34.19).

The hemoglobin was 13.4 g/dl (slightly less than the lower limit of normal of 14), the white blood cell (WBC) count 13,500/μl (normal 5,000 to 10,000), with 68% polymorphonuclear leukocytes, 20% band forms, 7% lymphocytes, and 5% monocytes. (A high total WBC with increased percentage of immature granulocytes indicates an acute inflammatory process.) The platelet count was 91,000/μl (normal 140,000 to 400,000). Serum aspartate aminotransferase (AST) was 273 (normal up to 40), and serum alanine aminotransferase (ALT) was 198 (normal up to 45). (The abnormal transaminases are consistent with an inflammatory process of the liver.) The chest film was normal. Blood cultures drawn at the time of admission to the hospital were ultimately sterile.

Because of the season during which this illness occurred, and because of its involvement of several systems (skin, muscles, liver, alimentary canal), the physicians caring for this man suspected Rocky Mountain spotted fever and began therapy with doxycycline (a long-acting tetracycline). One day after institution of this treatment, he became paraplegic and stuporous, recovering, with physical therapy, over the next several weeks. The doxycycline was continued for a total of ten days.

34.11 The diagnosis of Rocky Mountain spotted fever is ordinarily confirmed by which of the following tests:

    A. blood cultures.

    B. Weil-Felix ("febrile") agglutinins.

    C. antibodies against *Rickettsia rickettsii*.

    D. antibodies against *Rickettsia prowazekii*.

    E. antibodies against *Salmonella typhi*.

The correct answer is **C** (antibodies against *Rickettsia rickettsii*). *R. rickettsii* is the microbial etiology of Rocky Mountain spotted fever. **A** (blood cultures) is incorrect. In clinical practice, because rickettsiae are obligate intracellular pathogens, ordinary liquid blood culture media, which are cell-free, cannot support their growth. In addition, laboratory accidents that have resulted in aerosolization of rickettsial cultures have caused fatalities, and most clinical laboratories are unwilling to work with these organisms in culture. **B** (Weil-Felix ("febrile") agglutinins), which are antibodies directed against Proteus OX-19 and OX-2 antigens, are not specific enough, cross-reacting with antigens of other rickettsial species. Thus B is wrong.

> **D** (antibodies against *Rickettsia prowazekii*) is not correct because *R. prowazekii* is the etiology of epidemic typhus, not Rocky Mountain spotted fever. **E** (antibodies against *Salmonella typhi*) is incorrect because *S. typhi* is one of the etiologies of enteric fever, not Rocky Mountain spotted fever. The name "typhoid" fever may make one think about a possible relationship to a rickettsia species that causes "typhus" but the two should never be confused.

Complement-fixing antibody titers against *Rickettsia rickettsii* were positive at a dilution of 1:32 on day 10 of illness and 1:128 three weeks later. This four-fold rise in specific antibody confirms that the illness that this young man suffered was Rocky Mountain spotted fever.

**Discussion:** There is much about this patient's story that is very typical of Rocky Mountain spotted fever, and therefore very instructive. He became ill at the height of the summer, when ticks are most active. He spent time in a grassy area of a state which is well within the range of *Dermacentor variabilis*, the dog tick, which is a competent vector of *R. rickettsii*. The cell that *R. rickettsii* infects is the vascular endothelial lining cell. Thus it makes sense that Rocky Mountain spotted fever involves many different organ systems (which all have a blood supply), and causes the kind of leakiness of blood vessels that leads to edema and petechial hemorrhages. The vascular injury, together with certain immune-mediated events, may result in disseminated intravascular coagulation, consuming platelets and leading to the low platelet count that was seen in this patient. Any tissue can be involved, but the skin and central nervous system seem to be preferred targets of *R. rickettsii*, explaining the extent of his rash and the complication of paraplegia.

The onset of paraplegia after appropriate therapy was begun warrants special comment. In addition to causing blood vessels to leak, vasculitis may also result in occlusion of blood vessels. It is probable that, prior to the administration of the doxycycline, infection of this patient's spinal cord vessels had progressed to the point that spinal cord ischemia (impaired blood supply) was inevitable, causing injury and even death of enough motor neurons to lead to paraplegia. One of the reasons that Rocky Mountain spotted fever is such a frightening disease is its potential to cause infarction of tissue.

## Case 9: Woman with fever

This 28-year-old woman developed fever the day after the birth of her second child. She had always been well and had emigrated to the United States from India seven years earlier. Her first pregnancy, four years later, resulted in a healthy baby girl, who was well at home throughout the patient's second pregnancy. The patient was admitted to the hospital in active labor at the term (that is, after the full nine months) of her second pregnancy. Vaginal examination revealed amniotic fluid stained with meconium, and so

the patient was taken to the operating room for emergency cesarean section. (Meconium is fetal feces, and when it is present in the amniotic fluid prior to birth, it indicates that the baby is in enough distress to warrant quick delivery.) Prior to the administration of anesthesia, labor had progressed to the point that a healthy, full-term female infant was delivered vaginally.

The mother developed a temperature of 102°F on the first postpartum (after delivery) day. She was treated with oral ampicillin 500 mg every 6 hours. Temperature maxima of 101 to 102°F continued. She complained of mild headache and a sense of chilliness each evening, when her temperature reached its maximum. (This is not unusual in patients with fever.)

Further questioning at the time of the consultant's visit indicated that the patient is a vegetarian and had, during the week prior to parturition, consumed several meals consisting of pizza with extra Mexican-style cheese. Her three-year-old daughter had had otitis media (a middle ear infection) two weeks before the patient went into labor, but was well at home at the time the patient was admitted to the obstetric unit.

Physical examination done in the early afternoon of the third postpartum day revealed an alert woman in no distress. The temperature was 99°F. The general physical examination was within normal limits. The uterus was enlarged as expected following a delivery. The lochia (the normal bloody vaginal discharge that follows the birth of a baby) was normal in amount and appearance and did not have a foul smell.

The blood count was within normal limits, as was the chest film. Blood cultures, taken at the onset of fever, yielded a gram-positive bacillus, morphologically identical to that shown in Figure 34.20. Aerobic subculture on blood agar yielded colonies that were β-hemolytic. Further subculture revealed the organism to be motile.

**Figure 34.20**
Gram stain of blood culture shows gram-positive diphtheroid-like rods, many of which are at angles to one another. The material in the background is debris from the red cells in the blood inoculated into the liquid blood culture medium.

34.12 The most likely etiology of this patient's bacteremia is:

    A. *Streptococcus pyogenes*.

    B. *Escherichia coli*.

    C. *Propionibacterium acnes*.

    D. *Clostridium perfringens*.

    E. *Listeria monocytogenes*.

> The correct answer is **E** (*Listeria monocytogenes*). It is a gram-positive rod that may easily be mistaken for a diphtheroid. However, its β hemolysis and motility distinguish it from diphtheroids, which are much less likely to be hemolytic, and are nonmotile. Whereas **A** (*Streptococcus pyogenes*) and **B** (*Escherichia coli*) may cause postpartum bacteremia, both are incorrect answers to the question, because *Streptococcus pyogenes* is a gram-positive *coccus* and not a bacillus and *Escherichia coli*, while a bacillus, is gram-*negative* and not gram-positive. Although **D** (*Clostridium perfringens*) is a gram-positive bacillus, it is a wrong answer because it is anaerobic, and would be most unlikely to grow in aerobic subculture. The absence of a foul smell from the lochia, while not entirely ruling out anaerobic infection, lessens the probability that anaerobes are present.

The organism that grew from the cultures was *Listeria monocytogenes*. Ampicillin was continued, but the route was changed from oral to intravenous, and the dose raised to 3 g every 6 hours. (The reason is that high blood levels of ampicillin are required to eradicate a bacteremia due to an organism susceptible to this drug. Such high blood levels could not be achieved with oral administration of ampicillin.) Fever resolved rapidly, and the remainder of the postpartum course was uneventful for the patient. However, her baby became quite ill on its second day of life, and had to be transferred to a neonatal intensive care unit, requiring assisted ventilation for several days. Blood cultures from the baby grew out the same gram-positive bacillus. After much intensive care and many days of antibiotics, the baby also recovered.

**Discussion:** This patient had perinatal listeriosis. *Listeria monocytogenes* is an especially important pathogen among immunocompromised individuals, pregnant women, and newborns. The portal by which *Listeria monocytogenes* entered the mother's bloodstream was shown by cultures of her lochia to be her genital tract. It is probably from there that it entered the baby as well. The most likely source from which she acquired *Listeria monocytogenes* was the cheese on her pizza. While *Listeria monocytogenes* is present in a number of different foods, dairy products are among the most important sources of food-borne listeriosis. The association is so strong that pregnant women, especially in the third trimester, and immunocompromised individuals are advised not to eat soft cheeses. Because of its superficial resemblance to commensal diphtheroids, it is easy to miss *Listeria monocytogenes* in cultures. The combination of β-hemolysis and the motility it exhibits in special agar tubes when cultured at 20 to 25°C serve to distinguish this important pathogen from nonpathogenic look-alikes, allowing appropriate treatment of patients and rewarding vigilance in the clinical laboratory.

## Case 10: Man in coma

This 52-year-old man was found unresponsive at home on the day of admission. He had had a long history of alcoholism, complicated by a seizure disorder. For several days prior to admission he had been drinking heavily. He was found by relatives at home, unresponsive, with continuous epileptiform movements. (He did not regain consciousness between seizures.) In the Emergency Room his temperature was 105°F. His neck was stiff. Chest examination suggested pneumonia involving the upper and middle lobes of the right lung. A chest X-ray was taken (Figure 34.21). There was no response to verbal stimuli. (He was in a coma.)

Because of the fever and unconsciousness, lumbar puncture was done promptly to examine the cerebrospinal fluid (CSF). The CSF was very cloudy. There were 561 WBC/μl (98% polymorphonuclear leukocytes (PMNs). The protein concentration was 380 mg/dl, the glucose concentration 5 mg/dl. (These findings are typical for acute bacterial meningitis.)

34.13 The test that will yield the most rapidly available information about the presumptive bacterial cause of this patient's infection is:

    A. blood culture.

    B. CSF culture.

    C. CSF Gram stain.

    D. urine culture.

    E. sputum Gram stain.

> The correct answer is **C** (the CSF Gram stain). Although the Gram stain does not tell the exact genus and species of an organism, it narrows down the choices so that an intelligent guess regarding the probable microbial etiology is possible, considering the morphology and the overall clinical situation. Since the Gram stain takes only minutes to perform, precious time is saved in initiating therapy that is as specific as possible. **A** (blood culture) and **B** (CSF culture) are both wrong answers because of the time required for visible growth to appear in cultures, and the additional time required to identify organisms that do grow. Also, sometimes organisms may be so fastidious that they do not grow easily, further increasing the time it takes to identify them. **D** is wrong because the site of the clinically evident infection is not the urinary tract. **E** is wrong primarily because it may be difficult to obtain reliable sputum from an unconscious patient, resulting in unnecessary delays. Also, in patients whose infection involves the meninges, regardless of the source, defining the central nervous system process takes priority over most other diagnostic considerations and is most likely to lead to the most specific possibility because of the absence of "normal" resident flora in the CSF.

**Figure 34.21**
Chest film. The white areas are "liquid density," and the black areas are "air density." The central shadow represents the patient's heart. The wedge-shaped white areas on the left are the radiographic appearance of pneumonia involving the middle and upper lobes of the right lung.

Gram stain of the cerebrospinal fluid showed scant PMNs, and very large numbers of gram-positive cocci in pairs (Figure 34.22). The chest film confirmed pneumonia of the right upper and middle lobes. The peripheral WBC count was 4,700/ml (73 percent PMNs, 19 percent bands). (For a patient with this degree of illness due to infection, this WBC count is unusually low, and reflects his inability to mount appropriate defenses against his infection.)

**Figure 34.22**
Gram stain of the sediment of cerebrospinal fluid, showing a single polymorphonuclear leukocyte and large numbers of gram-positive cocci in pairs.
.

34.14 In this patient with lobar pneumonia and CSF that has a heavy concentration of gram-positive cocci in pairs (diplococci), the most likely microbial etiology of his infections is:

    A. *Neisseria meningitidis.*

    B. *Staphylococcus haemolyticus.*

    C. *Streptococcus pneumoniae.*

    D. *Listeria monocytogenes.*

    E. *Cryptococcus neoformans.*

The correct answer is **C** (*Streptococcus pneumoniae*), which is a gram-positive coccus that often occurs in pairs and is a notorious cause of community-acquired pneumonia, especially in heavy alcohol users. It has a propensity to invade the central nervous system, causing meningitis. **A** (*Neisseria meningitidis*) is incorrect because it is a gram-negative diplococcus, albeit an important cause of meningitis in adults. **B** (*Staphylococcus haemolyticus*) is wrong because this organism, indeed a gram-positive coccus, is not likely to be arrayed in pairs, but rather in clusters. Moreover, it is not often associated with lung infections, or with meningitis unless there is an antecedent break in the meninges, as with surgery or trauma. **D** (*Listeria monocytogenes*) is wrong because the organism is a gram-positive bacillus and not a coccus, although it is a well-known cause of meningitis, especially in heavy alcohol users. **E** (*Cryptococcus neoformans*) is wrong because, in spite of its name, it is not a coccus but a yeast, which is considerably larger than a coccus. (Cryptococcus, by the way, appears gram-positive in Gram stains, and can cause both pneumonia and meningitis, but you would never mistake it for a bacterium, both because of its size and because it has the morphologic property of budding.)

Penicillin (which when this patient was treated, was the drug of choice for *Streptococcus pneumoniae* infections) in very high doses was given within minutes of the lumbar puncture. The patient never regained consciousness, continuing to have seizures almost constantly for the next two days, despite aggressive anticonvulsant treatment. His heart rate slowed and his blood pressure became immeasurably low. Resuscitation attempts failed and he was pronounced dead on his third hospital day.

An α-hemolytic, gram-positive coccus, morphologically identical to the organism that was seen in the CSF Gram stain, grew from cultures of blood and CSF. It was identified as *Streptococcus pneumoniae*.

**Discussion:** *Streptococcus pneumoniae*, commonly known as the pneumococcus, is the most frequent cause of meningitis in adults, and usually enters the bloodstream (and from there the central nervous system) via the lungs. Occasionally, even with the most intensive supportive care and the earliest possible specific antimicrobial treatment, patients with pneumococcal infections die. This patient was at a particular disadvantage because his heavy alcohol use diminished his ability to fight many types of infection by reducing the capacity of his bone marrow to mount a response of the types of cells, polymorphonuclear leuko-

**Figure 34.23**
Wright stain of this patient's peripheral blood smear, revealing a spiral-shaped organism among (but not within) the circulating blood cells.

cytes, needed to engulf pneumococci and destroy them. The relatively small number of PMNs in his CSF were unable to keep up with the rapid proliferation of pneumococci in his subarachnoid space (where the CSF is located). Ordinarily, when CSF is cloudy in meningitis, it is because of a large number of PMNs in it. This patient's CSF was cloudy more from the massive numbers of pneumococci it contained. (Note: When this patient was seen, penicillin-resistant pneumococci were very rare; nowadays, empiric therapy would be vancomycin.)

## Case 11: Man with recurrent fever

This 21-year-old male university student had fever intermittently for several weeks. The patient had always been well, and was a varsity football player at an East Coast university. Shortly after the end of the school year he spent six weeks in North Carolina at an encampment on a military base. During this time he recalled multiple tick bites. He personally removed a number of ticks that had been embedded in his skin. He spent the remainder of the summer at his family's home in eastern Washington, and at their summer cabin in Idaho. After several weeks in the West, he developed fever as high as 105°F, accompanied by headache, myalgias (muscle pains), arthralgias (joint pains), nausea, and occasional vomiting. After five days his symptoms abated and he felt well. Ten days after the resolution of these symptoms he had them again, but they were less severe and only lasted about two days. Ten days after the second febrile illness he had a third, similar episode that also resolved after about two days.

He returned to his university at the end of the summer, and about two weeks after his last febrile episode, he again developed fever, this time mild, and accompanied by generalized malaise. When he was examined his temperature was 98°F, and his pulse 72 beats per minute. His physical examination was completely within normal limits except that his spleen tip was palpable about 4 cm below his left costal margin with deep inspiration. His hemoglobin concentration was 12.6 g/dl (lower limit of normal 14), his white blood cell

count was normal at 4500/μl, his platelet count 135,000/μl (lower limit of normal 140,000). An incidental observation was made by the laboratory technician who examined the patient's peripheral blood smear for the blood count. What was seen is shown in Figure 34.23.

34.15 Which of the following tick-borne infections is compatible with the microbial morphology shown in Figure 34.23.

   A. Rocky Mountain spotted fever (*Rickettsia rickettsii*)
   B. Colorado tick fever (*Coltivirus*)
   C. Ehrlichiosis (*Ehrlichia* species)
   D. Relapsing fever (*Borrelia* species)
   E. Babesiosis (*Babesia microti*)

The correct answer is **D** (relapsing fever), which is caused by a spirochetal organism of the genus *Borrelia*. Spirochetes do not appear on Gram stain but those that cause relapsing fever may be seen in Wright stain smears of peripheral blood. **A** (Rocky Mountain spotted fever) is incorrect because *Rickettsiae* are not visible with ordinary stains, and they do not have the spiral morphology seen in Figure 34.23. **B** (Colorado tick fever) is a wrong answer because viruses are generally too small to be seen with light microscopy. Pathologic changes that some viruses cause (for example, inclusion bodies) are visible with light microscopy, but the virus itself is not. **C** (Ehrlichiosis) is not caused by a spirochete. The abnormality that it creates is seen in circulating leukocytes and, because of its fancied resemblance to a mulberry, is called a morula. **E** (Babesiosis) also is not caused by a spirochete. The etiologic agent, a protozoan that resembles malarial forms, may, however, be seen in Wright stain preparations of peripheral blood.

The patient was treated with doxycycline 200 mg per day for ten days. Shortly after his first dose of doxycycline he had severe fever and chills. He subsequently felt better and recovered completely. Of note is the fact that six of his family members, who also spent time at the home in Idaho, also had an illness characterized by recurrent episodes of fever and other constitutional symptoms.

**Discussion:** This young man had a very typical case of relapsing fever, an illness that is transmitted by lice or ticks. Ticks are responsible for endemic disease. Those ticks that transmit *Borrelia* species that cause relapsing fever prefer humid environments and altitudes of 1500 to 6000 feet. Although this patient remembered tick bites in North Carolina, it is probable that he acquired relapsing fever in Idaho, since several family members who were with him in Idaho, and not North Carolina, had a similar illness. Tick-borne disease is generally not as severe as disease spread by lice, probably because of species differences in virulence among borreliae. Slightly fewer than half the people with tick-borne relapsing fever have an enlarged spleen. The symptoms are nonspecific, although the relapsing course may suggest the diagnosis. However, other tick-borne diseases, such as malaria and babesiosis, may present with similarly nonspecific symptomatology that may occur in episodes. Several tick-borne diseases may have characteristic manifestations visible in peripheral blood smears. The need to pay attention to findings seen in peripheral blood is well illustrated by this patient.

His apparent exacerbation of symptoms with the initial treatment is also typical of relapsing fever (and a few other spirochetal diseases). Rapid lysis of spirochetes causes endotoxin release and the attendant symptoms, which may be severe, including fever, chills, hypotension, and leukopenia. This "Jarisch-Herxheimer" reaction is clinically similar to an exaggeration of the febrile episodes observed with untreated disease.

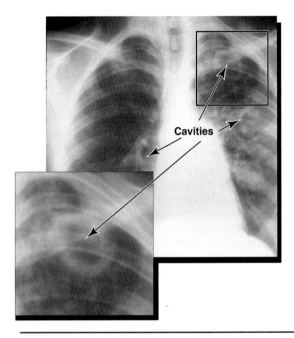

**Figure 34.24**
Chest radiograph reveals infiltrates in both lungs, with two cavities in the left upper lobe and probably another in the right lung.

## Case 12: Woman from Ecuador with cough

This 23-year-old woman had been having pain in her left anterior and posterior chest for one month. A native of Ecuador, the patient had been in the United States for 4 years, and had always been well. Two months prior to the current visit, she developed cough productive of whitish sputum, worse in the early morning. There was no attendant shortness of breath, and she had not noted any particular odor of the sputum. She had not had hemoptysis (the coughing up of blood). About one month after the onset of the cough, she began to have intermittent pleuritic (worse with coughing or deep breathing) left chest pain. In the one-and-one-half months leading up to the current visit, she had noted increasing fatigue and weight loss of ten pounds, but no loss of appetite. There was no history of fever or night sweats.

The patient had never injected drugs. She had had a total of two sexual partners, her last sexual contact having occurred two years earlier.

The physical examination revealed a well developed, well nourished young woman in no distress, with a temperature of 98°F, a pulse of 98 beats per minute, respiratory rate of 18 per minute, and blood pressure 102/60. There was no significant lymphadenopathy (no swollen lymph nodes). The chest revealed fine crackles in the suprascapular areas bilaterally, greater on the left than on the right. (There was probably fluid in the alveoli of the upper lobes.) The left upper lobe area was dull to percussion. (There was probably enough fluid in at least most of the alveoli in this area to cause the lungs to seem solidified ("consolidated") on the physical examination.) The remainder of the physical examination was unremarkable. The patient's chest film (Figure 34.24) shows infiltrates of both upper lobes, with at least two cavities in the left upper lobe and a probable cavity of the right lung (arrows).

34.16 Because of the history of productive cough and weight loss in a woman from South America, with cavitary pulmonary infiltrates seen on the chest film, the physicians caring for this patient suspected tuberculosis. Which of the following studies will give the most rapid presumptive support to the diagnosis of active pulmonary tuberculosis?

   A. Tuberculin (PPD) skin test

   B. Sputum culture for acid-fast bacilli (AFB)

   C. Sputum Gram stain

   D. Sputum acid-fast stain

   E. Sputum assay for *Mycobacterium tuberculosis* by polymerase chain reaction (PCR)

The correct answer is **D** (sputum acid-fast stain), which takes just minutes to perform and, when positive in a compatible clinical setting (which this patient certainly provides), is very strong presumptive evidence of active tuberculosis. **A** (PPD skin test) is not correct because a positive tuberculin reaction indicates infection with tuberculosis, but not necessarily active disease. **B** (sputum culture for AFB) is incorrect because cultures may take up to 6-8 weeks to yield growth of organisms. Cultures are important to confirm the diagnosis of tuberculosis, and to provide an isolate whose susceptibility to antituberculous drugs can be tested, but sputum cultures do not contribute to rapid presumptive diagnosis. **C** (sputum Gram stain) is incorrect because tubercle bacilli (and other AFB) are not visualized with Gram stain. **E** (PCR assay of sputum) takes several hours and is not usually available in ordinary community-based clinical laboratories. When it is positive (see below) it is very helpful, but at the present time, it is not practical for use with expectorated sputum.

The physicians caring for this patient obtained sputum for AFB stain and culture. The AFB stain (Figure 34.25) showed large numbers of acid-fast bacilli, some of which had the typical beaded appearance of *Mycobacterium tuberculosis*.

**Figure 34.25**
Acid-fast stain of sputum, showing many acid-fast bacilli. Beaded appearance of several of the AFB (inset) is characteristic, although not definitively diagnostic, of *Mycobacterium tuberculosis*.

34.17 The "classic" solid medium that is used to cultivate *Mycobacterium* species is:

    A. Sabouraud agar.

    B. Lowenstein-Jensen medium.

    C. MacConkey agar.

    D. Thayer-Martin medium.

    E. sheep blood agar.

> The correct answer is **B** (Lowenstein-Jensen medium), an egg-based solid medium that supports the growth of *Mycobacterium* species, including *M. tuberculosis*. **A** (Sabouraud agar) is used to cultivate fungi, not AFB. **C** (MacConkey agar) is a medium that is selective for gram-negative bacilli, not AFB. **D** (Thayer-Martin medium) is chocolate agar to which certain antibiotics have been added, and is a medium selective for *Neisseria gonorrhoeae* in specimens taken from nonsterile sites, such as genital secretions. **E** (sheep blood agar) is a general-purpose medium for bacteria that does not support the growth of *Mycobacteria*.

This patient's sputum was cultured in a liquid medium that produced fluorescence in the presence of actively respiring *Mycobacteria*, allowing growth to be detected in nine days. The presence of *Mycobacterium tuberculosis* in this culture was confirmed by DNA probe. The organism was later found to be susceptible to all antituberculous medications tested. On the basis of the positive AFB stain of her sputum, the patient was treated with isoniazide, rifampin, pyrazinamide, and ethambutol. She gained weight and stopped coughing shortly after the onset of treatment. She continued to respond very well to her treatment. Laboratory studies later confirmed that she was **not** co-infected with human immunodeficiency virus (HIV).

**Discussion:** One could hardly ask for a more classical presentation of pulmonary tuberculosis. The patient comes from an area of high endemicity for tuberculosis, and the constellation of weight loss, productive cough, and cavitary pulmonary infiltrates is extremely characteristic of tuberculosis. (Note: If she had had fever and night sweats, her presentation would have been "classic.") Although it is possible that she acquired tuberculosis after coming to the United States, it is likely that her active disease represents recrudescence (reactivation) of an infection that she acquired many years earlier. Sound cell-mediated immunity (CMI) has been found to be of great importance in containing tuberculous infection. It is not surprising, therefore, that tuberculosis is one of the infections that is especially severe in patients whose CMI is impaired by HIV infection. The association between active TB and HIV disease is so strong that the presence of active TB is felt to be a reason to look for concomitant HIV infection. That is why this patient was tested for HIV.

## Case 13: Woman with headache

This 68-year-old, right-handed woman was admitted to the hospital because of headaches that began about one month earlier.

She was in good general health. About one month prior to admission she developed progressively severe headaches and vertigo (a sensation that her environment was spinning around her). Shortly after the onset of these complaints, she noted photophobia (discomfort from light, to the extent that room lighting caused her eyes to hurt). The photophobia increased to the point that she had to wear sunglasses to cope with Christmas tree lights indoors. She was observed by her family to become increasingly lethargic (drowsy) and forgetful, prompting her hospitalization.

Physical examination revealed a lethargic woman who was oriented to person and place but not to time. (She knew her name and where she was, but not the month or the year or that Christmas and New Year's Day had just passed.) The temperature was 98.9°F. There was moderate resistance to anterior flexion of her neck beyond 60°. The lungs had crackles at both bases (consistent, in this instance, with findings described below in the chest X-ray). Neurologic examination revealed pain when her straightened legs were raised beyond 45° (evidence, with the resistance to neck flexion, that there was at least moderate inflammation of the meninges). In addition, when reaching for objects with her hands, she consistently over-reached and missed them ("past-pointing," indicative of cerebellar dysfunction). This latter finding was worse on the left than on the right.

Computerized tomography of the head revealed only mild cerebral atrophy (shrinkage—probably age-related). Because of the signs of meningeal irritation, a lumbar puncture was performed shortly after admission to the hospital.

The peripheral white blood cell count was 11,800/µl (normal between 5000 and 10,000), with 83 percent polymorphonuclear leukocytes, 9 percent band forms, 4 percent lymphocytes, and 4 percent monocytes (a slight increase in imma-ture granulocytes, suggesting an acute inflammatory pro-cess somewhere within the patient). The chest X-ray revealed diffuse interstitial infiltrates of both lower lobes (that is, increased fluid in the septa separating very minute air spaces).

The cerebrospinal fluid (CSF) obtained during the lumbar puncture was clear and colorless, with a total white blood cell count of 18/μl (normal up to 4), with 75 percent poly-morphonuclear leukocytes and 25 percent lymphocytes. (Polymorphonuclear leukocytes are never normally present in CSF.) The CSF glucose was 28 mg/dl with simultaneous blood glucose of 119 mg/dl. (The blood glucose was within normal limits; but CSF glucose considerably less than 50 percent of blood glucose suggests that a viable micro-organism is present in the subarachnoid space.) The CSF protein concentration was 58 mg/dl (very slightly above the upper limit of normal for this patient's age).

While performing the white blood cell count on the CSF, an alert laboratory technician observed structures that did not resemble white blood cells. A sample of CSF was cen-trifuged and the sediment resuspended in India ink. Under the microscope, in dramatic relief among the India ink parti-cles, were the organisms shown in Figure 34.26.

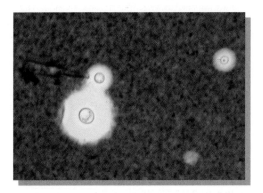

**Figure 34.26**
India ink preparation of CSF. A cell and its clear zone appears to be separating from a larger, similar cell. This process, called "budding," is characteristic of yeast cells. The clear zone surrounding the cells is actually a polysaccharide capsule displacing the India ink particles.

34.18  The most likely etiology of this patient's meningitis is:

    A. *Streptococcus pneumoniae.*

    B. *Candida albicans.*

    C. *Histoplasma capsulatum.*

    D. *Clostridium perfringens.*

    E. *Cryptococcus neoformans.*

The correct answer is **E** (*Cryptococcus neoformans*). It is a yeast that reproduces by budding and is characterized by a polysaccharide capsule. The presence of the polysac-charide capsule is very helpful for rapid diagnosis in microscopic examination of clinical specimens such as CSF. The capsule may appear gram-negative, and the yeast cell itself gram-positive, in Gram stains. But India ink very dramatically brings the capsule into view under the microscope. **A** (*Streptococcus pneumoniae*) is incorrect because, being a bacterium, it is much smaller than yeast and it does not manifest budding. *S. pneumoniae* progeny are the same size as its parent cell. It also does not dis-play its polysaccharide capsule in ordinary preparations. **B** (*Candida albicans*) is a yeast that manifests budding but it is not encapsulated. Hence this cannot be a correct answer. **C** (*Histoplasma capsulatum*) is incorrect for the same reason—it does not display a polysaccharide cap-sule in clinical specimens. **D** (*Clostridium perfringens*) is incorrect because, while larger in size than many bacteria, it is still much smaller than a yeast cell. Also, clostridia are not encapsulated and are not round, as are yeast cells.

The organism that grew from cultures of CSF and blood was *Cryptococcus neoformans*. Despite very aggressive therapy with amphotericin B, both intravenously and instilled directly into a lateral cerebral ventricle, the patient followed a relentless downhill course and died on the eighth day of treatment. Autopsy confirmed severe meningitis due to *Cryptococcus neoformans*.

**Discussion:** Invasive disease due to this organism is strongly suggestive of a defect in cell-mediated immunity, and its presence in this patient caused the clinicians caring for her to suspect that she had a malignant lymphoma. (This patient was treated in the early 1980s, prior to the emergence of human immunodeficiency virus (HIV) as a significant cause of severely impaired cell-mediated immu-nity. Moreover, she had none of the known risk factors that might lead to HIV infection.) In addition to the cryptococcal disease itself, autopsy revealed a clinically inapparent malignant lymphoma that was limited to the patient's uri-nary bladder and fallopian tubes.

The lymphoma did not cause this patient's death the way many cancerous tumors do, that is, by causing failure of a vital organ. Instead, the profound defect in cell-mediated immunity that accompanies lymphomas (as well as a num-ber of other clinical entities) created in this patient a predis-position to infection with an organism whose progression she could not resist. As *Cryptococcus neoformans* often does, it attacked her central nervous system preferentially. By the time this infection created clinical symptoms of headache, photophobia, and vertigo, it had passed the point of reversibility, and caused her death.

It is characteristic of malignancies that are accompanied by an immune defect that death is the result of an overwhelming infection. By correlating the immune defect with the underlying disease, one may often anticipate the complicating infection, and intervene in time to enjoy a favorable clinical outcome. Or, as with this patient, the presence of an opportunistic infection (one that takes particular advantage of individuals with an immune compromise) may herald the clinical onset of an immune-compromising disease. It is therefore quite important to be able to match an organism with the list of illnesses associated with the corresponding immune defect.

## Case 14: Hematuria in an Egyptian-born man

This 34-year-old man had always enjoyed good health. Several months before this visit he began to notice gross hematuria (he could see blood in his urine). The hematuria was unaccompanied by fever, pain, or burning on urination or by any increased sense of urgency to void. He had not had unexplained weight loss.

Born in Cairo, Egypt, he spent his childhood summers on his grandparents' farm in the Nile Delta. He recalled swimming in the Nile twice, the last time when he was in his early 20s. He finished college in Egypt and was well enough to complete military service there. His only infirmity was loss of vision in his right eye since childhood, for reasons unknown to the patient. He had not been back to Egypt since entering the United States ten years before the onset of the hematuria. He was working as a computer technician. There was no history of exposure to toxins either at work or during recreational activities.

The physical examination was completely within normal limits, except for a red opacity of the lens of the right eye, which was blind. His hemoglobin, 13.5 g/dl, was just below the lower limit of normal of 14. The rest of the laboratory studies were all normal.

Because of concern that the hematuria might herald a malignancy, the patient underwent fiberoptic cystoscopy (an examination that directly visualizes the inside of the urinary bladder). A mass was noted in the fundus of the bladder, biopsy of which is shown in Figure 34.27.

34.19 The part of the history that is most specifically connected with the diagnosis of infection with *Schistosoma haematobium* is which of the following?

 A. The presence of gross hematuria

 B. The patient's origin in Egypt

 C. Swimming in the Nile

 D. Concurrent blindness

 E. The mild anemia (hemoglobin 13.5 g/dl)

The correct answer is **C** (swimming in the Nile). *Schistosoma haematobium* is a fluke that requires a very specific snail to complete its life cycle. This snail is found only in certain bodies of water in Africa, most notably the Nile River. **A** (gross hematuria) is a symptom that results from the propensity of *S. haematobium* to invade bladder veins, where adult flukes lay their eggs. However, gross hematuria may occur with many conditions, and thus is not as specifically connected with *S. haematobium* infec-

**Figure 34.27**
Biopsy of the urinary bladder shows areas of inflammation, some containing an ovum with a terminal spine. The presence of this spine at the end of the ovum ("terminal" spine) identifies *Schistosoma haematobium*.

tion as is exposure to the snail vector caused by swimming in the Nile. **B** (being from Egypt) is of itself not enough to suspect schistosomiasis, since Egyptians who have not swum in water that is infested with the specific snail vector are not at risk of acquiring this parasite. **D** (blindness) is part of another parasitic infection associated with fresh water, onchocerciasis ("River blindness"). The roundworm *Onchocerca volvulus* is transmitted to humans by the bite of the black fly, which frequents the fresh water rapids of certain rivers, including some in Africa. **E** (anemia) is part of many disease processes and so is not necessarily a hint to the diagnosis of *S. haematobium* infection.

A person from the Nile Valley who has gross hematuria should be suspected of having infection with *S. haematobium* regardless of what other diagnoses may need to be entertained by the rest of the history. The fluke's life cycle illustrates why this is true. Infected humans inevitably excrete *S. haematobium* eggs in their urine, which finds its way into the water. Once thus excreted, these eggs develop into a very motile form called a miracidium that "homes in" on the intermediate host, which is a snail. In the snail, the fluke metamorphoses into a form called a cercaria, which swims freely in the water, waiting to penetrate the intact skin of a person who may be swimming or wading in this water. Once in the human, *S. haematobium* develops into adults, which migrate to the veins of the vesical plexus around the bladder. The female lays eggs, which create an inflammatory response that leads to bleeding, which is perceived by the infected individual as gross hematuria. The passage of these eggs, in urine, into water inhabited by the correct species of snail, completes the life cycle.

This patient was treated with praziquantel, a potent drug that is effective against a number of helminths, including schistosoma species. His hematuria resolved, and repeat cystoscopy revealed resolution of the infective process. He was warned not to swim in the Nile if he should return to Egypt.

## Case 15: Multisystem illness with skin changes

This 35 year-old man was well fifteen days prior to admission, when he underwent a right inguinal hernia repair. His subsequent course was uneventful until the fifth post-operative day. On that day he developed fever, chills, and diarrhea consisting of 5 to 6 watery stools per day. The diarrhea was accompanied by nausea and vomiting. There was no abdominal pain. These gastrointestinal symptoms lasted for four days, and were accompanied by what the patient described as total anuria (the complete suppression of urinary secretion by the kidneys). He also reported what he perceived to be delusions, especially when trying to fall asleep at night. At about the same time he developed generalized erythroderma (redness of the skin that blanches when the red areas are pressed), which lasted a few days. His wife, a nurse, observed petechiae (pinpoint intracutaneous hemorrhages) on his lower legs. With all of these symptoms, he refused to consider visiting a physician.

One week after the onset of the fever his herniorrhaphy wound opened and sersanguineous (mixed blood and serum) fluid began to ooze from it. He continued to feel malaise. The day prior to admission he was seen by his surgeon, who began treatment with oral tetracycline (because of a history of serious allergy to β-lactam drugs, manifest as urticaria). However, because of the severity of his symptoms and because of abnormal blood tests, he was admitted to the hospital the next day.

The temperature was 100.8°F, the pulse regular at 90 per minute, and the blood pressure 130/75. The herniorrhaphy wound was open, with tender, indurated (hardened), erythematous (red, with blanching on pressure) margins. Serosanguineous material was oozing from it.

After debridement of his wound and one day of treatment with clindamycin and tobramycin, he noted distinct improvement in his sense of well-being His temperature fell to normal. Intravenous clindamycin was continued for a total of seven days, followed by another three days orally. On about the fifth hospital day, sixteen days after the onset of his fever, he noted peeling of the skin of the palmar surfaces of his thumbs. This was followed, over the next three days, by generalized desquamation of the skin of his hands and knees, and, to a lesser extent, his feet (Figure 34.28).

34.20 An organism grew from the serosanguineous wound drainage, but not from the blood cultures. From the list below, the most likely organism to cause this constellation of clinical and laboratory findings is:

   A. *Escherichia coli*

   B. *Neisseria gonorrheae*

   C. *Pseudomonas aeruginosa*

   D. *Staphylococcus aureus*

   E. *Clostridium perfringens*

**Figure 34.28**
Desquamation of skin (knee).

The correct answer is D (Staphylococcus aureus). This patient has a classical presentation of the staphylococcal toxic shock syndrome (see below). There is nothing specific about this patient to suggest that A (E. coli) has caused his illness, and that organism would be somewhat unusual as a cause of a cutaneous wound infection in an otherwise healthy person. The skin lesions of B (N. gonorrheae) are isolated pustules, not desquamation, and these are associated with infection that is disseminated through the bloodstream, which is often accompanied by positive blood cultures. C (P. aeruginosa) is incorrect also because this organism is not associated with desquamation. The skin lesion that may suggest P. aeruginosa is a necrotic area called ecthyma gangrenosum. While E (C. perfringens) is associated with a skin manifestation, this is gas gangrene, and involves both muscle and skin.

S. aureus can elaborate a number of pyrogenic exotoxins called superantigens. These include toxic shock syndrome toxin-1 (TSST-1) and staphylococcal entertoxins. These superantigens bypass the usual activation of the immune system, with activation of a very large percentage of T cells, with massive release of cytokines. This results in a shock state similar to that from endotoxin. This patient had fever, diffuse erythroderma, and involvement of his liver (elevated transaminase and alkaline phosphatase), blood (anemia and very high white blood cell count that was out of proportion to the inflammation of his wound—which did not have purulent drainage), kidneys (elevated creatinine that was not corrected with hydration), diarrhea, and abnormal mental status. His platelet count was probably low at the time that he was noted to have petechiae, further evidence of a transient blood dyscrasia. And his wound grew out S. aureus which was later shown to produce staphylococcal enterotoxin B.

Staphylococcal toxic shock syndrome gained notoriety in the early 1980's, with its association with the use of super-absorbency tampons. However, the syndrome was first described in children with staphylococcal osteomyelitis, and, with the withdrawal of super-absorbency tampons from the commercial market, non-menstrual staphylococcal toxic shock syndrome is much more common than that associated with menstrual products. The reduced inflammation of the wound is probably from the TSST-1 itself, which interferes with migration of phagocytic cells into the wound. Desquamation of skin during convalescence is also a characteristic of staphylococcal toxic shock syndrome.

## Case 16: Diarrhea acquired in South America

This 18 year-old woman was admitted to the hospital seven days after the onset of severe diarrhea. Always in good health, the patient had emigrated to the United States from Ecuador several years earlier. She returned to her native country to enter a university in the capital. About eight days prior to admission she ate in a restaurant. All who were with her ate fish, as she did; but she was the only one who ate fresh vegetables.

Two days later she developed severe watery diarrhea, passing voluminous stool several times per day. Two days after that she began to vomit. These symptoms persisted until her departure for the United States a few days later. She described her stools as "rice water." At no time did she experience fever or chills.

When she was examined, her temperature was 98.4°F, her blood pressure low at 88/50, and her pulse was 72 per minute. Her skin was dry, with decreased turgor. Her eyes appeared to be sunken into their orbits and her oral mucosal surfaces were dry. The remainder of the physical examination was within normal limits.

The hemoglobin was 15.8 g/dL (normal 12-18 g/dL), the white blood cell count 16,300/mL (normal to 10,000). A specimen of arterial blood revealed the pH to be 7.32 (normal 7.40), the $PO_2$ 103 torr (normal), and the $PCO_2$ 25.4 torr (abnormally low). The blood urea nitrogen was 36 mg/dL and the serum creatinine 3.1 mg/dL (normal about 1.0). The concentration of bicarbonate in venous blood was 14 mEq/L (normal 22 – 28). Wright stain of stool revealed no leukocytes. The stool was negative for occult blood.

34.21 Culture of stool yielded an organism. The most likely organism to cause this illness, taking into consideration all of the clinical and laboratory data, is:

A. Escherichia coli O157:H7

B. Salmonella typhi

C. Clostridium difficile

D. Shigella sonnei

E. Vibrio cholerae

The correct answer is E (Vibrio cholerae). It causes disease by elaborating a toxin that greatly increased in influx of ions and water into the lumen of the intestine. As a

secretory, and non-inflammatory diarrhea, it is not characterized by fecal leukocytes or blood. A (E. coli O157:H7) causes hemorrhagic colitis, with copious stool as this patient had; but patients with this infection usually have very bloody stools. The reservoir is beef, and not fish or vegetables. B (S. typhi) causes enteric fever (this patient was never febrile) and when there is diarrhea, it is often preceded by constipation. It is an inflammatory process, so that there are fecal leukocytes. C (C. difficile) usually, but not always, causes disease in relation to health care, especially during or after administration of antibiotics. The associated diarrhea is intensely inflammatory, with very numerous fecal leukocytes. D (Shigella sonnei) is also a cause of extremely inflammatory diarrhea, with so many fecal leukocytes that pus may be visible in stool without magnification.

This patient had moderately severe cholera. It had been absent from the Western Hemisphere for some 70 years, until the early 1990's, when it entered Peru in shipments of fish from Asia. Once introduced to an area in which safe drinking water was not widely available, it spread, over the next few years, throughout South and Central America. This patient violated a cardinal rule of food safety in the developing world by eating uncooked vegetables. (V. cholerae persists in nature in aquatic environments; when contaminated, uncooked water is consumed, infection is transmitted. It is almost impossible to avoid infection when fresh vegetables, that have been either irrigated or rinsed with contaminated water, are consumed.) Because cholera is a toxin-mediated non-inflammatory process, constitutional symptoms such as fever are uncommon. Stool volume may be so great that it may be difficult to keep up with fluid losses. For this patient, dehydration was so severe that she had mild renal failure, with a creatinine of 3.1 mg/dL. Her acid-base balance was affected as well, perhaps in part by the renal failure, which causes metabolic acidosis. However, it is more likely that her metabolic acidosis was caused not by accumulation of hydrogen ions, but rather by extreme bicarbonate losses. Stool is alkaline, and when there is massive, prolonged diarrhea such as that experienced by this patient, the result can be metabolic acidosis, just as this patient had.

Among the various ways to categorize diarrhea, one that is useful clinically is inflammatory and non-inflammatory. A simple, inexpensive screening test is the microscopic examination of stool for leukocytes. When they are present, diarrhea is described as "inflammatory" and when they are absent it is "non-inflammatory." Four of the five proposed answers in this case discussion are causes of inflammatory diarrhea. The absence of fecal leukocytes virtually ruled them out. The epidemiologic setting, and the large volumes of watery stool, further supported the diagnosis of a non-inflammatory diarrhea, such as cholera. The links to South America and to fresh vegetables added credence to this diagnosis. This patient illustrates the importance of the history in making a clinical-microbiological correlation.

She was treated with doxycycline and intravenous hydration. She rapidly recovered and returned to university in Ecuador—after reinforcement of her understanding of safe food practices there.

# Review Questions

# 35

## Choose the ONE best answer

35.1 Which one of the following is the most common cause of infections associated with prosthetic heart valves, intravenous catheters, and intracranial shunts?

   A. *Escherichia coli*

   B. *Streptococcus pyogenes*

   C. *Pseudomonas aeruginosa*

   D. *Staphylococcus epidermidis*

   E. *Actinomyces israelii*

> Correct answer = D. *Staphylococcus epidermidis* is a gram-positive, coagulase-negative, novobiocin-sensitive bacterium. It is the most common cause of infections involving prosthetic devices. Other infections caused by *Staphylococcus epidermidis* include infective endocarditis in intravenous drug users, infection of intravenous peritoneal dialysis catheters and intracranial shunts, and urinary tract infections. *Escherichia coli*, *Pseudomonas aeruginosa*, *Actinomyces israelii*, and *Streptococcus pyogenes* are not commonly associated with any of the above infections.

35.2 The most common bacterial infection associated with intravenous drug abuse is

   A. skin and soft tissue infections

   B. osteomyelitis

   C. infective endocarditis

   D. embolic strokes that produce cerebral abscesses

   E. pneumonia

> Correct answer = A. The high incidence of skin and soft tissue infections is caused by many factors, including "skin popping" (injecting drugs subcutaneously); escape of drugs into soft tissue intravenous injection by extravasation; presence of adulterants in the injection material; sharing contaminated needles; and the presence of pathogenic organisms on the skin. Group A streptococci and *Staphylococcus aureus* are the most commonly isolated organisms.

35.3 Which of the following is more likely a feature of atypical pneumonia rather than a pneumonia caused by *Streptococcus pneumoniae*?

   A. High fever

   B. Nonproductive cough

   C. Gram-positive sputum stain

   D Sudden onset

   E. Rust-colored sputum

> Correct answer is B. *Mycoplasma pneumoniae* is the most common cause of atypical pneumonia. Atypical pneumonia is characterized by low-grade fever; an insidious onset; constitutional symptoms such as malaise, headache, and anorexia; a nonproductive cough; a gram-negative sputum stain; a patchy, interstitial infiltrate on a chest radiograph; and myalgias and arthralgias. *Streptococcus pneumoniae* (Pneumococcus) pneumonia would most likely present with sudden onset; chills and high fever; a gram-positive sputum stain; a parenchymal or lobar consolidation on a chest radiograph; and a cough that produces rust-colored sputum. Pneumococcus is the most common cause of community acquired pneumonia.

35.4 Bacteria with tumbling "end-over-end" motility are isolated from the cerebrospinal fluid of a 2-day-old infant with meningitis. This organism is likely to be

   A. *Escherichia coli*

   B. β-Hemolytic streptococcus

   C. *Listeria monocytogenes*

   D. *Haemophilus influenzae*

   E. *Neisseria meningitidis*

Correct answer = C. *Listeria monocytogenes*, a short, gram-positive rod, has an unusual tumbling "end-over-end" motility at 22°C, but not at 37°C. This property is useful in laboratory diagnosis because it rapidly differentiates the organism from all other gram-positive rods. In addition, the organisms produce a small zone of β-hemolysis around and under colonies grown on blood agar. *Listeria monocytogenes* can cause perinatal listeriosis. When symptoms are manifested early, the organisms are thought to have been transmitted *in utero*. In the early-onset syndrome, the infants are either born dead or die shortly after delivery. The late-onset syndrome is manifested as meningitis within the first 3 weeks after delivery. Adults, especially those who are immunocompromised, can occasionally develop meningoencephalitis and bacteremia caused by the organisms. The organisms are believed to be acquired primarily by ingestion of contaminated foods. Recent outbreaks of listeriosis have been linked to raw vegetables, raw and pasteurized milk (the milk was contaminated after pasteurization), and cole slaw. The organisms can invade and multiply within intestinal epithelial cells, as well as in phagocytes. The presence of neutrophils, low glucose, and increased protein in cerebrospinal fluid is suggestive of a bacterial etiology.

35.5 Dysphonia (changes in the voice) in a 2-year-old child with a grayish exudate in the posterior pharynx and massive, tender cervical lymphadenitis is most likely caused by

A. *Corynebacterium diphteriae*
B. *Neisseria meningitidis*
C. Group A streptococcus
D. *Propionibacterium* species
E. *Erysipelothrix rhusiopathiae*

Correct answer = A. *Corynebacterium diphteriae*, an aerobic gram-positive rod, is the cause of diphtheria. A hallmark feature of the disease is the development of a grayish "pseudomembrane" over the tonsils, larynx, and pharynx, which can obstruct breathing and cause cyanosis (a bluish color of skin and mucous membranes due to excessive concentration of deoxygenated haemoglobin in the blood). The membrane is not a true membrane. It consists of fibrin, red and white blood cells, and the organisms. It is deeply embedded and attempts to remove it may cause extensive

bleeding. Intubation or tracheostomy may be required to prevent suffocation. Children with the disease often have dysphonia or difficulty in speaking. *Corynebacterium diphtheriae* secretes a potent toxin, which is absorbed into the mucous membranes of the respiratory tract. This toxin causes inflammation, sore throat, and fever. Difficulty in breathing (dyspnea) and prostration follow shortly thereafter. Damage to the heart may occur, leading to cardiac arrhythmia. It may also cause problems with vision, speech, and swallowing. Some individuals may experience difficulty in moving arms or legs. These manifestation generally subside spontaneously.

35.6 An 8-year-old girl presents to the emergency room with high fever, nuchal rigidity (stiff neck), widespread ecchymoses (effusion of blood beneath the skin) scattered over her body, and clinical evidence of hypovolemic shock. A spinal tap reveals increased neutrophils, increased protein, and low glucose. The patient has diffuse bleeding from all venipuncture and intravenous sites. She dies 24 hours later. An autopsy reveals bilateral adrenal hemorrhage and a purulent meningitis. Which of the following results would be expected from the Gram stain of cerebrospinal fluid collected in the emergency room?

A. Gram-positive diplococci
B. Gram-negative rods
C. Gram-negative cocci in clumps
D. Gram-positive rods
E. Gram-negative diplococci

Correct answer = E. The child has the Waterhouse-Friderichsen syndrome, which is most commonly secondary to *Neisseria meningitidis* septicemia. This syndrome is characterized by: meningitis, septicemia, ecchymoses (effusion of blood beneath the skin), oozing of blood from puncture sites (disseminated intravascular coagulation), and hypovolemic shock secondary to acute adrenal insufficiency from bilateral adrenal hemorrhage. *Neisseria meningitidis* first colonizes the posterior nasopharynx. From this location, it enters the bloodstream and disseminates throughout the body. Meningitis is usually secondary to septicemia. Sepsis is a precipitating factor for disseminated intravascular coagulation.

35.7 A 45-year-old tourist returned from a trip to South America and abruptly began having cramps and diarrhea. The watery bowel movements came rapidly, one after another, and contained small bits of grayish-white stool. The man was sweaty and nauseated. Upon admission to the hospital, 2 liters of fluid were administered intravenously, which was supplemented by oral fluid. The patient was discharged 48 hours after admission. A gram-negative rod with the O1 antigen was isolated. Which of the following organisms produces these symptoms?

A. *Vibrio cholerae*
B. *Vibrio parahaemolyticus*
C. *Campylobacter jejuni*
D. *Campylobacter fetus*
E. *Helicobacter pylori*

Correct answer = A. The tourist is most likely to have been infected with *Vibrio cholerae.* Following an incubation period of approximately 1 to 4 days, the onset of symptoms (nausea, vomiting, diarrhea, and abdominal cramps) is abrupt. Stools, which contain large numbers of vibrios, epithelial cells, and flecks of mucus, have the appearance of rice water (that is, the grayish-white stool in the case history). In severe cases, massive amounts of fluid, sometimes 15 to 20 liters per day, can be lost, which leads to profound dehydration, electrolyte imbalance, anuria, (the complete suppression of urinary secretion by the kidneys) and circulatory collapse. *V. cholerae* is not invasive. After ingestion, it attaches to the microvilli of the brush border of the intestinal tract and secretes the cholera toxin. *V. cholerae* are spread by direct contact with an infected person and by contaminated water, food, and flies. The organisms are naturally pathogenic only for humans.

Correct answer = D. *Salmonella typhimurium* is the most common cause of enterocolitis in the United States. Many salmonellae, but not shigellae, produce $H_2S$ in media containing an inorganic sulfur source (for example, triple sugar iron agar). The symptoms and the course of the disease as described in the case history are typical for enterocolitis, but not for enteric fever, which is a life-threatening systemic illness caused by *Salmonella typhi*. Enterocolitis caused by *Salmonella* is an infection of the colon that usually begins approximately 18 to 24 hours after ingestion of the organisms. Diarrhea, fever, and abdominal pain are typical for the disease. Most cases are thought to go unreported, because the infection is usually not severe and is self-limiting within approximately 2 to 3 days. Dehydration and electrolyte imbalance are the major threats. The salmonella organisms associated with enterocolitis have been recovered from milk (including ice cream and cheeses), shellfish, dried or frozen eggs, poultry, beef, and water contaminated with feces. Meat products can be contaminated by animal fecal material during slaughter. Undercooling and improper storage at warm temperatures allow the organisms to proliferate to large numbers. Temperatures above 140°F will kill the organisms. The source of the Salmonella at the picnic could have been the potato salad, the chicken, or the hamburgers. Ingestion of a relatively large number of Salmonella is required in order for symptoms to appear. Dogs, pet turtles, and other cold-blooded animals can carry the organisms for extended periods of time. There are now restrictions on the import and sale of turtles in pet shops. Salmonella infections cause three distinct diseases: enterocolitis, enteric fever (typhoid fever), and septicemia.

35.8 An all-day family reunion was held on a summer day when the temperature soared to 103°F. The picnic food included potato salad, chicken, and hamburgers. The next morning, five family members experienced diarrhea, fever, and abdominal pain, which lasted for several days. One person was eventually hospitalized, and gram-negative $H_2S$-producing rods were isolated from the stool. Which of the following bacteria was most likely the cause?

A. *Shigella dysenteriae*
B. *Shigella sonnei*
C. *Shigella flexneri*
D. *Salmonella typhimurium*
E. *Salmonella typhi*

35.9 A 4-year-old child attending a day care center developed abdominal pain, a low-grade fever, and watery diarrhea. The next day his condition became worse and the mother took him to a pediatrician. Microscopic examination of the stool revealed the presence of numerous red and white blood cells and mucus. Blood cultures were negative, but a lactose negative, nonmotile gram-negative rod was isolated from the stool. Which of the following is the most likely causative organism?

A. *Escherichia coli*
B. *Enterobacter* species
C. *Klebsiella* species
D. *Salmonella typhi*
E. *Shigella sonnei*

Correct answer = E. The most likely causative organism is *Shigella sonnei*. Shigella should be suspected when a nonmotile, gram-negative rod that does not ferment lactose is isolated from a case of diarrhea. An important additional clue in the case history is the presence of blood in the stool. Shigellosis is a bacillary dysentery typified by the presence of blood and mucus in the stool. The organisms are capable of local invasion. They infect epithelial cells lining the intestinal tract, multiply within their cytoplasm, and spread to adjacent cells. Microabscesses form in the large intestine and terminal ileum, leading to necrosis, ulceration, and bleeding. Granulation and scar tissue may form at the ulcerative sites as the infection subsides. Shigellae almost never invades the blood circulation, unlike *Salmonella typhi* (a motile, lactose-negative rod), which does so routinely. *Escherichia coli*, *Enterobacter*, and *Klebsiella* are lactose positive. Shigella is transmitted from person-to-person via the "four Fs": food, fingers, feces, and flies. There are no known animal reservoirs. The organisms are highly contagious. Approximately one-half of all Shigella-positive stool cultures are from children under the age of 10 years. The incubation period is short (that is, only 1 to 2 days). Shigella dysentery produces a heat-labile exotoxin that acts as a neurotoxin, as well as an enterotoxin. Its action as a neurotoxin is associated with rectal spasms, pain and excitation in the meningocortical region of the brain, and coma. Shigella dysentery is not prevalent in the United States. It is found in individuals returning from countries where the organisms are more common.

Correct answer = C. Brucellosis is also known as undulant fever. Thus the daily periodicity of fever and chills is an important clue. Undulation of the fever is seen primarily with *Brucella melitensis*, which is found in goats and sheep. In addition, the slow insidious onset of symptoms and granulomatous lesions in the liver are classic manifestations. Farmers, veterinarians, and abatoir (slaughterhouse) workers are at greatest risk. The other two major species involved in human infections are *Brucella abortis* (cattle) and *Brucella suis* (swine). Brucella is transmitted primarily by direct contact with tissues of infected animals or by ingestion of raw, unpasteurized milk (and cheeses that are made from the milk). Aerosol transmission has been documented in meat-packing plants. The organisms can remain viable in dry soil for 40 to 60 days. Person-to-person transmission is rare. Brucellae are intracellular parasites. In animals, Brucella can cause contagious abortion. The organisms may be carried for years and shed in the milk of apparently healthy hosts. They localize in the mammary glands and in the pregnant uterus. Other animals who eat, or even lick, aborted fetuses can become infected. Brucellae are highly invasive. *Francisella tularensis*, *Salmonella typhi*, and *Mycobacterium bovis* are unlikely to be correct because the case history does not fit the diseases caused by these organisms. Most infections with brucellae remain asymptomatic; however, after an incubation period of 1 to 6 weeks, the disease may be acute, subacute, or chronic.

35.10 A previously healthy, 53-year-old sheep farmer is admitted to the hospital. Two months prior to admission, he developed swollen lymph nodes and myalgia. Approximately one week prior, he began having daily fevers, chills, and night sweats. Blood cultures were positive for a bacterium after prolonged incubation. Histologic examination of a liver biopsy revealed the presence of noncaseating granulomatous lesions. Which of the following microorganisms is the most likely cause?

A. *Francisella tularensis*
B. *Salmonella typhi*
C. *Brucella melitensis*
D. *Brucella canis*
E. *Mycobacterium bovis*

35.11 A gram-negative rod is isolated from the sputum of a 22-year-old woman who is hospitalized with cystic fibrosis. Laboratory tests show that the bacterium is aerobic and does not ferment glucose or any other sugar. The bacaterium is highly resistant to numerous antibiotics. The organism is most likely

A. *Escherichia coli*
B. *Klebsiella pneumoniae*
C. *Mycoplasma pneumoniae*
D. *Pseudomonas aeruginosa*
E. *Mycobacterium*

Correct answer = D. *Pseudomonas aeruginosa* is an aerobic, gram-negative rod that does not ferment glucose or any other sugar; thus, it is known as a "nonfermenter"; The organisms colonize within the respiratory tract of patients with cystic fibrosis and other chronic respiratory tract diseases. Respiratory diseases caused by the organisms range from relatively benign tracheobronchitis to severe necrotizing bronchopneumonia. *P. aeruginosa* is a ubiquitous, opportunistic pathogen. In addition to its involvement in the respiratory tract, it is associated with other nosocomial infections. In debilitated individuals, it can cause bacteremia, particularly in patients with diabetes, extensive burns, hematologic malignancies, or neutropenia; endocarditis; and urinary tract infections. Ear infections caused by the organisms include external otitis ("swimmer's ear") and malignant external otitis. *P. aeruginosa* is hardy and can grow in environments that are often hostile to other bacteria. It has few nutritional requirements and survives extremes of temperature. In hospitals, it can often be isolated from respiratory therapy equipment, sinks, water, bed pans, and floors. *Escherichia coli* and *Klebsiella pneumoniae* ferment glucose, and *Mycoplasma pneumoniae* and *Mycobacterium* species are not gram-negative rods.

35.12  A 49-year-old woman is bitten by her cat on the dorsal aspect of her right index finger at 8:00 A. M. By 4:30 P. M. she has a temperature of 38°C, and the finger and the dorsum of her right hand are red, swollen, and painful. An oxidase- and catalase-positive, gram-negative rod with bipolar staining is recovered from an aspirate of the abscess on her finger. The organism most likely responsible is

A. *Brucella canis*
B. *Pasteurella multocida*
C. *Haemophilus influenzae*
D. *Francisella tularensis*
E. *Yersinia pseudotuberculosis*

Correct answer = B. *Pasteurella multocida* is probably the most common bacteria that is isolated from wounds inflicted by cat bites, and to a lesser extent, dog bites. It is found worldwide in the upper respiratory tract of many domestic and wild animals. *P. multocida* causes a local cellulitis at the site of the bite, which evolves rapidly. Complications are common and include osteomyelitis of the underlying bone, necrotizing synovitis (inflammation of the synovial membrane), and suppurative arthritis. More than 90% of cellulitis cases that do not involve animal bites are caused by *Staphylococcus aureus* and group A streptococci. *Haemophilus influenzae* type B is an important cause of cellulitis in children.

35.13 A 35-year-old man who enjoys hunting jackrabbits has a sudden onset of headache, fever, chills, and swollen lymph nodes. He also experiences nausea, vomiting, and abdominal discomfort. A painful papule on his left hand heals over a period of about 6 weeks, and his lymphadenopathy subsides approximately 4 months later. No microorganisms are seen in lymph node aspirates, and routine blood cultures are negative. Which of the following organisms is the most likely causative agent?

A. *Yersinia pestis*
B. *Yersinia enterocolitica*
C. *Francisella tularensis*
D. *Pasteurella multocida*
E. *Brucella melitensis*

Correct answer = C. This patient's case is a typical presentation of ulceroglandular tularemia caused by *Francisella tularensis*. The ulceroglandular form of this disease, which is acquired by direct contact with tissues of infected animals (for example, jackrabbits, muskrats, squirrels), represents approximately 75% of tularemia cases in the United States. Systemic symptoms appear abruptly, and an ulcerating papule at the entry site of the organisms develops within 2 to 6 days. Regional lymph nodes may become extremely large, painful, and necrotic. Convalescence from tularemia is slow, and lymphadenopathy often persists for several months. *F. tularensis* is highly infectious. The organisms are very small, pleomorphic, intracellular gram-negative rods. Because of these characteristics, they are rarely observed in clinical specimens.

35.14 An elderly patient is placed on ampicillin and develops acute diarrhea with blood and mucus accompanied by fever and leukocytosis. Which one of the following organisms is the most likely cause of this patient's diarrhea?

A. *Staphylococcus aureus*
B. *Streptococcus pyogenes*
C. *Clostridium difficile*
D. *Clostridium perfringens*
E. *Bacillus cereus*

Correct answer = C. *Clostridium difficile* causes antibiotic-associated pseudomembranous enterocolitis. *C. difficile* is a part of the normal flora of the gastrointestinal tract in approximately 3% of the general population. When broad-spectrum antimicrobials (for example, ampicillin) are used, the drug-sensitive normal flora are killed. *C. difficile* is relatively resistant to many of these antibiotics, leading to bacterial overgrowth. It produces exotoxin A (an enterotoxin), which causes a watery diarrhea, and exotoxin B, a cytotoxin that damages the gut mucosa, leading to an accumulation of inflammatory cells and fibrin (pseudomembrane). Pseudomembranous enterocolitis is not an invasive enterocolitis. Although *Staphylococcus aureus* is also relatively resistant to broad-spectrum antibiotics and can cause diarrhea and fever, there is less damage to the gut mucosa. Blood loss and leukocytosis would not usually be observed, except in neonates. *C. perfringens* and *Bacillus cereus* can cause diarrhea, but the diarrhea is associated with food poisoning, not antibiotics. *Streptococcus pyogenes* does not cause diarrhea.

35.15 Which of the following diseases associated with anal intercourse causes visible but painless lesions in the anus or anal canal?

A. Human papillomavirus
B. *Treponema pallidum*
C. *Herpes genitalis*
D. *Neisseria gonorrhoeae*
E. Hepatitis A

Correct answer = B. The primary chancre of syphilis, caused by to *Treponema pallidum*, is visible on proctoscopic exam. However, the lesion commonly goes unnoticed, because it is painless. The patient may then progress into secondary syphilis. Human papillomavirus may produce condyloma acuminata (that is, veneral warts), squamous cell carcinoma in the anus, or both. Herpes genitalis causes visible vesicular lesions, which break down into painful ulcers in the perianal area. *Neisseria gonorrhoeae* produces an inflammatory proctitis as does *Chlamydia trachomatis*. Hepatitis A would have no visible lesions in the anus. However, it may be transmitted by anal intercourse, because the virus is shed in the stool.

35.16 Pathogenic bacteria enter the body by various routes, and entry mechanisms are critical for understanding the pathogenesis and transmissibility of each agent. Which one of the following is a correct association between a pathogen and its common entry mechanism?

A. *Neisseria meningitidis*—sexually transmitted entry
B. *Corynebacterium diphtheriae*—food-borne entry
C. *Rickettsia rickettsii*—entry by contamination of wound with soil
D. *Clostridium tetani*—inhalation entry
E. *Borrelia burgdorferi*—;arthropod vector-borne entry

Correct answer = E. *Borrelia burgdorferi* is spread by ticks and is the cause of Lyme disease. *Rickettsia rickettsii* also is usually spread by ticks. *Clostridium tetani* enters the body through wounds. *Neisseria meningitidis and Corynebacterium diphtheriae* both enter via the respiratory tract.

35.17 An executive in an office in Philadelphia has a window air conditioning unit that is a favorite roost for pigeons. She and her secretary both develop lung disease. What is the most likely causative agent?

A. *Candida albicans*
B. *Coccidioides immitis*
C. *Cryptococcus neoformans*
D. *Chlamydia trachomatis*
E. *Histoplasma capsulatum*

Correct answer = C. Pulmonary cryptococcosis can be caused by the inhalation of *Cryptococcus neoformans*, which grows abundantly in pigeon excretions. The birds are reservoirs for, but are not infected by, the fungus. Most cases of cryptococcosis are opportunistic infections in immunocompromised patients. In tissue, the yeast forms produce a granulomatous reaction if host immunity is intact, but no inflammatory reaction occurs if the host is immunocompromised. This is particularly true in the central nervous system (CNS). *Candida albicans*, *Coccidioides immitis*, *Chlamydia trachomatis*, and *Histoplasma capsulatum* are not associated with pigeon excreta.

35.18 A 44-year-old African-American woman presents to her physician in Tempe, Arizona, with the following symptoms: chest pain, fever, cough, and malaise. A few weeks ago this fourth-grade teacher took her class on a rock-hunting trip. A few of the students have also recently become ill. A chest radiograph showed hilar adenopathy, and a biopsy contained spherules. Which one of the following is the most likely diagnosis?

A. Candidiasis
B. Aspergillosis
C. Coccidioidomycosis
D. Histoplasmosis
E. Blastomycosis

Correct answer = C. Coccidioidomycosis is endemic to the American southwest and other arid climates. It is caused by the fungus *Coccidioides immitis*, which is found in soil. Often, several people may become infected when soil is disturbed and the dust carries the fungus. Symptoms include those common to other pulmonary diseases, as well as possible hypersensitivity reactions and dissemination to the central nervous system, skin, and joints. Frequently the disease is progressive in African Americans, Native Americans, and Filipinos. Infiltrates, hilar adenopathy, and pleural effusion may be been seen on radiograph, and spherules may be seen on biopsy. Candidiasis and aspergillosis are rare in immunocompetent people. Histoplasmosis is endemic to regions with moist soil, such as the Midwest. Blastomyces is also rare in the Southwest; it is more common in the Southeast, Midwest, and in men rather than in women.

35.19 Use of certain antibiotics (for example, tetracycline) may result in a disturbance of the normal flora of the mouth and subsequent predominance of which one of the following organisms?

A. *Haemophilus influenzae*
B. *Nocardia asteroides*
C. *Candida albicans*
D. *Treponema pallidum*
E. *Cryptococcus neoformans*

Correct answer = C. Opportunistic fungi fail to induce disease in most normal persons but may do so in those with impaired host defenses. *Candida albicans* causes thrush, vaginitis, and chronic mucocutaneous candidiasis. Considered to be part of the normal flora, candida infections are considered to be endogenous. Relative numbers of *C. albicans* are naturally kept to a low level by the overriding effort of normal bacterial flora being able to grow more quickly and compete more successfully for available nutrition. *C. albicans* is relatively resistant to broad spectrum antibiotics (for example, tetracycline) and may become the predominant organism after such use. *Nocardia asteroides*, *Treponema pallidum*, and *Cryptococcus neoformans* are not considered to be part of the normal flora.

35.20 An avid gardener developed a painless nodule in the finger that, over the ensuing weeks, spread up the arm, leaving a series of subcutaneous nodules. Some of these were draining pus. The most likely diagnosis in this patient is

A. mucormycosis
B. mycetoma
C. *Trichophyton rubrum* infection
D. *Trichophyton schoenleinii* infection
E. sporotrichosis

Correct answer = E. *Sporothrix schenckii* is a dimorphic fungus that lives on vegetation. Usually introduced into the skin by thorn puncture, it causes a local pustule or ulcer with nodules along the draining lymphatics. There is little systemic illness, but lesions may become chronic. Diagnosis is made by seeing round or cigar-shaped yeasts. Mycetoma occurs when soil organisms enter through wounds and cause abscesses, with pus discharged through sinuses. *Dermatophytoses* (*Trichophyton*) species infect only superficial keratinized structures. Mucor infections invade tissues of immunocompromised hosts. They proliferate in the walls of blood vessels and other tissues and result in necrosis.

35.21 A 9-month-old child develops a high fever associated with febrile convulsions. The fever ends abruptly after 3 days and is followed by a maculopapular rash. What is the most likely diagnosis?

A. Rubella

B. Rubeola

C. Roseola

D. Fifth disease

E. Varicella

Correct answer = B. [Note: rubella = German measles; rubeola = measles; fifth disease = erythema infectiosum; varicella = chickenpox.] Measles is accompanied by characteristic Koplik spots, which are bright red lesions with a white center that develop on the buccal mucosa. In a few days, the patient develops a generalized, blanching, erythematous maculopapular rash (viral-induced immune vasculitis), which begins at the hairline and extends down over the body. It gradually resolves with some desquamation over 1 or 2 weeks. Unlike German measles, rubeola is not associated with fetal congenital anomalies. The rubella virus is an RNA virus in the Togavirus family. It is the cause of German measles. It has an incubation period of 2 to 3 weeks. Painful lymphadenopathy, fever and malaise occur 5 to 10 days before the onset of the rash. The rash is maculopapular and, like rubeola, represents an immune complex-induced vasculitis. It begins on the face and progresses downwards to involve the extremities. The rash disappears in 3 days, thus the term "3 day measles". The immune complexes may produce a polyarthritis, particularly in adults. Rubella contracted during pregnancy produces teratogenic effects in the developing fetus, the most common of which is nerve deafness. Parvoviruses are the smallest of the DNA viruses. They produce erythema infectiosum, or fifth's disease, as well as a number of other disorders. Erythema infectiosum is characterized by a confluent rash usually beginning on the cheeks (slapped face appearance) which extends centripetally to involve the trunk. Varicella, or chickenpox, is primarily a childhood disease, whereas Herpes zoster, the cause of shingles, is due to reactivation of a latent varicella/zoster infection in the sensory ganglia. The incubation period of chickenpox is 14 to 16 days. The disease is highly contagious 2 days before the vesicles appear until the last lesion dries up. Varicella presents with generalized skin lesions, which begin as macules and progress into a vesicular and pustular stage. The rash spreads centrifu-

gally to the face and out to the extremities. Unlike smallpox (variola) vesicles which have the same appearance, varicella vesicles appear in varying stages of development as successive crops of lesions appear. Pneumonia is more likely to occur in adults and is the most common cause of death in the disease. It is frequently a fatal disease in immunocompromised patients.

35.22 A febrile 28-year-old heroin addict who is HIV positive presents with tachypnea and severe hypoxemia. The patient most likely has pulmonary disease caused by

A. *Streptococcus pneumoniae*

B. *Haemophilus influenzae*

C. *Mycoplasma pneumoniae*

D. *Pneumocystis jiroveci*

E. *Legionella pneumophila*

Correct answer = D. *Pneumocystis jiroveci* (formerly *Pneumocystis carinii*) is the classic opportunistic infectious agent associated with AIDS. At least one episode of *P. jiroveci* pneumonia occurs in approximately 75% of patients who do not receive prophylactic therapy. This fungus, which was formerly classified as a protozoan, was the leading cause of AIDS-related deaths before the development of effective drugs.

35.23 A 21-year-old male visits a sexually transmitted disease (STD) clinic with complaints of a purulent urethral discharge and dysuria. Pus cells, but no bacteria, are noted on the Gram stain examination of the exudate. Which of the following organisms are the most likely cause of this infection?

A. *Neisseria gonorrhoeae* and *Gardnerella vaginalis*

B. *Neisseria gonorrhoeae* and *Treponema pallidum*

C. *Haemophilus ducreyi* and *Neisseria gonorrhoeae*

D. *Ureaplasma urealyticum* and *Chlamydia trachomatis*

E. *Mycoplasma hominis* and *Neisseria gonorrhoeae*

Correct answer = D. The condition described is nongonococcal urethritis. Although *Neisseria gonorrhoeae* routinely causes urethritis in males, the gram-negative diplococci would be readily observed in a Gram stain examination of the exudate. The organisms are often found within white blood cells. Such observation would be sufficient to assume gonococcal infection and treatment. *Gardnerella vaginalis* is normally found in the female genitourinary tract and is associated with vaginitis. *Ureaplasma urealyticum* and *Chlamydae trachomatis* are the best choices for the described condition. The agents are quite small and would not be seen by microscopic examination. *Ureaplasma urealyticum* requires 10% urea for growth and is responsible for some cases of nongonococcal urethritis. *Chlamydae trachomatis*, however, probably causes the majority of such cases. *Mycoplasma hominis*, like *Ureaplasma*, lacks a cell wall. It is considered to be a normal flora organism that may be opportunistic, and is more often associated with disease in women than men. *Haemophilus ducreyi* is a sexually transmitted pathogen that causes chancroid (soft chancre). It is a small gram-negative rod that can be obtained from the chancroid lesion, which is a ragged ulcer on the genitalia accompanied by marked swelling and tenderness.

35.24 A midstream, "clean-catch" urine culture from an asymptomatic 24-year-old pregnant woman yields numerous bacteria that are lactose positive, motile, and susceptible to many common antibiotics. Which organism is most likely causing the infection?

A. *Serratia marcescens*
B. *Escherichia coli*
C. *Klebsiella pneumoniae*
D. *Pseudomonas aeruginosa*
E. *Proteus vulgaris*

Correct answer is B. *Escherichia coli* is the most common organism isolated from urinary tract infections. In young women, *E. coli* is involved in approximately 90% of these cases. The organisms are also the most common cause of gram-negative sepsis. Pyelonephritis (infection of the kidney) can be very painful and is among the most serious consequences of urinary tract infection. *Proteus vulgaris* is also a relatively common cause of urinary tract infections in patients with kidney stones or calculi (staghorn calculi). *Klebsiella pneumoniae* is an occasional cause. *Serratia marcescens* and *Pseudomonas aeruginosa* generally are associated with complicated urinary tract infections (that is, patients with structural abnormalities of the urinary tract) and other types of hospital-acquired infections.

35.25 A 25-year-old man complains of a urethral discharge and painful urination. A gram stain smear of the discharge shows many neutrophils but no bacteria. Of the following organisms, the one most likely to cause the discharge is

A. *Treponema pallidum*
B. *Neisseria gonorrhoeae*
C. *Candida albicans*
D. *Ureaplasma urealyticum*
E. *Staphylococcus aureus*

Correct answer = D. *Ureaplasma urealyticum* is one of several causes of nongonococcal urethritis in men. *Ureaplasma* can be distinguished from mycoplasma by its ability to produce the enzyme urease. The only other organism that could cause this man's symptoms is *Neisseria gonorrhoeae*; however, if *N. gonorrhoeae* were the causative agent, a gram stain of the urethral discharge would demonstrate gram-negative diplococci, often within white blood cells. *Treponema pallidum*, *Candida albicans*, and *Staphylococcus aureus* would be unlikely to cause nongonococcal urethritis.

35.26 Which organism listed below is regarded as the classic cause of atypical ("walking") pneumonia, characterized by an insidious onset, headache, nonproductive cough, and cold agglutinin formation?

A. *Chlamydia psittaci*
B. *Chlamydia trachomatis*
C. *Klebsiella pneumoniae*
D. *Mycoplasma pneumoniae*
E. *Streptococcus pneumoniae*

Correct answer = D. *Mycoplasma pneumoniae* infection is the classic cause of primary atypical pneumonia, characterized by an insidious onset, headache, nonproductive cough, and cold agglutinin formation. Immunity appears complete, but second episodes of the disease can occur. Autoantibodies against red blood cells (cold agglutinins) are produced, as well as antibodies against brain, lung, and liver cells. *M. pneumoniae* accounts for 5–10% of community pneumonias and is treated with erythromycin or doxycycline. *Chlamydia trachomatis* respiratory tract involvement is usually seen in 2- to 12-week-old infants. Infection is characterized by a paroxysmal cough, absence of fever, and eosinophilia. Radiographic examination may demonstrate lung consolidation and hyperinflation. Systemic erythromycin is an effective treatment. *Chlamydia psittaci* infections cause a patchy inflammation of the lungs in which consolidated areas are sharply demarcated. An exudate containing mononuclear cells is usually present. The sudden onset of illness in a person exposed to birds is suggestive of psittacosis, which presents with fever, anorexia, a sore throat, and severe headache. Tetracyclines are the drugs of choice. *Klebsiella pneumoniae* causes approximately 3% of bacterial pneumonias and produces an extensive hemorrhagic necrotizing consolidation of the lung. Sensitivity testing is necessary for effective antibacterial treatment. *Streptococcus pneumoniae* causes 75–80% of bacterial pneumonias and produces disease by multiplying in the lung. The polysaccharide capsule resists phagocytosis, and infection causes an outpouring of fibrinous edematous fluid into the alveoli, followed by red blood cells and leukocytes, resulting in consolidation of the lung. Eventually, antibody production against the capsules and mononuclear phagocytosis eliminate the infection. Expectoration of bloody sputum and a high fever are characteristic of early disease. Penicillins are the drugs of choice, but recently some resistance has been seen. None of these organisms, except M. pneumoniae, causes cold agglutinins to be formed.

35.27 A 68-year-old woman suddenly develops a fever of 38.2°C and a severe headache one evening. The following morning she also experiences a stiff neck and uncharacteristic drowsiness. At the emergency room, her temperature is 38. 8°C, and there is pain and resistance on flexion of her neck. The patient is noted to be mentally competent although lethargic. A cerebral spinal fluid sample is obtained by lumbar puncture. On the basis of the history and physical examination of this patient, what is the most probable diagnosis?

A. Viral meningitis
B. Fungal meningitis
C. Bacterial meningitis
D. Viral encephalitis
E. Brain abscess

Correct answer = C.

35.28 On the basis of the age of the patient described above, the probable etiologic agent is

A. *Staphylococcus aureus*
B. *Haemophilus influenzae*
C. *Streptococcus pneumoniae*
D. *Neisseria meningitidis*
E. none of the above

Correct answer = C. The findings of fever, headache, nuchal rigidity, and lethargy with an acute onset and the lack of dramatic neurologic manifestations suggest acute bacterial meningitis. Viral meningitis causes much of the same symptomatology, but the onset typically is more insidious and the patient usually is less acutely ill. Patients with viral encephalitis display the same general symptomatology as those with viral meningitis, but encephalitis is differentiated by dramatic neurologic manifestations and a much poorer prognosis. Fungal meningitis is more chronic and frequently is seen with other systemic signs of mycotic disease. Brain abscess usually is seen with other foci of infection, and the patient typically has deficits that reflect the location of the lesion. *Streptococcus pneumoniae* is the most common cause of bacterial meningitis among the elderly. *Haemophilus influenzae* type B is the most common cause of bacterial meningitis overall. Its incidence is highest in infants 6 to 12 months old and decreases with age; the incidence of meningitis caused by *H. influenzae* is low in adults. Meningococcal meningitis occurs primarily among young adults, and *Neisseria meningitidis* serogroups A, B, C, and Y cause most cases. *Staphylococcus aureus* occasionally causes meningitis but is a common cause of brain abscess.

"*See*" cross-references direct the reader to the synonymous term. "*See also*" cross-references direct the reader to related topics. [Note: Positional and configurational designations in chemical names (for example, "3-", "α-", "N-", "D-") are ignored in alphabetizing.]

# Figure Sources

**Fig. 2.1:** Courtesy of Bernard A. Cohen, MD, Christoph U. Lehmann, MD, DermAtlas, Johns Hopkins University.

**Fig. 4.1** Meridian Diagnostics, Inc, Cincinnati, Ohio.

**Fig. 4.1:** Forbes, B. A., Sahm, D. I. F., and Weissfeld, A. S. *Baily & Scott's Diagnostic Microbiology*. Mosby, Inc. 1988. Fig. 14-11, p. 200.

**Fig. 4.4:** Wistreich, G. *Microbiology Perspectives: A Photographic Survey of the Microbial World*. Prentice-Hall, Inc. 1999. Fig. 193, p. 86.

**Fig. 4.6:** Bottone, E. J., Girolami, R., and Stamm, J. M., *Schneierson's Atlas of Diagnostic Microbiology*, Ninth Edition, Abbott Laboratories, 1984, p. 49.

**Fig. 4.7:** Becton-Dickinson Microbiology Systems.

**Fig. 4.8:** Mahon, C. R. and Manuselis, G., *Textbook of Diagnostic Microbiology*, W. B. Saunders Company, 1995. Fig. 9-2A, p. 310.

**Fig. 4.9:** Alexander, S. K. and Strete, D. *Microbiology: A Photographic Atlas for the Laboratory*. Benjamin Cummings, 2001. Fig. 5.6, p. 71.

**Fig. 4.9:** Cappuccino, J. G. and Sherman, N., *Microbiology: A Laboratory Manual*, Fourth Edition, Benjamin/Cummings Publishing Company, Inc, 1996. Color plate 28.

**Fig. 4.9:** de la Maza, L. M., Pezzlo, M. T. and Baron, E. J., *Color Atlas of Diagnostic Microbiology, Mosby, 1997*. Fig. 8-16, p. 61.

**Fig. 4.9:** Forbes, B. A., Sahm, D. I. F., and Weissfeld, A. S. *Baily & Scott's Diagnostic Microbiology*. Mosby, Inc. 1988. Fig. 13.8, p. 173.

**Fig. 4.9:** Gillies, R.R. and Dodds, T.C., *Bacteriology Illustrated*, Third Edition, Williams and Wilkins Company, 1973, p. 41.

**Fig. 4.13:** Forbes, B. A., Sahm, D. I. F., and Weissfeld, A. S. *Baily & Scott's Diagnostic Microbiology*. Mosby, Inc. 1988. Fig. 15-6, p. 212.

**Fig. 6.10:** Lim, D. *Microbiology*, Second Edition. MCB/McGraw-Hill, 1998. Fig. 3.13, p. 55.

**Fig. 8.6:** Visuals Unlimited.

**Fig. 8.7:** Couresty of Dr. Gary E. Kaiser.

**Fig. 8.11:** Peters, G., Gray, E. D., and Johnson, G. M. in Bisno, A. L. and Waldvogel, F. A. *Infections Associated with Indwelling Medical Devices*. American Society for Microbiology, 1989. Fig. 1, p. 62.

**Fig. 8.12 (middle row, left):** Courtesy of The Canadian Infectious Diseases Society

**Fig. 8.12 (middle row, center):** Courtesy of Dr. John Bezzant.

**Fig. 8.12 (middle row, right):** Courtesy of Dr. John Bezzant.

**Fig. 8.12 (bottom row, left):** Costerton, J. W. and Lappin-Scott, H. M. ASM News 55

(12):653,

**Fig. 8.12 (bottom row, center):** Schenfeld, L. A. *N Engl J Med*. 342:1177 (2000).

**Fig. 8.12 (bottom row, right):** Courtesy of Dr. John Bezzant.

**Fig. 9.5:** Meltzer,D. L. and Kabongo, M. *American Family Physician*, July, 1997; pp. 145, 147.

**Fig. 9.10:** MacFaddin, J. F. *Biochemical Tests for Identification of Medical Bacteria*. Lippincott Williams & Wilkins, 2000. Fig. 3.1, p. 806.

**Fig. 9.10** Gillies, R.R. and Dodds, T.C., *Bacteriology Illustrated*, Third Edition, Williams and Wilkins Company, 1973, p. 58.

**Fig. 9.10:** Hart, T. and Shears, P., *Color Atlas of Medical Microbiology*, Mosby-Wolfe. 1996. Fig. 123, p. 97.

**Fig. 9.14:** Courtesy Dr. David Rayner, University of Alberta Lab Med & Pathology.

**Fig. 9.15 (top row, left):** Courtesy of Dr. Donna Duckworth.

**Fig. 9.15 (top row, right):** Courtesy of Dr. Donna Duckworth.

**Fig. 9.15 (bottom row, left):** Bisno, A. L. and Stevens, D. L., *N Engl J Med*. 334: (#4), 241 (1996).

**Fig. 9.15 (bottom row, middle):** Peterson, P. K. and Dahl, M. V., *Dermatologic Manifestations of Infectious Diseases*. The Upjohn Company, 1982. Fig. 48-1, p. 105.

**Fig. 9.15 (bottom row, right):** Mir, M. A., *Atlas of Clinical Diagnosis*, W. J. B. Saunders Company Ltd., 1995. Fig. 2.103; p. 86.

**Fig. 10.3:** 2000 Red Book: Report of the Committee on Infectious Diseases, American Academy of Pediatrics.

**Fig. 10.4:** Public Health Image Library, Centers for Disease Control and Prevention.

**Fig. 10.5 (left):** Alexander, S. K. and Strete, D. Microbiology: *A Photographic Atlas for the Laboratory*. Benjamin Cummings, 2001. Fig. 2.7, p. 13.

**Fig. 10.5 (right):** Courtesy Harriet CW Thompson, M.S., Department of Microbiology, Immunology &, Parasitology, Louisiana State University Health Sciences Center, New Orleans,

**Fig. 10.5 (bottom):** Farrar, W. E., Wood, M. J., Innes, J. A., Tubbs, H., *Infectious Diseases*. Second Edition, Gower Medical Publishing, 1992. Fig. 1.35. p. 1.11.

**Fig. 10.7 (upper left):** Bottone, E. J., Girolami, R., and Stamm, J. M., *Schneierson's Atlas of Diagnostic Microbiology*, Ninth Edition, Abbott Laboratories, 1984. p. 5.

**Fig. 10.7 (upper right):** Bottone, E. J., Girolami, R., and Stamm, J. M., *Schneierson's Atlas of Diagnostic Microbiology*, Ninth Edition, Abbott Laboratories, 1984. p. 5.

**Fig. 10.7 (bottom):** Public Health Image Library, Centers for Disease Control and Prevention.

**Fig. 11.2:** Bottone, E. J., Girolami, R., and Stamm, J. M., *Schneierson's Atlas of Diagnostic Microbiology*, Ninth Edition, Abbott Laboratories, 1984. p. 37.

**Fig. 11.2:** Sherris, J. C., Editor. *Medical Microbiology*, Second Edition, Appelton & Lange, 1990. Fig. 19.3, p. 349.

**Fig. 11.4:** Schaechter, M., Engleberg, N. C., Eisenstein, B. I., and Medoff, G. *Mechanism of Microbial Disease*, Third Edition. Williams and Wilkins, 1998. Fig. 14.6, p. 166.

**Fig. 11.5:** Hoeprich, P. D., Jordan, M. C. and Ronald, A. R., *Infectious Diseases, a Treatise of Infectious Processes*, Fifth Edition, J.B. Lippincott Company, Philadelphia, 1994. Fig. 70-6, p. 681.

**Fig. 11.7:** Bottone, E. J., Girolami, R., and Stamm, J. M., *Schneierson's Atlas of Diagnostic Microbiology*, Ninth Edition, Abbott Laboratories, 1984. p. 37.

**Fig. 11.8:** Images in Clinical Medicine. *N Engl J Med*, 336:707 (1997).

**Fig. 11.11:** Beeching, N.J. and Nye, F.J., *Diagnostic Picture Tests in Clinical Infectious Disease*, Mosby- Wolfe, 1996. Fig. 61, p. 33.

**Fig. 11.14 (left):** Bottone, E. J., Girolami, R., and Stamm, J. M., *Schneierson's Atlas of Diagnostic Microbiology*, Ninth Edition, Abbott Laboratories, 1984. p 37.

**Fig. 11.140 (right):** Bottone, E. J., Girolami, R., and Stamm, J. M., *Schneierson's Atlas of Diagnostic Microbiology*, Ninth Edition, Abbott Laboratories, 1984. p. 37.

**Fig. 11.14 (left, center row) :** McMilan, A. and Scott, G. R. *Sexually Transmitted Diseases*. Churchill Livingstone, 1991. Fig. 17, p. 12.

**Fig. 11.14 (right, center row):** Brown, T. J., Yen-Moore, A., and Tyring, S. K. *Journal of the American Academy of Dermatology*. Volume 41, Number 4. October 1999. Fig. 10.

**Fig. 12..5 (top, left):** Atlas, R. M. *Microorganisms in our World*. Mosby, 1995, p. 41.

**Fig. 12.7:** Wistreich, G. *Microbiology Perspectives: A Photographic Survey of the Microbial World*. Prentice-Hall, Inc. 1999. Fig. 131, p. 59.

**Fig. 12.8:** Koneman, E. W., Allen, S. D., Janda, W. M., Schreckenberger, P. C. and Winn, W. C., *Color Atlas and Textbook of Diagnostic Microbiology*, Fifth Edition, J. B. Lippincott Company, 1997. Plate 6-1A.

**Fig. 12.10 (left):** Koneman, E. W., Allen, S. D., Janda, W. M., Schreckenberger, P. C. and Winn, W. C., *Color Atlas and Textbook of Diagnostic Microbiology*, Fourth Edition, J. B. Lippincott Company, 1992. Plate 5-1A.

**Fig. 12.10 (right):** Varnam, A. H. and Evans, M. G. *Foodborne Pathogens*. Mosby-Yearbook, Inc. 1991. Fig. 170, p. 228.

**Fig. 12..12 (right):** Leboffe, M. J. and Pierce, B. E. *A Photographic Atlas for the Microbiology Laboratory*. Morton Publishing Company. 1999. Fig. 11-35, p.137.

**Fig. 12.14:** Copyright Dennis Kunkel Microscopy, Inc.

**Fig. 12.15:** Public Health Image Library, Centers for Disease Control and Prevention.

**Fig. 12.17 (top, left):** Leboffe, M.J. and Pierce, B. E. *A Photographic Atlas for the Microbiology Laboratory.* Morton Publishing Company. 1999. Fig. 11-21, p. 131.

**Fig. 12.17 (top, right):** Xia, H.X., Kean, C.T., and O'Morain. *European J. Clin. Microbiol. & Inf. Dis.* 13: 406 (1994).

**Fig. 12..17 (bottom):** Genta, R. M., and Graham, D. Y. *N Engl J Med.* 335:250 (Number 4) 1996.

**Fig. 13.2:** Musher, D. *J. Infectious Diseases,* 149:4, 4/84.

**Fig. 13.5 (left):** Quintiliani, R. and Bartlett, R. C., *Examination of the Gram-Stained Smear.* Hoffman-La Roche Inc., 1994. Fig. 7.

**Fig. 13.5 (bottom):** Farrar, W. E., Wood, M. J., Innes, J. A., Tubbs, H., *Infectious Diseases.* Second Edition, Gower Medical Publishing, 1992. Fig. 3.3, p. 3.4.

**Fig. 13.9 (upper left):** Alexander, S. K. and Strete, D. *Microbiology: A Photographic Atlas for the Laboratory.* Benjamin Cummings, 2001. Fig. 9.2, p. 123.

**Fig. 13.9 (upper right):** Koneman, E. W., Allen, S. D., Janda, W. M., Schreckenberger, p. C. and Winn, W. C., *Color Atlas and Textbook of Diagnostic Microbiology,* Fourth Edition, J. B. Lippincott Company, Philadelphia, 1992. Plate 7-2 E.

**Fig. 13.9 (bottom):** NIBSC/Science Photo Library/Photo Researcher, Inc.

**Fig. 13.11 (left):** Leboffe, M. J. and Pierce, B. E. *A Photographic Atlas for the Microbiology Laboratory.* Morton Publishing Company. 1999. Fig. 11-23, p. 132.

**Fig. 13.11 (right):** Koneman, E. W., Allen, S. D., Janda, W. M., Schreckenberger, P. C. and Winn, W. C., *Color Atlas and Textbook of Diagnostic Microbiology,* Fourth Edition, J. B. Lippincott Company, 1992. Plate 8-1 E.

**Fig. 13.11 (bottom):** Farrar, W. E., Wood, M. J., Innes, J. A., Tubbs, H., *Infectious Diseases.* Second Edition, Gower Medical Publishing, 1992. Fig. 2.29, p. 2.11

**Fig. 13.12:** Kassirer, J. P., *Images in Clinical Medicine,* Massachusetts Medical Society, 1997. p. 203.

**Fig. 13.15 (left):** Leboffe, M.J. and Pierce, B. E. *A Photographic Atlas for the Microbiology Laboratory.* Morton Publishing Company. 1999. Fig. 11-7, p. 124.

**Fig. 13.15 (right):** de la Maza, L. M., Pezzlo, M. T. and Baron, E. J., *Color Atlas of Diagnostic Microbiology, Mosby,* 1997. Fig. 9-18, p. 77.

**Fig. 13.16:** Volk, W. A., Gebhardt, B. M., Hammarskjold, M. and Kadner, R. J., *Essentials of Microbiology,* Fifth Edition, Lippincott-Raven, Philadelphia, 1996. Fig. 27-5, p 393.

**Fig. 13.17:** Courtesty of Dr. Sellers, Emory Uuniversity, Public Health Image Library,

Centers for Disease Control and Prevention.

**Fig. 13.18 (top, left):** Koneman, E. W., Allen, S. D., Janda, W. M., Schreckenberger, P. C. and Winn, W. C., *Color Atlas and Textbook of Diagnostic Microbiology,* Fifth Edition, J. B. Lippincott Company, 1997. Plate 8-3H.

**Fig. 13.18 (top, right):** Koneman, E. W., Allen, S. D., Janda, W. M., Schreckenberger, P. C. and Winn, W. C., *Color Atlas and Textbook of Diagnostic Microbiology,* Fourth Edition, J. B. Lippincott Company, 1992. Plate 7-2J.

**Fig. 13.18 (bottom):** Center for Disease Control, Atlanta.

**Fig. 13.20:** Wistreich, G. *Microbiology Perspectives: A Photographic Survey of the Microbial World.* Prentice-Hall, Inc. 1999. Fig. 140, p. 63.

**Fig. 13.21:** Leboffe, M. J. and Pierce, B. E. *A Photographic Atlas for the Microbiology Laboratory.* Morton Publishing Company. 1999. Fig. 11-44; p. 142.

**Fig. 13.23:** Hart, T. and Shears, P., *Color Atlas of Medical Microbiology,* Mosby-Wolfe. 1996. Fig. 221, p. 150.

**Fig. 13.23:** Krammer, T. T. *Comparative Pathogenic Bacteriology* (Filmstrip). W. B. Saunders Company 1972. Slide: 34.

**Fig. 14.4** Stephens, M. B. *Postgraduate Medicine,* Vol 99, No. 4, April 1996. p. 218.

**Fig. 14.5:** Bottone, E. J., Girolami, R., and Stamm, J. M., *Schneierson's Atlas of Diagnostic Microbiology,* Ninth Edition, Abbott Laboratories, 1984. p. 9.

**Fig. 14.8:** Courtesy of Dr. Gary E. Kaiser, The Community College of Baltimore County.

**Fig. 14.9 (top, right):** Finegold, S. M. and Sutter, V. L., *Anaerobic infections.* The Upjohn Company, 1986. Fig. 60, p. 51.

**Fig. 14.9 (bottom, left):** Finegold, S. M., Baron, E. J. and Wexler, H. M. *A Clinical Guide to Anaerobic Infections.* Star Publishing Company, 1992. Fig. 70, p. 69.

**Fig. 14.9 (bottom, center):** Finegold, S. M., Baron, E. J. and Wexler, H. M. *A Clinical Guide to Anaerobic Infections.* Star Publishing Company, 1992. Fig. 86, p. 82.

**Fig. 14.9 (bottom, right):** Kelly, C. P., Pothoulakis, C., and LaMont, J. T. *N Engl J Med.* 330:257-262 (1994).

**Fig. 15.3:** McMilan, A. and Scott, G. R. *Sexually Transmitted Diseases.* Churchill Livingstone., 1991 Fig. 63, p. 42.

**Fig. 15.4:** Brown, T. J., Yen-Moore, A. and Tyring, S. K. *Journal of the American Academy of Dermatology.* Volume 41, Number 4. October 1999. Fig. 1.

**Fig. 15.4:** Brown, T. J., Yen-Moore, A. and Tyring, S. K. *Journal of the American Academy of Dermatology.* Volume 41, Number 4. October 1999. Fig. 4.

**Fig. 15.4:** McMilan, A. and Scott, G. R. *Sexually Transmitted Diseases.* Churchill Livingstone, 1991 Fig. 63, p. 42.

**Fig. 15.4:** Brown, T. J., Yen-Moore, A. and Tyring, S. K. *Journal of the American Academy*

*of Dermatology.* Volume 41, Number 4. October 1999. Fig. 8,

**Fig. 15.5:** McMilan, A. and Scott, G. R. *Sexually Transmitted Diseases.* Churchill Livingstone., 1991. Fig. 136, p. 92.

**Fig. 15.7 (left):** McMillan, A. and Scott, G. R. *Sexually Transmitted Diseases.* Churchill Livingstone, 1991. Fig. 64, p. 42.

**Fig. 15.7 (right):** Brown, T. J., Yen-Moore, A. and Tyring, S. K. *Journal of the American Academy of Dermatology.* Volume 41, Number 4. October 1999. Fig. 1.

**Fig. 15.9:** Verdon, M. E., Sigal, Leonard H., *American Family Physician.* August 1997. p. 429,

**Fig. 15.9:** Department of Dermatology, Uniformed Services University, Bethesda, Maryland.

**Fig. 15.12 (next to bottom):** American Society Microbiology (Microbelibrary.org). Jeffrey Nelson, Rush University.

**Fig. 15.12 (bottom):** Ledbetter, L. S., Hsu, S., and Less, J. B., *Po*

**Fig. 15.14:** Wistreich, G. *Microbiology Perspectives: A Photographic Survey of the Microbial World.* Prentice-Hall, Inc. 1999. Fig. 72, p. 39.

**Fig. 15.14 (bottom):** Farrar, W. E., Wood, M. J., Innes, J. A., Tubbs, H., *Infectious Diseases.* Second Edition, Gower Medical Publishing, 1992. Fig. 13.40., p. 13.15

**Fig. 16.5 (top, right):** Michael Gabbridge/Visuals Unlimited.

**Fig. 16.5 (top, left):** Kassirer, J. P., *Images in Clinical Medicine,* Massachusetts Medical Society, 1997, p. 38.

**Fig. 16.5 (bottom):** Farrar, W. E., Wood, M. J., Innes, J. A., Tubbs, H., *Infectious Diseases.* Second Edition, Gower Medical Publishing, 1992. Fig. 2.25, p. 2.8.

**Fig. 17.2:** Cutlip, R. C., National Animal Disease Center. United States Department of Agriculture. Agricultural Research Service.

**Fig. 17.5:** Courtesy of Dr. Umberto Benelli, Online Atlas of Ophthalmology

**Fig. 17.8 (top center):** Wistreich, G. *Microbiology Perspectives: A Photographic Survey of the Microbial World.* Prentice-Hall, Inc. 1999. Fig. 158-B, p. 71.

**Fig. 17.8 (middle row, center):** Courtesy of Dr. Umberto Benelli, Online Atlas of Ophthalmology.

**Fig. 17.8 (middle row, right):** Courtesy of Vanderbilt University Medical Center, Department of Emergency Medicine.

**Fig. 17.8 (bottom row, left):** McMillan, A. and Scott, G. R. *Sexually Transmitted Diseases.* Churchill Livingstone, 1991. Fig. 25, p. 16.

**Fig. 17.8 (bottom row, middle):** Courtesy of Dr. Umberto Benelli, Online Atlas of Ophthalmology.

**Fig. 17.8 (bottom row, right):** McMillan, A. and Scott, G. R. *Sexually Transmitted Diseases.* Churchill Livingstone, 1991. Fig. 24, p. 18.

**Fig. 18.2:** Courtesy Dr. George P. Kubica, Public Health Image Library, Centers for Disease Control and Prevention.

**Fig. 18.2:** Alexander, S. K. and Strete, D. *Microbiology: A Photographic Atlas for the Laboratory.* Benjamin Cummings. Fig. 2.17, p. 15.

**Fig. 18.3:** Center for Disease Control, Atlanta, 1999.

**Fig. 18.4:** Tortora G. J., Funke, B. R. and Case C. E. *Microbiology, An Introduction.* Addison Wesley Longman, Inc. 1998. Fig. 24.10, p. 639.

**Fig. 18.5:** Iseman, Michael D., S/M Infectious Diseases Division. National Jewish Medical Research Center.

**Fig. 18.7:** Talaro, K. P. and Talaro, A. *Foundations in Microbiology, 3rd Edition.* WCB/McGraw-Hill, 1999. Fig. 19.19, p. 612.

**Fig. 18.9:** Courtesy Dr. George P. Kubica, Public Health Image Library, Centers for Disease Control and Prevention.

**Fig. 18.13:** Binford, C.H and Connor D.H. *Pathology of Tropical and Extraordinary Diseases: An Atlas*, Washington, D.D. 1976, Armed Forces Institute of Pathology.

**Fig. 18.14 (top, left):** Wistreich, G. *Microbiology Perspectives: A Photographic Survey of the Microbial World.* Prentice-Hall, Inc. 1999. Fig. 193, p. 86.

**Fig. 18.14 (top, right):** Center for Disease Control, Atlanta.

**Fig. 18.14 (bottom, left):** WebPath, courtesy of Edward C. Klatt MD, Florida State University College of Medicine.

**Fig. 18.14 (bottom, right):** Hogeweg, M. *Tropical Doctor* Suppl. 1, p. 15-21, 1992.

**Fig. 18.15:** Public Health Image Library, Centers for Disease Control and Prevention.

**Fig. 19.2:** Volk, W. A., Gebhardt, B. M., Hammarskjold, M. and Kadner, R. J., *Essentials of Microbiology*, Fifth Edition, Lippincott-Raven, Philadelphia, 1996. Fig. 34-1, p. 459.

**Fig. 19.3:** Public Health Image Library, Centers for Disease Control and Prevention.

**Fig. 19.5:** Greer, Ken/Visuals Unlimited.

**Fig. 20.2(A):** Larone, D. H. *Medically Important Fungi. A Guide to Identification.* Third Edition. American Society for Microbiology, 1995. p. 71.

**Fig. 20.2(B):** Schaf, David /Peter Arnold, Inc.

**Fig. 20.3(A):** Champe, S. P. and Simon, L. D. Cellular Differentiation and Tissue Formation in the Fungus Aspergillus nidulan, in *Morphogenesis.* Edited by Rossomando, E. F. and Alexander, S. Marcel Dekker, Inc. 1992. Fig. 2.

**Fig. 20.3(B):** Champe, S. P. and Simon, L. D. Cellular Differentiation and Tissue Formation in the Fungus Aspergillus nidulan, in *Morphogenesis.* Edited by Rossomando, E. F. and Alexander, S. Marcel Dekker, Inc. 1992. Fig. 3.

**Fig. 20.4:** Volk, W. A., Gebhardt, B. M., Hammarskjold, M. and Kadner, R. J.,

*Essentials of Microbiology*, Fifth Edition, Lippincott-Raven, Philadelphia, 1996. Fig. 35-3, p.477.

**Fig. 20.5(A):** Habif, Thomas p. *Clinical Dermatology, A Color Guide to Diagnosis and Therapy.* Mosby. 1996. Fig. 13-7, p. 367.

**Fig. 20.5(B):** Habif, Thomas p. *Clinical Dermatology, A Color Guide to Diagnosis and Therapy.* Mosby. 1996. Fig. 13-21, p. 374.

**Fig. 20.5(C):** Habif, Thomas p. *Clinical Dermatology, A Color Guide to Diagnosis and Therapy.* Mosby. 1996. Fig. 13-38, p. 383.

**Fig. 20.5(D):** Habif, T. P. *Clinical Dermatology, A Color Guide to Diagnosis and Therapy.* Mosby. 1996. Fig. 13-16, p. 371.

**Fig. 20.5 (E):** Mir, M. A., *Atlas of Clinical Diagnosis*, W. J. B. Saunders Company Ltd., 1995. Fig. 10.21; p. 203.

**Fig. 20.6(A):** Dr. Lucille K. Georg, Public Health Image Library, Centers for Disease Control and Prevention..

**Fig. 20.6(C):** Courtesy of Prince Leopold Institute of Tropical Medicine.

**Fig. 20.7:** Rubin, E. and Farber, J. L. *Pathology*, Second Edition. J. B. Lippincott Company, 1994. Fig. 9-60, p. 419.

**Fig. 20.8 (A):** Rubin, E. and Farber, J. L. *Pathology*, Second Edition. J. B. Lippincott Company, 1994. Fig. 9-57, p. 416.

**Fig. 20.8 (B):** Rubin, E. and Farber, J. L. *Pathology*, Second Edition. J. B. Lippincott Company, 1994. Fig. 9-58.

**Fig. 20.8(C):** Dr. Libero Ajello, Public Health Image Library, Centers for Disease Control and Prevention.

**Fig. 20.8(D):** Koneman and Roberts, *Practical Laboratory Mycology.* Williams and Wilkins.

**Fig. 20.9:** Center for Disease Control, Atlanta.

**Fig. 20.10:** Murray, p. R., Kobayashi, G. S., Pfaller, M. A. and Rosenthal, K. S., *Medical Microbiology, Second Edition*, Mosby, 1994. Fig. 44-3, p. 418.

**Fig. 20.10:** Murray, P. R., Kobayashi, G. S., Pfaller, M. A. and Rosenthal, K. S., *Medical Microbiology, Second Edition*, Mosby, St. Louis, 1994. Fig. 44-3, p. 418.

**Fig. 20.11:** Goldman, M., Johnson, p. C. and Sarosi, G. A.. *Clinics in Chest Medicine.* W. B. Saunders Company, 1999. Fig. 3. Volume 20, Number 3, September 1999.

**Fig. 20.13:** Kassirer, J. P., *Images in Clinical Medicine*, Massachusetts Medical Society, 1997. p. 44.

**Fig. 20.14:** Rubin, E. and Farber, J. L. *Pathology*, Second Edition. J. B. Lippincott Company, 1994. Fig. 9-51, p. 409.

**Fig. 20.15:** Rubin, E. and Farber, J. L. *Pathology*, Second Edition. J. B. Lippincott Company, 1994. Fig. 9-55, p. 414.

**Fig. 20.16:** McGee, J., Isaacson, P. G., and Wright, N. A. *Oxford Textbook of Pathology.* Oxford Press, 1992. Fig. 6.30.

**Fig. 20.18:** Volk, W. A., Gebhardt, B. M., Hammarskjold, M. and Kadner, R. J., *Essentials of Microbiology*, Fifth Edition,

Lippincott-Raven, 1996. Fig. 35-18, p. 492.

**Fig. 20.20:** Emond, R. T. D., Rowland, H.A.K. and Welsby, P. D., *Color Atlas of Infectious Diseases*, Third Edition, Mosby-Wolfe. 1995. Fig. 339. p. 283.

**Fig. 21.3:** Gillies, R. R. and Dodds, T. C., *Bacteriology Illustrated*, Third Edition, Williams and Wilkins Company, 1973. p. 194.

**Fig. 21.4** CDC – DPDx – Laboratory Identification of Parasites of Public Health Concern.

**Fig. 21.5:** Public Health Image Library, Centers for Disease Control and Prevention.

**Fig. 21.7:** Gillies, R. R. and Dodds, T. C., *Bacteriology Illustrated*, Third Edition, Williams and Wilkins Company, 1973. p. 198.

**Fig. 21.12:** Sun, T. *Parasitic Disorders. Pathology, Diagnosis and Management*, Second Edition. Williams and Wilkins, 1999. Fig. 5.7, p. 23.

**Fig. 21.14:** Public Health Image Library, Centers for Disease Control and Prevention.

**Fig. 22.2:** de la Maza, L. M., Pezzlo, M. T. and Baron, E. J., *Color Atlas of Diagnostic Microbiology, Mosby, 1997.* Fig. 15-104, p. 170.

**Fig. 22.4:** H. Zaiman. *A Pictorial Presentation of Parasites.* Slide 16.

**Fig. 22.6:** Kassirer, J. P., *Images in Clinical Medicine*, Massachusetts Medical Society, 1997. p. 295.

**Fig. 22.9:** Kassirer, J. P., *Images in Clinical Medicine*, Massachusetts Medical Society, 1997. p. 306.

**Fig. 24.4(B):** Ordoukhanian, E. and Lane, Alfred T., *Postgraduate Medicine*, 101, February, pp. 223-232, 1997.

**Fig. 24.4(C):** Ordoukhanian, E. and Lane, Alfred T., *Postgraduate Medicine*, 101, February, pp. 223-232, 1997.

**Fig. 24.7:** Arthur, R. R, Shah, K.V. *Papovaviridae* In: The Polyomaviruses. In Lennette E.H., Halonen P., Murphy, F. A., eds. *Laboratory Diagnosis of Infectious Diseases: Principles and Practices*, vol. II, Springer-Verlag 1988: 317-332.

**Fig. 24.8(B):** Ginsberg, H. S. *The Adenoviruses*, Plenum Publishers,1984.

**Fig. 24.8(C):** Volk, W. A., Benjamin, D. C., Kadner, R. J. and Parsons, J. T., *Essentials of Microbiology*, Fourth Edition, J. B.Lippincott Company,1991. Fig. 41.4, p. 563,

**Fig. 24.11:** Kassirer, J. P., *Images in Clinical Medicine*, Massachusetts Medical Society, 1997, p. 19.

**Fig. 25.2:** Volk, W. A., Gebhardt, B. M., Hammarskjold, M. and Kadner, R. J., *Essentials of Microbiology*, Fifth Edition, Lippincott-Raven, Philadelphia, 1996. Fig. 38-4A, p. 522. lippincott book.

**Fig. 25.4:** Courtesy of Bernard A. Cohen, MD, Christoph U. Lehmann, MD, DermAtlas, Johns Hopkins University.

**Fig. 25.5 (top):** Public Health Image Library, Centers for Disease Control and Prevention.

**Fig. 25.5(bottom):** Public Health Image Library, Centers for Disease Control and Prevention.

**Fig. 25.11:** Habif, T. P. *Clinical Dermatology, A Color Guide to Diagnosis and Therapy*. Mosby. 1996. Fig. 12-34, p. 345.

**Fig. 25.12:** Stephen K., *Hospital Practice*. July 15, 1996. Fig. 2, p. 139.

**Fig. 25.14:** Courtesy of Joan Barenfanger, Laboratory Medicine, Memorial Medical Center, Springfield, IL

**Fig. 25.15:** Ball, A. P. and Gray, J. A., *Colour Guide Infectious Diseases*, Churchill Livingstone, Edinburgh, 1992. Fig. 56, p. 40.

**Fig. 25.18:** Custom Medical Stock Photo.

**Fig. 25.23:** Public Health Image Library, Centers for Disease Control and Prevention.

**Fig. 25.24:** WebPath, courtesy of Edward C. Klatt MD, Florida State University College of Medicine.

**Fig. 25.26:** Henderson, D. A., et al. *Journal American Medical Association* 281:2130, 1999.

**Fig. 26.3:** Volk, W. A., Benjamin, D. C., Kadner, R. J. and Parsons, J. T., *Essentials of Microbiology*, Fourth Edition, J. B.Lippincott Company,1991. Fig. 45-1, p. 601.

**Fig. 26. 7:** Murray, P. R., Kobayashi, G. S., Pfaller, M. A. and Rosenthal, K. S., *Medical Microbiology, Second Edition*, Mosby, St. Louis, 1994. Fig. 68-12, p 714.

**Fig. 27.2:** Volk, W. A., Benjamin, D. C., Kadner, R. J. and Parsons, J. T., *Essentials of Microbiology*, Fourth Edition, J. B. Lippincott Company,1991. Fig. 46-1, p. 608.

**Fig. 27.7:** Moyer, L., Warwick, M., and Mahoney, F. J. *American Family Physician*. Fig. 2, 54: (Number 1) p. 112 (1996).

**Fig. 28.5:** Cotras, *Robbins Pathologic Basis of Disease*, Sixth Edition, W. B. Saunders Company, 1996. Fig. 7-38.

**Fig. 28.6:** Talaro, K. P. and Talaro, A. *Foundations in Microbiology, 3rd Edition*. WCB/McGraw-Hill, 1999. Fig. 25.12, p.801.

**Fig. 28.15:** Antman, K. and Change, Y. *N Engl J Med*. 342 (number 14) 1027 (2000).

**Fig. 28.19:** Armstrong, D. and Cohen, J., *Infectious Diseases*. Mosby 1999. Fig. 10.5, p. 8.10.4.

**Fig. 28.20:** Katayarma, C. Y. Li and Yam, L.T. *American Journal of Pathology*, 67:361, 1972. J. B. Lippincott Company.

**Fig. 29.2(A):** Fields, B. N., Knipe, D. M. and Howley, P. M.. *Virology, Third Edition*, Lippincott Williams and Wilkins, 1996. Fig. 1, p. 1140.

**Fig. 29.2(B):** Fields, B. N., Knipe, D. M. and Howley, P. M.. *Virology, Third Edition*, Lippincott Williams and Wilkins, 1996.

**Fig. 29.4:** http://www.pathguy.com/lectures/rabies.jpg

**Fig. 29.6:** Center for Disease Control, Atlanta.

**Fig. 29.7:** Courtesty Dr. Heinz F. Eichenwald, Public Health Image Library, Centers for Disease Control and Prevention.

**Fig. 29.8:** Mir, M. A., *Atlas of Clinical Diagnosis*, W. J. B. Saunders Company Ltd., 1995. Fig. 1.211, p. 42.

**Fig. 29.10(A):** Fields, B. N., Knipe, D. M. and Howley, P. M.. *Virology, Third Edition*, Lippincott Williams and Wilkins, 1996. Fig. 2, p. 1401.

**Fig. 29.12:** Fields, B. N., Knipe, D. M. and Howley, P. M. *Virology, Third Edition*, Lippincott Williams and Wilkins, 1996. Fig. 2, p. 1357. Photo courtesy of George Leser, Northwestern University, Evanston, Il.

**Fig. 29.15:** Jensen, M. M., Wright, D. N., and Robison, R. A. *Microbiology for the Health Sciences*. Prentice Hall, 1995. Fig. 33-2, p. 420.

**Fig. 29.16:** Treanor, J., et al., *Journal American Medical Association*, 283:1016-1024 (2000). Fig. 2, p. 1020.

**Fig. 29.17:** Courtesy Cynthia Goldsmith,Public Health Image Library, Centers for Disease Control and Prevention.

**Fig. 30.2:** Kapikian, A. Z., Kim, H. W., and Wyatt, R. G. Science 185:1049-1053, 1974.

**Fig. 31.2:** Hart, T. and Shears, P., *Color Atlas of Medical Microbiology*, Mosby-Wolfe. 1996. Fig. 16, p. 16.°

**Fig. 33.2 (B):** Connie Celum, Walter Stamm, Seattle STD/HIV Prevention Training Center.

**Fig. 33.2 (C):** Courtesty Diane P. Yolton, Pacific University.

**Fig. 33.2 (D):** Beeching, N.J. and Nye, F.J., *Diagnostic Picture Tests in Clinical Infectious Disease*, Mosby- Wolfe, London, 1996.Fig. 83, p. 46.

**Fig. 33.2 (E):** Courtesty Diane P. Yolton, Pacific University.

**Fig. 33.2 F:** Armstrong, Donald, and Cohen, Jonathan. *Infectious Diseases*. Mosby 1999. Fig. 25.9, p. 8.25.6.

**Fig. 33.2 (G):** CDC – National Center for HIV, STD and TB Prevention Division of Sexually Transmitted Diseases – STD Prevention – Syphilis Fact.

**Fig. 33.2 (H):** CDC – National Center for HIV, STD and TB Prevention Division of Sexually Transmitted Diseases – STD Prevention – Syphilis Fact.

**Fig. 33.2 (I):** MacMilan, A., Scott, G. R. *Sexually Transmitted Diseases*, Churchill Livingstone. 1991. Fig. 52, p. 34.

**Fig. 33.2 (K):** Salkind, M. R. *A Slide Atlas of Common Diseases*, Parthenon Publishing Group, 1994. Fig. 175.

**Fig. 33.2 (L):** Salkind, M. R. *A Slide Atlas of Common Diseases*, Parthenon Publishing Group, 1994. Fig. 183.

**Fig. 33.2 (M):** Gillies, R. R. and Dodds, T.C., *Bacteriology Illustrated*, Third Edition, Williams and Wilkins Company, Baltimore, 1973. p.198. 59.

**Fig. 33.2 (N):** Salkind, M. R. *A Slide Atlas of Common Diseases*, Parthenon Publishing Group, 1994. Fig. 172.

**Fig. 33.2 (O):** Brown, T. J., Yen-Moore, A. and Tyring, S. K. *Journal of the American Academy of Dermatology*. Volume 41, Number 5. November 1999. Fig. 1.

**Fig. 33.2 (Q):** Kassirer, J. P., *Images in Clinical Medicine*, Massachusetts Medical Society, 1997. p. 28.

**Fig. 33.2 (R):** Stone, D. R. and Gorbach, S. L. *Atlas of Infectious Diseases*. W. B. Saunders Company, 2000. Fig. 6-26, p. 103.

**Fig. 33.2 (S):** Salkind, M. R. *A Slide Atlas of Common Diseases*, Parthenon Publishing Group, 1994. Fig. 59.

**Fig. 33.2 (T):** Courtesy of Dr. Umberto Benelli, Online Atlas of Ophthalmology

**Fig. 33.2 (U):** Copyrighted image used with permission of the authors, Virtual Hospital (TM), www.vh.org

**Fig. 33.2 (V):** Salkind, M. R. *A Slide Atlas of Common Diseases*, Parthenon Publishing Group, 1994. Fig. 25.

**Fig. 33.2 (W):** Salkind, M. R. *A Slide Atlas of Common Diseases*, Parthenon Publishing Group, 1994. Fig. 60.

**Fig. 33.10 (A):** Wistreich, George. *Microbiology Perspectives: A Photographic Survey of the Microbial World*. Prentice-Hall, Inc. 1999. Fig. 199, p. 87.

**Fig. 33.10 (B):** Katz, D. S. and Leung, A. N. Radiology of Pneumonia. *Clinics in Chest Medicine*. Fig. 2. Volume 20. Number 3, September 1999. W. B. Saunders Company.

**Fig. 33.10 (C):** Katz, D. S. and Leung, A. N. Radiology of Pneumonia. *Clinics in Chest Medicine*. Fig. 4. Volume 20. Number 3, September 1999. W. B. Saunders Company.

**Fig. 33.10 (D):** Public Health Image Library, Centers for Disease Control and Prevention.

**Fig. 33.10 (E):** Goldman, M., Johnson, P. C. and Sarosi, G. A. Pneumonia: Fungal Pneumonias. *Clinics in Chest Medicine*. Volume 20, Number 3, September 1999. W. B. Saunders Company. Fig. 1.

**Fig. 33.10 (F):** Salkind, M. R. *A Slide Atlas of Common Diseases*, Parthenon Publishing Group, 1994. Fig. 59.

**Fig. 33.10 (G):** Courtesty Dr. David Ellis, University of Adelaide.

**Fig. 33.10 (H):** Emond, R. T. D., Rowland, H. A. K. and Welsby, P. D., *Color Atlas of Infectious Diseases*, Third Edition, Mosby-Wolfe. 1995. Fig. 339. p. 283.

**Fig. 33.10 (J):** Center for Disease Control, Atlanta.

**Fig. 33.10 6(K):** Salkind, M. R. *A Slide Atlas of Common Diseases*, Parthenon Publishing Group, 1994. Fig. 25.

**Fig. 33.10 (L):** Salkind, M. R. *A Slide Atlas of Common Diseases*, Parthenon Publishing Group, 1994. Fig. 9.

**Fig. 33.10 (N):** Arthur, R. R, Shah, K.V. *Papovaviridae* In: The Polyomavirues. In Lennette E.H., Halonen P., Murphy, F. A., eds. *Laboratory Diagnosis of Infectious Diseases: Principles and Practices*, Vol. II, Springer-Verlag 1988: 317-332.